MW01480009

theclinics.com

Agnes E. Rupley, DVM, Dipl. ABVP–Avian
CONSULTING EDITOR

VETERINARY CLINICS OF NORTH AMERICA

Exotic Animal Practice

Emergency and Critical Care

GUEST EDITOR
Marla Lichtenberger, DVM, Dipl. ACVECC

May 2007 • Volume 10 • Number 2

SAUNDERS

An Imprint of Elsevier, Inc.
PHILADELPHIA   LONDON   TORONTO   MONTREAL   SYDNEY   TOKYO

W.B. SAUNDERS COMPANY
A Division of Elsevier Inc.

Elsevier, Inc., 1600 John F. Kennedy Blvd., Suite 1800, Philadelphia, PA 19103-2899

http://www.vetexotic.theclinics.com

VETERINARY CLINICS OF NORTH AMERICA:　　　　　　　　　　Volume 10, Number 2
EXOTIC ANIMAL PRACTICE　　　　　　　　　　　　　　　　　　　ISSN 1094-9194
May 2007　　　　　　　　　　　　　　　　　　　　　　　ISBN-13: 978-1-4160-4380-5
Editor: John Vassallo; j.vassallo@elsevier.com　　　　　　　ISBN-10: 1-4160-4380-2

Copyright © 2007 by Elsevier Inc. All rights reserved. No part of this publication may be reproduced or transmitted in any form or by any means, electronic or mechanical, including photocopy, recording, or any information retrieval system, without written permission from the publisher.

Single photocopies of single articles may be made for personal use as allowed by national copyright laws. Permission of the publisher and payment of a fee is required for all other photocopying, including multiple or systematic copying, copying for advertising or promotional purposes, resale, and all forms of document delivery. Special rates are available for educational institutions that wish to make photocopies for nonprofit educational classroom use. Permissions may be sought directly from Elsevier's Rights Department in Philadelphia, PA, USA: phone: (+1) 215 239 3804, fax: (+1) 215 239 3805, e-mail: healthpermissions@elsevier.com. Requests may also be completed on-line via the Elsevier homepage (http://www.elsevier.com/locate/permissions). In the USA, users may clear permissions and make payments through the Copyright Clearance Center, Inc, 222 Rosewood Drive, Danvers, MA 01923, USA; phone: (978) 750-8400; fax: (978) 750-4744, and in the UK through the Copyright Licensing Agency Rapid Clearance Service (CLARCS), 90 Tottenham Court Road, London W1P 0LP, UK; phone: (+44) 171 436 5931; fax: (+44) 171 436 3986. Others countries may have a local reprographic rights agency for payments.

Reprints. For copies of 100 or more of articles in this publication, please contact the commercial Reprints Department, Elsevier Inc., 360 Park Avenue South, New York, New York 10010-1710. Tel: (212) 633-3813 Fax: (212) 633-1935, e-mail: reprints@elsevier.com.

The ideas and opinions expressed in *Veterinary Clinics of North America: Exotic Animal Practice* do not necessarily reflect those of the Publisher. The Publisher does not assume any responsibility for any injury and/or damage to persons or property arising out of or related to any use of the material contained in this periodical. The reader is advised to check the appropriate medical literature and the product information currently provided by the manufacturer of each drug to be administered to verify the dosage, the method and duration of administration, or contraindications. It is the responsibility of the treating physician or other health care professional, relying on independent experience and knowledge of the patient, to determine drug dosages and the best treatment for the patient. Mention of any product in this issue should not be construed as endorsement by the contributors, editors, or the Publisher of the product or manufacturers' claims.

Veterinary Clinics of North America: Exotic Animal Practice (ISSN 1094-9194) is published in January, May, and September by Elsevier, Inc.; Business and Editorial offices: 1600 John F. Kennedy Blvd., Suite 1800, Philadelphia, PA 19103-2899. Customer Service Office: 6277 Sea Harbor Drive, Orlando, FL 32887-4800. Subscription prices are $146.00 per year for US individuals, $253.00 per year for US institutions, $76.00 per year for US students and residents, $173.00 per year for Canadian individuals, $292.00 per year for Canadian institutions, $184.00 per year for international individuals, $292.00 per year for international institutions and $92.00 per year for Canadian and foreign students/residents. To receive student/resident rate, orders must be accompanied by name of affiliated institution, date of term, and the *signature* of program/residency coordinator on institution letterhead. Orders will be billed at individual rate until proof of status is received. Foreign air speed delivery is included in all *Clinics* subscription prices. All prices are subject to change without notice.

POSTMASTER: Send address changes to *Veterinary Clinics of North America: Exotic Animal Practice*; Elsevier Periodicals Customer Service, 6277 Sea Harbor Drive, Orlando, FL 32887-4800. **Customer Service: 1-800-654-2452 (US). From outside of the US, call 1-407-345-1000.**

Veterinary Clinics of North America: Exotic Animal Practice is covered in *Index Medicus*.

Printed in the United States of America.

EMERGENCY AND CRITICAL CARE

CONSULTING EDITOR

AGNES E. RUPLEY, DVM, Diplomate, American Board of Veterinary Practitioners–Avian; Director and Chief Veterinarian, All Pets Medical & Laser Surgical Center, College Station, Texas

GUEST EDITOR

MARLA LICHTENBERGER, DVM, Diplomate, American College of Veterinary Emergency and Critical Care, Mequon, Wisconsin

CONTRIBUTORS

HEATHER BOWLES, DVM, Diplomate, American Board of Veterinary Practitioners-Avian; Hunt Valley Animal Hospital, Cockeysville, Maryland

WILL CHAVEZ, DVM, Private Practice, West Hills, California

LEIGH ANN CLAYTON, DVM, Diplomate, American Board of Veterinary Practitioners-Avian; Director, Department of Animal Health, National Aquarium in Baltimore, Baltimore, Maryland

RYAN DE VOE, DVM, MSpVM, Diplomate, American College of Zoological Medicine; Diplomate, American Board of Veterinary Practitioners-Avian; Senior Veterinarian, North Carolina Zoological Park, Asheboro, North Carolina

DANIEL DOMBROWSKI, MS, DVM, Veterinarian and Coordinator of Living Collections, North Carolina Museum of Natural Sciences, Raleigh, North Carolina

M. SCOTT ECHOLS, DVM, Diplomate, American Board of Veterinary Practitioners-Avian; Director of Avian Medical and Surgical Services, Westgate Pet and Bird Hospital, Austin, Texas

STACEY R. GORE, DVM, Veterinary Intern, Department of Animal Health, National Aquarium in Baltimore, Baltimore, Maryland

JENNIFER E. GRAHAM, DVM, Diplomate of American Board of Veterinary Practitioners-Avian; Affiliate Assistant Professor, Department of Comparative Medicine, University of Washington, Seattle, Washington; Staff Veterinarian, Avian and Exotic Medicine, Angell Animal Medical Center, Boston, Massachusetts

CATHERINE A. HADFIELD, MA, VetMB, MRCVS, Associate Veterinarian, National Aquarium in Baltimore, Baltimore, Maryland

MICHELLE G. HAWKINS, VMD, Diplomate, American Board of Veterinary Practitioners-Avian; Assistant Professor, Department of Medicine and Epidemiology, School of Veterinary Medicine, University of California, Davis, Davis, California

J. JILL HEATLEY, DVM, MS, Diplomate, American Board of Veterinary Practitioners-Avian; Clinical Assistant Professor, Zoological Medicine, and Attending Veterinarian, Zoological Medicine Service, Southeastern Raptor Center, Auburn University College of Veterinary Medicine, Auburn, Alabama

STEPHEN J. HERNANDEZ-DIVERS, BVetMed, DZooMed (Reptilian), MRCVS, RCVS, Specialist in Zoo & Wildlife Medicine, Diplomate, American College of Zoological Medicine; Associate Professor of Exotic Animal, Wildlife & Zoological Medicine, Department of Small Animal Medicine and Surgery, College of Veterinary Medicine, University of Georgia, Athens, Georgia

JEFF KO, DVM, MS, Diplomate, American College of Veterinary Anesthesiologists; Professor of Anesthesiology, Department of Veterinary Clinical Sciences, School of Veterinary Medicine, Purdue University, West Lafayette, Indiana

ANGELA M. LENNOX, DVM, Diplomate, American Board of Veterinary Practitioners-Avian; Avian and Exotic Animal Clinic of Indianapolis, Indianapolis, Indiana

MARLA LICHTENBERGER, DVM, Diplomate, American College of Veterinary Emergency and Critical Care, Mequon, Wisconsin

DAVID MARTINEZ-JIMENEZ, LV MSc, Intern of Exotic Animal, Wildlife and Zoological Medicine, Department of Small Animal Medicine and Surgery, College of Veterinary Medicine, University of Georgia, Athens, Georgia

JOANNE PAUL-MURPHY, DVM, Diplomate, American College of Zoological Medicine; Clinical Professor, Special Species Health, Department of Surgical Sciences, School of Veterinary Medicine, University of Wisconsin, Madison, Wisconsin

CHRISTAL POLLOCK, DVM, Diplomate, American Board of Veterinary Practitioners-Avian; Cleveland Heights, Ohio

BRENT R. WHITAKER, MS, DVM, Deputy Executive Director for Biological Programs, National Aquarium in Baltimore; Research Associate, Center of Marine Biotechnology, University of Maryland, Baltimore, Maryland

EMERGENCY AND CRITICAL CARE

CONTENTS

Preface   xi
Marla Lichtenberger

**Shock and Cardiopulmonary-Cerebral Resuscitation
in Small Mammals and Birds**   275
Marla Lichtenberger

    Small mammals and birds present unique challenges for the clinician in treatment of life-threatening conditions. Numerous books have been written on shock, critical care, and cardiopulmonary resuscitation in small animals. The basic protocols can be adapted for use in small mammals and birds. A general review of the pathophysiology of shock is important to the understanding of fluid therapy plans discussed in this article. Using the general principles of cardiopulmonary-cerebral resuscitation in small animals, protocols are discussed for use in birds and small mammals.

Anesthesia and Analgesia for Small Mammals and Birds   293
Marla Lichtenberger and Jeff Ko

    This article should help the veterinarian to assess pain in small mammals and birds. The focus is on a multimodal approach to anesthesia and analgesia using opioids, nonsteroidal anti-inflammatory drugs, α_2-agonists, dissociatives, and local anesthetics as injectables, constant rate infusions, local blocks, and epidurals. Drugs used for induction, intubation techniques, and inhalant anesthesia are discussed. Protocols for critical patients and doses of common analgesics are covered.

Critical Care Monitoring   317
Marla Lichtenberger and Jeff Ko

    The use of various monitoring techniques in small mammals and birds has helped to advance the field of emergency medicine and improved the safe anesthetic management and critical care of the exotic pet. Monitoring techniques are used to detect changes in the cardiovascular and respiratory systems so that the clinician is aware of abnormalities before the problem becomes irreversible. The first part of this article discusses cardiovascular monitoring, which is divided into perfusion parameters, blood pressure, central venous pressure, and cardiac evaluation. The second part of the discussion is focused on respiratory monitoring, which includes basic principles and monitoring using pulse oximetry, an end-tidal gas monitor, other respiratory monitor devices, blood gas analysis, and lactate measurements.

Emergency and Critical Care of Pet Birds 345
Heather Bowles, Marla Lichtenberger, and Angela Lennox

Critically ill birds must be assessed accurately and provided with immediate supportive care. This article reviews the assessment and diagnostics required for evaluating the critical avian patient. The most common emergencies seen in pet birds are discussed. Diagnostics and treatments protocols are provided to help direct the practitioner toward a complete recovery.

Emergency Care of Raptors 395
Jennifer E. Graham and J. Jill Heatley

Raptors may present with a variety of conditions, such as trauma, debilitation, and disease, that necessitate emergency care. Emergency treatment should prioritize stabilization of the patient. Diagnostic testing should be delayed until feasible based on patient status. This article reviews emergency medicine in raptors, including appropriate handling and restraint, hospitalization, triage and patient assessment, sample collection, supportive care, and common emergency presentations.

Bandaging, Endoscopy, and Surgery in the Emergency Avian Patient 419
Will Chavez and M. Scott Echols

This article is divided into three parts and describes procedures used in avian medicine after initial stabilization. The first part includes the application of bandages and splints for fractures. The second part describes the use of endoscopy to examine the choana, oral cavity, trachea, and, to a lesser extent, internal organs. The last part discusses equipment required and techniques used for esophagostomy tube placement, air sac cannulation, and surgery, with approaches to the coelomic cavity and a select number of surgical procedures. This article is intended to provide the emergency animal clinician with knowledge necessary to provide basic stabilization for avian patients and knowledge of procedures that can be performed by the experienced clinician.

Critical Care of the Rabbit 437
Joanne Paul-Murphy

Emergency and critical care principles are similar for all mammals. However, because they are stressed easily, rabbits require specialized handling techniques. Rabbits must be evaluated efficiently and stabilized quickly before moving into the definitive diagnostic phase of their care. A thorough clinical history, systematic physical examination, and multiple diagnostic tests are ideal, but when a rabbit is in critical condition, emergency stabilization and fluid resuscitation must take priority. Common emergency presentations include gastrointestinal disorders, such as prolonged anorexia, respiratory distress, neoplasia, neurologic symptoms, exposure to toxins, trauma, and urinary tract infections or obstruction.

Emergency Medicine of the Ferret 463
Christal Pollock

Common emergency conditions seen in the ferret include insulinoma, cardiomyopathy, and urethral obstruction. When developing a diagnostic and therapeutic plan, the ferret veterinarian must seek a balance between species-specific information and information extrapolated from cat and dog medicine. The therapeutic plan must always include close and careful monitoring. Significant changes in the status of these small patients can occur extremely quickly in the course of providing basic supportive care, such as intravenous fluids or supplemental heat.

Emergency and Critical Care of Rodents 501
Michelle G. Hawkins and Jennifer E. Graham

Rodents may be presented on an emergency basis with various conditions causing debilitation and disease. Common causes of emergent presentations include trauma, respiratory disease, dental disease, gastrointestinal disease, reproductive disorders, and urinary tract obstruction. Emergency treatment should always include immediate stabilization of the patient until the patient is able to tolerate diagnostic testing and additional therapeutics. Rodent patients benefit from supportive care, including thermal, fluid, and nutritional support. Administration of cardiopulmonary resuscitation, antibiotics, and analgesics through various routes is also appropriate. This article presents an overview of emergency medicine in rodents, including emergency procedures, handling and restraint, triage and patient assessment, sample collection, and supportive care procedures. The most common emergency presentations for rodents are also discussed.

Emergency and Critical Care Procedures in Sugar Gliders (*Petaurus breviceps*), African Hedgehogs (*Atelerix albiventris*), and Prairie Dogs (*Cynomys spp*)   533
Angela M. Lennox

Less common exotic pet mammals are gaining in popularity. The Australian Sugar Glider, African Hedgehog, and prairie dog are seen regularly in exotic animal practices. They are subject to the same types of medical emergencies as more traditional pets, with the unfortunate addition of all too common underlying nutritional and husbandry-related disorders. Emergency stabilization and critical care are important first steps before collection of diagnostic test samples and administration of definitive medical care.

Emergency Care of Reptiles   557
David Martinez-Jimenez and Stephen J. Hernandez-Divers

Most reptile emergencies are the result of improper husbandry and nutrition. Reptiles are good at masking disease, and owners, failing to recognize early signs of illness, only seek veterinary assistance when issues are advanced and near terminal. The veterinarian should be familiar with reptile species-specific husbandry and nutritional requirements and basic clinical techniques. The same principles and techniques used in small animal medicine can be applied to reptile emergencies. This article reviews general emergency principles that apply to the reptilian patient and common emergency presentations. The main areas of discussion focus on cardiopulmonary resuscitation, fluid therapy, and analgesia.

Amphibian Emergency Medicine   587
Leigh Ann Clayton and Stacey R. Gore

General concepts of amphibian emergency medicine are presented, including a review of patient selection, appropriate history, and helpful equipment. Physical examination procedures, general treatment, and diagnostic techniques are discussed. This is followed by a review of conditions commonly observed in amphibians and specific treatment options.

Emergency Care of Invertebrates   621
Daniel Dombrowski and Ryan De Voe

Invertebrate species are commonly kept as pets as well as display and research animals. Clinicians interested in zoologic medicine should be prepared to provide veterinary care for these interesting creatures. This article provides an overview on the critical care of commonly encountered invertebrate species.

Emergency and Critical Care of Fish 647
Catherine A. Hadfield, Brent R. Whitaker, and Leigh Ann Clayton

Most fish emergencies are the result of inappropriate environmental conditions and primary or secondary infectious disease or trauma. The immediate response should be to increase aeration, provide suitable water, and decrease stressors. A thorough history, evaluation of the fish and their environment, and some rapid diagnostic tests (particularly direct and stained cytology) often provide the information needed to make a diagnosis and render appropriate treatment. When cohorts are at risk and the patient is unlikely to recover, euthanasia and necropsy are recommended to reach a definitive diagnosis. Some common emergencies include ammonia and nitrite toxicity; low dissolved oxygen; copper and chlorine toxicity; gas supersaturation; and certain bacterial, protozoal, and viral diseases.

Index 677

FORTHCOMING ISSUES

September 2007
   Neuroanatomy and Neurodiagnostics
   Lisa A. Tell, DVM, Dipl. ABVP–Avian
   and Marguerite F. Knipe, DVM,
   Dipl. ACVIM (Neurology),
   Guest Editors

January 2008
   Endocrinology
   Anthony A. Pilny, DVM, Dipl. ABVP

RECENT ISSUES

January 2007
   Cytology
   Michael M. Garner, DVM, Dipl. ACVP
   Guest Editor

September 2006
   Case Reports: The Front Line in Exotic Medicine
   Robert J.T. Doneley, BVSc, FACVSc,
   Guest Editor

May 2006
   Common Procedures
   Chris Griffin, DVM, Dipl. ABVP–Avian
   Guest Editor

The Clinics are now available online!

Access your subscription at
www.theclinics.com

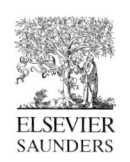

Preface

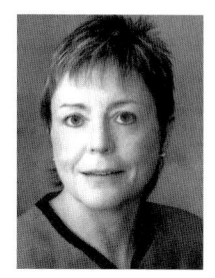

Marla Lichtenberger, DVM, DACVECC
Guest Editor

I am pleased to introduce the second edition of the *Veterinary Clinics of North America: Exotic Animal Practice* on emergency and critical care. This second edition retains the purpose of the original text: to provide new advances in critical care for the exotic pet. It has been 9 years since the publication of the first issue covering the topic of critical care. This new edition provides the most current information on emergency and critical care medicine for exotics. It integrates our current knowledge and understanding of clinical and research experiences into a practical and accessible publication.

Increasing numbers of exotic animals are being kept as pets, and owners want to receive the same high quality medical care as given to dogs and cats. I feel that all emergency veterinarians should learn basic emergency and critical care for exotics. Unless another veterinarian within the area will see exotic emergencies, it is the emergency veterinarian's duty to provide all pet animals and birds with basic emergency care. The field of emergency and critical care is developing rapidly; this issue focuses on clinically relevant and comprehensive information, in addition to new advances and application to therapy. It represents a completely rewritten version of the original issue, with updated information and references. The first three articles are new and they discuss shock, fluid therapy, anesthesia, analgesia, monitoring techniques, and cardiopulmonary-cerebral resuscitation in small mammals and birds. These topics are discussed separately in each article on reptiles, amphibians, invertebrates, and fish because of the differences in these species. Much of the information in the first article originates from a decade of practice and research in critical care medicine in exotic small mammals and birds at the Animal Emergency Center in Glendale, Wisconsin. I would like to express my deepest gratitude to Rebecca Kirby for her help, enthusiasm, and interest in the field of emergency and critical care of the exotic pet. Her mentoring helped develop and lay the groundwork for the research in shock and fluid therapy for the exotic animal patient, which is presented in the first article.

The primary emphasis in the following articles is on treatment of the most life-threatening problems first. Therefore, each article on the different species of exotic pets may refer back to the first articles on initial stabilization with fluid therapy, heat support, and analgesia. The author puts emphasis on understanding the pathophysiology of shock and fluid therapy to help the clinician understand that stabilization on initial presentation is more important than a definitive diagnosis. Oxygen, fluid therapy, heat support, and analgesia save more exotics than other drugs or treatments. The clinician will develop skills on when to put the exotic pet back in the cage, using the stepwise approach to diagnostics and treatments. Anticipating complications before they occur is imperative. Topics vital to the stabilization of each species are presented in a style interesting to the reader and practical to the clinician. The clinician should stop making a judgment on an exotic pet's worth, and recognize the bond that exists between owner and pet, regardless of species involved. The old sayings, "All exotic pets die in the hospital," and "It's only an exotic pet," are no longer acceptable.

The use of multiple authors was guided by the desire to present information from experts in the field of exotic pets. Much of the information is accompanied by published works listed at the end of each article, and anecdotal tales are held to a minimum.

Thank you very much to all who contributed. Your contribution of the latest advances will aid the veterinary exotic pet field, pet owners, and the pets themselves. Your knowledge and years of experience have resulted in new advances in emergency and critical care techniques for exotic pets. We want to encourage the exotic practitioner always to learn more and help bring this field to the next step. I appreciate all the time and effort you gave to make this issue the most recent and up-to-date publication for critical care medicine in exotics.

Marla Lichtenberger, DVM, DACVECC
11015 North Mequon Square Drive
Mequon, WI 53092, USA

E-mail address: marlavet@aol.com

Shock and Cardiopulmonary-Cerebral Resuscitation in Small Mammals and Birds

Marla Lichtenberger, DVM, DACVECC

11015 North Mequon Square Drive, Mequon, WI 53092, USA

Increasing numbers of exotic animals are being kept as pets, and owners want to receive high-quality medical care for these pets. Treatment of hypovolemic shock and cardiopulmonary arrest in exotic small mammals and birds is complicated by small patient size, physiologic diversity, and lack of research and clinical data on their response to therapy. Despite these impediments, the same principles and techniques of monitoring used in domestic animals can be applied to the bird and small mammal patient. The goal of this article is to provide an overview on the principles of shock, shock resuscitation methods, and cardiopulmonary-cerebral resuscitation (CPCR) in rabbits, ferrets, small mammals, and birds (pet birds and raptors).

Shock pathophysiology

Shock is defined as poor tissue perfusion from either low blood flow or unevenly distributed flow. This results in an inadequate delivery of oxygen to the tissues. This definition applies to all species of animals. Although there are many types of shock (eg, cardiogenic, distributive, or septic), this article concentrates on the pathophysiologic characteristics of hypovolemic shock.

Hypovolemic shock is caused by either an absolute or a relative inadequate blood volume. Absolute hypovolemia occurs as a result of actual loss of blood by arterial bleeding, gastrointestinal ulcers, or coagulopathies. In relative hypovolemia, there is no direct blood loss (hemorrhage) from the intravascular space. Examples of relative hypovolemia include severe dehydration from gastrointestinal tract loss, significant loss of plasma (burns), or extensive loss of intravascular fluids into a third body space, such as the

E-mail address: marlavet@aol.com

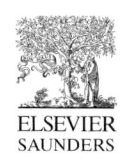

peritoneal cavity. When a small mammal or bird begins hemorrhaging or there is significant loss of body fluid, there is a decrease in blood volume and a decrease in venous return to the right side of the heart. This causes a decrease in return to the left side of the heart and therefore a decrease in cardiac output. With a substantial hypovolemia (ie, greater than 30% blood or plasma volume), blood pressure decreases below a mean arterial pressure of 60 mm Hg or a systolic pressure of less than 90 mm Hg. The carotid and aortic artery baroreceptors detect a decrease in stretch caused by the decrease in cardiac output. This sends a neural signal to the vasomotor center in the medulla oblongata, which results in inhibition of the vagal parasympathetic center and stimulation of the sympathetic center. This causes vasoconstriction of the veins and arterioles throughout the peripheral circulatory system and increases heart rate and strength of heart contraction. The humoral response, an increase in adrenal circulating catecholamines, stimulates renin release by way of adrenergic receptors on cells of the juxtaglomerular apparatus (specialized smooth muscle cells in the afferent arterioles). The release of rennin stimulates activation of the rennin-angiotensin-aldosterone system [1]. These combined effects lead to a restoration of blood pressure, increased cardiac performance, and maximal venous return in the face of blood loss.

Hypovolemic shock: three phases

Early or compensatory phase

The early or compensatory stage of shock occurs as a result of the baroreceptor-mediated release of catecholamines. Blood pressure increases because of the increase in cardiac output and systemic vascular resistance. This is the stage seen commonly in birds (as in dogs) with blood loss less than 20% of their total body weight. Small mammals, as is true in cats, rarely present with this stage of shock. Clinical signs in the bird include an increase in heart rate, normal or increased blood pressure, and normal or increased flow (bounding pulses and capillary refill less than 1 second). The increased heart rate and normal or increased blood pressure are key indicators of compensatory shock. Volume replacement at this stage is usually associated with a good outcome. This phase is rarely seen in small mammals and cats, as discussed later.

Early decompensatory phase

The second stage of shock is called the middle or early decompensatory stage of shock. This stage occurs when fluid losses continue. There is a reduction in the blood flow to the kidneys, gastrointestinal tract, skin, and muscles. There is an uneven distribution of blood flow.

Clinical signs of early decompensatory shock in birds and small mammals include hypothermia, cool limbs and skin, tachycardia, normal or decreased blood pressure, pale mucous membranes, prolonged capillary refill time, and mental depression. This stage of shock is seen in birds with a blood volume loss of greater than 25% to 30% of their total blood volume. In the author's experience, rabbits, ferrets, and other small mammals commonly present in early decompensatory stage of shock. Signs of early decompensatory shock in the small mammal patient (as in the cat) are bradycardia, hypothermia, and hypotension. Signs seen in the avian patient are increased heart rate and hypotension. Aggressive fluid therapy using crystalloids and colloids to support blood pressure and heart rate is required in this stage.

Decompensatory shock

When a large blood volume is lost (greater than 60% in avian species and 40% in small mammals) the neuroendocrine responses to hypovolemia become ineffective, and irreversible organ failure begins [1]. The late decompensatory stage of shock is the final common pathway of all forms of shock in all species.

The pathophysiologic profile of terminal shock is a continuum of that described for the early decompensatory stage, except that the damage has overwhelmed the body's natural protective mechanisms and multiple organ failure has occurred. The clinical signs are bradycardia with low cardiac output, severe hypotension, pale or cyanotic mucous membranes, absent capillary refill time, weak or absent pulses, hypothermia, oliguria to anuric renal failure, pulmonary edema, and a stupor to comatose state. Cardiopulmonary arrest commonly occurs.

Fluid resuscitation plan

A fluid therapy plan involves the type, quantity, and rate of fluid to be administered. Fluid therapy is used to correct life-threatening abnormalities in volume, electrolyte, and acid–base status. The primary goal is to give the least amount of fluids possible to reach the desired end points of resuscitation. Clinical markers are the most frequently used end points of resuscitation. The markers used are those parts of the initial survey that suggest a patient is in shock and include the following: altered mentation, prolonged capillary refill time (CRT), weak and thready pulse/hypotension, tachycardia/bradycardia, tachypnea, cold extremities, weakness, reduced urine output, and pale mucous membranes.

The fluid therapy plan typically has a resuscitation (correction of perfusion deficits), a rehydration (correction of interstitial deficits), and a maintenance phase [2]. Resuscitation implies an urgent need to restore tissue perfusion and oxygenation. Intravascular volume must be replaced first. The type, quantity, and rate of fluid administration required to reach the desired resuscitation end points are determined based on the phase of shock

[2]. Re-evaluation of hydration status after the resuscitation phase is necessary before planning the rehydration phase.

Interstitial volume deficits are typically associated with a decrease in skin turgor and dry mucous membranes. Rehydration of the interstitial compartment is best accomplished using an isotonic replacement fluid. The rate of fluid administration depends primarily on the rate of fluid losses and clinical status of the animal, as indicated by the physical examination and laboratory parameters. For animals with evidence of interstitial dehydration on physical examination but stable cardiovascular parameters, fluid deficits can be replaced over 12 to 24 hours. If the interstitial volume is rapidly lost, then the interstitial fluid deficit should be rapidly replaced (4–6 hours). Isotonic replacement fluids are administered according to the patient's estimated dehydration, maintenance needs, and anticipated ongoing losses. The maintenance phase provides fluids and electrolytes to replace ongoing losses, meet metabolic demands, and restore intracellular water balance until the patient is eating and drinking on its own. Maintenance requirements are higher in small mammals and birds because of their high metabolic rate.

Types of fluids

Individual characteristics of fluids influence type and volume of fluid administered. Crystalloid solutions are commonly used together with colloids in the resuscitation phase. The four basic groups of fluids (ie, crystalloids, synthetic colloids, hemoglobin-based oxygen carriers, and blood products) are discussed.

Crystalloids

Isotonic crystalloid solutions can be used together with colloids during the resuscitation phase. Crystalloids are the mainstay of the rehydration and maintenance phases of fluid therapy. Crystalloids (also called replacement fluids) are fluids containing sodium chloride and other solutes that are capable of distributing to all body fluid compartments. The most commonly used replacement fluids are 0.9% saline (Baxter; Deerfield, IL), lactated Ringer's solution (Abbott Laboratory; North Chicago, IL), and Normosol-R (CEVA Laboratories; Overland Park, KS) or Plasmalyte-A (Baxter).

Hypertonic saline is a hyperosmolar crystalloid fluid used for resuscitation of hypovolemia. It is usually given as a 7.5% solution (2600 mOsm/L). The hyperosmolarity leads to rapid intravascular volume expansion by drawing fluids from the interstitial and intracellular spaces into the intravascular space. Synthetic colloids (hetastarch) provide a synergistic effect when added to hypertonic saline resuscitation, as the duration (in excess of 3 hours) and extent of volume resuscitation (improvement of cardiac output and blood pressure) are greater than would be achieved with either agent alone [2,3]. It is administered in small volumes at 3–5 mL/kg over 10 minutes. The animal can be given 3–5 mL/kg of hetastarch with 3–5 mL/kg of 7.5% hypertonic saline (not mixed in the same syringe) each given over 10 minutes. The advantage is that rather than infusing three times the shed volume of isotonic crystalloids (eg, 90 mL/kg in a dog and bird and 60 mL/kg in small mammals), only a limited portion of the volume deficit needs to be administered when using hypertonic saline [3,4]. Recent research focuses on the effects that hypertonic saline has on the microcirculation, inflammatory response, and cellular function. These findings are intriguing evidence for its use in the veterinary patients that have hypovolemic/hemorrhagic shock, septic shock, and traumatic brain injury [3,4]. Potential side effects include hypernatremia, hyperchloremia, hypokalemia, and dehydration. This movement of intracellular fluid points to one of the feared complications of hypertonic saline resuscitation: cell dehydration. Hypertonic saline should be avoided in dehydrated patients, because the extravascular fluid compartment is volume-depleted before therapy.

Resuscitation of hypovolemic shock is performed using crystalloids along with colloids. This is because 80% of the volume of crystalloid fluid infused re-equilibrates and leaves the intravascular space within 1 hour of administration. On a short-term basis crystalloids expand the intravascular space, but this effect is short-lived. Crystalloids thus should be thought of as interstitial rehydrators, not intravascular volume expanders. This increase in interstitial fluid can lead to tissue edema (thus decreasing the ability of oxygen to diffuse to the cells). Interstitial edema may be extremely detrimental in cases of cerebral edema and pulmonary edema.

Colloids

Colloids are fluids containing large molecular-weight substances that generally are not able to pass through capillary membranes. Colloids can be considered intravascular volume expanders. The three types of colloids are natural colloids (ie, blood products as whole blood), synthetic colloids including hetastarch (Braun Medical Inc.; Irvine, CA), and hemoglobin-based oxygen carriers (ie, Oxyglobin, Biopure; Cambridge, MA).

Hetastarch

This synthetic colloid fluid contains large molecular-weight particles that effectively increase the colloid osmotic pressure (COP) beyond what can be obtained with blood product infusion alone. They maintain intravascular osmotic pressure because their molecular size is too large to pass through the normal capillary pores. They expand volume by approximately 1.4 times the volume actually infused. Synthetic colloids are administered with isotonic crystalloids to reduce interstitial volume depletion. The dose of crystalloid administered is only 40% to 60% of what it would be if crystalloids were used alone during resuscitation.

The standard daily dose of hetastarch is 20 mL/kg. The dose is given as an intravenous bolus (more slowly in small mammals over 10 minutes) for shock resuscitation, titrated in doses of 5 mL/kg to the desired effect. When used for COP support the dose should be administered over 24 hours.

Oxyglobin

Oxyglobin is a hemoglobin-based oxygen carrier (HBOC). HBOC are indicated during resuscitation when increased oxygen delivery to tissues is desired. Although HBOC are colloids, they have the added advantage of carrying oxygen to the tissues. Oxyglobin is a purified, polymerized bovine hemoglobin that is in a modified lactated Ringer's solution approved for use in dogs [5].

Oxyglobin can be administered by way of intravenous administration sets, and standard intravenous infusion pumps can be used for delivery. Because it contains no antigens, cross-matching is not required and there is no possibility of transfusion reactions. Filters are not required. It can be kept at room temperature and has a 3-year shelf life, which makes it useful for hospitals that cannot keep blood products readily available. Once opened, the bag must be discarded within 24 hours because of the production of methemoglobin. The disadvantage to its use is that availability is limited.

Oxyglobin is up to 10 times more effective than blood when given during fluid resuscitation to animals in hemorrhagic shock [5]. For this reason, low volumes of Oxyglobin can be used effectively to treat hemorrhagic shock. In hypovolemic ferrets, rabbits, and small mammals, Oxyglobin is infused at 2 mL/kg over 10 to 20 minutes as a bolus (as in the cat). This is in contrast to the bird, in which Oxyglobin has been infused by the author as a rapid bolus at 5 mL/kg over a few minutes.

Blood transfusion (natural colloids)

If promoting cardiac output is the first priority in the management of acute hemorrhage, then blood is not the ideal resuscitation fluid for acute blood loss, because blood products do not promote blood flow as well as some acellular fluids (eg, hetastarch). Blood is rarely used for initial resuscitation unless the patient is exsanguinating or there is excessive loss of clotting factors secondary to warfarin toxicity. The density of erythrocytes impedes the ability of blood products to promote blood flow (a viscosity effect). The availability of blood products in sufficient quantities to meet the needs of exotic patients is often the limiting factor in survival. Most hospitals do not have readily available donors and commercial blood banks do not carry exotic pet blood products except for ferret blood.

Blood products are administered when albumin, antithrombin, coagulation factors, platelets, or red blood cells are required. Most fluid-responsive shock patients tolerate acute hemodilution to a hematocrit of 20%. Most animals can tolerate an acute blood loss of 10% to 15% of their blood volume without requiring a blood transfusion. Acute hemorrhage exceeding 20% of the blood volume often requires transfusion therapy in addition to initial fluid resuscitation. In animals that have acute blood loss requiring transfusion therapy, fresh whole blood or packed red blood cells should be used in an attempt to stabilize the clinical signs of shock, maintain the hematocrit at greater than 25%, and sustain the clotting times within the normal range. Whole blood can be administered at 10–20 mL/kg intravenously or intraosseously.

Blood groups have not been identified in ferrets. Repeated attempts to identify naturally occurring erythrocyte antibodies or to experimentally induce erythrocyte antibodies were unsuccessful [6,7]. Blood groups have not been studied in rabbits, but transfusions have been administered successfully from donor rabbits in the author's clinic. A cross-match is recommended [6]. Blood groups have not been studied in birds. Homologous transfusions with species-specific blood is recommended [6,7]. Until controlled studies are performed, it is valid to assume that homologous transfusions are preferable to heterologous transfusions. A cross-match is recommended before transfusion [6,7].

Blood should be warmed at least 15 minutes before administration to prevent hypothermia. Warming can be done in a warm-water bath (42°C). The blood-administration set must include a filter to remove most of the aggregated debris. Administer the donor blood by slow bolus or by infusion with a syringe pump (Infusion Pump, Baxter Health Care; Deerfield, IL) into a catheter placed in the jugular, saphenous, or cephalic vein, or into an intraosseous catheter. Blood transfusions should be administered within 4 hours to prevent the growth of bacteria, according to standards set by the American Association of Blood Banks [10]. In cases of massive hemorrhage, blood can be given within minutes.

Fluid therapy plan for the avian patient

The avian patient with a blood volume loss of greater than 25% to 30% of their total blood volume presents in early decompensatory shock similarly to the dog. The heart rate is elevated, mucous membranes are pale, and hypotension is present.

Any sick, debilitated bird presenting for emergency care should immediately be placed in a warm incubator (temperature at 85°F–90°F [29.4°C–32.1°C]) with oxygen supplementation for 8 to 12 hours. When active external hemorrhage is present, this must be stopped immediately. Most birds benefit from the administration of warmed crystalloids at 3 mL/100 g body weight intravenously, intraosseously, or subcutaneous (SQ). Birds should be offered food and water during this time. When the bird seems stable (alert, responsive) and can be safely anesthetized with mask isoflurane (Abbott Laboratory) or sevoflurane (Abbott Laboratory), diagnostics and treatment for hypovolemia and dehydration can be performed. Blood pressure monitoring using Doppler and an ECG should be used during these procedures. External heat should be provided throughout, using a heating pad or forced warm heating blanket.

The Doppler cuff can be placed on the distal humerus or femur and the Doppler probe on the medial surface of the proximal ulna or tibiotarsus, respectively. The blood pressures of various avian species under isoflurane or sevoflurane anesthesia at the author's clinic is 90 to 140 mm Hg systolic. When blood pressures are less than 90 mm Hg systolic, birds are treated for hypovolemia as described below. Bolus administration of crystalloids (10 mL/kg) and colloids (hetastarch (HES) or Oxyglobin at 5 mL/kg) can be given intravenously or intraosseously until blood pressure is greater than 90 mm Hg systolic. In the author's experience, one or two bolus infusions are usually required. When hypotension cannot be corrected after using three boluses of hetastarch and isotonic crystalloids, the author recommends that the clinician use Oxyglobin at 5 mL/kg intravenously or intraosseously. Usually one to two boluses are required to increase the blood pressure in refractory cases. Oxyglobin has oxygen-carrying capacity and vasoconstriction properties. When Oxyglobin is not available, the author has used 7.5% hypertonic saline at 5 mL/kg bolus given slowly over 10 minutes to refractory hypotensive birds.

Blood pressure monitoring helps the veterinarian identify cardiovascular problems in patients under anesthesia earlier than when using an ECG only. Immediate correction of hypotension (systolic blood pressure less than 90 mm Hg) with a fluid bolus helps correct hypovolemia and prevents cardiovascular collapse and death.

Fluid therapy for the surgical patient is necessary to replace losses during the surgical procedure. After mask anesthesia induction using isoflurane or sevoflurane, the patient is intubated. An intraosseous or intravenous catheter is placed during surgical induction and the patient is maintained on a crystalloid infusion at 5 to 10 mL/kg/h. The patient is placed on an external heat source during the surgery. Doppler blood pressure and ECG monitoring should be used. Blood pressure is recorded every 5 minutes. If the blood pressure decreases to less than 90 mm Hg systolic, the patient is given a bolus of crystalloids at 10 mL/kg and colloids at 5 mL/kg. These boluses are repeated until the blood pressure is greater than 90 mm Hg systolic. This protocol helps identify hypotension and allows correction early. Dehydration deficits are calculated after correction of perfusion deficits.

Fluid therapy for shock in small mammals

In the author's experience, rabbits, ferrets, and other small mammals with hypovolemia commonly present in the early decompensatory stage of shock. The earlier compensatory stages of shock commonly seen in the dog and bird are not seen in the cat and the small mammal patient. Signs of early decompensatory shock in the small mammal patient (as in the cat) are bradycardia, hypothermia, and hypotension.

The blood volume in the ferret and rabbit is 50 to 60 mL/kg, in contrast to 90 mL/kg in the dog. When intravascular volume deficits result in poor perfusion, it has been recommended in the past that crystalloids be administered quickly in volumes equivalent to the animal's blood volume. Resuscitation with crystalloids alone, however, can result in significant pulmonary and pleural fluid accumulation. The resultant hypoxemia contributes to the shock pathophysiology.

Rabbits, ferrets, and small mammals are difficult to resuscitate from hypotensive episodes. In the rabbit, when baroreceptors have detected inadequate arterial stretch, it has been found that vagal fibers are stimulated simultaneously with sympathetic fibers [5,8–12]. As a result, the heart rate may be normal or slow instead of the typical tachycardia demonstrated by the dog. This baroreceptor response may be similar in the ferret and in other small mammals. In the author's experience, normal ferrets and rabbits have heart rates between 180 and 240 beats per minute (bpm), systolic blood pressures between 90 and 120 mm Hg, and temperatures between 100°F and 102°F (37.7°C–38.8°C).

Most ferrets, rabbits, and small mammals presented for hypovolemic shock demonstrate heart rate lower than 200 bpm, hypotension (systolic blood pressure less than 90 mm Hg), and hypothermia (temperature less than 98.0°F [36.6°C]). Because cardiac output is a function of contractility and rate, the compensatory response to shock normally seen in dogs and birds is most likely blunted in ferrets, rabbits, and small mammals. The hyperdynamic signs of shock seen in the dog and bird are not typically seen in the cat, ferret, rabbit, and small mammals. Shock in the cat, rabbit, ferret, and small mammal is most commonly decompensatory, manifested by normal heart rate or bradycardia (less than 180 bpm), hypothermia (temperature lower than 98.0°F [36.6°C]), weak or nonpalpable pulses with hypotension, and profound mental depression. The mucous membranes are gray or white and capillary refill is not evident. The bradycardia and low cardiac output contribute to hypothermia, and hypothermia accentuates the bradycardia.

Resuscitation from hypovolemic shock can be safely accomplished with a combination of crystalloids, colloids, and rewarming procedures. In the hypovolemic ferret, rabbit, and small mammal, a bolus infusion of isotonic crystalloids is administered at 10 to 15 mL/kg. Hetastarch is administered at 5 mL/kg intravenously over 5 to 10 minutes. The blood pressure is checked, and once it is greater than 40 mm Hg systolic, only maintenance crystalloids are given while the patient is aggressively warmed. The warming should be done within 1 to 2 hours with warm water bottles, forced air heating blankets, and warming the intravenous fluids. Intravenous fluid warmers facilitate core temperature warming (Elltec Warmel WL-1, Gaymar Industries Inc.; Oakland Park, NY).

Once the rectal temperature approaches 98.0°F, it seems that the adrenergic receptors begin to respond to catecholamines and fluid therapy. Temperatures during this rewarming phase must be checked frequently in all exotic species (especially ferrets) to prevent hyperthermia. Once the animal's rectal temperature has increased to 98.0°F, the blood pressure is rechecked, and crystalloid (10 mL/kg) with hetastarch at 5 mL/kg increments can be repeated over 15 minutes until the systolic blood pressure increases to greater than 90 mm Hg (systolic). The rectal temperature must be maintained as needed by a warm incubator and warmed fluids. When the systolic blood pressure is greater than 90 mm Hg, the rehydration phase of fluid resuscitation begins. A continuous rate infusion (CRI) of hetastarch at 0.8 mL/kg/h is continued during the rehydration phase. If end point parameters (normal blood pressure, heart rate, mucous membrane color, and CRT) are still not obtained, the animal is evaluated and treated for causes of nonresponsive shock (eg, excessive vasodilation or vasoconstriction, hypoglycemia, electrolyte imbalances, acid–base disorder, cardiac dysfunction, hypoxemia).

If cardiac function is normal, and glucose, acid–base, and electrolyte abnormalities have been corrected, treatment for nonresponsive shock is continued. Oxyglobin has not been approved for use in the cat, ferret, rabbit, or small mammal, but it has been used successfully at the author's hospital when given in small-volume boluses. Titrate 2-mL/kg boluses given over 10 to 15 minutes until normal heart rate and blood pressure (systolic blood pressure greater than 90 mm Hg) are obtained. This is followed by a continuous-rate infusion of Oxyglobin at 0.2 to 0.4 mL/kg/h. When Oxyglobin is not available the author has used the vasopressor dopamine at 5 to 10 mcg/kg/min. When Oxyglobin is not available for treatment of refractory hypotension, the author has used 7.5% hypertonic saline at 5 mL/kg bolus given slowly over 10 minutes. Vasopressors such as dopamine or norepinephrine can be used to treat refractory hypotension; however, when using the protocol mentioned, the author has never had to use these drugs in small mammals.

Dehydration deficits are assessed when perfusion parameters are normal. Replacement of dehydration deficits is done with the use of isotonic crystalloids. This is discussed in the rehydration section that follows.

Glucocorticoids in shock

The use of glucocorticoids in the treatment of shock is controversial. These drugs have been extensively investigated in the shock syndrome. Although they have repeatedly shown promise in some experimental studies, they have not shown consistent efficacy in clinical shock syndromes. The side effects of immunosuppression, increased risk for infection, hyperglycemia, and gastric ulceration, may outweigh their benefits. Their use in hemorrhage and hypovolemia is not currently recommended.

Sodium bicarbonate in shock

The most important method of correction of severe metabolic acidosis is aimed at increasing the pH through increasing the extracellular fluid pH. Crystalloid fluids containing lactate, acetate, and gluconate (eg, Plasma-Lyte, Normasol R, lactated ringers solution (LRS)) are considered an important means of increasing the alkalinity of the extracellular fluid. Correction of acidemia initially begins with correction of the patient's perfusion and hydration status through the use of fluid therapy.

When faced with severe acidemia resulting from lactic acidosis and when aggressive measures to improve oxygen delivery and reverse tissue hypoxia have already been initiated without improvement (ie, optimal fluid resuscitation), cautious use of sodium bicarbonate may be used. Blood gas parameters should be carefully monitored if bicarbonate therapy is deemed necessary.

Fluid therapy for dehydration deficits in small mammals and birds

Once immediate life-threatening perfusion deficits are corrected, provide additional fluid based on estimated percentage of dehydration and maintenance needs. The percentage of dehydration can be subjectively estimated based on the presence and degree of loss of body weight, mucous membrane dryness, decreased skin turgor, sunken eyes, and altered mentation. These parameters are largely subjective because they can also be affected by decreased body fat and increased age. Four percent to 6% dehydration is estimated based on increased skin tenting, dry oral mucous membranes, and normal pulses. Ten percent dehydration is evidenced by severe skin tenting, very dry mucous membranes, and dry eyes. Greater than 10% dehydration is also accompanied by signs of hypovolemic shock.

To determine the volume of fluid required for rehydration, use the formula: Volume (L) = hydration deficit × body weight (kg) × 1000 mL. For example, a 2-kg rabbit that is 10% dehydrated requires 0.1 × 2 × 1000 mL, or 200 mL of fluids for rehydration. Dehydration deficits are added to daily maintenance fluid requirements; then estimate ongoing losses. Maintenance requirements for the small mammal and bird are higher than those required for dogs and cats because of their high metabolic rate, and are estimated at 3 to 4 mL/kg/h. The small mammal and bird require larger maintenance volumes because of their high metabolic rates. Eighty percent of the calculated fluid deficit can be replaced in the first 24 hours. Usually acute losses are replaced over 6 to 8 hours and chronic losses over 12 to 24 hours. After successfully treating hypovolemic shock and replacing fluid deficits estimated based on the percentage of dehydration, one should administer maintenance fluids until the mammal or bird can maintain hydration on its own, provided no ongoing losses are present. The adage, "As soon as the gut works, use it," is recommended for early enteral feeding. Enteral feeding decreases intestinal cellular death and subsequent bacterial translocation leading to sepsis. Enteral feeding amounts can be used as part of the animal's maintenance requirements and should be included in the calculation of fluid volumes required. Enteral feeding is discussed in the articles in this issue for each species.

Cardiopulmonary-cerebral resuscitation

The goal of cardiopulmonary resuscitation (CPR) is the restoration of spontaneous circulation. In the 2000s, the American Heart Association changed the guidelines to include the preservation of neurologic function as a goal of successful resuscitation. The term *cardiopulmonary-cerebral resuscitation* was adopted. The most recent International Heart Association guidelines for CPCR and emergency cardiac care in humans were published in 2004. Basic life support consists of the ABC approach (airway, breathing, circulation). Advanced life support consists of electrocardiographic identification of the arrest rhythm, defibrillation, fluid and drug administration, and postresuscitative care. A crash cart should be readily available with supplies (ie, drugs on Table 1) to maximize the chances of a successful outcome. There are anatomic differences in avian species and small mammals, and therefore guidelines for CPCR are discussed for each species. This section reviews the American Heart Association's CPCR guidelines of 2000 and extrapolates these principles to small mammals and birds.

Table 1
Quick reference chart for avian and small mammal CPCR drugs

Drug (conc.)	Weight (g) Weight (kg) Dose	25 mL	50	100	1	2
Epi low (1:10,000) (0.1 mg/mL)	0.01 mg/kg	0.0025	0.005	0.01	0.1	0.2
Epi high (1:1000) (1 mg/mL)	0.1 mg/kg	0.0025	0.005	0.01	0.1	0.2
Atropine[a] (0.54 mg/mL)	0.02 mg/kg	0.001	0.002	0.004	0.037	0.074
Glycopyrrolate (0.2 mg/mL)	0.01 mg/kg	0.0025	0.005	0.01	0.1	0.2
Glucose (50%)	1 mL/kg dilute 50% with saline	0.025	0.05	0.1	1	2
Calcium (100 mg/mL)	50 mg/kg	0.01	0.025	0.05	0.5	1
Doxapram (20 mg/mL)	2 mg/kg	0.0025	0.005	0.01	0.1	0.2
Vasopressin (20 U/mL)	0.8 u/kg	0.001	0.002	0.004	0.04	0.08
External defib	2–10 J/kg	n/a	n/a	1	2	4

[a] Atropine (onset of action, 15–30 s) is not recommended in rabbits, because many possess serum atropinesterase and dose is unpredictable. Increasing the dose of atropine increases the risk for severe tachycardia and increases the risk for ventricular arrhythmias. Use glycopyrrolate (onset of action, 30–45 s) in rabbits.

Effectiveness of cardiopulmonary-cerebral resuscitation

The presence of palpable pulses is not an indication of adequate blood flow. Although palpable pulses may evaluate the response to CPR, they do not indicate the adequacy of organ perfusion during CPR. Two measurements described in the article by Lichtenberger and Ko in this issue on monitoring, end-tidal CO_2 and blood gas measurements, can provide a more accurate assessment of organ perfusion.

The excretion of carbon dioxide in exhaled gas is a function of pulmonary blood flow (cardiac output), and thus the level of CO_2 in exhaled gas changes in direct proportion to changes in cardiac output. End-tidal CO_2 should be used to monitor cardiac output during CPR. A steady increase in end-tidal CO_2 during CPR is more likely to be associated with a successful outcome. When end-tidal CO_2 does not increase to greater than 10 mm Hg after a resuscitation time of 15 to 20 minutes, the resuscitative effort is unlikely to be successful [13]. The common practice of monitoring arterial blood gases during CPR should be abandoned in favor of monitoring venous blood gases. Venous blood gases represent the oxygenation and acid–base status of the peripheral tissues [13–17]. Arterial blood can show a respiratory alkalosis, whereas venous blood shows a metabolic acidosis during CPR [13–17].

Failure to regain consciousness in the first few hours after CPR is not a harbinger of prolonged or permanent neurologic impairment [13–17]. Coma that persists longer than 4 hours after CPR, however, carries a poor prognosis for full neurologic recovery.

Several brainstem reflexes can have prognostic value in patients that do not regain consciousness after CPR, but none can match the predictive value of the papillary light reflex (PLR). Absence of the PLR after 1 or more days of coma indicates little or no chance for neurologic recovery. This reflex has no prognostic value in the first 6 hours after CPR, because it can be transiently lost and then reappear [13–17]. Finally, the resuscitation drugs atropine and epinephrine can produce papillary dilation, but these agents do not interfere with the pupillary response to light [13–17].

Cardiopulmonary-cerebral resuscitation in birds

The prognosis for respiratory arrest, especially when caused by isoflurane anesthesia overdose, is good. Cardiac arrest in birds carries a poor prognosis, because direct compression of the heart is not possible because of the overlying sternum. Because birds do not have a diaphragm, closed-chest compressions cannot use the thoracic pump mechanism to increase overall negative intrathoracic pressure. Anesthetized birds should always be monitored using an electrocardiogram and Doppler blood pressure (BP) measurement. Early recognition of cardiovascular instability is imperative in avian species. If cardiopulmonary arrest occurs when a bird is anesthetized, administration of anesthesia should be stopped immediately. If the bird is masked, intubate and initiate positive-pressure ventilation with 100% oxygen. Alternatively, positive-pressure ventilation can be achieved by way of placement of an air sac cannula. Administer doxapram (0.2 mL for a large bird and 0.1 mL for a small bird intramuscularly) to stimulate the respiratory centers. In the author's experience, birds commonly become bradycardic before a cardiac arrest.

Use atropine (see Table 1) for a vagolytic effect to increase the heart rate. Epinephrine (0.01 mg/kg 1:10,000 solution = 0.1 mg/mL) and atropine (0.02 mg/kg) can be given intravenously, intraosseously, or by way of the endotracheal route (using a tom cat catheter inserted down the endotracheal tube and doubling the dose used for intravenous administration). Also dilute the drug with sterile saline to a volume of 1 mL per 100 g body weight.). Intracardiac injections are no longer recommended by the American Heart Association because of the risk for lacerating coronary vessels, causing hemopericardium or intractable arrhythmias [18].

Vasopressin is a nonadrenergic agent that causes pronounced vasoconstriction by way of direct stimulation of vasopressin (V1) receptors on vascular smooth muscle [18]. It has been suggested that a single dose of vasopressin (see Table 1) may be considered in veterinary CPCR for pulseless electrical activity or asystole. Although the pharmakinetics of this drug have been explored in mammals, there are currently no data available for the avian species. Fluids should be administered to hypovolemic patients but avoided in euvolemic patients. There are no studies documenting the efficacy of electrical defibrillation, and therefore it must be used with caution. An electrocardiogram and Doppler BP measurement help determine rhythm and pulse quality, respectively.

Intracardiac injections should be avoided because of the risk for lacerating coronary vessels. An electrocardiogram, Doppler BP measurement, and end-tidal CO_2 levels can be used to evaluate the effectiveness of cardiopulmonary resuscitation (Fig. 1).

Cardiopulmonary-cerebral resuscitation in small mammals

Anesthesia-related arrests represent one of the more treatable causes of arrest in veterinary patients. Doxapram is given as a respiratory stimulant with respiratory arrest.

In the author's experience, most small mammals become bradycardic before respiratory arrest while under inhalant anesthesia. The inhalant anesthesia should be turned off and the animal should be intubated or if intubated, start ventilating with 100% oxygen. Most small mammals other than the ferret are difficult to intubate (see intubation methods in another article by Lichtenberger and Ko in this issue), and therefore the author recommends the following considerations:

1. If you are unable to intubate, consider forced high-flow oxygen ventilation using a tight-fitting mask over the nose and mouth.

Positive-pressure ventilation should be provided using 100% oxygen at a rate of 20 to 30 breaths per minute. The disadvantage of this technique is accumulation of gastric air and bloating that can limit diaphragm movement.

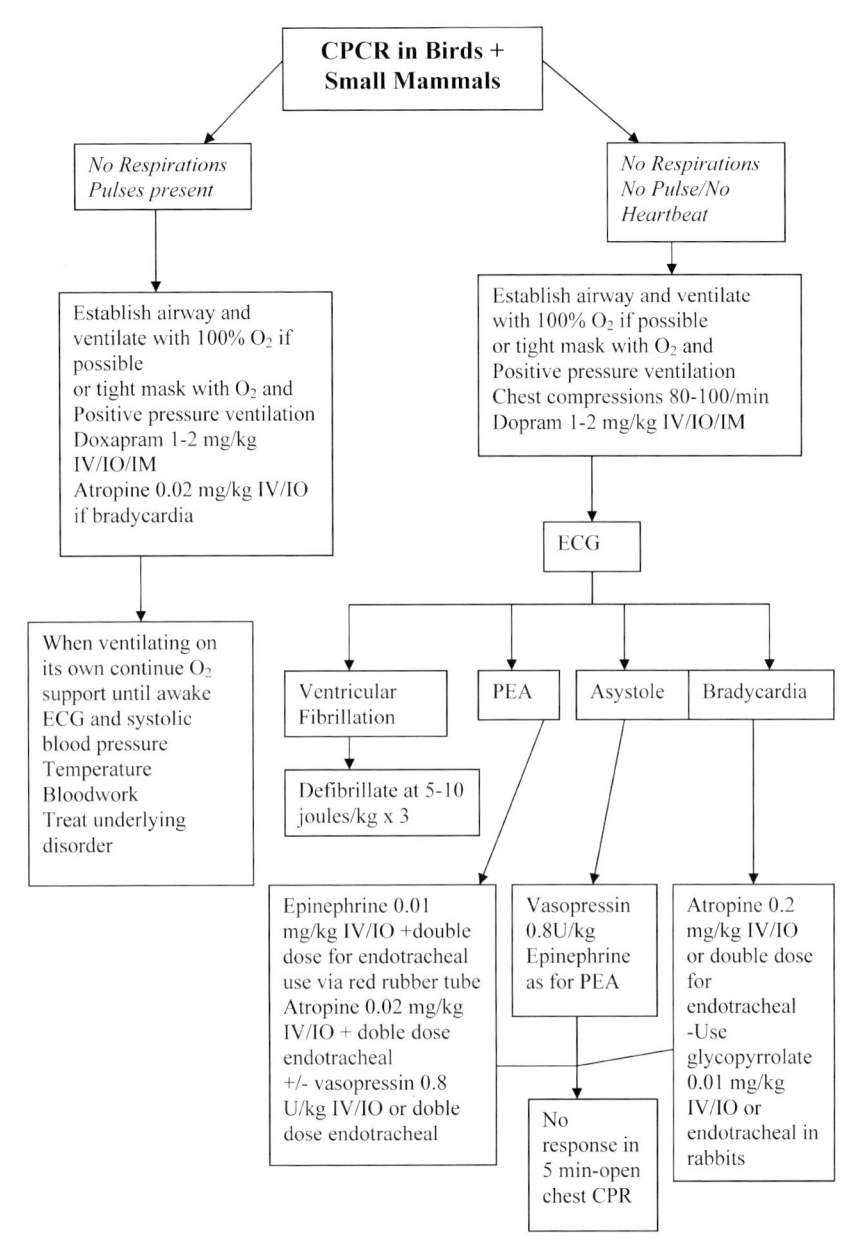

Fig. 1. Cardiopulmonary-cerebral resuscitation in birds and small mammals.

2. The second technique is to perform a tracheotomy. This procedure is similar to that described in dogs and cats [19].

Cardiac arrest involves cessation of effective circulation and is recognized by the loss of consciousness and collapse. A palpable pulse is not felt, the mucous membranes are pale or cyanotic, and respirations commonly cease (ie, cardiopulmonary arrest). Immediate basic life support principles (ie, ABCs) should be initiated. The animal is intubated and ventilated with 100% oxygen. The chest compressions of 80 to 100 times per minute directly compress the myocardium, which leads to increased cardiac output. It is important that both hands be placed on each side of the chest with compressions done at the widest portion of the chest. The duration of the compression should take up half of the total compression–release cycle.

The team should continually assess their efforts at CPR. Check to see if the efforts are generating a palpable pulse. If no pulse is felt, increase the force of chest compressions and assess the electrocardiogram. Different cardiac arrhythmias may require specific treatments. During cardiac arrest and resuscitation, progressive ischemia and acidosis are present. Epinephrine has routinely been the vasopressor of choice for ventricular fibrillation, asystole, and pulseless electrical activity (PEA); however, epinephrine and other catecholamines lose much of their effectiveness as vasopressors in the hypoxic and acidotic body state. Successful resuscitation depends on coronary perfusion being adequate. Coronary perfusion pressure greater than 15 mm Hg is believed to be a predictor of return of spontaneous circulation. The use of vasopressin is today used as a possible consideration for asystole, PEA, and ventricular fibrillation. The addition of vasopressin is first given during the acidotic state and then epinephrine is added soon after. This may improve rates of restoration of spontaneous circulation and survival. Vasopressin is inexpensive. The use of vasopressin in the treatment of shock states and for CPCR should be considered in the veterinary patient. The author has used the drug in small-animal CPCR during asystole in a case of cardiac arrest in a rabbit. There was an immediate return of a heart beat and blood pressure. One dog lived to discharge. The rabbit did eventually die from other chronic disease processes. The author recommends that the clinician consider administering vasopressin during asystole in small mammals and birds. Consider vasopressin use during CPCR with other rhythms (ventricular fibrillation, PEA) refractory to epinephrine, defibrillation, and atropine.

References

[1] Astiz ME. Pathophysiology and classification of shock states. In: Fink MP, Abraham EA, Vincent J-L, et al, editors. Textbook of critical care. Philadelphia: Elsevier/Saunders; 2005. p. 897–918.
[2] Rudloff E, Kirby R. Colloid and crystalloid resuscitation. In: Dhupa N, editor. Philadelphia: W.B. Saunders; 2001;31(6):1207–29.

[3] Smith GJ, Kramer GC, Perron PR, et al. A comparison of several hypertonic solutions for resuscitation of bled sheep. J Surg Res 1985;39:517–28.
[4] Velasco IT, Rocha e Silva M, Oliveira MA, et al. Hypertonic and hyperoncotic resuscitation from severe hemorrhagic shock in dogs: a comparative study. Crit Care Med 1989;17:261–4.
[5] Lichtenberger ML. Principles of shock and fluid therapy in special species. In: Fudge AM, editor. Seminars in avian and exotic pet medicine, emergency medicine. St Louis (Mo): W.B. Saunders; 2004. p. 142–53.
[6] Morrisey J. Transfusion medicine in birds: Western Veterinary Conference 2004. Veterinary Information Network Online Proceedings. Accessed May 1, 2006.
[7] Finnegan M, Daniel G, Ramsay E. Evaluation of whole blood transfusions in domestic pigeons (*Columba livia*). J Avian Med Surg 1997;11(1):7–14.
[8] Jenkins JR. Avian critical care and emergency medicine. In: Altman R, Clubb S, Dorrestein G, et al, editors. Avian medicine and surgery. Philadelphia: W.B. Saunders; 1997. p. 839–64.
[9] Rupley A. Critical care of pet birds. In: Rupley A, editor. The veterinary clinics of North America—exotic animal practice. Philadelphia: W.B. Saunders; 1998. p. 11–42.
[10] Quesenberry K, Hillyer E. Supportive care and emergency therapy. In: Ritchie B, Harrison G, Harrison L, editors. Avian medicine: principles and application. Lake Worth (FL): Wingers Publishing, Inc.; 1994. p. 406–7.
[11] Lichtenberger M, Orcutt C, DeBehnke D, et al. Mortality and response to fluid resuscitation after acute blood loss in Mallard Ducks (*Anas platyrhynnchos*). Proc Annu Conf Assoc Avian Vet 2002;23:65–70.
[12] Sturkie PD. Body fluids: blood. Avian physiology. New York: Springer-Verlag; 1986. p. 102–21.
[13] Marino PR. Cardiac arrest. In: Marino PL, editor. The ICU book. Philadelphia: Lippincott Williams and Wilkins; 1997. p. 260–98.
[14] Wenzel V, Russo S, Arntz HR, et al. The new 2005 resuscitation guidelines of the European Resuscitation Council: comments and supplements. Anaesthesist 2006;55(9):958–66.
[15] Crowe DT. Cardiopulmonary resuscitation in the dog: a review and proposed new guidelines (Parts 1 and 2). Semin Vet Med Surg (Small Anim) 1988;3:321–48.
[16] Curro TG. Anesthesia of pet birds. Semin Avian Exotic Pet Med 1998;7:10–21.
[17] Orcutt CJ. Emergency and critical care of ferrets. Vet Clin North Am 1998;1:99–126.
[18] Costello MF. Principles of cardiopulmonary cerebral resuscitation in special species. Semin Avian Exotic Pet Med 2004;13(3):132–41.
[19] White RN. Emergency techniques. In: King L, Hammond R, editors. Manual of canine and feline emergency and critical care. Dorset (UK): UK Lookers; 1999. p. 307–40.

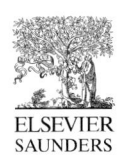

Anesthesia and Analgesia for Small Mammals and Birds

Marla Lichtenberger, DVM, DACVECC[a],*, Jeff Ko, DVM, MS, DACVA[b]

[a]*11015 North Mequon Square Drive, Mequon, WI 53092, USA*
[b]*Department of Veterinary Clinical Sciences, School of Veterinary Medicine, Purdue University, West Lafayette, IN 47908, USA*

Pain is present with many diseases as well as in association with surgical and traumatic conditions. The demonstration of pain is not always obvious; therefore, an animal should be assumed to be experiencing pain in any condition expected to produce pain in human beings. The assessment and control of pain is an art as well as a science. Human beings and animals express three types of opioid receptors: μ, κ, and δ [1–5]. The authors have used this information for the clinical use of opioids in small mammals. Clinicians should keep in mind that the art of pain management is a continual learning experience requiring assessment and therapeutic adjustment for individual animals, even when they are undergoing similar surgical procedures. Therefore, standard or rule-of-thumb analgesic and anesthetic protocols are not always appropriate.

There are ongoing studies in the avian species to investigate opioid receptors in the brain and spinal cord. In the past, investigations led to the belief that psittacines possess primarily κ-receptors [6]. Recommendations for κ-receptor agonists, such as butorphanol, are given for the avian species. In a recent study, an amphibian model for the investigation of opioid analgesia has provided novel data on the mechanisms of opioid receptors, adding an evolutionary perspective [1–5]. There is an apparent receptor type of selectivity during evolution, although all three receptors exist even in the amphibian species. Future studies in the avian species may lead to further investigation for use of μ-receptor agonist drugs for analgesia.

If animals can experience pain, how do we assess pain in ferrets, rabbits, or birds? It is likely that the tolerance of pain by these animals varies greatly

* Corresponding author.
E-mail address: marlavet@aol.com (M. Lichtenberger).

from individual to individual. Furthermore, these animals' innate ability to mask significant disease and pain makes it difficult for us to assess their degree of pain. Compared with dogs and cats, pain in ferrets, rabbits, and birds is far more difficult to assess. As in cats, the mainstay of pain assessment in ferrets, rabbits, and birds seems to be behavioral.

Behaviors that are commonly seen in ferrets, rabbits, and birds with acute trauma or postoperative pain include a depressed, immobile, or silent demeanor, and they seem to be distanced from their environment. They may stand with their eyes half-closed and do not groom themselves. Rabbits and ferrets may exhibit bruxism. They do not respond normally to petting or attention; ferrets, rabbits, and birds tend to hide when experiencing pain.

Multimodal analgesia in all species of birds and small mammals

The process of nociception and pain involves multiple steps and pathways; thus, a single analgesic agent is unlikely to alleviate pain completely. An effective pain management plan should include drugs of different classes, with each acting at a different step of the pathway; this is termed *multimodal analgesia*. For example, a ferret can be premedicated with an opioid, which modulates pain; ketamine can be used as part of the induction protocol to reduce wind-up; a local anesthetic block could be incorporated to inhibit pain transmission; and a nonsteroidal anti-inflammatory drug (NSAID) can be added before or after surgery to alter pain transduction. This approach also allows smaller doses of each drug to be used, because the effects are additive or synergistic and reduce any undesirable side effects from larger doses of individual drugs.

Pain management options in the rabbit, ferret, and bird

There is no doubt that pain management in the ferret, rabbit, and bird in clinical practice is presently inadequate. Traditional belief is that the ferret, rabbit, and bird have adverse respiratory depression after opiate treatment; however, in the authors' opinion, the ferret, rabbit, and bird become comfortable and sleep normally after administration of opioids after surgery. Birds have mainly κ-receptors for pain, and therefore respond well to κ-agonist opioids for pain relief. Rabbits are more sensitive to the side effects of most opioids. Ferrets are deficient in the glucuronidation pathway, as are cats, and inappropriate dosing of NSAIDs can lead to toxicity [7].

Fear of these adverse effects has resulted in many ferrets, rabbits, and birds not receiving analgesics after surgery or trauma. Drugs used in rabbits and ferrets are discussed in the next section, followed by treatment for pain in birds. The avian species are discussed separately, because pain receptor research in birds defining receptors centrally and peripherally is currently underway. New research should bring us new desperately needed injectable analgesia choices in birds. The use of only butorphanol and isoflurane for general anesthesia and analgesia for procedures in birds may become obsolete in the future. The current protocols for analgesia and anesthesia in birds are discussed at the end of this section.

Anesthetic or analgesic drugs used in small mammals

The five major classes of analgesics used for acute pain management are opioids, nonsteroidal anti-inflammatory drugs, local anesthetics, alpha-agonists, and dissociatives. Drugs and doses used by the authors in ferrets, rabbits, and birds are discussed. All doses used by the authors are given in Table 1.

Opioids

Ferrets, rabbits, and birds were suspected to have "respiratory depression" after administration of opioid drugs when they were indeed resting quietly without pain. When used appropriately, opioids can be administered to small mammals and are safe and effective for alleviating pain. Opioids generally have a wide margin of safety and excellent analgesic properties. In veterinary medicine, the most commonly used opioids are fentanyl, hydromorphone, morphine, buprenorphine, and butorphanol. Some animals may respond better to one opioid over another, depending on individual variability, breed, species, and source of pain. Opioids act centrally to limit the input of nociceptive information to the central nervous system (CNS), which reduces central hypersensitivity [8]. Opioids are commonly used in the critically ill patient because they have a rapid onset of action and are safe, reversible, and potent analgesics. There are four classes of opioids: pure agonists, partial agonists, agonist-antagonists, and antagonists. Their use as a constant rate infusion (CRI) is discussed elsewhere in this article. Combination anesthetic protocols are commonly used in small mammals for the multimodal approach to analgesia. In a study using different combinations of intramuscular drugs (medetomidine and ketamine; medetomidine, fentanyl, and midazolam; and xylazine and ketamine), the quality of surgical anesthesia was greatest with the medetomidine and ketamine. All combinations allowed recovery of similar duration. The advantage of the combination of medetomidine, fentanyl, and midazolam is to be able to antagonize each component of the combination [5].

1. Butorphanol (Dolorex; Intervet, Millboro, Delaware) continues to be the most commonly used opioid in small mammals despite recent questioning of its analgesic properties. Described as an agonist-antagonist agent, its agonist activity is exerted at the κ-receptors and its antagonist actions are demonstrated at the μ-receptors. Opioid drugs in this class exert a "ceiling" effect, after which increasing doses do not produce any further analgesia. Butorphanol seems to be an effective visceral

Table 1
Analgesia drugs used in small mammals

Drug	Preoperative dose for rabbit or ferret	Induction dose for ferret or rabbit	Constant rate infusion dose or postoperative dose for rabbit or ferret
Tranquilizers			
Diazepam	0.5 mg/kg IV	—	—
Midazolam	0.25–0.5 mg/kg IM or IV	—	—
Opioids			
Butorphanol	0.2–0.8 mg/kg SQ, IM, or IV	—	0.1–0.2 mg/kg loading dose, then 0.1–0.2 mg/kg/h
Fentanyl	5–10 µg/kg IV	—	During surgery: 5–20 µg/kg/h with ketamine CRI After surgery: 2.5–5 µg/kg/h with ketamine CRI
Hydromorphone	0.05–0.1 mg/kg IV	—	0.05 mg/kg IV loading dose, then 0.05–0.1 mg/kg/h
Tramadol	—	—	After surgery: 10 mg/kg PO q 24 hours
NMDA antagonists			
Ketamine	—	4–10 mg/kg IV	During surgery: 0.1 mg/kg IV loading dose, then 0.3–0.4 mg/kg/h with fentanyl CRIAfter surgery: 0.3–0.4 mg/kg/h with fentanyl CRI
Propofol	—	4–6 mg/kg IV	—
Etomidate	—	1–2 mg/kg IV with benzodiazepine	—

α_2-agonists		
Medetomidine	1–2 μg/kg IM or IV	1–2 μg/kg q 4–6 hours IV
NSAIDs		
Carprofen	—	4 mg/kg PO q 24 hours
Ketoprofen	—	After surgery: 1–2 mg/kg q 24 hours
Meloxicam	—	0.2 mg/kg (first dose) SQ, IV, or PO and then 0.1 mg/kg q 24 hours (rabbit: 0.3 mg/kg q 24 hours)
Local anesthetics		
Lidocaine	—	Local infiltration during surgery: 1 mg/kg at incision site or ring block
Bupivacaine	—	Local infiltration during or after surgery: 1 mg/kg at incision site or ring block
Epidurals		
Morphine preservative-free	—	0.1 mg/kg epidural with or without bupivacaine before surgery
Bupivicaine 0.125%	—	0.1 mg/kg epidural with or without morphine

The drug doses in this table are those that are used by the author in small mammals. Few pharmacologic studies have been done with regard to the listed drugs in the ferret and rabbit.

Abbreviations: CRI, continuous rate infusion; IM, intramuscular; IV, intravenous; NMDA, N-methyl-D-aspartate; NSAIDs, nonsteroidal anti-inflammatory drugs; PO, by mouth; q, every; SQ, subcutaneous.

but poor somatic analgesic. It is a poor analgesic choice for surgical patients in which there is somatic and visceral pain. Its ceiling effect limits its use to minor procedures, and the frequent dosing required is inconvenient and relatively expensive. When used in the authors' clinic for treatment of pain in the ferret and rabbit, they prefer to use it as a CRI instead of administrating repeated doses. The drug seems to have a duration of only 2 to 4 hours after administration of a single bolus in most animals. Butorphanol can also be used to antagonize the respiratory depression of the μ-receptor agents without reversing the analgesic effect.

2. Buprenorphine is a mixed agonist-antagonist. Pharmacokinetic and pharmacodynamic data have suggested that 2- to 4-hour dosing intervals may be required for buprenorphine administration in most species of mammals. Buprenorphine is a slow-onset long-acting opiate in mammals that possesses a unique and complex pharmacologic profile. Buprenorphine may exhibit a plateau or ceiling analgesic effect. In rats, once buprenorphine reached its maximal effect, administration of additional drug produced detrimental effects or no additional analgesia, although the higher dose may prolong the duration of analgesia [9]. This ceiling effect of dosing has also been demonstrated in mice [10]. Analgesic effects at the same dosage can also be variable among different strains of rodents [9]. Gastrointestinal side effects are the most commonly reported adverse effect with buprenorphine; thus, lower doses are recommended when treating gastrointestinal stasis [11]. One adverse effect of buprenorphine administration that has recently been reported in rats is the ingestion of certain types of bedding, especially sawdust or wood chips [12]. This "pica behavior" was not demonstrated when the rats were on a paper pellet type of bedding, and it is recommended that rats be housed on other materials after administration of this drug. Buprenorphine is most commonly administered subcutaneously, intramuscularly, or intravenously. The opioid buprenorphine has the disadvantage of being difficult to reverse (using naloxone) because the drug is difficult to displace at the receptor [13]. Buprenorphine can be used for reversal of μ-receptor opioid respiratory depression while maintaining postoperative analgesia for 420 minutes in rabbits [14].

3. Hydromorphone (hydromorphone hydrogen chloride [HCl] injection, *United States Pharmacopeia* [USP]; Baxter Healthcare Corporation, Deerfield, Illinois) and fentanyl (fentanyl citrate injection, USP; Abbott Laboratories, North Chicago, Illinois) are μ-receptor agonists. They are excellent analgesics for visceral and somatic pain. CRIs are necessary when using rapidly metabolized opioid, such as fentanyl, for operative and postoperative analgesia. Table 1 lists doses used by the authors. Fentanyl and hydromorphone can be reversed using naloxone or partially reversed with butorphanol (reverse the respiratory depression and sedation without completely reversing analgesia).

4. Naloxone is a μ- and κ-antagonist. Naloxone can reverse sedation, respiratory depression, and bradycardia, but the reversal of sedation and analgesia can cause pain, excitement, delirium, and hyperalgesia [15]. Low-dose naloxone (0.04 mg/kg titrated slowly intravenously) can be used to reverse CNS depression without affecting analgesia [15]. The duration of naloxone is short; therefore, the authors recommend administering butorphanol to reverse μ-antagonist CNS depression without antagonizing κ-antagonist analgesia effects.
5. Tramadol (opioid type drug) is another drug that can be used orally for postoperative pain control. No studies have been done on use of this drug in small mammals. Tramadol binds to opiate receptors and also inhibits reuptake of norepinephrine and serotonin. The agent thus activates two endogenous antinociceptive mechanisms in the spinal cord and brain stem. The doses that are currently being used by the authors, as suggested in Table 1, have been extrapolated from human medicine.

Nonsteroidal anti-inflammatory drugs

NSAIDs are another option for alleviation of acute postoperative and traumatic pain. As in other species, there are concerns about preoperative use of NSAIDs in small mammals. The main concerns relate to inhibition of prostaglandin synthesis, which may lead to gastrointestinal erosion, impaired renal function, and bleeding. The limited ability for glucuronide conjugation in ferrets can prolong the duration of action of NSAIDs; however, with appropriate changes in dose and dosing intervals, they can be used safely. The advantages of this category of drugs are their long duration of action and that they are not a controlled substance. In young ferrets with no evidence of renal disease, this group of drugs is a good choice.

Injectable and oral carprofen is available in the United States, but it is unlikely to be labeled for use in ferrets. Carprofen is not a potent inhibitor of prostaglandin synthetase and has proved to be a safe agent in ferrets. Ketoprofen (Ketofen; Fort Dodge Animal Health, Fort Dodge, Iowa) is available as an injectable agent, but because of its cyclooxygenase (COX)-1 inhibition, it should be reserved for postoperative administration. Meloxicam (Metacam; Boehringer Ingelheim Vetmedica, St. Joseph, Missouri) is available in injectable and oral forms and is the most commonly used NSAID in small mammals. It primarily has COX-2 inhibition. Doses are given in Table 1.

NSAIDs should not be used in animals with preexisting renal disease, hypovolemia, or bleeding disorders or if severe surgical hemorrhage is anticipated. The authors do not recommend that NSAIDs be used as a preanesthetic drug in the critically ill patient. The drug can be used after surgery in stable normovolemic small mammals when they start eating. Renal values are always checked before use.

Flunixin meglumine is a potent inhibitor of COX-1 and COX-2. Recommendations for its use in rabbits with gastric stasis and septic shock are common in literature. This is most likely attributable to its use in horses with colic. The authors warn against NSAID use when any gastric ulceration is present or suspected. To date, no safety or toxicity studies of NSAIDs have been conducted in small mammals.

Local anesthetic agents

Local anesthetic agents can be used successfully in ferrets. The two most commonly used agents are lidocaine (Lidocaine HCl Oral Topical Soln, USP 2%; Hi-Tech Pharmacal Company, Amityville, New York) and bupivacaine (Bupivacaine HCl, 0.5%; Abbott Laboratories). Suitable dosages and anticipated duration of action are shown in Table 1.

Use of local anesthetics for incisional line blocks, wound infiltration, nerve ring blocks, epidural anesthesia or topically is recommended by the authors. For incisional line blocks before surgery, the authors use a 25-gauge 0.25-inch needle to infiltrate the subcutaneous tissue and skin. The local anesthetics are used as part of the multimodal approach to analgesia. The calculated dose of the drugs should not exceed the doses listed in Table 1. Local analgesic protocols (eg, ring blocks, incisional blocks) are commonly combined with other drugs (ie, opioids, CRIs) for multimodal analgesia (Fig. 1).

An advantage of local anesthetics is their low cost and noncontrolled drug status. A complete sensory block prevents nerve transmission, making the use of these agents attractive for practical preemptive techniques. Local anesthetics can be infiltrated into the surgical skin site, or discrete nerve blocks can be performed. The addition of an opioid to the mixture of local anesthetics for local blocks potentially lengthens the median duration of analgesia (addition of morphine to the lidocaine-bupivacaine mixture

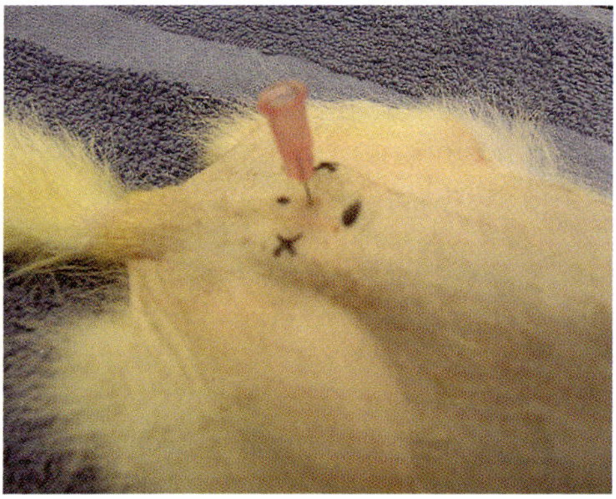

Fig. 1. Epidural anesthesia in a ferret. For epidural anesthesia, a 25-gauge needle is placed in the distal two thirds of the LS space. The black line indicates the seventh lumbar vertebrae. The "x" marks indicate the wings of the ilium. The black dot indicates the first sacral vertebrae.

prolonged analgesia 10 hours longer with the morphine and 9 hours longer with the buprenorphine) [15,16], with the conclusion being that adding an opioid to the local anesthetic mixture lengthens the duration of analgesia. In the authors' experience, the analgesia is prolonged significantly when adding an opioid to the local block. In another study, a buprenorphine–local anesthetic axillary perivascular brachial plexus block provided postoperative analgesia lasting three times longer than a local anesthetic block alone and twice as long as buprenorphine given by intramuscular injection plus a local anesthetic-only block. This supports the concept of peripherally mediated opioid analgesia by buprenorphine. This study was performed in human patients, and the dose of buprenorphine was 0.003 mg mixed with the lidocaine-bupivacaine as given in Table 1 for local anesthetics.

Dental blocks

There are five important dental blocks for small mammals. All five blocks incorporate the lidocaine-bupivacaine mixture as discussed previously for the ring block. The total dose of the mixture is drawn up into a syringe, and one fifth of the total dose is given into each of five sites. A 25- to 27-gauge needle is used with a 0.5- to 1-cc syringe.

The following techniques can be used to provide regional anesthesia for rabbits and other small mammals (Dale Kressin, personal communication, 2007). Kressin recommends the following protocols for dental blocks.

Infraorbital nerve block. The infraorbital nerve arises from the maxillary branch of the trigeminal nerve. This nerve provides sensory fibers to the upper incisor teeth, upper lip, and adjacent soft tissues. The zygomatic nerve also arises from the maxillary nerve just proximal to the infraorbital nerve. This nerve also supplies sensory fibers to the lateral aspect of the face.

The infraorbital foramen is located approximately 5 to 12 mm dorsal to the crestal bone adjacent to the upper first premolar (cheek) tooth at the lateral aspect of the skull. The foramen is not as easily palpated as in the dog. The facial tuber is a palpable bony prominence at the mesial (rostral) aspect of the zygomatic bone and is approximately 4 to 10 mm ventral to the infraorbital canal. The infraorbital nerve can be blocked by infusion of local anesthetic at this foramen (Fig. 2).

Mental nerve block. The mental nerve arises from the mandibular nerve as it extends into the mental foramina to form the mental nerve. The mental nerve supplies sensory fibers to the ventral and lateral aspect of the mandible, lip, and lower incisor and motor fibers to local muscles.

The mental nerve exits the mental foramen located at the dorsal lateral aspect of the body of the mandible. The foramen is rostral (2–4 mm) to the first mandibular premolar (cheek) tooth and is located ventrally in the dorsal one third of the body of the mandible. The mental nerve can be blocked by infusion of local anesthetic at this foramen (see Fig. 2).

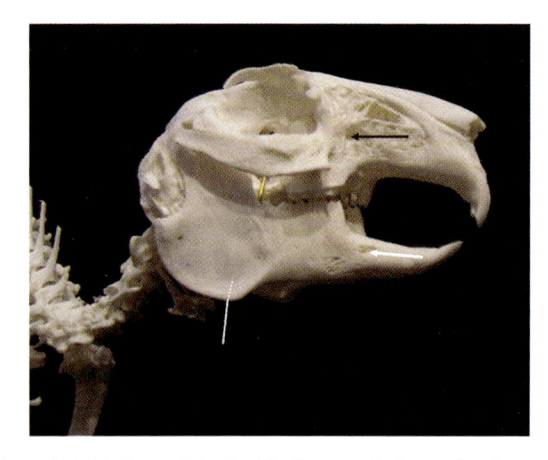

Fig. 2. Oblique lateral skull of a rabbit. The black arrow indicate the placement for the needle for an infraorbital nerve block (deep) and maxillary nerve block (superficial). The white arrow indicates the placement for a mental nerve block. The white line indicates the placement of the needle for a mandibular nerve block (dotted white line indicates that placement is medial to the mandible).

Mandibular nerve block. The mandibular nerve arises from the trigeminal nerve and supplies sensory and motor fibers to the ventral mandible as well as to the muscles of mastication. The mandibular nerve provides sensory fibers to the mandibular molar and premolar (cheek) teeth as well as to adjacent tissues.

The mandibular nerve enters the mandibular foramen on the medial surface of the mandible. An intraoral approach to block this nerve is not practical in the rabbit as in other species because of the limited access to the oral cavity. An extraoral approach should be made with great care to avoid neurovascular structures (facial vessels and nerves) at the ventral aspect of the mandible. The mandibular foramen is approximately midway between the distal aspect of the last molar (cheek) tooth and the ventral aspect of the mandible. Additionally, the foramen is approximately 2 to 5 mm distal to the third molar tooth. After this location is determined, an infusion needle of appropriate length can be "walked along" the medial aspect of the mandible to the mandibular foramen for infusion of the local anesthetic. This effectively blocks the mandibular premolar and molar (cheek) teeth (see Fig. 2).

Maxillary nerve block. The maxillary nerve supplies sensory fibers to the upper premolar and molar (cheek) teeth and adjacent tissues.

Intraoral approaches to the maxillary nerve have not been attempted by the authors because of the limited access to the oral cavity. In large-breed rabbits, the maxillary nerve can be blocked using a "caudal infraorbital" strategy. A 27-gauge needle is advanced 1 to 2 cm into the infraorbital canal. The syringe is aspirated to ensure that the needle is not in a vessel lumen. Firm digital pressure is placed over the rostral end of the infraorbital canal while slowly infusing the local anesthetic. This block anesthetizes all ipsilateral premolar and molar (cheek) teeth and the adjacent periodontal tissues. In small rabbits and other small mammals, it may not be possible to thread the needle into the infraorbital canal. It these cases, the authors place the needle at the rostral entrance to the canal, apply firm digital pressure, and infuse the local anesthetic. Application of "splash blocks" of the local anesthetics to the periodontal ligament and adjacent soft tissues may also augment regional anesthesia (see Fig. 2).

Palatine nerve block. The sphenopalatine nerve ends within the sphenopalatine ganglion. Three nerves extend from the ganglion to regional tissues. The nasal cavity is innervated by the nasal rami, the rostral or anterior hard palate by the nasopalatine nerve, and the posterior hard palate by the anterior palatine nerve. The oral cavity of the rabbit limits easy visualization; however, the anterior palatine nerve can be blocked as it exits the larger palatine foramen. This foramen is located halfway between the palatal aspect of the third upper premolar (cheek) tooth and the palatal midline. Infusion of a local anesthetic blocks this nerve and the palate of the ipsilateral side (Fig. 3).

Intratesticular block

The authors recommend that castration in small mammals be performed with an intramuscular preoperative injection of buprenorphine (0.02 mg/kg) with midazolam (0.25 mg/kg). Mix bupivacaine (0.5%) at a rate of 0.1 mg per 100 g of body weight and lidocaine (2%) at a rate of 0.1 mg per 100 g body weight with buprenorphine at a rate of 0.0003 mg per 100 g

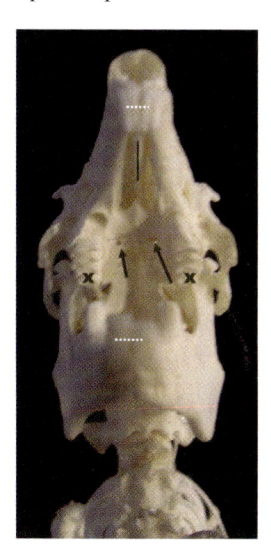

Fig. 3. Open-mouth skull of a rabbit. The black arrows indicates the placement for a palatine nerve block. The white dotted line indicates the top and bottom incisors. The black solid line indicates the palatal midline.

of body weight. This can be diluted in saline to have a final volume of 1 mL. Use a 25-gauge 0.625-inch needle for guinea pigs or rabbits and a 27-gauge 0.625-inch needle for a mouse or gerbil. Place the needle through the testicle, starting from the caudal pole and aiming for the spermatic cord. It is desirable for the needle to exit the testicle proximally, because it is the spermatic cord that is going to be ligated. Aspirate before injection. Inject, expressing firm back-pressure, while withdrawing the needle. Expect to use approximately one third of the drug volume per testicle, leaving the organ firmly turgid. Repeat for the other testicle, and the remaining drug can be used to place a dermal incisional block. This should provide analgesia for 22 hours (B. Stein, personal communication, 2006).

α_2-agonists

The α_2-agonists, such as medetomidine (Domitor; Pfizer Animal Health, Exton, Pennsylvania), possess analgesic, sedation, and muscle-relaxant properties. The higher dose (30 µg/kg) drugs are usually reserved for healthy animals because of the cardiopulmonary depression that accompanies their use. One study in healthy rabbits found that the combination of medetomidine and ketamine showed the best sedation, whereas the medetomidine-fentanyl-midazolam combination had the least cardiovascular effects and the xylazine-ketamine combination had the greatest cardiovascular side effects [17].

Microdose medetomidine (1–3 µg/kg) minimally affects the blood pressure in animals with normal cardiac output and provides good analgesia, sedation, and muscle relaxation when used with a tranquilizer and opioid. Medetomidine requires only slight α_2-adrenoceptor availability to decrease noradrenaline turnover [18], and extremely low doses of medetomidine result in sympatholysis. Therefore, patients who require a high level of sympathetic tone to maintain blood pressure may not tolerate medetomidine (ie, animals in shock or in compensated heart failure). In conscious dogs, intravenous medetomidine at a rate of 1.25 µg/kg increased blood pressure by 15% and decreased heart rate by 26% and cardiac output by 35% [19].

In postoperative patients, sympathetic tone was not entirely abolished by medetomidine. Only the unwanted increases in heart rate and blood pressure were attenuated. Medetomidine has no effect on cortisol levels [20]. The α_2-agonists are commonly used in human medicine to decrease the stress response. Their use in small mammals for inhibition of the stress response may be warranted. The authors recommend the microdose of medetomidine for use in small mammals but warn the clinician not to use this drug in any animal with a compromised cardiovascular system.

Ketamine

Ketamine is commonly used for induction of anesthesia in small mammals. Reports in human and veterinary medicine indicate variable patient response after ketamine administration, which is related to the status of the cardiovascular system at the time of ketamine administration. Ketamine used for induction is well tolerated in the stable patient. Patients that exhibit significant preexisting stress or a patient with hypertrophic cardiomyopathy has an increased risk of cardiovascular destabilization after ketamine administration. Ketamine increases sympathetic tone, causing an increase in heart rate, myocardial contractility, and total peripheral vascular resistance. The authors think that high-dose ketamine used for induction of anesthesia in a stressed small mammal (especially the rabbit) may cause an increased risk of destabilization. The authors avoid using ketamine as an induction agent for the stressed critically ill rabbit. The N-methyl-D-aspartate (NMDA) receptor plays an important role in central sensitization, and there is much interest in developing drugs that can inhibit this receptor. In veterinary medicine, a commonly used NMDA antagonist is ketamine (Vetaket; Lloyd Laboratories, Shenondoah, Iowa), which may be effective at preventing, or at least lessening, wind-up at subanesthetic doses. When used with inhalant anesthesia and opioids, there is a reported opioid-sparing and inhalant anesthetic–sparing effect seen. The interesting perspective about ketamine is that minute amounts used by way of a CRI route induce an analgesic effect. Microdose ketamine does not cause an increase in sympathetic tone and is frequently used for analgesia with a CRI.

Constant rate infusions

CRIs have several advantages over bolus delivery when treating with an analgesic. When using a CRI, a drug can be titrated to effect, resulting in a reduction of the total amount of drug used, fewer side effects, less "rollercoaster" analgesia, fewer hemodynamic effects, and improved cost-effectiveness. One disadvantage to a CRI is a slow rise in drug plasma concentration to therapeutic levels, which is why a loading dose of the drug is frequently given before starting a CRI. Another disadvantage of a CRI is the need for a pump, which is the easiest way to administer a CRI. Syringe pumps, most of which use a 1- to 60-cc syringe for drug delivery through an intravenous extension set, allow constant-rate delivery of small volumes of drug. When these CRIs are combined, there is an overall inhalant anesthetic–sparing effect. A common side effect of inhalant anesthesia is hypotension, which is avoided when inhalant anesthesia is combined with ketamine or opioid CRIs. The dose of fentanyl used by the authors is much lower than previously reported for use in small mammals. The authors do see a much greater depressive effect in small mammals when using the high-dose ranges of fentanyl. They have not seen fentanyl-induced ileus or other gastrointestinal side effects in small mammals when using the lower end of the dose given in Table 1, when combined with ketamine. The multimodal approach of using two or more drugs combined allows for lower doses with fewer side effects of both drugs than when either drug is used alone. The authors commonly use the lower CRI doses for butorphanol-ketamine CRIs or fentanyl-ketamine CRIs in rabbits with gastric stasis pain (see Table 1). Ketamine is an excellent adjunct to opioid therapy and frequently allows a reduction in the opioid dose being administered.

Anesthesia induction agents in rabbits and ferrets

1. Etomidate (Amidate; BenVenue Laboratories, Bedford, Ohio) is an imidazole derivative that undergoes rapid redistribution and hepatic metabolism, resulting in rapid recovery after a single bolus [21,22]. Etomidate induces minimal cardiovascular depression with a wide margin of safety. It has a respiratory depressant effect but is dose dependent. The drug is given to effect, using the lower end of the dose range (1–2 mg/kg administered intravenously). Patients should preferably be intubated, or at least provided an oxygen mask. Etomidate is frequently used in one of the authors' clinics in patients that have poor cardiovascular function and is the most common drug that author (ML) uses for induction of anesthesia for minor procedures or surgery in small mammals. The authors routinely combine diazepam with etomidate induction in compromised patients. The recommended dose of etomidate after premedication with diazepam (Diazepam inj, USP; Abbott Laboratories; Valium at a rate of 0.5 mg/kg administered intravenously) is 1.0 mg/kg. The combination of diazepam allows lower doses of etomidate as well as minimal myoclonic twitching during induction.
2. Propofol (PropoFlo; Abbott Laboratories) is chemically unrelated to other anesthetic drugs. It has a fast onset and short duration of action. Apnea after administration of propofol is seen with rapid injection of the drug. The authors use propofol as an induction agent in stable ferrets at a dose of 2 to 4 mg/kg administered intravenously and combined with diazepam or midazolam (0.25–0.5 mg/kg administered intravenously), so that the lowest dose of propofol is used. The propofol is given over 1 to 2 minutes as a slow intravenous bolus, and oxygen is administered with a mask. Endotracheal intubation should be done when apnea occurs. The animal may be ventilated until spontaneous breathing resume. Propofol induction has been studied extensively in the rabbit as an induction agent. There are numerous studies in healthy rabbits documenting the safety of medetomidine or midazolam preoperative sedation when used with propofol intravenously [18,23,24]. The authors do not recommend using medetomidine or propofol in the unstable cardiovascular patient.
3. The combination of ketamine and diazepam (4–10 mg/kg and 0.25–0.5 mg/kg, respectively, administered intravenously) is commonly used for induction in ferrets and rabbits. This dose of ketamine does cause an increase in sympathetic response, and the authors recommend avoiding high-dose ketamine in any animal with heart disease or a heart murmur.

The ferret and rabbit (not unlike the cat) can have occult cardiac disease without outward clinical signs. The increase in sympathetic response with ketamine in an already stressed animal increases myocardial oxygen demand. A normal stable animal can handle this sympathetic response, but for the occult cardiomyopathy or a critically ill patient, this drug may prove detrimental.

Inhalants

Based on available research in dogs, cats, and ferrets, there are advantages of sevoflurane and isoflurane [25], depending on the circumstances. Isoflurane has an advantage if cost is an issue. Sevoflurane may have an advantage if mask induction is necessary or if the anesthetist needs to adjust the depth of anesthesia. Mask induction and changing the depth of anesthesia are important in exotics. Sevoflurane has a much less pungent odor. No differences in the speed of recovery were noted in ferrets in a controlled study. In most animals and birds, the maximum allowable concentration (MAC) for isoflurane is between 1.28 and 1.63; for sevoflurane, the MAC is between 2.10 and 2.60. Isoflurane and sevoflurane have dose-dependent vasodilation properties leading to hypotension. Neither drug has any analgesic properties after termination of anesthesia.

Epidural anesthesia or analgesia in small mammals

Epidural drugs achieve pain relief with less or no systemic effects as compared with drugs administered intramuscularly or intravenously. This factor is important in small mammals when the administered drug has negative side effects, such as cardiac and respiratory depression. Epidural drugs may decrease recovery time, which is always an advantage when working with ferrets, rabbits, and other small mammals. The short recovery time occurs because of the inhalant-sparing effect induced with an epidural anesthetic.

The local anesthetics lidocaine and bupivacaine are most commonly used for epidural analgesia. Using local anesthetics can result in sensory, motor, and autonomic blockade. This may be prevented by administering the diluted dose and lower dose recommended by the authors and given in Table 1. When placing an epidural needle, the clinician should lower the local anesthetic dose by one half when cerebrospinal fluid (CSF) fluid is seen in the hub (CSF fluid may only fill the hub with use of a stylet).

In most small mammals, after epidural injection of lidocaine, analgesia develops within 10 to 15 minutes and lasts from 60 to 90 minutes Bupivacaine can provide between 4 and 8 hours of surgical analgesia. It may exert analgesic effects with minimal motor blockage when used in a dilute concentration. This dilution may be obtained by mixing one part of 0.25% bupivacaine (0.125% bupivacaine at a rate of 0.1 mg/kg) with one to three parts of an opioid by volume administered at the desired opioid dose. The principle advantages of local anesthetics are the potential for complete regional anesthesia and marked potentiation of the analgesic effect of the epidural opioids. Morphine (Morphine Sulfate inj preservative free, USP; Baxter Healthcare, Cherry Hill, New Jersey) at a rate of 0.1 mg/kg administered into the epidural space provides prolonged postoperative analgesia for up to 24 hours. Morphine is the least soluble opioid, and this characteristic delays the epidural and systemic absorption of the drug [8]. The peak analgesic effects may be delayed for 90 minutes after injection, and some analgesia may be present for 6 to 24 hours. It is important to administer it immediately after induction of anesthesia because of the relatively long latency to peak analgesia. Bupivacaine or lidocaine can be administered with morphine epidurally so that the onset of analgesia is shortened to 15 to 30 minutes, with a duration of 8 to 24 hours. In human patients, postoperative neural blockage has also been associated with attenuation of the stress response, improved respiratory function, and improved hemodynamic stability [8]. We notice marked improvement in postoperative recovery in small mammals after they receive epidural analgesia before abdominal surgery or surgery on the rear limbs. When included as part of a patient management strategy, these epidural analgesic techniques, as part of the multimodal approach, may reduce morbidity and mortality.

The lumbosacral (LS) space is the preferred site of injection because of the relatively large space between L7 and S1. In most ferrets, the dural sac terminates just cranial to that location (L7–S1). The absence of a complete dural sac at the LS junction reduces the likelihood of subdural injections. The dural sac of many rabbits extends to the sacrum, and attempts at epidural injection of the LS space in this species may result in subdural injections. Most subdural injections are also subarachnoid, and injected medications enter the CSF. Possible complications of subarachnoid injection include leakage of CSF, mitigation of the drug to the brain stem, and complete spinal blockage when using local anesthetics. We recommend the use of a 25-gauge hypodermic needle for epidural injections in small mammals and find that the length of the needle rarely enters past the epidural space. A stylet can be cut from orthopedic wire or wire sutures and then sterilized. It is important to have a stylet because it prevents a skin plug from clogging the needle. This would prevent you from seeing CSF fluid, and if a skin plug were injected into the epidural space, it could serve as a nidus for infection and inflammation. The disadvantage of using a hypodermic needle versus a spinal needle is that the bevel is longer, with cutting edges on the hypodermic needle, and this does not allow you to sense the "pop" when the needle passes through the ligamentum flavum. Care should be taken to avoid cutting and traumatizing the spinal cord during insertion. The authors recommend aspiration with a syringe after placement of the needle. If CSF is seen in the hub of the needle, half of the dose that was intended for epidural administration should be administered instead.

The procedure for epidural anesthesia is similar to that described for dogs and cats. A 25-gauge needle is advanced transcutaneously at an angle of 90° to the skin in the center of the LS junction. If bone is encountered, the needle is walked cranially or caudally to find the LS space. In small mammals, when using a sharp 25-gauge needle, the resistance or pop through the ligamentum flavum is minimal. Confirm epidural placement with the use of a syringe and negative suction. There should be no CSF in the hub of the needle.

Intubation techniques for inhalation anesthesia in all species

Ferrets

Endotracheal intubation in the ferret is done in the same way as described for cats. Holding the head perpendicular to the table facilitates intubation.

Rabbits

Intubation of the rabbit trachea is challenging because of the small oral commissure, fleshy tongue, and deeply seated larynx. The larynx is also easily traumatized by aggressive intubation techniques, and care must be taken for gentle introduction of the endotracheal tube (ET) into the larynx. An uncuffed 1- to 2-mm ET is recommended for rabbits weighing less than 2 kg. An uncuffed 2- to 3-mm ET can be used in rabbits weighing more than 3 kg. Rabbits can be intubated blindly with a small-diameter ET orally or nasally. It is preferable to use a clear uncuffed ET so that the condensation of respiration is visible on the interior of the tube when the tip of the ET is dorsal to the larynx. Anesthesia is induced using mask inhalation with isoflurane, sevoflurane, or intravenously administered propofol, ketamine-midazolam, or etomidate. The anesthetized rabbit is placed in sternal recumbency, and the head is extended so that the trachea is perpendicular to the table surface. The tip of the tongue must be gently drawn out of the mouth, but excessive tension on the tongue may cause a vagal response. A small drop of topical lidocaine gel applied to the glottis or end of the ET can decrease this effect. Advance the ET to the proximal larynx. At the beginning of inspiration, condensation of respiration disappears in the tube, and the tube is gently inserted into the trachea. Rabbits can be intubated entering the glottis from the nasopharynx and using the same principles of observing condensation in the ET before advancing the tube into the trachea. Do not use positive pressure and chest excursions to test placement of the ET tube, because air going into the stomach often mimics a true chest excursion. Alternatively, another method for confirming correct placement of the ET is to use capnography. Excessive force should be avoided when placing the ET. Laryngeal swelling and postoperative death have occurred with multiple attempts at placement of the ET with force.

The glottis can be visualized using a laryngoscope with a number 1 Miller blade, with the rabbit in a sternal position and the head and neck extended. The laryngoscope can be used to depress the tongue and free the epiglottis from its position dorsal to the soft palate. The oral cavity is often too small to maintain visualization of the glottis when the ET tube is inserted into the oropharynx. A 5- or 8-French, 56-cm-long, polypropylene urinary catheter can be advanced between the arytenoid cartilages and into the trachea as a guide. The laryngoscope blade is removed after the guide catheter is in place, and the ET tube is advanced over the guide catheter and directed into the trachea.

Direct visualization of the glottis allows placement of a larger diameter ET tube. Endoscopic endotracheal intubation can be accomplished after anesthesia is induced by placing the rabbit in a dorsoventral position. A rigid endoscope can be placed within the lumen of a 4.5-mm ET tube to advance under direct visualization through the glottis and into the lumen of the trachea. Once in the trachea, the ET tube is advanced over the endoscope. The endoscope should be withdrawn quickly, and the ET is attached to the anesthetic machine with a breathing circuit.

A semiflexible fiberoptic endoscope may be inserted into the ET (inner diameter of 2.0–2.5 mm) from its adapter end, and the tip of the scope is positioned to within 1 to 2 mm of the beveled end of the tube. The semiflexible endoscope has a portable handheld light source. The endoscope and ET are advanced over the base of the tongue until the tip of the epiglottis is visible through the soft palate. The tip of the endoscope is then advanced in a dorsocaudal direction, lifting the soft palate and allowing the epiglottis to fall forward. The tube is advanced into the laryngeal opening, and the ET is advanced over the scope into the trachea. The endoscope is then removed.

For nasotracheal intubation, the rabbit is held in extreme extension as in intubation blindly through the mouth. A 1-mm (small rabbits weighing <1 kg) or 2-mm ET is passed medially and ventrally into the nose. The ventral meatus is entered while the ET is passed into the larynx and trachea.

Other small mammals (eg, rodents, guinea pigs)

Small mammals may be intubated using the same technique described previously for rabbits using a flexible endoscope. When a flexible endoscope is not available, most small mammals are anesthetized and maintained with inhalant anesthesia using a tight-seal mask.

Birds

When the procedure takes less than 10 minutes and is noninvasive, such as blood collection or radiography, intubation is not usually necessary. When the procedure takes longer than 10 minutes, intubation of the patient can be crucial. Most birds weighing 100 g or more can be intubated with minimal difficulty. It is possible to intubate birds as small as 30 g in body weight, but they present a greater challenge because of the small tube size. For small birds, an ET can be made using a red rubber tube or catheter of the appropriate size. Small birds tend to produce mucous that clogs these small-diameter tubes. The clinician must be aware of this, because a clogged tube causes hypoventilation and hypercapnia. Frequent suction may required during the anesthesia to maintain the patency of the tube.

Anesthesia or analgesia drugs used in birds

Most seriously ill birds experience pain and anxiety during hospitalization. Administration of analgesics is strongly recommended in these birds. Studies in pigeons have demonstrated that they have more κ-opioid receptors in the forebrain than μ-opioid receptors. There are many conflicting reports on the effects of μ-receptor drugs in birds [26–29]. There is a major concern about interspecies differences in doses required for analgesia. This difference in response may be related to differences in opioid receptor populations within the spinal cord and CNS [6]. This may explain why not all birds respond to μ-agonists, such as morphine, fentanyl, and buprenorphine, in the same manner as mammals. Butorphanol at a rate of 1 to 2 mg/kg administered intramuscularly has been shown to be a useful analgesic is birds. We have used butorphanol CRI during surgery and after surgery in birds, and there seems to be an inhalant anesthetic–sparing effect with this route of administration.

The MACs for isoflurane and sevoflurane in birds are 1.44% and 2% to 3%, respectively. Sevoflurane in birds seems to be less irritating, and thus reduces the stress of mask inhalation. All inhalants produce dose-dependent decreases in cardiac performance. The mechanism varies between the two agents, with halothane showing dose-related decreases in cardiac output, blood pressure, and systemic vascular tone, whereas isoflurane better preserves cardiac output but alters systemic vascular tone and tissue perfusion. All inhalants potentially cause increases in intracranial pressure. In hypovolemic patients (hypovolemia commonly occurs during surgery with losses through hemorrhage or with an open body cavity), lower concentrations of these agents are necessary to prevent significant cardiovascular destabilization. For this reason, we always use inhalation agents in combination with opioids to produce a MAC-sparing effect or inhalation agent dose reduction during surgery. Butorphanol is commonly used as a premedication drug for surgery. When hypotension occurs during surgery because of inhalant-induced vasodilation, the clinician is left with few choices. Repeating the butorphanol dose is possible but rarely results in a significant reduction in the inhalant concentration. Intraoperative hypotension requires immediate attention. Anesthetic depth should be assessed, and the anesthetic dose should be reduced. If hypotension is caused by bradycardia, this can be treated with atropine. If hypotension occurs and the anesthetic concentration cannot be reduced, a crystalloid bolus with a colloid (hetastarch) bolus is administered. The boluses are repeated until the systolic blood pressure is greater than 90 mm Hg. In refractory hypotension, the clinician can consider using Oxyglobin (Biopure, Cambridge, MA) (2-mL/kg bolus) in place of hetastarch. The clinician should also check the packed cell volume (PCV) and blood glucose concentration. Hypoglycemia and anemia can lead to refractory hypotension and should be corrected if present. If blood pressure is normal, the bird should be continued on a CRI of crystalloids (10 mL/kg/h) and hetastarch (0.8 mL/kg/h) or Oxyglobin (0.2 mL/kg/h).

Intraoperative administration (20 minutes before the end of anesthesia) of NSAIDs may decrease the tissue sensitization that occurs as a result of surgical trauma and may reduce the dose of opioid drug required. NSAIDs like meloxicam (Metacam) administered intramuscularly at a dose of 0.5 mg/kg can be used for pain relief when perfusion parameters and kidney parameters are normal. NSAIDs are rarely used before surgery in long surgical procedures because of the risk of intraoperative bleeding and hypotension.

Local anesthetics block sodium ion channels, which interrupts the transmission of pain impulses. When used before surgery, local anesthetics block the site of tissue manipulation, which helps to prevent central sensitization.

The lidocaine 2% is mixed in the same syringe with bupivacaine 0.5% for a ring block or incisional block and is based on a dose of 1 mg/kg for each of the drugs. This total amount is given in multiple sites subcutaneously and intramuscularly. This incisional block is never used as the only analgesia. The multimodal approach is used and, as an example, can be combined with a preoperative opioid, epidural, inhalant, and postoperative NSAID.

Cesarean section analgesia and anesthesia protocols in small mammals

Preoperative drugs

The patient is sedated with midazolam administered intramuscularly, an intravenous catheter is placed, and the animal is started on crystalloids. In some of the smaller mammals (eg, guinea pig, hedgehog), intravenous catheterization is difficult. Inhalant mask anesthesia decreases the stress of this procedure. The ferret and guinea pig need a small cutdown (use a 22-gauge needle bevel to make a hole at catheter entrance) to avoid burring the catheter on entering the skin. Blood work, radiographs, and other diagnostics can be done at the same time. When an intravenous catheter cannot be placed, the use of an intraosseous catheter should be attempted.

Induction

Propofol or etomidate administered intravenously or intraosseously and an epidural injection of morphine and bupivacaine are given.

Maintenance

The animal is intubated or masked and maintained on oxygen. A lidocaine-bupivacaine incisional block is performed. After the fetuses are removed, the patient is started on isoflurane or sevoflurane inhalant. The patient is given buprenorphine or hydromorphone intravenously.

After surgery

One dose of NSAIDS can be given after surgery, and the animal may be sent home on tramadol (see Table 1).

Critically ill surgical patient

Preoperative resuscitation with fluids to correct perfusion deficits are discussed in another article in this issue. The small mammal is rehydrated, as discussed in that article, over 6 to 8 hours. The animal is treated with a sedative-analgesic combination (ie, opioid and midazolam) as required for pain during resuscitation. In some of the exotic patients, such as the guinea pig, intravenous catheters are difficult to place while the patient is conscious. Guinea pigs have short legs and pull away when the catheter is inserted into the skin. The mammal can be anesthetized with an inhalant using a mask. This decreases the stress on the mammal. The mammal's blood pressure can be taken at that time. The mammal is taken off anesthesia after catheter placement and stabilized on fluid therapy. Many critical mammals are hypothermic and need heat support. When its blood pressure is stabilized, the mammal is taken to surgery.

Preoperative drugs

Thirty minutes before surgery, the small mammal is given a preoperative loading dose of fentanyl intravenously along with a ketamine microdose (1–2 mg/kg administered intravenously). A CRI of fentanyl and ketamine is prepared.

Induction

The animal is induced with etomidate and midazolam administered intravenously and is intubated if possible; otherwise, it is maintained on a mask with an inhalant. An epidural injection of morphine with or without bupivacaine can be used in the painful animal.

Maintenance anesthesia

The CRI of fentanyl and ketamine is started at the lower CRI dose given in Table 1. The fentanyl-ketamine CRI requires that a loading dose of the drugs be given before starting the CRI (see Table 1). The dose can be mixed with saline in a syringe. The CRI can be piggy-backed with a Y-shaped connector to the crystalloids or colloids being administered during surgery.

The animal is maintained on sevoflurane at the lowest possible concentration. Using a CRI of fentanyl-ketamine lowers the inhalant concentration. The maintenance dose of isoflurane or sevoflurane is at 1% or 2%, respectively. A lidocaine and bupivacaine incisional block is used. Isotonic crystalloids (eg, lactated Ringer's solution, Plasma-Lyte-A, Normosol-R) are used as a CRI at a rate of 10 mL/kg/h with a colloid CRI at a rate of 0.8 mL/kg/h during surgery.

Hypotension during surgery

If hypotension occurs during surgery, the inhalant anesthesia is reduced first and the CRI is increased. The animal should also be treated for hypovolemia if there is blood loss or fluid deficits are suspected until the blood pressure is normal. Checking blood glucose, PCV, or total protein (TP) and blood gas analysis during surgery is recommended. Monitoring devices, such as the pulse oximeter, end-tidal carbon dioxide (CO_2), temperature, and electrocardiographic (ECG) rhythm and rate, are checked for abnormalities.

After surgery

Continue the CRI of fentanyl for 12 to 36 hours after surgery or until the patient is stable. NSAIDs can be given if perfusion, hydration, and gastrointestinal and renal function are normal.

References

[1] Stevens CW. Opioid research in amphibians: a unique perspective on mechanism of opioid analgesia and the evolution of opioid receptors. Rev Analgesia 2005;8(7):93–131.
[2] Stevens CW, Kendall K. Time course and magnitude of tolerance to the analgesic effects of systemic morphine in amphibians. Life Sci 1993;52(15):PL111–6.
[3] Brenner GM, Klopp AJ, et al. Analgesic potency of alpha adrenergic agents after systemic administration in amphibians. J Pharmacol Exp Ther 1994;270(2):540–5.
[4] Stevens CW, Brenner GM. Spinal administration of adrenergic agents produces analgesia in amphibians. Eur J Pharmacol 1996;316(2–3):205–10.
[5] Stevens CW. Relative potency of mu, delta and kappa opioids after spinal administration in amphibians. J Pharmacol Exp Ther 1996;276(2):440–8.
[6] Clyde L, Paul-Murphy J. Avian analgesia. In: Fowler ME, Miller RE, editors. Zoo and wild animal medicine: current therapy 4. Philadelphia: WB Saunders; 1999. p. 309–14.
[7] Quesenberry KE, Orcutt C. Basic approach to veterinary care. In: Quesenberry KE, Carpenter JW, editors. Ferrets, rabbits and rodents clinical medicine and surgery. 2nd edition. Philadelphia: WB Saunders; 2000. p. 13–24.
[8] Dobromylskyj P, Flecknell PA, Lascelles BD, et al. Management of postoperative and other acute pain. In: Flecknell P, Waterman-Pearson A, editors. Pain management in animals. Philadelphia: WB Saunders; 2000. p. 81–145.

[9] Jablonski P, Howden BO. Oral buprenorphine and aspirin analgesia in rats undergoing liver transplantation. Lab Anim 2002;36(2):134–43.
[10] Swedberg MD. The mouse grid-shock analgesia test: pharmacological characterization of latency to vocalization threshold as an index of antinociception. J Pharmacol Exp Ther 1994;269(3):1021–8.
[11] Liles JH, Flecknell PA, Roughan J, et al. Influence of oral buprenorphine, oral naltrexone or morphine on the effects of laparotomy in the rat. Lab Anim 1998;32(2):149–61.
[12] Jacobson C. Adverse effects on growth rates in rats caused by buprenorphine administration. Lab Anim 2000;34(2):202–6.
[13] Flecknell PA, Liles JH, Woolton R. Reversal of fentanylfluanison neuroleptanalgesia in the rabbit using mixed agonist/antagonist opioids. Lab anim 1989;23(3):147–55.
[14] Muir WW. Drug antagonism and antagonists. In: Gaynor JS, Muir WW, editors. Handbook of veterinary pain management. St Louis (MO): Mosby; 2002. p. 393–404.
[15] Candido KD, Winnie AP, Ghaleb Fattouh MW, et al. Buprenorphine added to the local anesthetic for axillary brachial plexus block prolongs postoperative analgesia. Reg Anesth Pain Med 2002;27(2):162–7.
[16] Bazin JE, Massoni C, Bruell P, et al. The addition of opioids to the local anesthetics in brachial plexus block: the comparative effects of morphine, buprenorphine and sufentanil. Anesthesia 1997;52(9):858–62.
[17] Henke J, Astner S, Brill T, et al. Comparative study of three intramuscular anesthetic combinations (medetomidine/ketamine, medetomidine/fentanylmidzazolam, and xylazine/ketamine) in rabbits. Vet Aanesth Anal 2005;32(3):1261–70.
[18] Aeschbacher G, Webb AI. Propofol in rabbits. Q. Determination of an induction dose. Lab Anim Sci 1993;43(4):324–7.
[19] Lamont L, Tranquilli W. Alpha2 agonists. In: Gaynor JS, Muir WW, editors. Handbook of veterinary pain management. St Louis (MO): Mosby; 2002. p. 199–220.
[20] Lamont LA, Tranquilli WJ, Mathews KA. Adjunctive analgesia therapy. In: Mathews KA, editor. The veterinary clinics of North America small animal practice. Philadelphia: WB Saunders; 2000. p. 805–13.
[21] Janssen PA, Niemegeers CJ, Marsboom RP. Etomidate, a potent non-barbituate hypnotic. Intravenous etomidate in mice, rats, guinea pigs, rabbits and dogs. Arch Int Pharmacodyn Ther 1975;214(1):92–132.
[22] Hughes KL, MacKenzie JE. An investigation of the centrally and peripherally mediated cardiovascular effects of etomidate in the rabbit. Br J Anaesth 1978;50(2):101–8.
[23] Aeschbacher G, Webb AI. Propofol in rabbits. 2. Long-term anesthesia. Lab Anim Sci 1993;43(4):328–35.
[24] Ko JC, Thurman JC, Tranquilli WJ, et al. A comparison of medetomidine-propofol and medetomidine-midazolam-propofol anesthesia in rabbits. Lab Anim Sci 1992;42(5):503–7.
[25] Lawson AK, Lichtenberger M, Day T, et al. Comparison of sevoflurane and isoflurane in domestic ferrets. Vet Ther 2006;7:3–8.
[26] Bardo MT, Hughes RA. Shock-elicited flight response in chickens as an index of morphine analgesia. Pharmacol Biochem Behav 1978;9:147–9.
[27] Curro TG, Brunson DB, Paul-Murphy J. Determination of the ED50 of isoflurane and evaluation of the isoflurane-sparing effect of butorphanol in cockatoos (Cacatua spp.). Vet Anesth 1994;23:429–33.
[28] Paul-Murphy JR, Brunson DB, Miletic V. Analgesic effects of butorphanol and buprenorphine in conscious African grey parrots (Psittacus erithacus erithacus and Psittacus erithacus timneh). Am J Vet Res 1999;60:1218–21.
[29] Hoppes S, Flammer K, Hoersch K, et al. Disposition and analgesic effects of fentanyl in white cockatoos (Cacatua alba). J Avian Med Surg 2003;17:124–30.

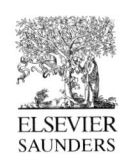

Critical Care Monitoring

Marla Lichtenberger, DVM, DACVECC[a],*, Jeff Ko, DVM, MS, DACVA[b]

[a]*11015 North Mequon Square Drive, Mequon, WI 53092, USA*
[b]*Department of Veterinary Clinical Sciences, School of Veterinary Medicine, Purdue University, West Lafayette, IN 47907, USA*

Critical care monitoring in the exotic patient is complicated by the small patient size, physiologic peculiarity, and limited information available for each species. Despite these impediments, the same principles and techniques of critical care monitoring used in domestic animals can be extrapolated to exotic small mammal and bird patients.

Critical care monitoring techniques are performed to help detect early homeostatic instability before damage becomes irreversible. The cardiovascular system, respiratory system, and central nervous system (CNS) form the essential body systems; failure of one usually results in failure of the others and the subsequent death of the patient. The most common systems monitored in veterinary medicine involve the cardiovascular and respiratory systems. Consequently, this article emphasizes monitoring of the cardiovascular and respiratory systems.

The routine use of critical care monitoring in exotic pet medicine has advanced the field of emergency and critical care in the past 10 years. Commonly used cardiovascular monitoring devices in clinical practice are the perfusion parameters demonstrated on physical examination (ie, mucous membrane color; capillary refill time; auscultation of heart rate; pulse rate, rhythm, and strength; mentation; temperature). Further evaluation of the cardiovascular system is presented using indirect blood pressure monitoring; central venous pressure (CVP); and cardiac evaluation using an electrocardiogram (ECG), echocardiogram, radiographs, and cardiac output monitoring. CVP measurement is ideal to acquire knowledge about the intravascular volume status. The avian emergency clinician must be familiar with the differences in the avian lungs compared with those of small mammals, which is discussed in the section on monitoring of the respiratory

* Corresponding author.
E-mail address: marlavet@aol.com (M. Lichtenberger).

system. Monitoring principles related to anesthesia are discussed, and such commonly used respiratory monitors as the pulse oximeter, end-tidal gas monitor, respiratory probe, respirometer, apnea monitor, and point-of-care blood gas analyzer are covered.

Monitoring the cardiovascular system using perfusion parameters

The transport of fluid and oxygen through the blood vessels to the capillaries is called perfusion. Tissue perfusion depends directly on adequate intravascular volume and a normally functioning cardiovascular system. What we would really like to know is that circulation or perfusion of tissues with blood is adequate to meet the tissues' metabolic needs, which involves supplying adequate oxygen and nutrients and removing excessive carbon dioxide and wastes. If we could easily measure oxygen delivery to tissues, that would be ideal. Oxygen delivery depends on cardiac output (perfusion) and the oxygen content of the blood. Unfortunately, few practices have the means to measure cardiac output or blood gases.

The intravascular volume status of a patient is difficult to assess accurately with a clinical test. An estimate can be made through multiple physical examination findings and CVP measurements. It is also important to understand the pros and cons of each monitoring parameter and their clinical implications. The physical examination findings are heart rate, mucous membrane color, capillary refill time, mentation, and body temperature.

Heart rate

The heart rate varies for each of the species of small mammals and birds. Heart rate is inversely related to body size [1]. The resting heart rate (minute^{-1}) for mammals is calculated from the allometric equation, Heart Rate = 241 × $M_b^{-0.25}$, where M_b is the body weight in kilograms. A heart rate 20% greater than or less than the calculated rate for an individual is considered tachycardic or bradycardic, respectively [2]. The heart rate is only part of the cardiac output equation (Cardiac Output = Stroke Volume × Heart Rate). Heart rate is under control of the sympathetic and parasympathetic nervous system.

The heart rate changes during the various stages of shock and is an important part of the sympathetic compensatory response. The heart rate initially increases in the early stages of compensatory hypovolemic shock (blood loss of 15%–25% of total blood volume) because of the baroreceptor sympathetic response. This stage is seen in birds but is often missed in small mammals, such as cats (see the article by Lichtenberger on shock resuscitation in small mammals and birds elsewhere in this issue), which is thought to be attributable to a vagal influence. In the early decompensatory state of hypovolemic shock (blood loss of 25%–40% of the total blood volume), the heart rate remains elevated in birds but is less than 180 beats per minute (BPM) in small mammals. In the late decompensatory stage of shock (blood loss >40% of total blood volume in the small mammal and >60% in birds), the heart rate decreases with loss of sympathetic nervous system compensation [3].

Mucous membrane color

This is an indirect measurement of peripheral tissue perfusion. Pink mucous membranes in living small mammals and birds indicate good peripheral tissue perfusion. Anatomic mucous membrane locations used are the gum and scleral or rectal mucosa (or cloacal mucosa in birds).

Capillary refill time

Capillary refill time is used concurrently with mucous membrane color as an indirect measurement of peripheral tissue perfusion. The mucous membrane is digitally compressed until blanched, and the time it takes to return to its original color is determined. This should be less than 2 seconds in birds and small mammals. A prolonged capillary refill time is indicative of poor perfusion of the tissue.

Mentation

Determine the level of consciousness and whether the animal is stuporous and arousable with noxious stimuli or comatose (eg, unconscious and not arousable with noxious stimuli). A decline in the level of consciousness implies brain injury or a decrease in cerebral perfusion. A complete neurologic examination must be performed to evaluate brain functions.

Body temperature

Normal body temperature is addressed in the articles on different species in this issue. Small mammals and birds frequently become hypothermic in early decompensatory stages of shock. Body temperature is easily recorded in most species of small mammals using a rectal thermometer. Cloacal temperature probes can be used to record body temperature in birds, but the results are rarely recorded in the conscious avian patient and are impractical in most cases. Avian body temperatures are higher than those of mammals. The normal cloacal temperature is 104°F to 107.6°F (40°C–42°C).

Monitoring of temperature during anesthesia is important in small mammals and avian patients. During the first 10 minutes of anesthesia, there is a rapid loss of heat because of the patient's small body size. Temperatures can be monitored using a rectal probe in small mammals or a cloacal probe in birds. Rectal temperatures may be difficult to maintain and are affected by stool content in the rectum. Temperatures can be monitored using an esophageal probe that records core body temperature, ECG recording, respiratory rate, and pulse oximetry (PC-Vetgard; DVM Solutions, San Antonio, Texas) (Fig. 1). Anesthetic drugs contribute to hypothermia because of

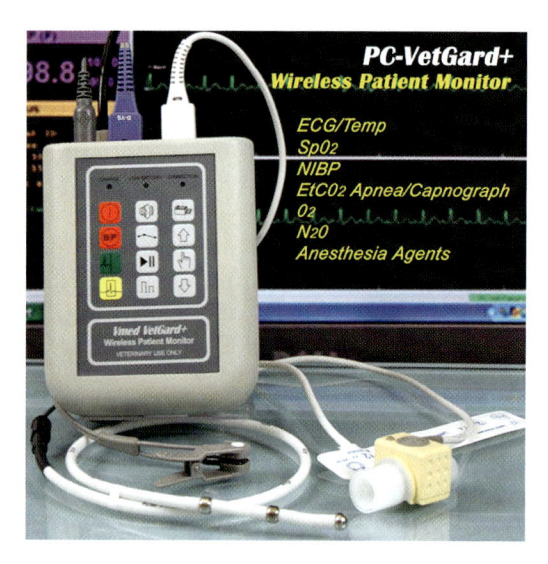

Fig. 1. Esophageal monitoring probe. The esophageal probe is inserted into the esophagus of the anesthetized small mammal or bird. The probe measures core body temperature, pulse oximetry, and heart rate and portrays an ECG tracing. (*Courtesy of* DVM Solutions, San Antonio, TX; with permission.)

vasodilation, which increases surface heat loss, and reduced muscle activity, which reduces heat production. Providing supplemental heat (water blanket or forced-air warming blanket) and core body temperature warming using warmed intravenous fluids is recommended. Warming the mammal or bird should start at the time of induction of anesthesia until the small mammal has fully recovered and its body temperature has been confirmed to be normal. Many prolonged recoveries are more often related to an animal's low body temperature (which reduces metabolism of the anesthetics and prolongs the anesthetic effects) than to the specific drugs used.

Hyperthermia can also occur and, if severe, can be even more detrimental. The ferret is prone to hypothermia during anesthesia and surgery, but it can become hyperthermic during recovery if kept wrapped in a warming blanket for longer than 15 to 20 minutes. Recovery of the ferret should involve in checking body temperature every 5 minutes until the ferret is awake and the temperature is 99°F to 100°F (37.2°C–37.7°C).

Measurement of blood pressure

Direct blood pressure measurement

The "gold standard" for measuring blood pressure is the direct method, which entails placing a catheter in an artery and connecting it to a monitor by means of a pressure transducer. Unfortunately, arterial catheterization of small mammals and birds is technically difficult, time-consuming, and expensive. Ideally, in the critically ill patient, direct blood pressure monitoring provides beat-to-beat monitoring of the blood pressure because of the dynamic nature of the patient. Invasive blood pressure monitoring is useful for arterial blood gas sampling, continuous real-time monitoring, intentional pharmacologic or mechanical cardiovascular manipulation, and in cases of failure of indirect blood pressure monitoring. Analysis of the arterial waveform can also give insight into the nature of the blood pressure problem. A rapid decline in the down stroke of the waveform frequently indicates rapid runoff of the blood, and hence decreased systemic vascular resistance (SVR) [4]. A slow decline in the down stroke of the arterial waveform may indicate increased SVR. A low end-diastolic pressure typically indicates hypovolemia [4].

Kinking of the arterial catheter or severe spasm of the artery can lead to dampening of the arterial waveform [4]. During arterial waveform dampening, the mean arterial pressure (MAP) frequently remains reliable even though the systolic and diastolic blood pressures cannot be relied on. Care needs to be taken never to inject anything except heparinized or nonheparinized saline through the arterial line. Air bubbles can lead to air embolism; thus, extra caution is necessary to avoid injecting air bubbles into the arterial catheter.

Indirect blood pressure monitoring

The indirect blood pressure monitor is most commonly used in veterinary medicine. The indirect method of blood pressure monitoring (whether using the Doppler or oscillometric method) is clinically useful in determining if a patient is hypotensive, normotensive, or hypertensive. In general, the MAP should be kept at greater than 60 mm Hg and the systolic pressure should be kept at greater than 90 mm Hg to ensure adequate organ perfusion in the conscious and anesthetized patient. Although there are several indirect or noninvasive methods (ie, oscillometric, Doppler) available, it is sometimes impossible to obtain a reading on exotic patients. Traditionally, oscillometric blood pressure monitors have been unreliable in the cat and small mammals. The Doppler method is more versatile than the oscillometric method and is the method of choice used by the authors for all exotic patients. Advantages of using the Doppler method include relatively low cost, portability, and better reliability in small and hypotensive animals compared with other indirect methods (ie, oscillometric blood pressure monitors). Disadvantages include the inability to determine diastolic pressure, and thus MAP. The ultrasonic Doppler flow probe (Parks Medical Electronics, Aloha, Oregon) uses ultrasonic waves to detect and make blood flow audible in an artery distal to the blood pressure cuff.

Materials for Doppler blood pressure monitoring

Materials for Doppler blood pressure monitoring include the following (Fig. 2): a (Classic Cuff Critikon; General Electric Health Care, Mexico),

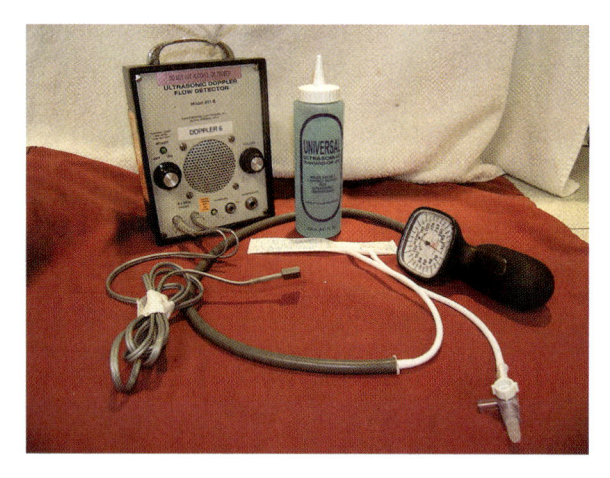

Fig. 2. Indirect Doppler blood pressure monitor. This shows the indirect Doppler blood pressure monitor with the cuff, sphygmomanometer, and gel.

a sphygmomanometer (Propper Manufacturing Company, Long Island City, New York), Ultrasource Transmission Gel (Graham-Field, Bayshore, New York), and a Doppler blood pressure monitor (Parks Medical; Parks Medical Electronics or Minidop; Jorgensen Laboratories, Burlington, Wisconsin).

The Doppler blood pressure cuff (Classic Cuff Critikon) is placed on the distal humerus and attached to the sphygmomanometer. The sphygmomanometer is attached to the tubing of the cuff.

Blood pressure monitoring in the ferret, rabbit, or small mammal

The ferret, rabbit, or small mammal is placed in lateral or sternal recumbency. A pneumatic cuff is placed above the carpus or tarsus, or on the tail in a ferret (Fig. 3) [5]. In rabbits and other small mammals, the cuff is placed above the elbow. The rear leg can be used for blood pressure recording but is less sensitive than the front leg in the authors' experience. The front limb was more reliable than the rear limb for blood pressure measurements in a study in rabbits [6]. The cuff size should ideally be approximately 40% of the circumference of the tarsus, carpus, humerus, or base of the tail. Unfortunately, the smallest cuff available is a number 1 cuff or an infant-sized cuff, which is usually too large for many exotic pets. A study in ferrets has shown that this larger cuff gives falsely lower indirect systolic blood pressures when compared with direct systolic blood pressures [5]. The indirect systolic blood pressure recordings were approximately 28 to 30 mm Hg less than the direct arterial blood pressure recordings in that study [5]. The clinician must keep this in mind when recording indirect systolic blood pressures in mammals. The discrepancy between direct and indirect blood pressure monitoring has been seen in other species (ie, rabbit, dog, cat) to

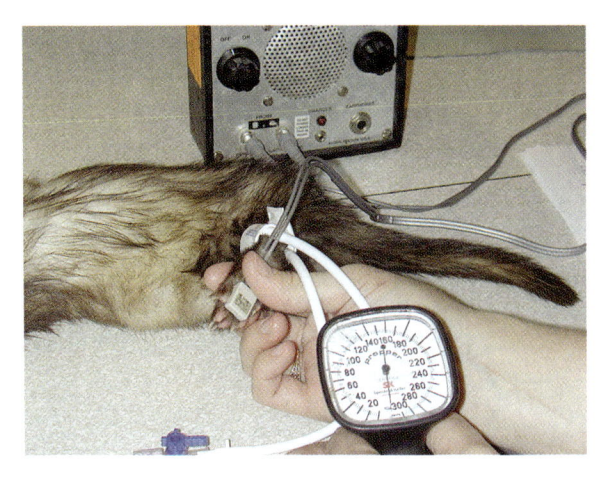

Fig. 3. Indirect blood pressure in a ferret. The indirect Doppler blood pressure is measured on the distal limb of a ferret. The cuff is placed above the tarsus, and the probe is placed above the pads of the feet.

various degrees and has been attributed to difficulty in correctly determining the appropriate cuff size, variability in cuff sensitivity, and variation in arterial waveforms between anatomic sites [5,6]. The authors suspect that this difference in direct versus indirect Doppler blood pressure in other small mammals and rodents is similar to that found in the ferret (eg, falsely lower blood pressures because of large cuff size).

For using the Doppler method to measure blood pressure, the hair is shaved on the ventral carpus or tarsus, or tail in the ferret, and on the medial midshaft of the radius-ulnar area in other small mammals. The transducer probe crystal is placed on the shaved area (radial artery on front leg or digital branch of the tibial artery on rear leg) in a bed of ultrasonic gel and taped or held in place. The cuff bladder is inflated to a pressure that exceeds systolic blood pressure. At this time, the Doppler signal of blood flow is diminished, and the blood pressure cuff is then deflated gradually. The first sound heard as the cuff is deflated denotes the systolic pressure.

With practice, the Doppler method, utilizing a sphygmomanometer and a Doppler flow probe, is fairly easy to use in small mammals. The Doppler method in all small mammals and birds is a good indicator of changes in trends of systolic blood pressure while treating hypovolemic shock or as a monitoring guideline during procedures or surgery. Normal systolic blood pressure in small mammals ranges from 80 to 120 mm Hg.

Blood pressure monitoring in the avian species

In birds, the cuff is placed on the proximal humerus or distal femur (Figs. 4 and 5). The proper cuff width size for different species is measured at 40% of the circumference of the humerus or distal femur. To the authors' knowledge,

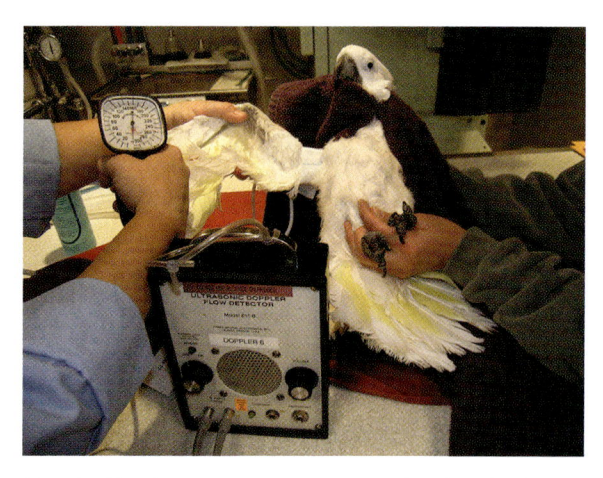

Fig. 4. Indirect Doppler blood pressure measurement on the wing of a bird. The cuff is placed on the distal humerus. The Doppler probe is placed on the radial-carpal bone to detect ulnar artery flow.

there have been no studies done documenting proper cuff size for measurement of blood pressure in birds. For birds weighing less than 100 g, a number 1 cuff is the smallest cuff available and is much too large. The clinician must take into account that the larger cuff size in birds weighing less than 100 g gives a falsely lower systolic blood pressure reading. Even with this disadvantage, indirect blood pressure monitoring is possible in birds as small as 30 g. The Doppler probe is placed on the distal ulnar artery (above the radial carpal bone of the wing), on the proximal ulnar artery (at the bend of the elbow of the wing), or on the medial tibial tarsal bone (measurement on the leg).

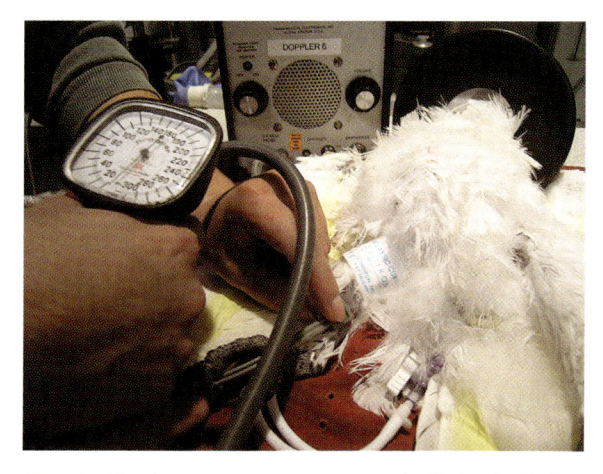

Fig. 5. Indirect Doppler blood pressure measurement on the limb of a bird. The cuff is placed above the stifle. The Doppler probe is placed on the medial midshaft of the tibial-tarsal bone.

The systolic pressure is measured as previously described. Although some clinicians believe that they can estimate diastolic pressure from a change in the pitch of the pulse, diastolic pressure cannot be reliably determined using this method. Systolic pressures obtained with the Doppler method have been found to correlate well with direct pressure measurements in anesthetized ducks [7]. The Doppler method of blood pressure measurement in birds has been found to correlate better with direct blood pressure measurements than in mammals. This is likely attributable to the fact that birds have thin skin with little subcutaneous tissue, which allows better contact of the probe and the artery.

Normal systolic blood pressure for birds under isoflurane anesthesia is between 90 and 150 mm Hg, and it is between 90 and 180 mm Hg in the conscious bird. The authors define hypertension in the psittacine bird as systolic blood pressure greater than 200 mm Hg. Raptors have a slightly higher systolic blood pressure than psittacine birds. In the authors' experience, systolic blood pressure measured indirectly in several species of raptors was between 150 and 240 mm Hg.

Central venous pressure

CVP is a measure of the hydrostatic pressure within the intrathoracic vena cava [8,9]. As long as no vascular obstruction exists, CVP is reflective of right atrial pressure (RAP). As a measure of RAP, CVP provides information concerning the adequacy of venous blood volume (or preload). Its measurement requires that the catheter tip, usually of a jugular catheter (ie, central venous catheter, which can be single, double, or triple lumen), be as close to the entry of the right atrium as possible. The catheter can be connected to a pressure transducer or a manometer. If the latter technique is used, the manometer (a plastic open-ended tube with centimeter markings) is attached by a three-way stopcock between a fluid bag and a catheter. The manometer is zeroed to the level of the right atrium in lateral recumbent animals (the level of the manubrium). The manometer is placed perpendicular to the ground, is first filled physiologic saline, and is then opened to the catheter (ie, central venous catheter) of the patient by turning the stopcock. The saline in the manometer should slowly drop to level out at the CVP. The measurement should be duplicated at least three times for validation.

The normal reference range for CVP in dogs and cats has been reported to be 0 to 10 cm H_2O, with the most common range cited being 0 to 5 cm H_2O [8,9]. The normal CVP values in small mammals are most likely similar to those in dogs and cats. Although CVP monitoring can be performed in small mammals, it is technically difficult. CVP monitoring in birds is likely not feasible. Values less than 0 cm H_2O are indicative of hypovolemia, and values greater than 12 to 15 cm H_2O are suggestive of volume overload. The trends in the CVP over time may provide vital information about an individual patient. For example, for a ferret with oliguric renal failure, when CVP values that have been steady at 6 to 7 cm H_2O for 3 days suddenly decrease to 0 cm H_2O, the ferret may be developing hypovolemia, perhaps secondary to newly developed polyuria. Similarly, a gradual rise to 12 cm H_2O in a rabbit receiving intravenous fluids for vomiting and anorexia may be a warning sign of impending volume overload.

Cardiac evaluation

The cardiac system must be evaluated in any critical patient in which the clinician identifies an arrhythmia or heart murmur or suspects heart disease. The identification of heart disease enables the clinician to change treatment and anesthetic plans for the avian or small mammal patient. Radiology, echocardiograms, and ECGs are commonly used. Cardiac output monitoring is a new tool available to the veterinarian.

Radiology

Normal values for the vertebral heart score have been reported in ferrets as 4.00 cm (range: 3.75–4.07 cm) for the right lateral projection and 4.08 cm (range: 3.85–4.15 cm) for ventrodorsal projections [10]. The ferret heart is located much more caudally than in the dog or cat (eg, between the sixth and eighth intercostal spaces). In other small mammals and the ferret, normal radiologic findings are reported in small mammal texts. In birds, measurements of cardiac size on radiographs are limited because of large size variation in different species.

Echocardiogram

An echocardiogram is indicated for assessment of cardiac function and structure of the heart. Standarized protocols for echocardiogenic examination in avian and small mammal patients have been established [11–15]. The examination can usually be performed in the conscious patient. The avian patient may be presented for weakness, syncope, or acute respiratory distress. The echocardiogram in these patients can be evaluated for pericardial effusion or cardiomyopathy (most myocardial dysfunction causing failure in birds is right-sided disease) [13]. Atherosclerosis (see the article on hypertension in birds in this issue) is reported commonly in the cockatoo and African Gray and Amazon Parrots, with nutritional deficiencies, obesity, limited exercise, and age playing a role in its development (see the article by Bowles, Lichtenberger, and Lennox in this issue) [12]. Common cardiac diseases seen in the ferret, rabbit, and small mammal are cardiomyopathies and valvular diseases. Any small mammal presented for acute respiratory distress, weakness, or syncope should have a full cardiac workup involving an ECG, blood pressure measurement, and echocardiogram.

Echocardiograms using B mode and M mode in mammals are similar to those done in dogs and cats [13,14]. Normal values have been published in ferrets and rabbits [13,14]. The normal shortening fraction in the ferret is approximately 33%, and it is approximately 39% in the rabbit. The left atrium/aorta (LA/Ao) ratio is approximately 1.3 in the ferret and rabbit [13,14].

Because of avian anatomy, suitable echocardiographic windows to the heart are limited. In psittacines and raptors, the ventromedian approach is routinely used. The scanner is placed on the midline directly behind the sternum, and the beam plane is directed craniodorsally (Fig. 6). In birds (eg, pigeons) with a larger space between the last ribs and pelvis, the parasternal approach can be used (Fig. 7). With the ventromedian approach, two longitudinal (comparable to the long axis in the mammal echocardiogram) views of the heart are obtained. The vertical view (corresponding to the two-chamber view) shows the heart lying on the inner surface of the sternum, and the frontal view or four-chamber views are produced by a counterclockwise 90° rotation of the scanner. Because only long-axis views are possible with the ventromedian approach, M-mode echocardiograms cannot be used in birds to evaluate chamber wall size and contractility. These measurements are taken from the two-dimensional views. Images are small, and small changes in size may not be detected. The normal chamber size in several bird species has been reported [10,12,13]. The normal width shortening

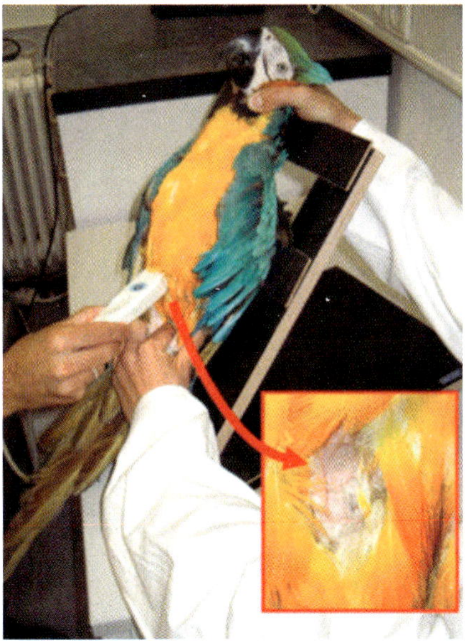

Fig. 6. Ultrasound transducer position for an echocardiographic examination in the psittacine bird. This shows the coupling of the transducer on the ventromedian approach using a normally featherless area (*inset*). (*From* Pees M, Krautwald-Junghanns ME. Avian echocardiography. Seminars in Avian and Exotic Pet Practice 2005;14(1):14–21; with permission.)

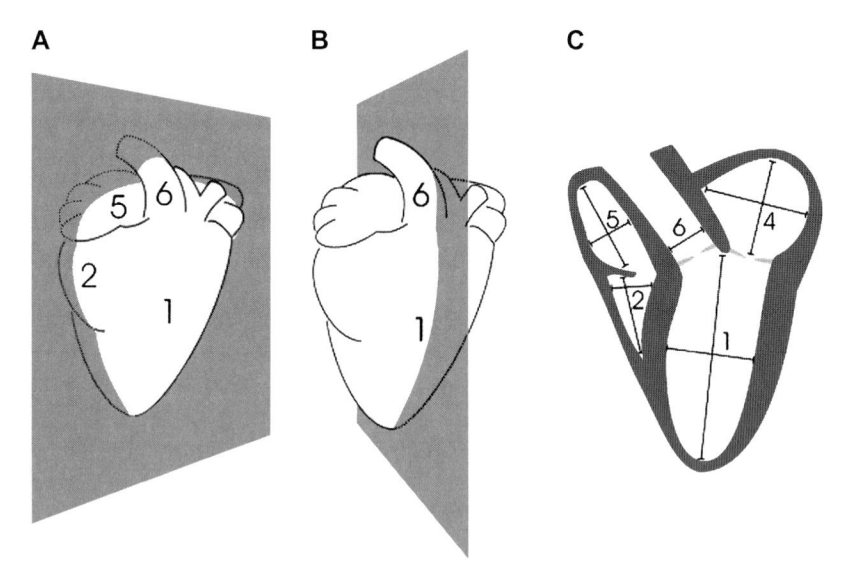

Fig. 7. Ventromedial approach to ultrasound examination in the psittacine bird. Using the ventromedian approach, the heart is presented in two views: the horizontal view (*A*) and the vertical view (*B*). (*C*) With the horizontal view, measurements can be taken from the following structures: left ventricle (1), right ventricle (2), interventricular septum (3), left atrium (4), right atrium (5), and aortic root (6). (*From* Pees M, Krautwald-Junghanns ME. Avian echocardiography. Seminars in Avian and Exotic Pet Practice 2005;14(1):14–21; with permission.)

fraction in some psittacine species in the left ventricle is approximately 22% to 27%, and it is approximately 30% to 52% in the right ventricle [10,12,13].

Electrocardiogram

An ECG is useful to detect and diagnose cardiac arrhythmias, but one should remember that electrical activity does not ensure mechanical (pumping) activity. The ECG can actually remain relatively normal in birds and small mammals with severe cardiopulmonary compromise or even cardiac arrest from anesthetic overdose. An ECG machine has little value as a monitor of anesthetic depth. One of the first signs of deterioration in your patient or the result of an anesthetic overdose may be bradycardia and ST segment depression. Diagnosis of cardiac disease in all species involves a thorough examination using an ECG, blood pressure assessment, radiographs, and echocardiographic examination.

The practitioner should be aware of the characteristics of the avian ECG, which are quite different from those of the mammalian ECG [15–20]. Avian heart rates vary between 150 and 1000 BPM. The normal ECG (Fig. 8) in birds starts with a P wave; however, in some groups of birds, it is followed by a depression called a Ta wave, representing atrial repolarization. This seems to be a physiologic phenomenon in pigeons [20] and in some

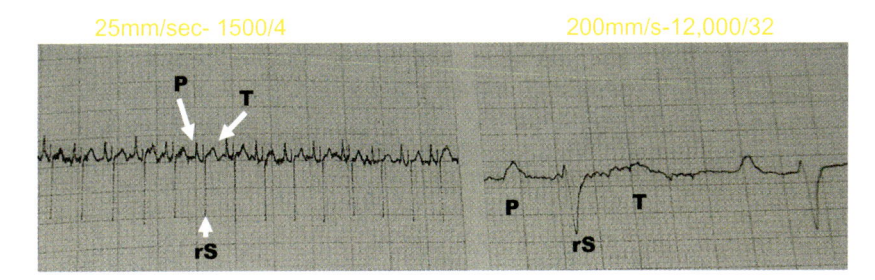

Fig. 8. Avian ECG. The normal sinus rhythm recording of the avian ECG at 25 and 200 mm/s. The P, rS, and T wave are shown in the recording.

gallinaceous [18] and psittacine birds [21]. The QRS complex is another difference, which is described as an rS complex in birds with a negative deflection. This is attributable to the fact that ventricular depolarization in birds starts subepicardial to the endocardium, whereas depolarization spreads from the endocardial side to the epicardial side in mammals. The ST segment is short or absent. When the ST segment is present, ST elevation is frequently present and is a normal waveform. ST segment elevation in mammals is associated with hypoxia or myocardial ischemia. The T wave is opposite the ventricular complex and is positive in lead II. The P-on-T phenomenon (P wave is superimposed on T wave) is a normal finding in Amazon Parrots and some Gray Parrots. Normal ECG measurements have been determined for various species of birds, rabbits, and ferrets [22–25]. The ECG recordings in small mammals are similar to those recorded in dogs and cats. Normal cardiac measurements have been determined for various species of birds, rabbits, and ferrets [22–25].

There is a lack of information correlating abnormal ECG recordings with cardiac pathologic findings in pet psittacine birds and small mammals. Recent studies have reported that heart disease in birds may occur more frequently than was once assumed [26]. The prevalence of heart disease in small mammals is unknown. Cardiomyopathy is seen commonly in ferrets. In the past 5 years, the rabbit has gained tremendous popularity as a pet. Today, the authors are seeing a larger population of rabbits with older age–related problems, including heart disease. It is important to identify significant arrhythmias clinically because they can degenerate into malignant beats and may lead to cardiac arrest and death. Arrhythmias associated with anesthesia, hypothermia, hypoxia, and metabolic and electrolyte abnormalities may occur without underlying heart disease. These arrhythmias are usually corrected with treatment of the underlying cause.

Recording the electrocardiogram

The most common lead used for determining these abnormalities is the lead II ECG. In emergencies, critical care monitoring, and monitoring of the surgical patient, the lead II ECG recording is primarily used to determine the presence of arrhythmias or in conjunction with other diagnostic tests to determine presence of cardiac disease. The lead II ECG recording should be used to determine the rate, rhythm, and conduction abnormalities. For ECG recordings in the conscious animal, use of atraumatic alligator clips is common. Sternal recumbency is commonly used to record the ECG, and there are minimal changes in measurements when compared with the ECG performed in right lateral recumbency. Birds are frequently recorded in dorsal recumbency. At a paper speed of 50 mm/s, it is difficult to detect arrhythmias and to measure the ECG waveforms in birds. A recording speed of 100 to 200 mm/s is recommended (because of the fast heart rate in small mammals and birds) for use in birds, and the machine is standardized at 1 cm equal to 1 mV. There are ECG machines commercially available that record at 100 to 200 mm/s (Vetspec and Vetronics, West Lafayette, Indiana). In the avian species, ECG clips are attached on the right wing (RA), left wing (LA), and left leg (LL), and the right leg is connected to the ground. Alternatively, for anesthetic monitoring, bipolar leads can be attached, with one cranial to the sternum and slightly paramedian to the right side of the body and the other attached caudally and to the left side of the sternum [15]. In small mammals, ECG clips are placed on the right and left arms and LL using modified painless clips [15] or are attached to 25-gauge needles penetrating through the skin [15].

Measurement of heart rate and general inspection

Measuring the heart rate gives clues to the cardiac rhythm and is determined first. Heart rate is calculated as the number of times the heart beats per minute. Heart rate usually implies ventricular rate (the number of QRS complexes per minute), but it can also refer to atrial rate (the number of P waves per minute). The recording paper has a series of marks at the top of the paper. At a paper speed of 50 mm/s, these marks are spaced so that they are 3 seconds apart, or the number of complexes can be multiplied by 20 at 50 mm/s. To estimate heart rate per minute at a speed of 100 mm/s, the number of complexes that occur in 3 seconds is counted and multiplied by 30. A second method of determining heart rate per minute at a paper speed of 100 mm/s is to count the number of small boxes from R to R (or S wave to S wave in birds) and divide into 6000 (divide the number of small boxes from R to R into 3000 when paper speed is 50 mm/s). The third method for calculating ECG heart rate is by multiplying the paper speed (mm/s) times 60 and dividing that by the distance in millimeters between two R waves, giving the frequency in BPM. The heart rate should be classified as rapid (tachycardia), slow (bradycardia), or normal [16].

Evaluate rhythm

Evaluate the distance between R or S waves to determine if the rhythm is regular. Use a piece of paper to mark the distance between R or S waves, and then move along the ECG strip to determine whether or not the marks correspond to the new R or S waves. The variation in the R-R or S-S interval should be less than 10% to be considered a regular rhythm.

Identification of P waves

Is the atrial activity regular and the shape uniform? Doubling the sensitivity of the ECG may be helpful in magnifying the P waves.

Recognition of QRS complexes

The QRS complexes should be characterized according to their morphology, uniformity, and regularity.

Relation between P waves and QRS complexes

Is there a P wave for every QRS complex?

Measuring the P-QRS-T complex

In small mammals, the R wave is similar to that seen in other small animals. In birds, the Q wave is the first negative deflection and the r or R wave is the first positive deflection. The Q waved is often absent in the avian ECG. The S wave is the first negative deflection after the R wave. When there is no R wave, the negative deflection is called a QS wave. The largest wave in the QRS complex is depicted with a capital letter (ie, Rs, rS). Rhythm abnormalities in small mammals and birds are similar to those reported in small animals. The authors' clinical experience indicates that the most common rhythm abnormality occurring in small mammals and birds during anesthesia before cardiac arrest is severe bradycardia, which becomes progressively slower before asystole occurs. ST depression also commonly occurs with hypoxia or ischemia. When bradycardia occurs, the anesthesia should be reduced or terminated and atropine should be given (glycopyrrolate is preferred in rabbits).

Cardiac output monitoring

Cardiac output has traditionally been impractical to perform routinely on anesthetized veterinary patients because of the necessity of placing a pulmonary artery catheter. Recently, a less invasive cardiac output monitoring system using a lithium dilution cardiac output monitor has been validated in anesthetized dogs. This system only requires an indwelling peripheral venous catheter and arterial catheter. It may be slightly impractical to use in small dogs or cats because of the amount of blood that is required for each measurement (approximately 4–8 mL per measurement). It can be used in larger dogs, however, and may be useful in pharmacologic manipulation of anesthetized patients. Further clinical studies need to be performed to determine its usefulness in clinical patients.

Other transpulmonary cardiac output monitors have been developed using cold thermodilution techniques. Minimally invasive cardiac output monitors have been developed that use the end-tidal carbon dioxide (CO_2) concentration to determine cardiac output. In addition, a novel noninvasive ultrasound device (USCOM; USCOM Ltd, Sydney, Australia) is available for real-time stroke volume and cardiac output measurements. The device is reliable for trends in stroke volume and cardiac output in rats [26] and is currently being investigated for use in birds by one of the authors. Further studies need to be performed in veterinary patients before it is validated for clinical use.

Monitoring the respiratory system during anesthesia

Avian respiratory system

The avian respiratory system is different than that in mammals. In birds, unlike mammals, inspiration and expiration require muscular activity. In mammals, expiration is passive. When the inspiratory muscles contract, pressure in the air sacs becomes negative relative to ambient atmospheric pressure and air flows from the atmosphere into the respiratory system. The air flows into the lungs for gas exchange and then into the air sacs. During contraction of expiratory muscles, the reverse process occurs, with air flowing from the air sacs across the lungs and out through the trachea. The avian trachea consists of complete cartilaginous rings throughout its length. Use of a noncuffed endotracheal tube is recommended for birds. The tracheal is also long in birds, which increases the tracheal dead space volume. Birds compensate for this with a deeper and slower breathing pattern.

The ventilation components are the larynx, trachea, syrinx, intra- and extrapulmonary primary bronchi, secondary bronchi, parabronchi (tertiary bronchi), air sacs, skeletal system, and respiratory muscles. There are usually nine air sacs present in most psittacine birds. There are two types of parabronchi (tertiary bronchi) in the avian lung, which are used for gas exchange. The parabronchi are long narrow tubes that have numerous openings into atria. The atria lead into air capillaries through ducts. Paleopulmonic parabronchial tissue is found in all birds and consists of parallel minimally anastomosing parabronchi. The direction of gas flow is unidirectional. Neopulmonic parabronchial tissue is a meshwork of anastomosing parabronchi located in the caudolateral portion of each lung of flying birds. There is bidirectional air flow throughout the respiratory cycle in the neopulmonic parabronchi. During positive-pressure ventilation (PPV), it is possible that the direction of gas flow within the avian lung, especially the paleopulmonic lung, may be reversed. Fortunately, this reversal of direction does not affect gas exchange, because the gas exchange efficiency of the avian lung does not depend on the direction of flow. The lungs do not expand or contract. The nature of the avian respiratory system makes it possible to ventilate birds with a continuous stream of oxygen containing a gas mixture introduced through the trachea and into the lungs. Alternatively, the gas mixture can be introduced through a cannula inserted into an air sac, allowing the gas to pass across the lungs and out the trachea.

The respiratory gas volume per unit body mass of the respiratory system in birds is two to four times that of small animals. The small animal lung has 96% of the volume of gas in the bronchi and alveoli, whereas only 10% of the total specific volume is in the parabronchi and air capillaries in the avian lung. This results in minimal functional residual capacity (FRC) in birds and makes periods of apnea critical. Apnea causes significant problems during anesthesia, thus requiring better control of oxygenation and ventilation, and necessitates the use of an endotracheal tube during anesthesia.

Anesthesia in small mammals and birds

Anesthetic induction

Mask induction techniques are used with birds and the small mammals without intravenous catheters or when intravenous catheterization is difficult in the conscious patient. The masks can range from commercially available small animal masks to homemade plastic bottles and syringe cases. The size and shape of the mask depend on the size and shape of the bird's beak and small mammal's face. The mask should be as small as possible. Disposable latex gloves can be placed over the mask opening, with a central hole cut for insertion of the head. The tight seal of the mask reduces the amount of waste gas released into the environment. Several induction techniques have been used, including slowly increasing the concentration of gas anesthetic agent until the desired effect has been attained. The disadvantage of this method is the longer time it takes to achieve loss of consciousness, and it may increase the excitement and stress level of the patient. The authors commonly use an induction mask with high oxygen flow rates (2–4 L/min) and adjust the anesthetic vaporizer concentration to a highest available concentration (5% for isoflurane and 7%–8% for sevoflurane), restraining the bird for approximately 20 to 25 seconds to achieve induction. The vaporizer setting is then reduced to a setting near the minimum anesthetic concentration (MAC). The MAC for isoflurane is approximately 1.3% to 1.44% in birds and 1.28% to 1.63% in small animals. The MAC for sevoflurane is between 2.21% in birds (chicken) and between 2.3% and 2.7% in small animals.

Breathing circuits and gas flow

Non-rebreathing circuits, such as the modified Jackson Rees and Bain circuits, are typically used during companion bird and small mammal anesthesia. These systems rely on a relatively high fresh gas flow rate to remove CO_2. They offer advantages over a rebreathing circuit, such as instant change according to adjustment of the vaporizer setting and lower resistance to breathing. Oxygen flow rates in non-rebreathing circuits should be two to three times the minute ventilation or 200 to 300 mL/kg/min.

Use of low-flow oxygen

In a small mammal or bird weighing less than 1 kg, a non-rebreathing or pediatric circle system is preferred. Oxygen flow rates used for standard small animal patients are suitable for most birds at 20 to 40 mL/kg/min when using a rebreathing system and at 200 to 300 mL/kg/min when using a non-rebreathing system (Ayres T-piece; Bain). For some vaporizers, the lower limit of oxygen flow rate required to maintain vaporizer accuracy is approximately 350 mL/min. This should be the lower limit regardless of patient size. Current recommendations for ventilatory support include two to six breaths per minute using tidal volumes ranging from 10 to 15 mL/kg, with a peak airway pressure less than 10 cm H_2O [27].

Positive-pressure ventilation

Ventilation is the act of tidal breathing to allow fresh gas (oxygen) to reach the alveoli and to allow exhaled gases (CO_2) to be removed from the lungs. During inhalation anesthesia, ventilation also facilitates inhalant gas delivery and removal from the lungs. The respiratory minute volume (RMV) is defined as the total volume of gas ventilated by the lungs in 1 minute. The RMV is technically the respiratory rate per minute multiplied by the tidal volume. Increases in RMV generally cause hyperventilation (decreased arterial CO_2), and decreases in RMV generally cause hypoventilation (increased arterial CO_2). Periodically provided PPV in birds, even during spontaneous breathing, can help to prevent the formation of endotracheal mucus plugs in small patients. Mucus plugs are common in birds and small mammals.

Normal RMV is approximately 200 mL/kg/min. This is derived from the fact that normal tidal volume is approximately 10 mL/kg and normal respiratory rate is approximately 20 breaths per minute. Some small mammals may require a high respiration rate. Most anesthesiologists use a tidal volume range for ventilation of 10 to 15 mL/kg. At greater than 15 mL/kg, peak inspiratory pressures (PIPs) may become excessive and barotrauma to the lungs may occur. Newer lung protective strategies used for long-term ventilation include using lower tidal volumes (6–8 mL/kg) and subsequently higher respiratory rates (30–80 breaths per minute) to maintain normal RMV. These newer strategies have been proven in human medicine to help prevent ventilator-induced lung injury. Because most anesthetic-related ventilation is short term, traditional tidal volumes and respiratory rates are still considered acceptable.

Most anesthesia ventilators are volume controlled or pressure controlled. Volume-controlled ventilators allow you to set a tidal volume and respiratory rate to achieve a targeted RMV. This type of ventilator distends the lungs with the preset tidal volume, resulting in a PIP. To prevent barotrauma to the lungs, the PIP should not exceed 15 to 20 cm H_2O. Poor lung compliance is frequently associated with high PIPs during volume-controlled ventilation. Volume-controlled ventilation is probably the most frequent type of ventilation available in the veterinary sector. A commercially available ventilator and anesthetic delivery machine (Anesthetic Workstation; Halowell EMC, Pittsfield, Massachusetts) has been specifically designed for use in exotic pets. Another ventilator (Vetronics) that employs a T-piece breathing system is also used for exotic pets.

Pressure-controlled ventilators allow you to set a PIP and a respiratory rate. This type of ventilator distends the lungs to the preset PIP, resulting in a tidal volume. In poorly compliant lungs, this type of ventilation may deliver extremely small tidal volumes; subsequently, the respiratory rate needs to be increased to maintain the RMV. Pressure-controlled ventilation is helpful to use in extremely small patients in which accurate tidal volumes may be difficult to set or in patients in which poor lung compliance could lead to dangerously high PIPS if volume-controlled ventilation were used. Problems frequently encountered with pressure-controlled ventilation include dangerously low tidal volumes if mucus plugs or endotracheal tube kinking occurs. Thus, gradual hypoventilation may result without the operator becoming aware. In contrast, if the endotracheal tube becomes occluded during pressure-regulated volume-limited ventilation (Halowell EMC system), the resulting high airway pressure triggers an alarm that alerts the clinician. Therefore, a low-RMV alarm is crucial in patient safety when pressure-controlled ventilation is used. The Bird Ventilator is a good example of a pressure controlled ventilator that is frequently used in veterinary medicine.

The clinician should practice caution when using the volume-cycled ventilator during surgical procedures in the coelomic cavity, with a large opening in the air sac. Volume-cycled ventilators deliver only a preset volume of anesthetic gas, making it difficult to control ventilation and anesthesia, because most of the gas leaks from the opening in the air sac. The pressure-limited ventilator under the circumstances of an open air sac continues to supply anesthetic gas until the preset pressure is achieved. There is a continuous flow from the ventilator through the respiratory system if there is a large opening in the air sac.

Mechanical ventilation is frequently necessary in the anesthetized patient because of the fact that most anesthetic agents are respiratory depressants; therefore, hypoventilation is a frequent problem encountered during anesthesia. Severe hypoventilation leads to respiratory acidosis, which may worsen hypotension, may increase the risk of cardiac arrhythmias, can cause CNS depression, may increase intracranial pressure, and frequently causes myocardial depression [28–30]. In addition to hypoventilation, hypoxemia frequently occurs in the anesthetized patient, which may require mechanical ventilation to help correct. A good rule of thumb to remember is that the Pao_2 should be approximately five to six times the fraction of inspired oxygen (FIo_2). For example, if a patient is breathing an FIo_2 of 100%, the Pao_2 should be approximately 400 to 500 mm Hg. If the Pao_2 is significantly lower than this, it should be recognized that the patient is having pulmonary dysfunction.

The five pathophysiologic causes of hypoxemia include ventilation-perfusion (V/Q) mismatching, alveolar hypoventilation, diffusion barrier, true shunt, and decreased FIo_2. V/Q mismatch from atelectasis or decreased cardiac output is the most common cause of hypoxemia under anesthesia. Alveolar hypoventilation is also a frequent cause of mild hypoxemia. Diffusion barrier and true shunt are rare causes of hypoxemia. Decreased FIo_2 is most commonly seen with hypoxic mixtures of nitrous oxide.

Respiratory monitoring

Pulse oximetry

The pulse oximeter works by emitting two different wavelengths of light (660 and 940 nm). Oxyhemoglobin (O_2Hb) absorbs most light at 940 nm, and deoxyhemoglobin absorbs most light at 660 nm. The amount of each wavelength of light that is absorbed, transmitted, and reflected is determined; placed into an algorithm; and displayed on the pulse oximeter as the oxygen saturation.

The pulse oximeter relies on the fact that there is pulsatile flow to work and to measure arterial oxygen saturation accurately. Therefore, it does not work well in poorly perfused or vasoconstricted regions. Most pulse oximeters provide a signal strength of pulsatile flow (a plethysmograph) to help the clinician assess whether or not the number that is being displayed is likely accurate.

Methemoglobin (MetHb) absorbs light at 660 and 940 nm. When MetHb is present and the level of MetHb in the blood approaches 40%, the pulse oximeter trends toward a reading of 80% to 85%. In the presence of MetHb, the pulse oximeter gives falsely low readings for saturations greater than 85% and gives falsely high readings for saturations less than 85%.

Carboxyhemoglobin (COHb) absorbs light at a spectrum similar to that of O_2Hb. When COHb is present, the pulse oximeter mistakes it for O_2Hb and the saturation on the pulse oximeter reads falsely high.

Pigmented skin, ambient light, and motion artifact interfere with pulse oximeter readings. Frequently during these situations, the pulse oximeter simply does not read, it displays its default setting (usually 85%), or the plethysmograph strength is low or absent.

A pulse oximeter is a noninvasive means of estimating arterial hemoglobin saturation for oxygen (Spo_2). Most pulse oximeters used in veterinary medicine use a clip that is applied to the patient's tongue, toe web, or pinna. The clip contains an infrared light transmitter/detector system, and by sensing the difference in the amount of light absorbed during arterial pulsations versus background absorption, the instrument reports the percent oxygen saturation of arterial hemoglobin. Most also report the pulse rate. The pulse oximeter gives assurance that blood is adequately oxygenated and the heart is beating and generating at least partial circulation and indicates pulse rate and rhythm.

Avian pulse oximetry. Pulse oximetry used in psittacine birds and pigeons was found to have poor accuracy when monitoring oxygen saturation and had a high incidence of motion artifact in such procedures as coelomic endoscopy. Spectrophotometric analyses revealed different photometric behavior between avian and human hemoglobin, which likely results in an underestimation of the actual oxygen saturation in birds. The authors recommend the use of pulse oximetry to maintain an SpO_2 greater than 90% in assisted and spontaneous ventilation as a trend-monitoring device. Remember that birds can be well oxygenated and at the same time be hypercapnic or hypocapnic, which demonstrates the importance of using capnography in birds.

Small mammals. Many things can interfere with the ability of a pulse oximeter to obtain an accurate SpO_2 reading, including decreased peripheral perfusion (whether from poor overall systemic circulation, peripheral vasoconstriction, or hypothermia), movement, bright ambient lighting, anemia, or dark skin pigmentation. Pulse oximeters only emit light at two wavelengths to detect O_2Hb and reduced hemoglobin (RHb). Any light-absorbing species other than O_2Hb and RHb (ie, COHb, MetHb) are not accounted for and, when present (ie, COHb in CO_2 poisoning, MetHb in Tylenol toxicity), produce erroneous readings.

It is important to recognize that pulse oximetry and PaO_2 are related to one another by means of the hemoglobin dissociation curve. A pulse oximeter reading of 98% to 100% may be associated with a PaO_2 of 100 to 600 (or higher) mm Hg. A normal PaO_2 on 100% oxygen should be approximately 500 mm Hg or higher. A PaO_2 of 100 mm Hg in patients breathing 100% oxygen reflects a major pulmonary problem. Unless an arterial blood gas measurement is obtained during anesthesia, the anesthetist could be misled that the patient who has an SpO_2 of 98% has normal pulmonary function. In this patient, detrimental consequences could occur if the patient is later recovered in room air. Alternatively, a pulse oximeter reading of 90% correlates to a PaO_2 of 60 mm Hg, which indicates moderate hypoxemia. This value would indicate severe pulmonary dysfunction if the patient were breathing 100% oxygen. Pulse oximeters are much more sensitive in detecting desaturation than is the naked eye, however. Most animals do not become cyanotic (ie, have observably bluish mucous membranes) until the SpO_2 reading is less than 70%, but the pulse oximeter is useful in indicating any decrease in SpO_2, allowing earlier detection of oxygenation changes or circulation problems.

Respiratory monitor

A temperature differential respiratory monitor consists of a temperature probe that extends into the airway by means of an adaptor placed between the endotracheal tubes and breathing circuit. Each time the animal exhales, the warm exhaled gas is detected by the temperature probe and is counted as a breath. Many respiratory monitors give an audible beep for each exhalation; some can be programmed to alarm if no exhalations are detected within a 30- or 60-second period (apnea alert). Respiratory monitors can be useful to count respiratory rate, particularly for tiny patients (small mammals and birds) with small tidal volumes (when chest wall or breathing bag movements cannot be easily seen). Respiratory monitors give no indication of adequacy of ventilation (removal of CO_2), however. Overall ventilation depends on respiratory rate and tidal volume, and the respiratory monitor does not measure tidal volume. An animal with a normal or high respiratory rate can hypoventilate significantly.

Respirometry

A respirometer is a mechanical device that allows precise measurement of the tidal volume of an intubated patient. It is useful under anesthesia as well as during recovery to determine if a patient is taking adequate tidal volumes. A progressive decrease in tidal volume, such as might occur with a pneumothorax slowly developing in an anesthetized trauma patient with a small pulmonary leak and PPV, can be detected early when a respirometer is used. The change in tidal volume precedes any changes in other monitored respiratory variables, often before any detrimental effects on cardiopulmonary function have taken place.

A Wright's respirometer is attached directly to the endotracheal tube or placed in the expiratory limb of the breathing circuit. The device can measure the volume of a single breath or be left "on" in place to measure the total of all breaths for a given time (eg, total volume over 1 minute, which is the minute volume).

Apnea monitors

Apnea monitors have been designed for use with human infants at risk of apnea, bradycardia, or other causes of sudden infant death syndrome. These devices consist of a small mattress pad or small arm and leg probes connected to a motion detector and alarm system. They are easy to use and simply monitor a small patient for the presence of regular small movements associated with breathing and life. The monitor alerts staff if no movement is detected in a set period (usually 15–30 seconds).

Capnometry and capnography

Capnometry and capnography are the measurement and graphic display, respectively, of the amount of CO_2 in exhaled gas. End-tidal carbon dioxide (ET_{CO_2}) refers to the amount of CO_2 measured at the end of exhalation, when the gas being sampled is presumably that originating from the alveoli. The amount of CO_2 in end-tidal or alveolar gas is theoretically nearly the same as the amount of CO_2 in blood perfusing the alveoli, which allows ET_{CO_2} to be used as an estimate of arterial Pa_{CO_2}. Because the equilibrium between arterial and alveolar CO_2 is not quite perfect, the normal ET_{CO_2} is usually 2 to 5 mm Hg less than the normal Pa_{CO_2}, which is 35 to 45 mm Hg in conscious small mammals and birds.

When using capnography in avian and small mammal patients, a sidestream capnograph can be used and the dead space associated with the endotracheal tube must be minimized [28,31]. The capnograph can be connected to the breathing circuit through an 18-gauge needle inserted into the lumen of the endotracheal tube adapter [28,31]. The needle should not obstruct the lumen of the endotracheal tube. The sidestream capnograph is invaluable for small exotic pets for assessing ventilation accurately. The disadvantage of the sidestream capnograph monitor is that when the gas sample volume requirements are too high, this may lead to artificially low ET_{CO_2} readings. The clinician should check the aspiration volume required for his or her sidestream capnography monitor. The ideal sidestream capnograph for use in the small exotic patient should require a small sample volume for evaluation or contain an infant/neonatal microstream system that uses 25 to 50 mL/min (Nellcor Puritan Bennett 70 or 75; Tyco Healthcare, Pleasaton, California). This aspiration volume of 25 to 50 mL/min should be accurate in exotics weighing greater than 100 g. The use of the capnograph in small mammals and birds weighing less than 100 g may not be reliable.

Monitoring of ET_{CO_2} gives an assessment of ventilation, which is often depressed during anesthesia and recumbency. Increases in ET_{CO_2} to greater than 45 mm Hg may indicate respiratory inadequacy, which could be caused by excessive anesthetic depth (depression of CNS respiratory center) or the limitations of positioning (inability to expand air sacs fully). The patient should be ventilated to restore a more normal ET_{CO_2}. This means that the rebreathing bag should be squeezed to deliver an inspiratory pressure of 15 to 20 cm H_2O. Never deliver an inspiratory pressure greater than 20 cm H_2O to small mammals or birds or a tidal volume of approximately 15 mL/kg. The cause of the increase in ET_{CO_2} should be investigated, and the clinician should adjust the position of the patient (inability to expand the lungs fully in small mammals or the air sacs in birds can cause an increase in ET_{CO_2}) or decrease the depth of anesthesia.

ET_{CO_2} measurement has another benefit in that detection of CO_2 in exhaled gas occurs only when the patient's trachea is properly intubated and there is adequate blood circulating through the alveoli. Thus, failure to detect ET_{CO_2} in a patient should be cause for alarm. It may indicate esophageal intubation, disconnection or obstruction of the breathing circuit, acute pulmonary thromboembolism, hypopulmonary circulation, or circulatory arrest.

As with the pulse oximeter, the reliability of the ET_{CO_2} reading can be evaluated by observing the graphic display of exhaled CO_2. The normal capnogram has a fairly steep "up" slope (corresponding to the beginning of exhalation), a flat plateau (when end-tidal or alveolar gas is exhaled and the maximum CO_2 is detected), and a steep "down" slope (inspiration).

Therefore, a capnogram without a plateau is not a reliable indicator of true ETco$_2$.

Capnography is not used when a celiotomy is performed on the avian patient. Once the abdomen is opened through the air sac, the capnograph is unable to measure ventilation in an open system.

Blood gas analysis

Arterial blood gas analysis allows measurement of the partial pressure of dissolved oxygen in the blood. Venous blood gas cannot be used to assess oxygenation, although low venous oxygen tension is associated with poor outcomes.

Arterial blood gases are the gold standard for assessing acid-base status (pH, bicarbonate, and base excess) and ventilatory status (Paco$_2$). Venous blood gases can be used as an estimate for acid-base status and ventilatory status if the perfusion is adequate to the vessel from which the blood sample was taken. Arterial CO$_2$ is always lower than venous CO$_2$ [28]. Therefore, if venous CO$_2$ is elevated, an assessment cannot be made about the ventilation status of the patient, and arterial blood gas should be measured to confirm the ventilatory status of the patient.

Adequate oxygen delivery to the tissues depends on cardiac output (stroke volume × heart rate) and arterial oxygen content. Arterial oxygen content is the summation of the Pao$_2$ and the Spo$_2$. The formula for oxygen content is as follows:

$$[SaO_2 \times Hb(g/dL) \times 1.34(ml/g)] + [PaO_2(mm\ Hg) \times 0.003(ml/dL)]$$

where Hb is hemoglobin. This formula takes into consideration the oxygen-carrying capacity of hemoglobin (1.34 mL of oxygen per gram of hemoglobin) and the fraction of dissolved oxygen in the blood (0.003 mL of oxygen dissolved per 100 mL of blood). Based on this formula, it can be seen that hemoglobin concentration is a major determinant of oxygen content. Therefore, to determine oxygen delivery correctly, the hemoglobin concentration, Spo$_2$, cardiac output, and Pao$_2$ are all necessary. Cardiac output cannot be easily measured, especially in small exotic pets and birds, but a general assessment of cardiac output can come from assessment of cardiovascular parameters (blood pressure measurement, heart rate and rhythm, pulse quality, mucous membrane color, and capillary refill time).

Point-of-care laboratory testing offers the obvious and much needed advantage of being able to perform pH, blood gas (Po$_2$ and Pco$_2$), and many clinical chemistry determinations at the patient's bedside. This means that accurate, reliable, and rapidly obtained laboratory data are immediately available to the clinician so that critical decisions can be made. Two different units (i-SSTAT and IRMA) have been evaluated in small animals (not exotics). Both have performed satisfactorily and are capable of determining pH, blood gases, and derived related variables (eg, Hco$_3$). They can determine sodium, potassium and Ca^{+2}. The i-STAT offers the extra advantage of being able to determine additional blood chemistry values, including blood urea nitrogen (BUN), glucose, SpO_2, anion gap, hemoglobin, and others.

Blood gases: the essentials. Blood gas analysis is the determination of the pH, Po_2, and Pco_2 of the blood. This information is used to assess the acid-base status and pulmonary function of a patient. This requires equipment for the analysis and skill to perform the collection. The utility of having such capabilities in a practice is determined by the number and types of cases that are seen at the practice and the ability to collect the samples and interpret the results.

A pH less than the normal range in a patient's blood sample is referred to as acidemia, and a pH greater than the normal range is referred to as alkalemia. Severe acidemia (<7.2) is associated with energy metabolism perturbations, neurologic alterations, and detrimental cardiovascular consequences (eg, decreased cardiac contractility). Clinical signs of alkalemia are rarely seen. Acidosis or alkalosis is a process that leads to an accumulation of acid or base, respectively, and is qualified by being respiratory or metabolic in origin. Hypoventilation leads to respiratory acidosis (by increasing Pco_2), whereas hyperventilation leads to respiratory alkalosis. Metabolic acid-base derangements occur in many disease processes. Some common conditions characterized by potentially serious metabolic acidosis in small animals include diabetic ketoacidosis, toxicities (eg, ethylene glycol, aspirin), renal failure, and shock.

Lactate. If shock is defined as a decrease in oxygen delivery to the tissue, resulting in anaerobic metabolism, resuscitation should be considered complete only when there is no evidence of ongoing anaerobic metabolism or tissue acidosis. It is now suggested that global markers of anaerobic metabolism (eg, lactate) may be sensitive markers of adequate resuscitation.

The normal lactate level in dogs and cats is <3 mmol/L on the Nova (Nova Biomedical, Walthum, Massachusetts), and Idexx (Idexx Laboratories, Westbrook, Maine) chemistry analyzers. Normal lactate in a recent study in rabbits (unpublished data, Lichtenberger and Schwartz, 2006) is approximately 7 to 10 mmol/L on the Idexx and Nova analyzers [29]. This is higher than that reported for dogs and cats. The authors are evaluating the possible mechanisms for these results in rabbits. There are no published data for normal lactate levels in other small mammals or birds at this time.

Avian anesthesia

If the procedure is to be longer than 30 minutes, the patient should be intubated (see the section on intubation in the article on analgesia in this issue).

Care should be taken during intubation to ensure that the trachea is not damaged. In birds, the endotracheal tube should provide a good seal with the glottis but should not fit tightly. If the tube is cuffed, the cuff should not be inflated or should be inflated with tremendous care. An overinflated cuff can cause damage to the tracheal mucosa because of the complete cartilaginous rings present in birds. Damage to the trachea may not become evident until as long as 5 to 7 days after intubation, when the healing process and subsequent fibrotic narrowing of the tracheal lumen cause signs of respiratory distress. Intubating small birds (ie, less than 100 g of body weight) has risks, because endotracheal tubes with small internal diameters can impose significant resistance to air flow, especially if mucus accumulates in the lumen of the tube. During anesthesia, mucus production can become copious, thick, and tenacious. Endotracheal tube obstruction can be detected by monitoring the bird's pattern of ventilation. As the airway becomes occluded, the duration of the expiratory phase becomes prolonged. Mechanically sighing the bird usually confirms the presence of an obstruction, because the air sacs fill in a relatively normal manner during inspiration but empty slowly or not at all during expiration [28]. An anticholinergic, such as atropine or glycopyrrolate, reduces mucus production and decreases plug formation but may also increase mucus viscosity, making it harder to clear [27]. These drugs also cause an increase in heart rate, thus increasing the work load of the heart and myocardial oxygen demand. The authors do not recommend the routine use of anticholinergic drugs except for treatment of bradycardia. Monitoring core body temperature, pulse oximetry, and ECG using an esophageal probe is ideal. PPV provided by means of a mechanical ventilator or by manually compressing the reservoir bag can be used effectively to maintain the avian patient with the help of capnography. During PPV, airway pressures should not exceed 15 to 20 cm H_2O to prevent volutrauma to the air sacs.

Small mammal anesthesia

Small mammals have similar anatomy and physiologic principles of the respiratory system as are seen in small animals. Anesthesia principles are applied to small mammals based on anesthesia in other small animals. Intubation is difficult (except in the ferret) and has been discussed previously. Most small mammals (except for the ferret and rabbit) require injectable analgesia used together with mask inhalation. Monitoring of core body temperature, ECG, and pulse oximetry using the esophageal probe is ideal.

Summary

The routine use of cardiovascular and respiratory monitoring in the critical care exotic patient is important to help detect instability before irreversible damage occurs. An understanding of cardiovascular monitoring of perfusion parameters in the critically ill exotic pet is necessary in understanding and treating shock. The importance of blood pressure monitoring in the avian and small mammal patient is emphasized. Cardiac evaluation is important in any unstable patient to determine the presence of cardiac disease or rhythm disturbances. CVP and cardiac output are discussed so that the reader is aware of the future trends of veterinary medicine. The avian respiratory system is unique, and it is essential to understand these differences when treating and monitoring the avian patient. Anesthesia principles of the breathing circuits, oxygen flow, and ventilation have been reviewed for use in the exotic pet.

Monitoring of the respiratory system by means of pulse oximetry, respiratory monitors, respirometers, apnea monitors, capnometry, and blood gas analysis may be used during anesthesia in avian and small mammal patients.

References

[1] Schmidt-Nielsen K. Scaling. Why is animal size so important? New York: Cambridge University Press; 1984.
[2] Sedgwick CJ. Allometrically scaling the data base for vital sign assessment used in general anesthesia of zoological species. Proc Am Assoc Zoo Vets 1991;360.
[3] Lichtenberger MK, Orcutt C, DeBehnke D, et al. Mortality and response to fluid resuscitation after acute blood loss in mallard ducks (Ana playrhynnchos). 2002 Scientific Proceedings, 22nd Annual Meeting of the Association of Avian Veterinarians. Monterey, CA; 2002. p. 65–7.
[4] Marino PL. Arterial blood pressure. In: Marino PL, editor. The ICU book. Philadelphia: Lippincott Williams & Wilkins; 1997. p. 143–53.
[5] Olin JM, Smith TJ, Talcott MR. Evaluation of noninvasive monitoring techniques in domestic ferrets (Mustela putorius furo). Am J Vet Res 1997;58(10):1065–9.
[6] Ypsilantis P, Didilis VN, Politou M, et al. A comparative study of invasive and oscillometric methods of arterial blood pressure measurement in the anesthetized rabbit. Res Vet Sci 78(3):269–75.
[7] Lichtenberger MK, Chavez W, Brunsen D, et al. Direct versus indirect blood pressure monitoring during acute blood loss in Peking ducks (Anas platyrhynchos domesticus). Proceedings of the Ann Avian Vet Conf. New Orleans, LO; 2004. p. 3–6.
[8] Aldrich J, Haskins S. Monitoring the critically ill patient. In: Bonagura JD, Kirk RW, editors. Current veterinary therapy, vol. XII. Philadelphia: WB Saunders; 1995. p. 98–105.
[9] Oakley RE, Olivier B, Eyster GE, et al. Experimental evaluation of central venous pressure monitoring in the dog. J Am Anim Hosp Assoc 1997;33:77–82.
[10] Petrie JP, Morrisey JK. Cardiovascular and other diseases. In: Quesenberry KE, Carpenter JW, editors. Ferrets, rabbits, and rodents: clinical medicine and surgery. St. Louis (MO): Saunners; 2006. p. 58–71.
[11] Pees M, Krautwald-Junghanns ME, Straub J. Evaluating and treating the cardiovascular system. In: Harrison GJ, Lightfoot TL, editors. Clinical avian medicine. Palm Beach (FL): Spix Publishing Inc; 2006. p. 379–94.
[12] Pilny AA. Retrospective of atherosclerosis in psittacine birds: clinical and histopathologic findings in 31 cases. Proceedings of AAV. 25th Annual Conference, New Orleans, LA; 2004. p. 349–51.
[13] Krautwald-Junghanns ME, Schulz M, Hagner D, et al. Transcoelomic two-dimensional echocardiography in the avian patient. J Avian Med Surg 1995;9:19–31.
[14] Plehn JF, Foster E, Grice WN, et al. Echocardiographic assessment of LV mass in rabbits: models of pressure and volume overload hypertrophy. Am J Physiol 1993;265:2066–72.

[15] Stepien RL, Benson KG, Wenholz LJ. M-mode and Doppler echocardiographic findings in normal ferrets sedated with ketamine hydrochloride and midazolam. Vet Radiol Ultrasound 2000;41:452–6.
[16] Schoemaker NJ, Zandvliet MM. Electrocardiograms in selected species. Sem in Avian and Exotic Pet Medicine 2005;14:26–33.
[17] Lumej JT, Richie BW. Cardiology. In: Richie BW, Harrison GJ, Harrison LR, editors. Avian medicine: principles and application. Lake Worth (FL): Wingers Publishing; 1994. p. 114–231.
[18] Lumeij JT, Stokhof AA. Electrocardiogram of the racing pigeon (Columba livia domestica). Res Vet Sci 1985;38:273–8.
[19] Zandvliet MM. Electrocardiography in psittacine birds and ferrets. Sem in Avian and Exotic Pet Medicine 2005;14:34–51.
[20] Smith F, West N, Jones D. The cardiovascular system. In: Whittow G, editor. Sturkie's avian physiology. San Diego (CA): Academic Press; 2000. p. 141–231.
[21] Bolulianne M, Hunter DB, Julian RJ, et al. Cardiac muscle mass distribution in the domestic turkey and relationship to electrocardiogram. 1992;36:582–9.
[22] Nap AM, Lumeij JT. Cardiology in birds. Tijdschr Diergeneeskd 1991;116(Suppl 1):82S–4S.
[23] Huston S, Quesenberry KE. Cardiovascular and lymphoproliferative diseases. In: Quesenberry KE, Carpenter JW, editors. Ferrets, rabbits and rodents: clinical medicine and surgery includes sugar gliders and hedgehogs. St Louis (MO): Saunders; 2003. p. 211–20.
[24] Richtarik A, Woolsey TA, Valdivia E. Method for recording ECGs in unanesthetized guinea pigs. J Appl Physiol 1965;20:1091–3.
[25] Casares M, Enders F, Montoya JA. Comparative electrocardiography in four species of macaws (genera Anodorhyncvhus ans Ara). J Vet Med A Physiol Pathol Clin Med 2000;47: 277–81.
[26] Oglesbee BL, Oglesbee MJ. Results of post-mortem examination of psittacine birds with cardiac disease: 26 cases 1991–1995. JAMA 1998;212:1737–42.
[27] Phillips RA, Sloniger JA, Scansen B, et al. Cardiac output measurements in animals using the non-invasive USCOM device [abstract]. Proc of Int Vet Emer and Crit care 2006;1023.
[28] Ko J. Oxygen flow rates 1. Proceedings of the West Vet Conf. Los Vegas, NV; 2006:22–8.
[29] Edling TM. Advances in anesthesia monitoring in birds, reptiles and small mammals. Exotic DVM 2003;5(3):15–20.
[30] Schwartz Z, Lichtenberger MK, Thamm DH, et al. Lactate normals in the healthy rabbits comparing three different analyzers [abstract]. Proc of Int Vet and Crit Care 2006;1038.
[31] Edling TM, Degernes LA, Flammer K, et al. Capnographic monitoring of anesthetized African grey parrots receiving intermittent positive pressure ventilation. J Am Vet Med Assoc 2001;219(12):1714–8.

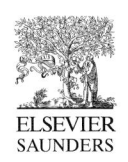

Emergency and Critical Care of Pet Birds

Heather Bowles, DVM, DABVP-Avian[a],*,
Marla Lichtenberger, DVM, DACVECC[b],
Angela Lennox, DVM, DABVP-Avian[c]

[a]*Hunt Valley Animal Hospital, 11206 York Road, Cockeysville, MD 21030, USA*
[b]*Thousand Oaks Pet Emergency Clinic, Thousand Oaks, CA, USA*
[c]*Avian and Exotic Animal Clinic of Indianapolis, Indianapolis, IN, USA*

Most birds do not show signs of illness in the early stages of disease. Often birds with chronic disease present as emergencies because of their ability to mask clinical signs of disease until their condition is severe. In virtually all cases, the authors advise the receptionist to recommend the bird be brought in for an examination. If the owner is concerned enough to call, then the bird is likely sick and needs to be seen. Although all signs reported by the client can be of concern, sitting at the bottom of the cage, bleeding, respiratory distress, regurgitation, and anorexia are considered true emergencies. The client should be instructed to bring the bird in a cage or suitable alternative, (eg, box, cat carrier). The water dish should be emptied, but the cage should not be cleaned before travel to the hospital.

This article discusses triage techniques, history, physical examination, and diagnostic procedures. Common treatment procedures are presented, such as catheterization, nebulization, air sac cannulation, and radiographic techniques. The importance of nutrition precedes discussion on common emergency presentations. The reader should be aware that shock, fluid therapy, cardiopulmonary–cerebral resuscitation, analgesia, and anesthetic monitoring techniques in birds are presented elsewhere in this issue. The clinician must stabilize all critically ill birds (see the article by Lichtenberger in this issue).

Triage

Once the bird has arrived, it is ideal to have a trained receptionist call for an immediate triage by an experienced technician, as prompt, accurate treatment is vital for a favorable outcome. In cases of bleeding, seizures,

---

* Corresponding author.
E-mail address: heatherdvm@gmail.com (H. Bowles).

head trauma, and respiratory distress, the bird should be evaluated immediately by the veterinarian. The veterinarian should proceed immediately to the section for treatment protocols. If the bird is depressed, weak, or sitting at the bottom of the cage, it should be placed immediately in a warmed incubator with oxygen. The optimum temperatures for ill birds are 85 to 90° F (29 to 30° C). Many birds will benefit from symptomatic treatment such as oxygen supplementation, fluid therapy, broad-spectrum antibiotics and antifungals, and nutritional support and observation for the first 2 to 8 hours in a warmed incubator before diagnostic testing is preformed.

History

Take a complete history while the bird is being stabilized in the incubator with oxygen. History should include information such as age, sex (if known) source of the bird, and presence of other birds in the household. Dietary history includes types and proportions of foods offered and consumed, and any changes in food or water consumption. Determine the length of illness and progression of signs and symptoms. Other important information includes exposure to trauma, toxins (plant, airborne, overheated nonstick cookware, metal, cleansers), and other pets in the household. Inquire about recent illness in other birds in the household. Other important information includes changes in droppings, reproductive activity including courtship behavior and oviposition, and other changes in behavior. Environmental history includes information on type of caging, and whether the bird is able to leave the cage unsupervised.

Preprinted history questionnaires are often extremely useful.

Examination

Initially the bird should be evaluated in its cage. Posture, ability to ambulate and perch, respiratory status, interest in the environment, and fluffing of the feathers are assessed. The cage can be examined for regurgitated material, blood, or other discharge. If the bird is presented in its regular cage, inspect it for potential sources of toxins. Examine the feces for color, volume, and consistency. Feces that are scant and green to black suggest anorexia. Urates are normally white to off white, but may take up color from food dye in the feces. Urine is normally scant and clear, but many birds display stress-related polyurea at presentation. Frank blood may be noted either from the gastrointestinal (GI) or urinary tract or from hemorrhaging masses in the cloaca.

Perform a complete physical examination as the condition of the bird allows. Work in a small room with low ceilings, closed window, and no fans, especially if the bird is flighted. Some birds, particularly finches and canaries, should be captured in a darkened room. Prior to restraint, have all equipment ready in advance to minimize handling time, and attempt to determine if the bird is stable enough for examination. Death during handling occurs most frequently in birds that are weak and in respiratory distress. In an authors' experience, other birds at risk include obese budgerigars on inappropriate (seed) diets. It is wise to advise owners of very ill birds that handling and treatment may result in worsening of condition and even death.

Physical examination must be complete and thorough as in any other species. Structures unique to birds include the crop, which is palpated for the presence of food and/or foreign material, and the choanal slit of the oropharynx, which is examined for the presence of inflammatory debris, foreign material, and blunted papillae suggesting hypovitaminosis A. Feathers of the rest of the body are parted carefully to examine the skin. The beak is inspected for bleeding, symmetry, and fractures. Examination of the basilic vein and determination of refill time is useful to evaluate perfusion status. Hydration is assessed by skin turgor. Auscultation is challenging in birds because of relatively small size, rigid lungs, and unique respiratory system. Auscultation may reveal abnormalities in heart rate, rhythm, murmur, and abnormal lung and/or air sac sounds. As respiratory sounds in birds are normally minimal, the detection of crackles, wheezes, and clicks are likely abnormal.

The palpable ceolomic space is the area between the ventral keel and pelvis. The space is normally small, and often the only normal palpable structure may be the ventral aspect of the ventriculus. Abnormalities that may be detected include: abdominal distension, intraceolomic fluid, palpable mass, caudoventrally displaced ventriculus, and/or an egg [1–3]. Overall body condition is evaluated through palpation of the pectoral muscle mass. Muscle is reduced and the keel readily palpable in underconditioned birds. In contrast, in overconditioned birds, the central keel bone often is obscured. and the pectoral muscle mass takes on a plump, rounded appearance. The vent and cloaca are inspected for the presence of lesions including masses, swelling, and prolapsed tissue. The feathers surrounding the vent normally are clean and not matted with feces or debris.

Complete neurologic examination is covered in detail in a later section in this article. Weigh the bird in grams and observe it in the incubator at the conclusion of the examination to determine the impact of handling on overall condition.

In cases where complete physical examination is not recommended because of poor patient condition, perform a rapid examination while transferring the bird from cage or carrier to the incubator. Quickly palpate the pectoral muscle mass and ceolomic space during transfer, and observe the bird carefully after releasing into the incubator.

Diagnostic testing

Blood work

Blood collection is preformed most commonly by venipuncture of the right jugular vein, although the medial metatarsal and basilic vein may be used in larger species. The amount of blood collected is never more than 1% of the bird's total blood volume. One of the authors (Lichtenberger) recommends that a good rule of thumb for the critically ill bird is to collect 0.4 to 0.5 mL/100 g body weight.

Routine hematology and chemistry analysis include a complete blood cell (CBC) count, and at a minimum aspartate aminotransferase (AST), creatine kinase (CK), glucose, uric acid, calcium, phosphorus, albumin, and electrolytes. Hematology and biochemistry tests are important in the diagnosis of infectious, metabolic, inflammatory, and some toxic diseases. A packed cell volume evaluates the patient for the presence of anemia. A blood smear should be evaluated for blood cell quantity and morphology, the presence of parasites, evidence of polychromasia, and presence of anisocytosis. It should be noted that birds have efficient mechanisms for compensation after blood loss, and begin regeneration within 12 to 36 hours [4].

A white blood cell (WBC) count may be performed with a Neubauer-ruled hematocytometer using the Eosinophil Unopette 5877 (Becton-Dickinson, Cockeysville, Maryland) or by using the Natt and Herrick method. Both methods require that samples be read in a timely fashion to prevent overstaining of cells. An estimated WBC count may be performed, particularly to corroborate results from the previous techniques or if cell quality is declining in a sample. A differential cell count in a monolayer blood smear under 40 × power is performed, and the total leukocyte count is estimated by dividing the raw leukocyte count by the number of fields counted and multiplying this number by 2000. Adjustments must be made in anemic patients, and counts may not be accurate if the sample quality is poor, for example, slides with excessive numbers of smudge cells or lacking an adequate monolayer region. A red blood cell count per microliter of whole, anticoagulated blood, may be performed using the Natt and Herrick method as well [5].

Heterophil morphology can give important information regarding underlying disease status. Although standards for evaluation of cell morphology have not been established, many authors recommend grading heterophil abnormalities from 1 to 4+. Cell abnormalities include basophilic cytoplasm and cytoplasmic granules, rounding of cytoplasmic granules, nuclear hypersegmentation, and cytoplasmic vacuolation. Monocytosis is commonly present with chronic inflammatory or infectious disease. Severe leukocytosis has been associated with chlamydiophila infection, mycobacteriosis, and aspergillosis, but is not always consistent. Stress alone may significantly raise heterophil counts in an otherwise healthy bird, especially in young macaws. Lymphocytosis typically is associated with significant immune stimulation. Lymphocytes may exhibit reactive change (darker cytoplasm, nuclear changes, prominent nucleoli, and cytoplasmic scalloping). These changes have been noted both in the presence of infection and in apparently normal birds [5].

Thrombocyte counts usually are reported as adequate or decreased. Normal numbers range from approximately 20,000 to 50,000/uL. Clumping of thrombocytes should be documented also. Reduced numbers may be associated with a coagulopathy. Morphologic changes, such as blebbing or enlargement of the cytoplasm, should be noted, and these may be associated with recruitment of cells for phagocytic defense [5].

Ancillary diagnostic tests are performed based on history, physical examination, and results of other diagnostic testing. These may include but are not limited to: blood lead level, plasma zinc level, protein electrophoresis, chlamydiophilia testing, and *Aspergillus* testing. Plasma protein electrophoresis (EPH) is useful in detecting inflammation associated with many diseases (eg, chlamydiophilia, aspergillosis, mycobacteriosis, ceolomitis, liver disease, and renal disease). There is significant controversy regarding various diagnostic tests for chlamydiophila and aspergillosis, and the reader is referred to the literature for a more thorough discussion.

Liver function

Enzyme profiles are routinely assessed to detect liver damage. Commonly measured enzymes include AST, ALP, CK, lactate dehydrogenase (LDH) and GGT, but it should be kept in mind that correlation of enzyme elevation with the true presence and severity of liver disease is often poor [6]. A recent study reported poor correlation between liver enzyme elevation and liver disease confirmed by means of biopsy in 30 psittacines [7].

The half-lives are 0.71 hours for LDH, 16 hours for alanine aminotransferase (ALT), and 8 hours for AST [8]. These enzymes are sensitive for liver disease but not specific. AST sources include liver, skeletal muscle, heart, kidney, and brain. Elevated levels are usually the result of liver or muscle damage. Marked increases in AST (greater than four times normal) usually indicate liver necrosis. Mild-to-moderate increases (two to four times normal) are usually the result of skeletal muscle injury. Elevation from skeletal muscle leakage can be differentiated from liver sources by measuring CK levels. Levels of CK will increase with skeletal muscle damage. Therefore, a mild-to-moderate increase in AST with an increase in CK is more likely caused by skeletal muscle injury. Marked increases in AST without increased CK suggest severe diffuse hepatic damage; however, hepatic damage and inadequate function may be present with normal levels of AST. The plasma half-life of AST in pigeons is 7 to 9 hours [8]. Bile acid evaluation may support the diagnosis of liver disease, but absolute confirmation, including evaluation of type and extent of disease is only possible with liver biopsy. LDH is not specific for liver disease, but the advantage is its very short half-life. Prolonged LDH elevation without CK elevation suggests that liver damage is more likely than skeletal muscle damage [6].

Serum calcium

Most laboratories report total serum calcium, which is a combination of ionized calcium, protein-bound calcium, and complexed calcium. It is a less precise estimate of true calcium status than ionized calcium alone.

Ionized calcium in normal individuals is maintained within a narrow range, and deviations are more likely to represent true disease than do deviations in total serum calcium [9]. Calcium concentration may decrease with inadequate calcium in the diet and excessive egg-laying; however calcium usually is mobilized from the bone to maintain calcium blood concentration within normal limits. Ovulating hens often have elevated calcium levels caused by calcium mobilization for egg production. Hens that suffer from chronic egg laying may develop osteoporosis despite a normal serum total calcium concentration. Other causes of hypocalcemia include hypovitaminosis D_3, hypoalbuminemia (only total calcium is affected), and hypoparathyroidism [9]. Calcium concentration elevations may occur with vitamin D toxicosis (dietary or other source) and hyperparathyroidism. Artifactual elevations in total serum calcium can occur with lipemia and hyperproteinemia [9].

Phosphorus and glucose

Phosphorus levels rise along with calcium during egg formation in female birds. In healthy individuals the calcium:phosphorus range is maintained above one. Marked deviations in phosphorus (hyperphosphatemia and hypophosphatemia) have been associated with renal disease in birds. Increased phosphorus elevations also may be associated with hyperparathyroidism [10]. Glucose may be the mammalian level (about 300 mg/dL). Hypoglycemia can be seen with starvation in small or very young birds, liver failure, neoplasia, and septicemia. Hyperglycemia is a common response to stress and should not be mistaken for diabetes mellitus. Persistent hyperglycemia can indicate diabetes mellitus and pancreatitis, and indicates the need for pancreatic biopsy [10].

Uric acid

Uric acid concentration may increase with renal disease, dehydration, or gout. Uric acids are the main avian nitrogenous waste product and are excreted through tubular secretion. Birds eliminate nitrogenous waste by tubular secretion; they respond to water deprivation by decreasing overall glomerular filtration rate (GFR), altering blood flow from reptilian-type nephrons to mammalian-type nephrons. This gradually increases their plasma osmolality to recover more water from the glomerular filtrate. Uric acid is mostly unaffected by GFR until GFR is severely reduced, and urine flow is insufficient to move the uric acid condensates through the tubules. Therefore uric acid levels only will be elevated in severely dehydrated birds [5].

Loss of two thirds of the functional mass of the kidney is required for uric acid increase greater than 15 mg/dL. Normal uric acid concentrations do not guarantee that the kidneys are healthy. When uric acid is greater than12 mg/dL, the authors recommend treatment for dehydration and re-evaluation. Persistent uric acid elevations despite rehydration and fluid therapy are indications for endoscopic biopsy of the kidney [11].

Hypoproteinemia

Hypoproteinemia may occur with malnutrition, chronic renal and hepatic disease, malabsorption, or blood loss. Plasma albumin and globulin (alpha, beta, and gamma levels) should be evaluated by serum protein EPH. An increase in beta globulins may occur with acute inflammation or infection (ie, nephritis, hepatitis, aspergillosis, chlamydiophila infection, mycobacteriosis, egg-related ceolomitis). Increase in gamma globulins is seen commonly with chronic inflammation and infection. More work needs to be done on improving the test methodology itself, and on correlation of EPH with clinical disease. Two independent laboratories in the United States found poor correlation on identical samples submitted to both laboratories [12]. Hypoalbuminemia is not a consistent finding in birds with renal failure [12]. This indicates that the disease process is typically not glomerular disease (ie, tubular nephritis or interstitial nephritis), is early stages of glomerular disease, or that birds do not lose protein with glomerular disease [11].

Bile acids

Bile acids assays are very sensitive and specific for liver disease. Normally over 90% of bile salts are reabsorbed by enterohepatic reuptake by the liver. Controlled studies show postprandial increases in plasma bile acids when normal birds are tested. Increases in postprandial samples in birds with liver disease, however, do not overlap with postprandial bile acid values in normal birds. Therefore a single postprandial can be used to evaluate birds with suspected liver disease. Presence or absence of a gall bladder in various bird species does not affect measurement of bile acids. Severe elevations tend to occur with gall bladder hyperplasia, hepatic fibrosis, and severe hepatic lipidosis. Mild-to-moderate elevations tend to occur with mild hepatic lipidosis, cholangiohepatitis, and infectious disease (ie, chlamydiosis). It should be noted that bile acid levels may be normal in the presence of significant liver disease [8].

Urinalysis

Urinalysis is problematic in birds because of normal mixing of urine and feces in the cloaca and voided sample, and because of natural intestinal reabsorption of water from urine [12]. Therefore urinalysis must be interpreted with care, and protein, inflammatory cells and red cells may originate from the GI tract. Urine protein electrophoresis may be a useful test for bird with glomerulonephritis, but no studies are available. Ureteral cannulation is possible, but this requires anesthesia and is technically difficult [11].

Evaluation of feces and crop specimens

Fecal wet mounts can reveal *Giardia* spp., *Trichomonas* spp. (crop wash), and *Macrorbabdus ornithogaster* (megabacterium or avian gastric yeast).

Fecal cytology and Gram's stain are commonly used screening tools, but they have a potential for overinterpretation. In most cases, the presence of large numbers of gram-negative bacteria, budding yeast or clostridium spores are considered abnormal. Some authors, however, believe that these findings in a normal bird are may be reflection of poor nutrition and/or husbandry. An abnormal Gram's stain in a bird with evidence of illness, especially GI disease, may be more significant, and culture and sensitivity are indicated. Treatment with appropriate antibiotics and/or antifungals can be initiated pending culture results [13].

Nasal flush

Sinusitis and disease of the nares commonly causes upper respiratory disease. Birds may sneeze, pick their nares with their toenails, or appear generally ill. There may or may not be a nasal discharge. A nasal flush with sterile saline is performed easily with physical restraint. Hold the patient with the head lowered and beak pointed toward a sterile collection container. Infuse sterile saline into one nare with a syringe while occluding the other nare with a finger, then repeat on the other side. The fluid is collected in the sterile container and used for cytology and culture. Holding the patient in this position allows the fluid to exit through the choanal slit and leave the mouth, thereby preventing the fluid from gaining access to the oropharynx. It may be difficult to flush the nares if there is a significant amount of material in the nasal and sinus passages. Diagnostic testing results should be interpreted with caution because of contamination of the sample from the oral cavity. After collection of diagnostic samples, flushing can be repeated with medication (antibiotics, antifungals) added to flush solution. The infraorbital sinus may be sampled as well. Sterile saline is infused into the sinus rostral to the orbit, aspirated and submitted for diagnostic testing. This technique prevents oral contamination; however, careful restraint or anesthesia is necessary, and sample sizes retrieved are limited.

Radiographs

Radiography is an integral part of avian medicine. The clinician must have knowledge of normal avian radiographic anatomy before attempting to interpret abnormal radiographs. Normal avian radiographs require proper positioning and may be stressful to the conscious avian patient. It is impossible to obtain proper positioning without anesthesia in most cases. In the ventral-dorsal position, stretch the neck out and extend all four limbs. Superimpose the keel over the spine. In the lateral view, stretch the neck out. Extend the wings above the body. Stretch and separate each leg. A common dilemma for veterinarians is that the emergency avian patient may not appear stable enough for anesthesia and radiographs, which requires careful consideration. It should be kept in mind that if the bird is to be anesthetized, other diagnostic procedures and treatments may be attempted including venipuncture, blood pressure, ECG, and intravenous (IV)/intraosseous catheterization (IO) catheterization. Radiographs are useful to identify ingested metal, GI obstruction, foreign body, presence of an egg, organ enlargement or displacement, and fractures. The lungs and air sacs may be evaluated for pathology also, such as changes in radiographic density and masses. Oral contrast media can help evaluate the size of the GI tract, and to identify GI tract displacement caused by the presence of a mass or organomegaly. Care must be taken to prevent aspiration of barium, which can occur both in the anesthetized or conscious patient. Anesthetized birds therefore should be intubated. Other options include horizontal beam radiography in the awake bird [14]. Barium sulfate is administered at 2 mL/100 g BW and radiographs taken at 20 minutes, 1 hour, and 3 hours, depending on patient size and the goal of the study [14].

Ultrasound

Ultrasonography uses the transmission and reflection of sound waves to produce an image. Sound waves cannot penetrate the gas-filled air sac system, and this limits organ visualization in the avian patient. Because of the small size of most birds and the limited window of accessibility, the ultrasound transducer must have a small contact area. The cranioventral approach to the heart and coelomic viscera is the most reliable approach to most psittacine birds. This acoustic window is located on midline just caudal to the sternum. A transducer frequency of 7.5 MHz or higher is recommended [15]. The bird is restrained in dorsal recumbency, with the head and cranial coelom elevated to assist in visualization. Feathers are wetted with a small amount of isopropyl alcohol. Acoustic coupling gel is applied to the skin. In the normal bird, liver, heart, and active gonads (usually the ovaries) are distinguishable. Spleen, normal kidneys, and inactive gonads are difficult to identify. The indications for ultrasound include investigation of soft tissue masses, hepatomegaly, cardiac disease (see the article by Lichtenberger in this issue), renomegaly, disorders of the reproductive tract, and identification of ascites. Ultrasound guided aspirates also can be performed [14].

Computed tomography (CT)

CT is a cross-sectional imaging modality that uses radiographs to create a digital image or slice that is reformatted into planes of view [16]. CT is used best for evaluating bone and air-filled structures (skull, sinuses, and lower respiratory tract). Soft tissue resolution is inferior to MRI. The major advantage of the CT scan is the short time required for the study; with a typical study can be performed in 10 minutes. General anesthesia is required.

MRI

MRI is performed using a strong external magnetic force to align certain atoms within the body about a desired axis. The magnetic field then is turned off, and the unit senses energy released as atoms returning to their resting state [16]. A cross-sectional image is produced. MRI is used for imaging soft tissue structures. MRI has been used to evaluate the diagnosis and management of chronic sinusitis in psittacines [16]. General anesthesia is required. The disadvantage of the MRI study compared with the CT scan is the longer time required. A typical study may require 30 minutes to 1 hour.

Procedures

Intraosseous catheterization

In many cases IO catheterization is a superior choice over IV catheterization, as the latter is often more technically difficult in terms of placement and maintenance, especially in small birds. If the bird removes an IV catheter unnoticed, significant blood loss could occur.

IO catheters can be placed in most birds in the distal ulna and in the proximal tibiotarsus (Fig. 1). Short spinal needles (20 to 22 G × 3.1 cm) can be used in larger birds, while 22 to 25 G injection needles can be used in smaller birds. Should the needle become occluded, appropriate-sized sterilized cerclage wire can be inserted into the needle to remove the obstruction. To place an ulnar catheter, palpate the dorsal tubercle of the distal ulna. Pluck the feathers over this area and aseptically prepare the area for better visualization of the landmark. Lidocaine 2% (0.2 mg/100 g diluted with saline) is used to block the skin and periosteum over the site. Grasp the ulna between the fingers of one hand. With the other hand, the spinal needle is positioned over the distal ulna and aimed between the fingers holding the

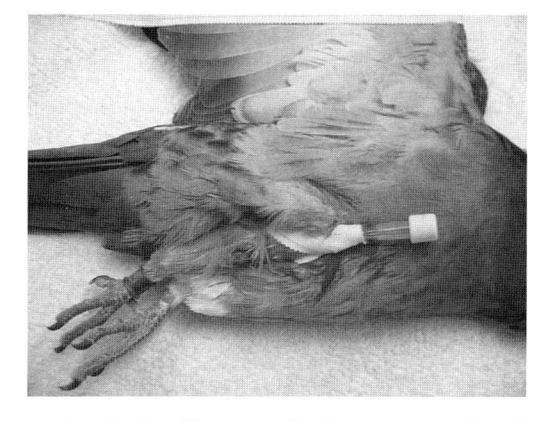

Fig. 1. Intraosseous catheterization. Placement of an intraosseous catheter in proximal tibiotarsus of a bird.

ulna. Apply a small amount of pressure as the needle is rotated through the cortex of the bone. Once the cortex is breached, slowly work the needle along the medullary canal of the bone until the needle is seated in the ulna. Use a tuberculin syringe and a small amount of heparinized saline to test the patency of the catheter. The ulnar vein should blanch as the fluid is injected. The IO space is not elastic (as is a vein), and so some resistance is expected. This resistance can be minimized by using small-volume syringes or by giving fluids by constant rate infusion. When the catheter is securely in place, attach a male adapter plug that has been flushed with heparinized saline. Some clinicians use injection caps or T ports. The catheter can be secured into the ulna by placing a small piece of tape at the hub in a butterfly fashion and suturing it to the skin. The catheter then is incorporated into a figure- eight wing bandage to minimize movement of the wing. Wing movement can cause the catheter to move and widen the perforation in the bone and cause fluid leakage from this site. For IO catheter in the proximal tibiotarsus, the cnemial crest is palpated easily at the cranial and proximal portion of the tibiotarsus. The leg is extended and flexed at the knee, and the area is plucked and aseptically prepared. The needle is inserted at the cnemial crest at the insertion of the patellar ligament. There is no vein in which to visualize blanching, so check for patency by injecting fluids, or if necessary, confirm by obtaining radiographs of the limb in two views [2,3].

Intravenous catheterization

IV catheters can be placed using short, small-gauge catheters in the right jugular, ulnar, and dorsal metatarsal veins. The jugular vein is a large vein that is easily to catheterize, but this can be difficult to maintain in an active bird.

Many birds do not tolerate the wrapping necessary to maintain the catheter. An IV jugular catheter can be placed in birds as small as 75 g. Usually, no feathers need to be plucked, because there is an area of apterylae over the jugular veins. Prepare the catheterization site aseptically. The vein is entered at the distal one-half to one-third with a 20 or 22 gauge catheter of sufficient length to reach the thoracic inlet [2,3].

The basilic vein is visualized easily for catheterization as is passes over the proximal ulna. Smaller catheters, such as 24 gauge, should be used for this vein. Once the catheter is stabilized, the wing is wrapped in a figure eight bandage to limit mobility. The dorsal metatarsal vein has the advantage of easy visualization of the catheter after placement. The tough lizard-like skin of the feet helps to hold the catheter firmly in place. This vein can be used in most birds over 300 g and can be seen as it courses along the dorsomedial aspect of the tarsometatarsus [2,3].

Nasal flush

Techniques for nasal flush are discussed under diagnostic testing.

Nebulization

Nebulizers are designed to convert liquids to appropriately sized aerosol particles for inhalation. The nebulizer consists of a disposable or reusable nebulizer and a pressurized gas (air or oxygen) source. A small volume of medication and a larger volume of diluent are placed into the nebulizer chamber. The aerosol particle size produced by a nebulizer is affected by the gas flow used to power it, the volume of solution, and the construction of the nebulizer.

Nebulization can be useful to deliver moisture or topical medications to the mucous membranes of the respiratory system. Inhalant delivery of aerosolized medication offers numerous theoretical benefits, including a large absorptive surface area across a permeable membrane, a low enzyme environment potentially resulting in low drug degradation, avoidance of hepatic first-pass metabolism, potential for high drug concentrations directly at the site of disease, and reduced potential for systemic toxicity [17]. In veterinary medicine, the literature on inhalant therapy is extremely sparse, and what does exist focuses more on aerosol drug delivery to horses than to small pet animal or exotic species. There are only single published studies in conscious, unsedated cats and rats demonstrating the ability to deliver particles to the lower airways by means of ultrasonic nebulization [18,19]. Regardless, aerosol delivery of medication has become popular for treatment of dogs, cats, small mammals, and birds with respiratory disease. The administration of nebulized particles using positive-pressure ventilation through an endotracheal tube may be the most efficient method for lower airway particle delivery, but this is not always practical in a clinical setting. Nebulization also has been administered to birds in a closed cage, induction chamber or aquarium, or by means of a face mask. Typically, the systemic drug dose has been empirically diluted in 5 to 10 mL of saline and delivered over a single 15- to 30-minute nebulization session. One of the authors (Lichtenberger) has anesthetized avian patients with severe small airway disease (eg, aerosol hypersensitivity, smoke inhalation), intubated, and nebulized a bronchodilator directly into the endotracheal tube.

The most frequently used antibiotic medications for nebulization are the aminoglycoside antibiotics, but there are no established guidelines for administration of these drugs by this route. Amphotericin B has been used effectively by means of nebulization for lower airway fungal disease in rats [10]. In the experience of one of the authors, other antifungals (itraconazole, terbinafine at 10 mg/kg twice daily diluted in 5 mL of saline) also can be nebulized. Parental bronchodilators such as terbutaline also have been used empirically by means of nebulization in birds with lower airway disease. In birds, terbutaline (0.01 mg/kg) often is given initially intramuscularly or subcutaneously while the bird is placed into an oxygen environment, and then terbutaline (0.01 mg/kg diluted in 5 to 10 mL of saline three times daily) is nebulized for subsequent treatment. Mucolytic therapy with N-acetylcysteine by means of nebulization also has been used by some clinicians to facilitate the clearance of respiratory secretions.

Because of its potential irritation to the airways, a bronchodilator should precede therapy with N-acetylcysteine, and nebulization with this drug should be considered with caution in small exotic animals. N-acetylcysteine also has been given at 150 mg/kg by mouth for the first dose followed by 70 mg/kg by mouth three times daily for 2 to 3 days (Lichtenberger).

Ultrasonic nebulizers generate an aerosol through ultrahigh-frequency vibration of a piezoelectric crystal at the bottom of a liquid. The advantages of an ultrasonic nebulizer include faster nebulization time, longer product life, smaller particle size (3 to 10 micros), and quieter operation compared with a jet nebulizer. The nebulizer can be connected to a cage or inhaled directly through a mask (Fig. 2). The apparatus also can be connected to an anesthetized bird with an endotracheal tube. The ultrasonic nebulizer can be purchased for a low cost ($150/unit); therefore it is affordable for both veterinarians, and in special circumstances, by owners for continued home therapy. Some ultrasonic nebulizers have been designed specifically for the veterinary market (DVM Pharmaceuticals, Inc., IVAX Corp, Miami, Florida) [18,19].

Other procedures

Air sac cannulation and nutrition (gavage tube feeding and esophagostomy tube placement) are discussed by Chavez and Echols in this issue.

Common diseases and syndromes

Respiratory distress

Acute respiratory distress is usually a life-threatening emergency. Every bird presenting with respiratory distress will require immediate stabilization

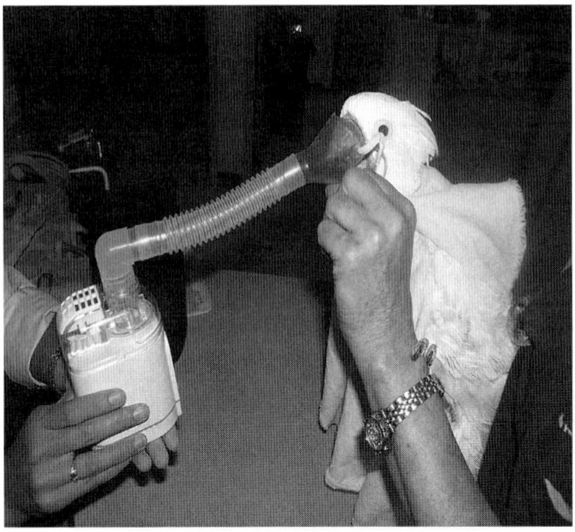

Fig. 2. Nebulization technique. Nebulization using an ultrasonic nebulizer and mask.

in a warmed oxygenated incubator (oxygen flow at 5 L/min delivers a oxygen concentration of 78% to 85% in most incubators. In the experience of one of the authors (Lichtenberger), a bronchial dilator, (eg, terbutaline 0.01 mg/kg intramuscularly every 6 to 8 hours; Brethine, Novartis Pharmaceuticals Corporation, East Hanover, New Jersey) and an analgesic with antianxiety properties, butorphanol (1 to 2 mg/kg intramuscularly every 2 to 3 hours; Torbutrol, Intervet Inc., Mibboro, Delaware) can be administered to birds in respiratory distress before placement into the oxygen-enriched incubator.

The dyspneic patient should be evaluated to determine if the disease condition involves the upper or lower airway. Typically history, auscultation, and physical evaluation will allow the clinician to determine this accurately. Birds also can develop significant dyspnea because of compression of the air sacs by either intraceolomic fluid or a space occupying mass. Palpation of the abdomen often will allow the clinician to assess if there is distension by fluid, a palpable mass, or displaced viscera.

After placing the bird in the incubator, observation of breathing pattern, respiratory sounds, and a quick, efficient physical examination are the most important tools for diagnosing and treating respiratory distress [20–24]. Auscultation of the lungs may not reveal subtle respiratory disease because of the rigidity of the avian lungs. Auscultation, however, can detect abnormal respiratory sounds such as wheezing or clicks and help localize them to upper or lower airways. Auscultation also is recommended to identify heart murmur, arrhythmia, and determine heart rate, which is frequently challenging in birds because of relatively rapid heart rates. The history and physical examination will help the clinician localize the lesion, which will facilitate immediate steps to stabilize the patient. The following discussion will give an anatomical and physiological overview of the five different areas of the respiratory system and describe history, physical examination, diagnosis, and treatment protocols for diseases occurring in each area. Respiratory distress may be caused by an upper airway disease (sinus), large airway disease (glottis to syrinx), small airway (primary bronchi), parenchymal disease (lungs or air sacs), or intraceolomic disease (fluid, organ enlargement or mass), resulting in compression of the air sacs.

Five areas of the respiratory system

Upper airway and infraorbital sinus

Anatomy and physiology

The cere is the area around the most dorsal surface of the maxillary rhampotheca or upper beak. It may be feathered or unfeathered in various species of psittacine birds. In adult male budgerigars, the cere is usually blue; in adult females, it is usually brownish-pink. In each species, it has a characteristic size and shape.

The nares or nostrils are located dorsally within the area of the cere in psittacine birds. The openings may be shaped abnormally as a result of chronic upper respiratory infection or trauma and should be noted on the physical examination. Air moves through the nares into the nasal cavity. In psittacines and many other pet birds, a rounded, keratinized structure called the operculum is found in the rostral-most extent of the nasal cavity. It acts as a baffle to deflect and prevent inhalation of foreign material [25].

The nasal cavity in most species is divided by a nasal septum. Within the lateral walls of the cavity are highly vascularized nasal conchae. Most birds have three conchae: the rostral, middle, and caudal nasal conchae. The middle nasal concha is the largest of the three. A clinically important anatomic feature is the relationship of this concha to the openings of the infraorbital sinus, the only true paranasal sinus of birds. This sinus opens dorsally into the middle and caudal nasal conchae. The caudal nasal concha drains only into the nasal cavity by its dorsal opening into the infraorbital sinus. As a result, the only passageway for drainage of mucopurulent material in the infraorbital sinus is the caudal nasal concha up through the dorsal opening, or over the middle nasal concha into the nasal cavity [25].

The infraorbital sinus is located ventromedial to the orbit and has numerous diverticuli. A rostral diverticulum extends into the maxillary rostrum or bill; a preorbital diverticulum lies rostral to the orbit. A postorbital diverticulum may be subdivided to surround the opening of the ear, and a mandibular diverticulum extends into the mandibulary rostrum. In addition to its communication with the nasal conchae, the infraorbital sinus also communicates with the cervicocephalic air sac at its caudal-most extent. Knowledge of the relationship of this sinus and air sac with the bones of the skull is important during examination of the upper respiratory system and during irrigation and surgical drainage procedures [25].

Sinusitis history

The owner often will describe sneezing, picking the nares with their toenails, nasal discharge, redness of the sinus area, and/or ocular discharge, and some birds will rub their beak on the perch. In some cases, nasal discharge is removed rapidly by the bird, and the only evidence is brownish discoloration of the feathers above the nares.

Pattern of breathing, respiratory sounds, and physical examination

There will be a soft audible breathing sound localized to the nasal cavity, with open-mouth breathing only with complete, bilateral nasal and/or sinus obstruction. There will be an increased respiratory rate but usually without an increased effort.

Etiology

Causes include infraorbital infection (bacterial, fungal, chlamydiophila), foreign body, neoplasia, abscess, granuloma, fibrinous plug [26], and avian pox [27,28]. Squamous metaplasia from nutritional hypovitaminosis A may affect the epithelium lining the nasal and sinus passages, facilitating opportunistic infection as well. Extension of an infection or inflammation of the nares into the sinus may cause redness and swelling of the peri-orbital area. The signs may be limited to the upper respiratory tract or may involve the lower respiratory tract.

Diagnostic tests

A nasal flush or infraorbital sinus aspiration and culture and sensitivity of the fluid are recommended. Endoscopy of the choanal area and biopsy of any lesions are the next diagnostic procedures that would be used to diagnose cases that are nonresponsive to initial treatment. Radiographs and CT or MRI scans of sinuses may be useful [15].

Treatment

Many times a nasal flush will help remove mucous and discharge so that the bird can breathe easier. Initial cytology of the fluid can help the clinician decide on treatment (antibiotics, antifungals) pending cultures and sensitivities. Nasal antibiotic drops (or ophthalmic drops) and therapeutic nasal flushes with antibiotic solutions may be used for minor infections and systemic antibiotics for more severe disease.

Large airway (glottis, trachea to the syrinx)

Anatomy and physiology

The larynx is composed of four almost ossified cartilages with an overlying mucosa or laryngeal mound. The larynx is not involved in sound production in birds. The rima glottis represents the laryngeal opening into the trachea and is not covered by an epiglottis as it is in mammals. The rima glottis and trachea are larger in diameter on a per weight basis than they are in mammals. This principle provides one reason why it is easier to intubate birds than mammals. This increased diameter directly reflects one physiologic adaptation of birds—the use of their beaks for the manipulation of objects. The increased length of the trachea is part of an adaptation in birds whereby the increased length of their necks allows use of their beak to manipulate objects. The increase in length causes an increased air resistance, however. A wider rima glottis, and a wider trachea, are necessary to reduce this resistance. To compensate for the wider and longer trachea and its corresponding increase in dead space, the respiratory rate of birds is less than that of mammals, with a larger tidal volume. These anatomic and physiologic differences are important when selecting endotracheal tubes for anesthetic procedures. In addition, the tracheal rings of birds are complete. They are shaped like a signet ring and overlap to form a more rigid trachea than that of a comparably sized mammal. These two facts are important to reduce the possibility of tracheal kinking when moving the neck. Overinflation of cuffed endotracheal tubes is potentially easier in a bird because of the less expansive nature of the trachea, and this can lead to mucosal edema and difficulty breathing. Whenever possible, uncuffed endotracheal tubes should be used [29].

The trachea often bifurcates immediately after entering the thoracic inlet. At this bifurcation is the syrinx, which represents the voice box of birds. The syrinx is highly variable among species but represents numerous cartilages, which may be ossified, and syringeal muscles and membranes. Most syringeal muscles are external to the tracheal birfurcation. Depending on the species, birds also may have internal syringeal muscles within the space of the trachea and/or bronchi. This narrowed internal diameter of the syrinx is a common site for tracheal granulomas and foreign bodies [29].

History

Owners may report a voice change and/or intermittent respiratory stridor increasing in intensity with time. Birds may present in respiratory distress, in some cases with no previous clinical signs.

The bird may have demonstrated a change in voice or intermittent respiratory stridor noise that has increased in intensity over weeks and presents with respiratory distress. Some birds present with sudden onset of respiratory distress with no previous clinical signs.

Pattern of breathing, respiratory sounds, and physical examination

There is loud inspiratory stridor and often an increased rate and effort with open-mouth breathing. The bird may have no other abnormal physical examination findings. In cases of near-complete obstruction, the bird may present in extreme dyspnea, gasping for air. If there is a complete obstruction, the bird will present gasping for air and eventually will fall over and go into respiratory arrest.

Etiology. The most common cause of large airway obstruction is foreign body inhalation, in particular seed hulls in smaller birds. Other causes of obstruction include *Aspergillus* granuloma (especially African gray parrots), and tracheal trauma, including fibrinous stenosis secondary to recent endotracheal intubation [29].

Diagnostic tests

Radiographs, blood work, endotracheal wash, and endoscopy can help diagnose the cause of airway obstruction. Foreign bodies rostral to the syrinx often can be visualized by means of transillumination of the trachea.

Treatment

Large airway obstruction requires rapid anesthetic induction with sevoflurane/isoflurane anesthesia and rapid intubation and ventilation with 100% oxygen. It should be noted that birds in extreme respiratory distress often breathe much easier under general anesthesia, likely because of reduction of fear and stress associated with dyspnea. Emergency air sac cannulation is performed (see article by Chavez and Echols in this issue). The cannula remains in place until the obstruction is relieved or removed medically or with surgery. Successful relief of airway obstruction can be tested by manually occluding the air sac cannula for several minutes while observing respirations. One of the authors (Lichtenberger) has maintained air sac tubes in place for 2 days to up to 5 weeks.

In larger birds, endoscopy can occasionally be used to successfully remove an obstruction. In some cases, a flexible feeding tube or catheter can be used to aspirate foreign material out of the trachea by using a syringe and applying negative pressure. Foreign material located rostral to the thoracic inlet can be flushed out of the trachea and into the mouth by inserting a needle through the trachea just below the foreign material and carefully introducing air or saline while holding the bird in an upside down position.

Surgical approaches to the trachea and syrinx have been described [20].

Small airway

Anatomy and physiology

The mainstem or primary bronchi represent the continuation of the syrinx. Each perforates the septal surface of the lung and continues into the lung parenchyma as the intrapulmonary primary bronchus. The portion of the bronchus is long as it continues to the caudal extremity of the lung. Its diameter is variable among species but is widest at its entrance into the lung tissue and then tapers progressively. The epithelium of the primary bronchus is pseudostratified with goblet cells, and there are areas with ridges carrying cilia. There are four groups of secondary bronchi that arise from the primary bronchus. Their anatomy are described with the description of the lung parenchyma [29].

History

History may include recent exposure to airborne toxins, including aerosols, smoke, or fumes from overheated nonstick cookware. Blue and gold macaws (*Ara ararauna*) may present with history of exposure to cockatoo dander.

Pattern of breathing, respiratory sounds, and physical examination

Birds present in variable stages of respiratory distress, often severe. Many present with a soft expiratory wheeze. Stress and handling often exacerbate clinical signs.

Etiology. Small airway disease includes exposure to inhalant respiratory irritants and toxins including overheated polytetrafluoroethylene or similar compounds in nonstick cookware or newly installed furnaces, smoke, aerosols, candles, or other potential airborne toxins [21,22]. A hypersensitivity syndrome has been identified in blue and gold macaws raised in close proximity cockatoos [25]. Infectious pneumonia (bacterial, fungal) is not uncommon in pet birds.

Diagnostic tests

Stabilize the bird for 12 to 24 hours with bronchodilators and oxygen before performing diagnostic tests. There are no specific tests for airborne toxins or allergic syndrome of blue and gold macaws. Diagnostic tests include complete blood count, serum chemistries, radiographs, endoscopy, aspergillus serology, and PCR. While these diagnostics are often unremarkable in cases of inhalant toxins, leukocytosis, polycythemia, increased lung and/or air sac density, granuloma, hyperinflation of air sacs may be evident in cases of infectious disease and hypersensitivity.

Treatment

The most effective bronchodilators are pharmaceutical agents that stimulate β-adrenergic receptors in bronchial smooth muscle and promote smooth muscle relaxation. For this reason they have become an authors' first line of treatment for bronchoconstriction causing acute respiratory distress. These β-receptor agonists are most effective and least toxic when they are given as an aerosol that is inhaled. β-agonists, such as terbutaline can be given intramuscularly in birds (0.01 mg/kg every 6 to 8 hours) initially for immediate effect (improvement seen within 5 minutes) and then continued by nebulization for 24 to 48 hours (see nebulization in procedures in this article). A sedative such as butorphanol can be used to reduce fear and anxiety associated with respiratory distress. Prior to beginning diagnostic testing or more invasive treatment, test the bird by turning off the oxygen and observe the breathing pattern. If the bird is able to breath normally at rest, test the bird's ability to withstand more aggressive handling. At this point, it is likely the bird can be anesthetized for radiographs and blood work to rule out other disease components.

Birds that improve with therapy and are stable can be sent home on oral terbutaline for 3 to 4 days. At-home nebulization may be beneficial in some cases. Advise the owner to remove the source of the aerosol toxin.

If no improvement is seen within 24 hours of therapy, one of the authors (Lichtenberger) places the bird under inhalant anesthesia and intubates. Tracheal and ceolomic endoscopy with biopsy as indicated is performed to help identify the severity of the disease. In the author's experience, smoke or Teflon toxins can cause the most significant damage to not only the small airways, but also to the lungs. Nonsteroidal anti-inflammatory drugs (NSAIDS) can be used if inflammation of the trachea is severe. The bird is nebulized (see nebulization methods) with terbutaline (0.01 mg/kg) and then followed in 5 minutes with acetylcysteine 100 mg/mL (Mucomyst, Bristol) nebulization (10 mL in 4 mL saline) by means of the endotracheal tube. This may be repeated twice a day until there is improvement. Broad spectrum antibiotics and/or antifungals should be initiated in those patients with evidence of infectious disease.

Coelomic cavity disease (mass, fluid, or organomegaly)

Anatomy and physiology

The coelomic cavities of birds are similar between species, and in general there are 16 distinct and separate cavities in the adult bird. Eight of the cavities are air sacs, and the remaining eight are cavities of the coelom proper, with five as peritoneal cavities, and the remaining three represented in mammals as well. The mammalian cavities include: the right and left pleural cavities and the pericardial cavity. The five peritoneal cavities of birds include the left and right ventral hepatic peritoneal cavities, the left and right dorsal hepatic cavities, and the intestinal peritoneal cavity [25].

History

There is often no prior history, and many birds will present with acute respiratory distress. In case of a large egg compressing the air sacs or egg ceolomitis, there may be a history of egg laying. Some birds may present with vague history of decreased appetite and lethargy before presentation.

Pattern of breathing, respiratory sounds, and physical examination

The bird will have increased respiratory rate and effort, which increases with stress and handling. There are usually no abnormal respiratory sounds. In many cases, the ceolomic space (space between the ventral keel and pelvis) is wider than normal, and there may be a palpable mass or fluid.

Etiology

Any ceolomic mass or disease producing organ enlargement or fluid can cause ceolomic distention. Common causes of coelomic distension are fluid accumulation, heart disease, hypoalbuminemia, liver disease, egg-related ceolomitis [30], or presence of a mass (neoplasia, abscess, egg).

Diagnostic tests and treatment

Ascites. Ascites resulting in coelomic distension and respiratory distress requires immediate coelomocentesis. Coelomocentesis may be performed on the right lateral coelom just cranial to the cloaca or on the ventral midline. Use a 25 to 22 gauge needle and 12 mL syringe (Fig. 3). Often, ultrasound can help guide coelomocentesis if the fluid is located within a specific loculated space and difficult to aspirate.

Save any fluid recovered for culture/sensitivity and cytology. Transudate is characterized by a clear to pale-yellow color, with a low specific gravity (<1.020), low protein (1 g/dL) and a low cellularity. The most common

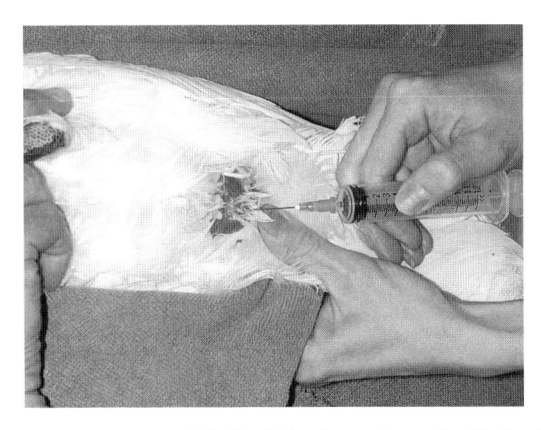

Fig. 3. Coelomocentesis. Removal of fluid within the coelom of a bird using a syringe and 22-gauge needle.

causes of a transudate are liver failure (eg, cirrhosis) or heart failure. Exudate is characterized by a high specific gravity (>1.020), a high protein content (>3 g/dL) and presence of inflammatory cells and mesothelial cells. Cytology of the septic fluid may show a large number of white cells with intracellular bacteria. One of the authors (Lichtenberger) uses comparison of ceolomic fluid and serum glucose to differentiate septic ceolomitis from nonseptic [31]. In cases of septic ceolomitis, ceolomic fluid glucose is usually lower than serum glucose. Turbid yellow, green or brown yolk-like fluid, or inspissated yolk material in the coelomic cavity is indicative of ectopic ovulation or a ruptured oviduct. Cytology reveals yolk material and fat particles. Small–to–moderate amounts of free yolk in the abdomen may be absorbed by the body, and associated inflammation is treated with NSAIDs. The presence of ceoloc bacteria indicates antibiotic therapy is necessary. Ectopic eggs and large amount of celomic yolk usually require exploratory surgery, removal, and often salpingohysterectomy. More information on treatment of reproductive-related disease is presented here.

Ceolomic neoplasia often produces fluid containing blood and occasionally exfoliated neoplastic cells on cytology. Abdominal ultrasound is performed to identify presence of an abdominal mass. A 22 gauge needle can be used for ultrasound-guided aspiration of the mass. Confirmation of and identification of ceolomic masses are also possible with endoscopy and/or exploratory surgery. Ideally, a coagulation profile should be performed prior to fine needle aspirate or surgery.

Careful auscultation is indicated for a heart murmur, gallop, or other arrhythmia, or crackles suggestive of cardiogenic edema. If heart failure is suspected, administer furosemide (2 to 4 mg/kg IV) and nitroglycerine ointment on the tongue and allow the bird to stabilize before further diagnostics. If there is ceolomic effusion, coelomocentesis is performed. A cardiac workup will require blood pressure measurements, radiographs, and an echocardiography. If there is significant coelomic fluid present secondary to heart disease, coelomocentesis should be performed (see section on coelomic enlargement in respiratory distress). There have been no reports of cardiac failure and documented hypertension (hypertension is discussed as a separate topic). The most common heart problems reported in psittacine birds are right-sided congestive heart failure with ascites and hydropericardium [15]. Pericardiocentesis is recommended when hydropericardium is present. Left-sided heart failure is less common in psittacines reported thus far. Reports of thickened mitral valve and left and right side failure have been reported [15]. Heart medications commonly used are enalapril at 2.5 mg/kg BID, and furosemide, 0.15-2.0 mg/kg PO, IM SID-BID [15]. The author (Lichtenberger) prefers benazepril at 0.5 mg/kg PO BID. If contractility is poor and/or dilated cardiomyopathy is identified on echocardiogram, digoxin has been recommended at 0.02-0.05 mg/kg BID [15]. No clinical studies on the toxicity of any cardiac drugs have been performed in birds.

Parenchymal disease (lungs and/or air sacs)

Anatomy and physiology

The lungs are paired and attached firmly to the ribs and dorsal body wall. They appear spongy on radiographs and are visualized best using a lateral view. The mainstem bronchi divide into secondary bronchi. These bronchi subsequently divide into parabronchi. All parabronchi anastomose freely with other parabronchi and have expansions within their walls, called atria, which allow gas exchange. Parabronchi maintain a constant mean diameter within a species [25,32].

The mediodorsal and medioventral secondary bronchi connect to form a functional unit. These bronchi terminate at the cranial pulmonary air sacs and form the basis of the paleopulmonic respiratory system. The parabronchi of the lateroventral secondary bronchi connect with the laterodorsal secondary bronchi, and they in turn are connected to the mediodorsal secondary bronchi. The cranial pulmonary air sacs are expandable sacs that are connected to the lungs by these bronchial arrangements and include the cervical, clavicular, and cranial thoracic air sacs. The lateroventral bronchi are connected with the caudal pulmonary air sacs of the lungs. These caudal air sacs are the caudal thoracic and abdominal air sac. This latter arrangement represents the neopulmonic respiratory system. Air sacs, in general, are similar histologically to a peritoneum, with squamous to columnar epithelium, a basement membrane, and an underlying connective tissue support. Only in the area immediately surrounding an opening of a parabronchus does the tissue change to ciliated columnar epithelium. The paleopulmonic and neopulmonic systems are defined best physiologically rather than anatomically [32].

Birds do not have a diaphragm and therefore rely on changes in pressure between their air sacs relative to the atmospheric pressure to move air through a nonexpandable lung. The pressure changes within the air sacs are the result of volume changes in the thoracoabdominal cavity. On inspiration, the ribs move cranioventrally, thereby increasing the thoracoabdominal space. This results in a lowering of the pressure in the air sacs. On expiration, the ribs move caudodorsally, thereby reducing the space in the chest and increasing the pressure in the air sacs. Expiration is an active process requiring skeletal muscle contraction. For this reason, it is extremely important during restraint that the sternum can move freely, or the bird may suffocate. It also should be noted that ventilation of the apneic bird can be accomplished by gently compressing the sternum and allowing it to recoil into normal resting position [32].

Gas exchange occurs in the walls of the parabronchi, the atria, and more importantly in the air capillaries, which are the avian equivalent of alveoli. The blood–gas barrier of birds is similar to that of mammals in that it consists of an endothelial capillary cell, a common basal lamina, and an air capillary epithelium of squamous cells. The difference is that the blood–gas barrier is much thinner in birds than in mammals. The diameter of the air capillaries of birds is much smaller than that of a mammalian alveolus, allowing for a much larger number of air capillaries in a given space when compared with mammals [32].

Because of the unidirectional continuous flow of air of the paleopulmonic system, birds are more efficient than mammals in capturing oxygen (O_2) and removing carbon dioxide (CO_2). The nonoxygenated blood enters at an approximately 90° angle from the parabronchus. This cross-current gas exchange enhances the ability to oxygenate the blood [32].

The epithelial cells of the lung act as fixed macrophages and transfer engulfed material to interstitial macrophages. Air that enters the caudal air sacs is filtered to a lesser degree than air in the cranial air sacs, making the caudal air sacs more susceptible to disease [25,32].

History

There is usually a history of not doing well, lethargy, and anorexia. These birds are usually sick with weight loss caused by the chronic disease process.

Pattern of breathing, respiratory sounds and physical examination

Birds often exhibit signs of increased respiratory rate and/or effort and are in general poor body condition. There are generally no respiratory sounds.

Etiology

Causes of parenchymal disease include: cardiogenic pulmonary edema (discussed in previous section on coelomic diseases), smoke inhalation, aspiration pneumonia, aspergillosis, chlamydophilosis, gram-negative bacteria, poxvirus, Pacheco's disease, reovirus, encephalitozoonosis [30], and neoplasia [31].

Diagnostics

Radiographs and an echocardiogram are performed to rule out cardiac disease and evaluate the lungs and air sacs. An endotracheal wash, culture, and sensitivity are useful in cases of bacterial infection. A chlamydiophila test should be performed. Ceolomic endoscopy with biopsy is useful to detect neoplasia and disease processes producing distinct lesions or granulomas. Complete blood count, serum chemistries, and aspergillus serology and PCR are also useful diagnostic tests.

Treatment

Parenchymal disease may benefit from use of parental or nebulization of bronchodilators and antibiotics. An air sac tube may improve respiration partially in birds with small airway and primary lung.

Birds with a history of regurgitation or vomiting and possible aspiration pneumonia may benefit from broad-spectrum antibiotics (eg, enrofloxacin, cephalosporins, trimethoprim sulfadiazine) and bronchodilators.

Birds suspected of aspergillosis (leukocytosis and pulmonary nodules) can be treated with terbinafine hydrochloride (Lamisil) or itraconazole at 10 to 15 mg/kg twice daily for 4 weeks. Itraconazole should be used with caution in African gray parrots.

Birds suspected of psittacosis (leukocytosis, clinical signs varying from chronic unthriftiness to acute anorexia, diarrhea and respiratory distress, and lime green feces) should be treated with drugs inhibiting the growth of *Chlamydiophila,* such as doxycycline, macrolides, chloramphenicol, and/or fluoroquinolones). Diagnosis of psittacosis is problematic in avian species. There is no gold standard that can be used to unequivocally determine if a particular test is accurate. One author recommends the use of two tests run simultaneously (eg, serology antibody test and a PCR test) to lessen chances of false-positive and false-positive results. Treat with doxycycline for 6 weeks. Many protocols are recommended (see psittacosis treatment later in this article under GI disease). There is no treatment for viral infections and many birds die within a short time.

Trauma

Traumatic injuries and fractures occur commonly in the avian pet bird and control of hemorrhage, oxygen and heat support, analgesics, and parental antibiotics are the initial treatment protocol for all birds with injuries.

Most common injuries are lacerations, bite wounds, self-mutilation, thermal wounds, or fractures. Lacerations and abrasions in birds are caused commonly by enclosure wires, inappropriate toys, collision during flight, other birds, or household pets. Birds sustaining bite wounds from dogs, cats, or other birds are encountered frequently. Injuries from metal leg bands are also common. Open-style steel bands may cause problems if the band gap is large enough to allow the bird to get hung up on the cage wire. Inappropriately sized bands may cause soft tissue swelling and vascular compromise to the distal leg and toes. Feather, toenail, and beak injuries can cause significant hemorrhage. Self-mutilation behavior may cause extensive soft tissue wound injuries. Thermal injuries most commonly occur in the crop of neonates fed improperly heated hand-feeding formula, in most cases heated in the microwave without proper mixing. Accidental burns may occur when birds come in contact with hot liquids, hot surfaces, or electrical wires. Fractures should be splinted to prevent further complication as soon as the bird's condition is stable. Simple bandaging techniques may be used to provide adequate stability until definite treatment is possible [3].

Treatment protocols

General emergency and supportive care
External hemorrhage must be stopped immediately. Birds with broken blood feathers often present as an emergency. The developing feather contains a rich blood supply, which retracts when the feather is mature. This shaft can bleed when fractured, especially if the feather is large. Pressure at the base of the follicle often will stop the bleeding. In some cases, larger feathers with fractured shafts must be removed. This is accomplished by grasping the feather at its base with a hemostat, and extracting the feather from the follicle. In the case of large primary wing feathers (remiges), it is important to support the bones of the wing during extraction to prevent fractures. Occasionally the follicle will continue bleeding, but this usually can be controlled with digital pressure or fine absorbable suture. Hemostatic agents such as silver nitrate may damage or destroy the feather follicle, resulting in feather loss or growth of abnormal feathers.

Excessive hemorrhage also may occur following nail or beak injury. Hemostatic agents or a hand-held cautery unit may be used to stop bleeding from the nail tip. It is difficult to stop bleeding of the beak in a conscious, struggling bird; therefore the authors recommend inhalant anesthesia. The tip of the beak can be cauterized with a hand-held or electric cautery unit. Hemostatic agents such as silver nitrate can be used also, but care should be taken to use these products sparingly to avoid ingestion after recovery from anesthesia.

Wounds and open fractures
Wounds and open fractures are commonly treated with beta-lactams (eg, piperacillin 100 to 200 mg/kg intramuscularly, IV every 6 to 8 hours), trimethoprim-sulpha, or fluoroquinolones [33].

Analgesics
Administration of analgesics is necessary in birds that have experienced a fracture or soft tissue trauma. Studies in pigeons have demonstrated

that they have more kappa opioid receptors in the forebrain than mu opioid receptors. This may explain why birds do not respond to mu agonists, such as morphine, fentanyl, and buprenorphine, in the same manner as mammals. Butorphanol has been shown as a useful analgesic is birds. Posttraumatic administration of NSAIDs may decrease soft tissue sensitization and may reduce the dose of opioid drug required. NSAIDs such as meloxicam, ketoprofen, and carprofen (Metacam,) at 0.5 mg/kg intramuscularly can be used for pain relief, when the bird is well perfused, and kidney function is normal [34,35].

Lidocaine can be used safely in birds at doses below 2 mg/kg. When giving 1 to 2 mg/kg to small birds, the commercially available concentration of lidocaine should be diluted at least 1:10. Lidocaine can be mixed with bupivicaine 0.5% (1 mg/kg). This mixed dose can be injected intramuscularly or infiltrated locally at the surgery or wound site [35].

Punctures and small contaminated wounds can be left open to drain

Large lacerations treated within a few hours are flushed with sterile saline solution and sutured partially closed. Older wounds should be cleaned, debrided, and bandaged twice daily, then closed as needed after the infection is minimized. Alternatively, 50% dextrose, sugar, and honey have been advocated as a wound dressing to treat large contaminated wounds. Sugar, honey, and 50% dextrose are readily available inexpensive materials that when applied to a wound are considered bactericidal because of their high osmolality. Additionally, they provide the wound with a local nutrient source to promote granulation tissue. This high osmolality is also responsible for moving edematous fluid out and drawing macrophages into the wound. The wound is debrided and flushed with saline. The sugar or honey is applied to the wound, and it is covered by a wet-to-dry bandage.

Topical wound treatments are products that are applied to wounds to stimulate wound healing. They promote wound healing by stimulating production of cytokines or growth factors within the wound. Topical preparations that have shown some effect on wound healing include acemannan, D-glucose polysaccharide, hydrolyzed bovine collagen, porcine collagen products, and tripeptide-copper complex [36,37]. Topically applied platelet derived growth factor (Regranex) has been shown to improve healing in chronic diabetic foot ulcers in people. It has also proven effective in healing a large defect in a fish suffering from lateral line disease (B. Whitaker, personal communication, 2004). Sugar and honey have been advocated as a wound dressing to treat large contaminated wounds. Sugar and honey are readily available inexpensive materials that when applied to a wound is considered bactericidal due to the high osmolality and provides the wound with a local nutrient source to promote granulation tissue. This high osmolality is also responsible for moving edematous fluid out and drawing macrophages into the wound.

Treatment for self-mutilation

Treatment for self-mutilation may include temporary collaring while treating the underlying cause, which may be pathological or behavioral. The area should be cultured and cleaned, treated with silver sulfadiazine cream, and bandaged with a moisture-permeable dressing if possible.

Scaly mites

Scaly mites (knemidoptes pilae) cause hyperkeratotic lesions on the feet and base of the beak in parakeets. The birds are brought in for treatment for rubbing their beak on the perch and/or for growths/wounds on the beak and feet. The mites are rarely seen on microscopic examination. Treatment involves placing 0.2 mg/kg ivermectin in a tuberculin syringe and dropping it over the right jugular vein. This is repeated in 2 to 3 weeks [33].

External burn injuries

External burn injuries are treated with cold compresses for a period of 20 to 30 minutes. Superficial burns should be cleansed gently using sterile saline. Partial or full-thickness burns should be cleansed gently and debrided daily and treated topically with a water-soluble antibiotic dressing as silver sulfadiazine (Silvadine cream 1%). This procedure is very painful, and it should be done under general anesthesia with appropriate analgesia.

Surgical repair of crop fistulas is performed only after complete granulation of the wound edges has occurred with clear demarcation between healthy and diseased tissue. Attempting to suture the necrotic infected tissue may result in dehiscence. The bird can continue eating or be tube-fed throughout this time. The bird should be started on antibiotics. Monitor until the wound contracts, and a fistula appears (7 to 14 days). When the wound heals and fistula forms, the scab is removed and necrotic skin and crop are excised surgically. Surgery before wound contraction is often unsuccessful because of the difficulty in distinguishing apparently healthy tissue from tissue that will ultimately necrose. Surgical glue can help seal the wound to prevent leakage of food until surgery is preformed. Surgical repair to cover affected areas may include techniques such as advancement flaps and skin grafts depending upon the location and extent of skin loss [38].

Fractures

Fractures are usually not life-threatening, and they may be supported with external coaptation depending upon the location. The patient should be evaluated thoroughly for any open or closed fracture and soft tissue trauma. If an open fracture is present, exposed tissues are treated with irrigation, debridement, and bandaging. The bone segment(s) should be protected by replacing it(them) under the skin or with appropriate bandaging. A figure-eight bandage is applied to stabilize fractures of the radius, ulna, or carpometacarpus (see surgery and endoscopy article in this issue, by Chavez and Echols). The wing is bandaged in a figure eight fashion and to the body for fractures of the humerus. Fractures distal to the knee are stabilized with a lateral splint, or in smaller species (less than 100 g body weight), a tape splint may be applied (see surgery and endoscopy article by Chavez and Echols in this issue). Femoral fractures may be stabilized using a spica splint or an off weight-bearing sling until surgery is possible (see surgery and endoscopy article by Chavez and Echols in this issue). If the patient is stable enough to perform immediate surgery, appropriate surgical repair may be performed after radiographs are performed. Immediate fracture repair offers the advantage of early stabilization and less postfracture muscle contracture, which facilitates surgical repair. Closed reduction and repair have been associated with significantly less soft tissue, nerve, and vascular damage [30,31,39–41].

Reproductive-related emergencies

Chronic egg laying

Chronic egg laying occurs when a hen lays repeated clutches or larger than normal clutch size without regard to the presence of a mate or accurate breeding season. This process often physically exhausts the reproductive tract and is a serious metabolic drain, particularly on calcium stores, all of which may predispose the hen to egg binding, yolk peritonitis, and osteoporosis. Commonly affected species include cockatiels, finches, and lovebirds; however, any species may be affected. Diagnosis of chronic egg laying is based on history and physical examination. There typically is a history of the hen laying large numbers of eggs with or without a pause period in between clutches. A thorough history of the home environment will often reveal several reproductive stimuli and a mate relationship with one or more members of the household or an inanimate object. Physical examination may reveal normal findings, a palpable egg in the coelom, or other secondary disease conditions such as a pathologic fracture secondary to osteoporosis. Serum chemistries may reveal hypercalcemia, hypercholesterolemia, and hyperglobulinemia supportive of an ovulating hen. There may be a hypocalcemia present if the hen's calcium stores are depleted, and particularly if she is consuming a low-calcium diet such as seed [42–44]. The owner should be instructed on methods to stop the chronic egg laying as decreasing the light cycle, removing the male bird, and/or changing location of the cage. Elimination of an inappropriate sexual bond and restoration of proper social bond often requires behavioral modification technique and cooperation from all members of the household. Other options include the use of drugs such as leuprolide acetate (Lupron, TAP Pharmaceuticals) or salpingohysterectomy with or without partial ovariectomy.

Egg binding

Cockatiels, canaries, and finches most commonly are reported to be affected and seem to present with more severe clinical signs, possibly because of their small size. Clinical signs associated with egg binding and dystocia vary according to severity, size of the bird affected, and degree of secondary complications. Common signs include acute depression, abdominal straining, persistent tail wagging, a wide stance, failure to perch, abdominal distension, dyspnea, and/or sudden death. An egg lodged in the pelvic canal may compress the pelvic blood vessels, kidneys, and ischiatic nerves, causing circulatory disorders, lameness, paresis, or paralysis. Pressure necrosis of the oviductal wall may occur. Dystocia may cause metabolic disturbances by interfering with normal defecation and micturition, and cause ileus and renal disease, respectively. The severity of the patient's condition can be estimated by the degree of depression and the length of time clinical signs have been present [42–44].

Diagnosis of egg binding or dystocia in a severely compromised patient may be made based on history and physical examination alone, and the patient may not be stable enough to survive other diagnostic procedures. Rapid diagnosis and therapy are crucial for a successful outcome. Physical examination may reveal depression, lethargy, a thin or normal body condition, and dehydration. There may be dyspnea or an increased respiratory rate caused by compression of the caudal thoracic and abdominal air sacs. The hen may not be able to perch, and may demonstrate pelvic limb paresis, paralysis, or cyanosis. Owners may report lack of recent stool production. An egg typically, but not always, is palpable in the caudal abdomen. Cranially located, soft-shelled, and nonshelled eggs may not be detected on abdominal palpation. Palpable, calcified eggs may be located within the oviduct or be free in the ceolom subsequent to uterine rupture. Careful celomic palpation, cloacal examination, radiographs, coelomic ultrasound, laparoscopy, and/or laparotomy may be required to determine the egg's position [42–44].

It should be kept in mind that the presence of palpable egg does not always represent an abnormal medical condition. A normal egg is palpable within the ceolomic cavity within up to 24 hours of normal oviposition.

Radiography and ultrasonography aid in evaluation of the position and characterization of the egg(s). General confirmation of the presence of an egg can be done with the bird simply standing awake on the radiographic cassette. There may be multiple eggs identified in the coelom because of an obstruction distally or secondary to motility disorders. Osteomyelosclerosis or hyperostosis of the femurs, tibiotarsi, radii, ulnas and/or spine is a common finding in birds with estrogenic stimulation, and appears as a general filling or calcification of the normally hollow bone cavity (Fig. 4). Other suggestive radiographic findings include suggestion of ovarian or uterine enlargement and displacement of other soft tissue structures by an enlarged uterus or eggs.

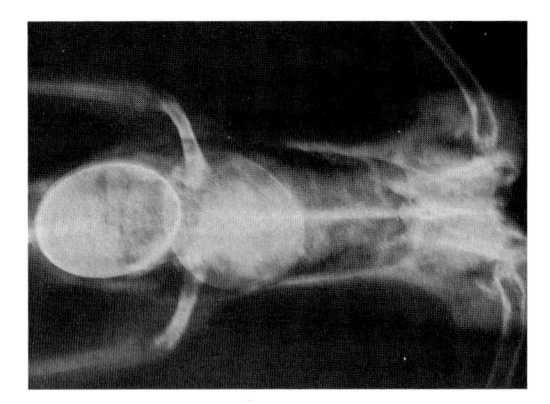

Fig. 4. Osteomyelosclerosis on a radiograph. These radiodense changes seen within the femurs of the bird are seen commonly before and during egg laying.

Coelomic ultrasound often will reveal an egg and may help identify a soft-shelled or nonshelled egg that may have been difficult to identify on radiographs. Again, there may be several eggs visible within the coelom. Follicles may be visible on the ovary, indicating the potential for further ovulation and egg formation.

A hematologic analysis and serum chemistries are useful to identify any predisposing and secondary diseases. A complete blood count may reveal a leukocytosis with a relative heterophil in the presence of concurrent inflammatory or infectious process. Serum chemistries may demonstrate elevated aminotransferase and creatinine phosphokinase caused by skeletal muscle enzyme leakage from tissue damage, or as a result of reduced food consumption and a hypermetabolic state. Hypercholesterolemia and hyperglobulinemia are supportive of ovulation. Elevated total and ionized calcium and may be indicative of calcium mobilization in a reproductively active bird. Conversely, hypocalcemia may be observed if the hen has been consuming a calcium-poor diet or has been laying excessive numbers of eggs, resulting in depletion of calcium stores [42–44].

Therapy varies with history, severity of clinical signs, and diagnostic test results. Supportive care should include elevated environmental temperature, parenteral calcium, fluid therapy, and nutritional support. Broad-spectrum antibiotics are indicated if an infectious etiology is suspected or if the integrity of the oviduct may be compromised. Analgesics often are indicated. Supportive care alone is often enough to facilitate oviposition, although the hen should be monitored closely for deterioration of condition, which may require further intervention [42–44].

Prostaglandin and hormonal therapy may be used to induce oviductal contractions. This may result in expulsion of the egg if the contractility of the oviduct is sufficient; the uterus is intact; the egg is actually within the oviduct, and there is no obstruction such as a neoplastic mass, granuloma, or egg adhered to the oviduct. Studies performed in poultry have found that prostaglandin E2 (PGE2) and prostaglandin F2alpha (PGF2alpha) bind at specific receptor sites in the uterus and vagina. The uterine myometrium appears to preferentially bind PGF2alpha, because it contains low-affinity and some high-affinity binding sites for PGE2, and specific high-affinity for PGF2alpha. Prostaglandin F2alpha binds at the shell receptor sites to cause a time- and dose-dependent mobilization of cellular calcium in the presence of extracellular calcium, thereby causing uterine muscle contraction. It has been demonstrated in vitro that PGE2 is itself ineffective in calcium ion mobilization, but will enhance PGF2alpha-induced calcium mobilization. This suggests that PGE2 may potentiate the ability of PGF2alpha to cause uterine contraction. In the vagina, high-affinity binding sites for PGE2 predominate. It is possible that a high PGE2 concentration in the vagina is needed to saturate high-affinity binding sites and block PGF2-alpha-binding sites. This allows relaxation of the uterovaginal sphincter and vagina. Because fewer PGE2 high-affinity binding sites are present in the uterus, they are not likely to interfere with PGF2alpha binding and may potentiate the action of PGF2 alpha. When an egg is present in the uterus, injections of PGF2alpha and PGE2 will cause the concentration of arginine vasotocin (AVT) to increase in systemic circulation; however, PGF2alpha is the more potent stimulator of AVT release. It is suggested that prostaglandins stimulate uterine contractions, which in turn stimulate the release of AVT from the neurohypophysis, and that AVT probably acts synergistically with PGF2alpha to increase uterine contractions. Oxytocin and AVT appear to specifically affect the uterus, inducing powerful contractions. It is important to note that PGF2alpha, oxytocin, and AVT do not cause relaxation of the uterovaginal sphincter while inducing oviductal contractions. This may result in reverse peristalsis, dilation of the uterovaginal sphincter, severe pain, and rupture of the uterus. Therefore, before use it is important to determine if the uterovaginal sphincter is indeed open. In addition, prostaglandin and hormonal therapy require exogenous calcium to be effective. As many of these patients are severely hypocalcemic because of either malnutrition or chronic egg laying, supplemental calcium may be required before administration of these medications [42–44].

PGE2 gel[g] may be applied to the uterovaginal sphincter, at a dose of 0.1 mL per 100 g bird. PGE2 causes relaxation of the uterovaginal sphincter while causing oviductal contractions, and it may be applied topically, thereby decreasing the incidence of systemic side effects. These contractions may expel the egg within 15 minutes. Contact with PGE2 gel may cause altered menses and induce spontaneous abortion in women. Therefore, it is important to flush any excess from the cloaca after egg expulsion, and precaution staff and clients regarding contact with any stool and/or urine produced. Prostaglandin F2alpha, oxytocin, and AVT also will cause powerful uterine contractions. Prostaglandin F2alpha is administered parenterally, rather than locally, and is more likely to cause systemic reactions such as hypertension, bronchoconstriction, and general smooth muscle stimulation [42–44].

If supportive care and medical therapy fail to induce oviposition, then manual manipulation may be necessary. Massaging the abdomen and vaginal opening may relax the vaginal sphincter and allow passage of the egg. It may be helpful to infuse lubricants into the cloaca to moisten the urodeum and vagina. Careful digital pressure applied to the cranial portion of the egg and directed caudally may encourage movement through the distal oviduct and cloaca. Using a cloacal speculum, the vaginal opening of the oviduct can be dilated by inserting a blunt probe (ie, lubricated cotton-tipped swab) that is advanced gently in a twirling motion. Potential complications may include retroperistalsis of the egg out of the oviduct into an ectopic position within the coelom, rupture of the egg, oviductal trauma, oviductal laceration, and displacement of the egg or fragments out of the uterus and into the ceolom. If fertilization may have occurred and the egg may be fertile, it may be incubated if successfully removed intact [42–44].

Ovocentesis may be performed to facilitate passage of an egg. Aspiration may be performed through the cloacal opening if the egg is located distally, or transcelomically if the egg is positioned more cranially. The egg is manipulated so that it is visible through the cloaca, and a needle is inserted into the egg through the cloaca. The contents of the egg are aspirated into a syringe, while the shell is collapsed manually and the pieces expelled through the cloaca. If the egg cannot be visualized through the cloaca because of a more cranial location, transabdominal ovocentesis may be performed. The egg is manually placed directly against the abdominal wall so that other abdominal organs are displaced and not damaged during aspiration. A needle is inserted through the skin and abdominal wall into the egg. The egg contents are aspirated into the syringe while the egg is collapsed manually. The eggshell remnants are expelled through the cloaca, either naturally or with clinical assistance. It is important to confirm radiographically that these eggshell pieces have been expelled completely. If these pieces are not expelled within a reasonable amount of time, approximately 36 hours, it may be necessary to irrigate the oviduct through the cloaca or laparotomy approach. A salpingohysterectomy may be performed if egg remnants are retained and the hen is not required for breeding. Some clinicians advocate flushing the uterus postoviposition with saline, chlorhexidine, or iodine to remove any shell fragments and decrease the incidence of metritis. Oviductal rupture, resulting in an ectopic egg, shell fragments, or yolk coelomitis, is a possible complication of ovocentesis [42–44].

Medical therapy to reduce reproductive hormone levels and reproductive activity should be used to temporarily prevent further egg production. Surgical removal of an egg is required in cases of ectopic eggs and dystocia, including oviductal rupture, oviductal torsion, or mechanical obstruction, or if medical treatment is not successful. If surgical intervention is necessary, bacterial culture and sensitivity and histopathology should be performed on oviductal tissue samples. Salpingohysterectomy may be considered to prevent further reproductive complications, and any predisposing and secondary diseases should be corrected [42–44].

Cloacal and oviductal prolapse

Cloacal prolapse may occur secondary to chronic straining from masturbation, egg laying, space-occupying abdominal masses, and inappropriate weaning and social behavior. Physical examination will reveal prolapsed tissue through the vent that may be intermittent or persistent. Careful cleaning, irrigation, and lubrication of prolapsed tissue are a necessity. Affected tissue should be examined for necrosis, and any adhered egg should be removed. Cytology and bacterial culture and sensitivity should be performed on prolapsed tissue to aid in antibiotic therapy. A complete blood count, serum chemistries, radiographs, ultrasound, and endoscopic examination of the ceolom and cloaca are useful to determine any other predisposing cause. Chronic reproductive-associated behavior and straining secondary to masturbation may respond to pharmacologic therapy such as leuprolide acetate, and/or environmental manipulation to decrease reproductive stimuli. Cloacopexy and the use of temporary stay sutures may be helpful in temporary or permanent reduction. Those procedures interfere with movement of the cloaca, however, and may alter defecation and micturition. Ventplasty may decrease the vent opening and prevent further prolapse if the vent has become flaccid. Clomipramine hydrochloride administration anecdotally has been reported to contract the vent orifice and assist in the resolution of prolapse of the cloaca. Salpingohysterectomy with partial ovariectomy or orchiectomy may be beneficial in those patients refractory to medical therapy. Broad-spectrum antibiotics should be initiated, pending bacterial culture and sensitivity, because primary and secondary bacterial infections are common [42–44].

Oviductal prolapse may occur secondary to any condition that causes chronic, excessive abdominal straining such as physiologic hyperplasia, egg laying or dystocia. An intraceolomic, space-occupying mass also may induce prolapse of the oviduct. Predisposing factors may include abnormal or soft-shelled eggs, malnutrition, obesity, salpingitis, and cloacitis. Typically, the uterus protrudes through the cloaca, often with a partial prolapse of the vagina and cloaca [42–44].

Rapid management is necessary to prevent necrosis of these tissues. Any egg that may be present should be removed, and all exposed tissues cleaned, irrigated, and kept well moistened to prevent desiccation. Topical anti-inflammatories such as dimethyl sulfoxide may be applied; any lacerations should be repaired, and all tissues should be replaced gently. Temporary stay sutures may be indicated to aid in preventing recurrence, as prolapse of the oviduct may recur, and repeated replacement often is required. Bacterial culture and sensitivity of the prolapsed tissue should be performed to aid in appropriate antibiotic therapy. Complete blood count, serum chemistries, radiographs, ultrasonography, and laparoscopy should be included in a complete diagnostic evaluation to identify any predisposing and secondary disease conditions. Treatment should be directed at clearing any bacterial infection, preventing further prolapse. It also is important to decrease reproductive hormone levels to prevent further egg formation, decrease the size of oviductal tissue, and allow the reproductive tract to rest. Broad-spectrum antibiotics and antifungal medication should be initiated while bacterial and fungal cultures are pending. Salpingohysterectomy may be considered to prevent recurrence, or in cases of severe uterine damage. Predisposing factors should be corrected to prevent recurrence and secondary diseases addressed [42–44].

Neurologic disease

Head trauma is common in free-flying birds. Seizures are common in pet birds because of heavy metal intoxication, hypoglycemia (neonates and raptors), or idiopathic epilepsy (cockatiels). Infectious disease such as proventricular dilatation disease (PDD) and paramyxovirus also may cause neurologic signs as weakness and ataxia. Weakness and falling off the perch can be seen in African gray parrots with hypocalcemia syndrome. The etiology is controversial and may be primary vitamin D3 deficiency. Neoplasia, egg yolk embolism, and other nonviral infectious diseases have been reported to cause neurological signs [45]. *Sarcocystis* spp. have been reported to cause ataxia and weakness. Infection has been reported in over 60 species of birds, with Old World psittacines apparently more susceptible [46]. One of the authors (Lichtenberger) has seen a chronic case of sarcocytis in a cockatoo in Wisconsin that presented with weakness and ataxia.

Signs of neurological disease include seizures, ataxia, paresis or paralysis, head tilt, circling, and blindness. A neurological examination should be performed to confirm if there is a neurological abnormality and to localize the lesion. An excellent review of the neurological examination has been written [46]. The basic neurological examination consists of observation, cranial nerve examination, postural reactions, and spinal reflexes. The bird initially is evaluated in the cage for mentation, posture, and gait. Seizures and abnormal behavior (changes in personality) are a function of the cerebrum. Change in consciousness is a function of the brainstem and cerebral cortex. The cranial nerves (CN) are evaluated as follows:

- Evaluation of menace test (CN 2 and 5)
- Evaluation of papillary light reflex (CN 2 and 3)
- Detection of strabismus (CN 3, 4, and 6)
- Evaluation of palpebral reflex (CN 5 and 7)
- Determination of beak tone (CN 5 and 7)
- Observation of oculocephalic or physiological nystagmus (CN 8 with CN 3, 4, and 6 responsible for eye movements)

Postural conscious proprioception is performed by placing the leg in an abnormal position to evaluate the bird's ability to correct it. Visual placing can be performed by asking the bird to step up to or from a perch, as normal motor tracts and motor cortex are required for this reaction. The patellar reflex can be performed on each leg. Hyper-reflexia demonstrates an upper motor neuron lesion (UMN), while hyporeflexia demonstrates a lower motor neuron (LMN) lesion. A pinch stimulus to the end of the wing evaluates the withdrawal reflex (brachial plexus integrity), while pedal reflex is demonstrated by pinching the toe. An intact vent reflex demonstrates integrity of the pudendal nerve. Evaluation of deep pain is reserved for birds showing evidence of spinal cord disease [46].

Collection of cerebral spinal fluid has been reported by means of an approach into the atlanto–occipital joint under general anesthesia; however, this procedure is difficult and not recommended because of high risk of puncture of the venous sinus [46]. CT and MRI also can be performed [46].

Diagnostics and treatment

Head trauma

Head trauma is common in birds, and this frequently occurs without direct observation by the owner. Many pet birds can become injured in their enclosures, or when they are not observed outside an enclosure. If MRI and CT are not available, practitioners must rely on history and clinical signs for diagnosis and treatment options. With the exception of fracture, radiographs are usually unrewarding. The mainstay of head trauma treatment is oxygen and maintenance of a normal blood pressure. The bird is to be kept in an incubator with heat and oxygen. Analgesics are provided if the bird is excitable or restless in the cage. Seizures are controlled with phenobarbital or potassium bromide (follow seizure protocol). In traumatic brain injury, it is documented that systemic hypotension in the face of intracranial hypertension (vascular bleed or mass) results in perpetuation of secondary neurology injury, and therefore worsened outcome. Hypotension is treated with small-volume fluid resuscitation (0.9% sodium chloride bolus IO or IV at 10 mL/kg until indirect systolic blood pressure is 90 to 120 mmHg). The small-volume resuscitation is used to bring the blood pressure to normal and to avoid hypertension and risk of disturbing the intracranial clot. Corticosteroids are controversial and no longer used in human or small animal medicine. The authors recommend that steroids not be administered to birds. Complications from steroids are immunosuppression, GI ulceration, and delayed healing. Mannitol can be considered only in the bird showing worsening of neurological status (ie, stupor to comatose).

Spinal disease

Paresis indicates the presence of reduced motor function in the limbs. Paralysis indicates complete loss of motor movement in the pelvic limbs.

The most common etiology is trauma. The clinician should rule out a pathological fracture caused by hypocalcemia in chronic egg layers. Other causes include neoplasia, degenerative disease (psittacine poliomyelomalacia), nutritional deficiencies (vitamin E, thiamine, riboflavin, pyridoxine), and inflammatory disorders including proventricular dilatation disease (PDD) and polioencephalomyelitis of rainbow parakeets. Other etiologies include aspergillosis, toxicities including heavy metal, organophosphates, botulism and tick paralysis, and vascular disease (fibrocartilaginous embolic myelopathy). Diagnostic tests include blood work, radiographs, MRI, and CT. Treatment for spinal trauma is almost always supportive, but can involve bandage support, or in select cases, surgery [47–50]. The neck can be stabilized using a rigid support bandage made out of tongue depressors, plaster, and/or bandage material.

Corticosteroids are controversial in human and small animal medicine. Supportive care is required for weeks, including nutrition and analgesia.

Seizure

The possible differentials for seizures include a toxin exposure, trauma, hypoglycemia, hypertension, or hypocalcemia. Idiopathic epilepsy has been diagnosed in peach-faced lovebirds, red-lored Amazons, double-headed Amazons, and mynah birds.

The work up for a bird presenting with seizures should include a complete physical examination and evaluation of blood glucose, calcium, and PCV/TP. When the patient is stable, consider CBC and complete biochemistry panel, radiographs, and heavy metal screening. Indirect systolic blood pressure should be measured. Ideal levels are less than 200 mm Hg after the seizure is controlled.

Any bird presenting in status epilepticus (seizure repeated at brief intervals for 30 minutes or more without complete recovery of consciousness between individual attacks) should be treated with an injection of midazolam (0.25 mg/kg intramuscularly) and therapy directed toward the underlying cause, if known. When seizures cannot be controlled with the use of midazolam, one of the authors (Lichtenberger) has used a phenobarbital load as described: anesthetize the bird with isoflurane or sevoflurane. Most birds will stop seizuring under general anesthesia. Administer phenobarbital intramuscularly every 15 minutes at 4 mg/kg intramuscularly for a maximum of two doses. Perform blood work, measurement of blood pressure, and radiographs while the bird is under anesthesia Recover the bird in a warm oxygenated incubator with the head elevated. Phenobarbital is continued at a daily oral maintenance dose (2 mg/kg by mouth) for 12 hours after the phenobarbital load.

Heavy metal. Metal intoxication includes ingestion of lead, zinc, or other poisonous metallic substances. The bird may present with a history of investigating or ingesting foreign objects, but many cases of heavy metal toxicity occur without history of known exposure. Common sources include drapery weights, stained glass windows, gunshot, pennies, linoleum, galvanized cage metal, and other sources including contaminated drinking water. Many older homes have lead paint or water pipes. Physical signs are often vague and may include polyuria and polydipsia, regurgitation, diarrhea, green urates, ataxia, lethargy, or stupor, and seizure. Amazon parrots commonly present with hematuria or hemoglobinemia. Radiographs may reveal metallic objects in the GI tract or the metal may already have been digested and/or passed. Blood lead and plasma zinc levels may be elevated; however, in suspected cases chelation therapy is initiated before receiving these results in the critically ill bird [1,46,51]. The hemogram may be completely normal, but might reveal anemia and erythrocytic ballooning (red blood cells that show bulges in the normal elliptical shape and often accompanied by areas of hypochromasia). Basophilic stipling is not seen in birds. Treatment includes fluid therapy, antiemetics, nutritional support, chelation, and anticonvulsants when indicated. Chelation options include calcium EDTA, D- penicillamine, and succimer (30 mg/kg by mouth every 12 hours for 14 days made by a compounding pharmacy at 25 mg/mL suspension). Injectable calcium EDTA offers a benefit of parenteral therapy, particularly in those patients that are regurgitating or those that may not absorb oral D- penicillamine effectively [1]. Barium sulfate or activated charcoal may help move lead particles through the digestive tract.

Proventricular dilatation disease (PDD). PDD is a disease of unknown etiology, but circumstantial evidence suggests one or more viruses cause it. Numerous clinical reports document spread of the disease through a collection, and therefore it is likely contagious. Clinical manifestations of the disease are the result of lymphoplasmacytic inflammation of the nerves of the GI tract and brain, spinal cord, and peripheral nerves [1]. The disease is seen most commonly in macaws, cockatoos, African greys, Amazon parrots, and conures, although all species are susceptible. Clinical signs include regurgitation, severe weight loss, anorexia, passing of whole seeds in the stool, weakness, ataxia, and other neurological signs. PDD should be a differential diagnosis with any bird with CNS disease. The onset of PDD is seen at 3 to 4 years, but birds as young as 10 weeks and as old as 17 years have been documented. Radiographs often reveal a dilated proventriculus, and barium contrast studies reveal slow transit. Confirm definitive diagnosis with crop or proventricular biopsies. Not all birds with PDD have crop lesions, so failure to find lesions in a biopsy does not rule out the disease. The biopsy must contain a blood vessel (nerves travel with blood vessels). Treatment involves supportive care and nutrition. Celecoxib (10 mg/kg every 24 hours) has been advocated as a treatment, although no controlled trials have been done.

Hypocalcemia syndrome. Hypocalcemia occurs commonly in parakeets, lovebirds, and cockatiels that are chronic egg layers (see chronic egg laying).

Large quantities of circulating calcium can be taken up by the shell gland during egg formation. An important predisposing cause is an unsupplemented all-seed diet. Clinical signs include tremors, weakness, and seizures. Chronic egg layers commonly present with multiple pathological bone fractures. An ionized calcium less than 1 mg/dL or total calcium less than 8 mg/dL is often suggestive of hypocalcemia. Total calcium should be interpreted with caution, because a hypoalbuminemia can lower the total calcium falsely. It is always ideal to use measurement of ionized calcium. The clinician should keep in mind that birds require exogenous vitamin D3 (100 IU/300 g every 7 days). Calcium is given (50 to 100 mg/kg intramuscularly). Change diet to allow for supplemental calcium. Sunlight or UV light should be supplied.

A syndrome of hypocalcemia and associated clinical signs has been described in African gray parrots. It appears to be caused by an abnormal calcium and vitamin D3 metabolism. The birds should be treated with IV or intramuscular calcium, vitamin D3, and exposure to full-spectrum UV lighting. Dietary improvement should be initiated.

Gastrointestinal disease

Chlamydophilosis

This disease will be discussed under GI disorders, although respiratory and GI signs are common. *Chlamydophilia psittaci* infections can occur in almost any species of caged birds. Clinical signs vary from mild respiratory sinusitis, rhinitis) or GI signs (diarrhea, regurgitation, yellow-green urates) to severe multisystemic signs [52]. Doves, pigeons, and cockatiels carry the disease without showing clinical signs except when stressed. A suspected case of chlamydiosis is defined as a bird with compatible clinical signs that is linked to a person or another bird that had chlamydiosis, a subclinical infection with a single high serological titer (ie, high elementary body agglutination or EBA in psittacines for anti-IgM; serum, cloacal, or choanal positive polymerase chain reaction [PCR] assays; complement fixation or CF anti-IgG for doves and pigeons; solid-phase enzyme-linked immunoassay [ELISA]-positive test which is not available in the United States) [44]. The PCR test has the advantage of identifying an early infection as early as 5 days from oral cavity, 10 days from the cloana and 15 days from the blood. No test is 100% sensitive. Supportive care initially is started with heat and fluids. Nutritional support is recommended. No protocol ensures safe treatment of complete elimination of infection in every bird. Doxycycline is presently the drug of choice for treating birds with avian chlamydiosis. There are numerous protocols recommended depending on the situation (ie, flock treatment, oral medication, or water treatments). The authors recommend that sick birds be treated with an injectable form of Vibramycin SF IV (European formulation that can be imported through www.NOIVBD.nl, info@NOIVBD.nl) and given at 75 to 100 mg/kg intramuscularly every

5 to 7 days for the first 4 weeks and then every 5 days for two more treatments. The injectable tetracycline formulation labeled for IV use in people can be used IV in birds. The bird can be given the initial dose IV and then continued on oral doxycycline medications [45].

Vomiting and regurgitation

Differentiation must be made between behavioral and pathological regurgitation. Behavioral regurgitation usually is directed at an object (mirror) or the owner. Birds also can vomit with the stress of traveling or after anesthesia. Pathological vomiting or regurgitation can lead to life-threatening dehydration, starvation, electrolyte imbalance, and aspiration pneumonia. It is difficult for an owner to differentiate passive regurgitation versus active vomiting. Most clinicians use the terms interchangeably. Often food material is adhered to the feather on the head or nares. Decreased body condition must be attributed to a specific disease. Birds that have a history of vomiting or regurgitation may suffer from aspiration pneumonia or sinusitis. Etiology includes neonates with crop stasis (improper formula temperature and consistency), dietary indiscretion (toxins, plants, spoiled food), infections (PDD, bacterial, fungal, gastric yeast), goiters in budgerigars, chlamydiophilia, heavy metal intoxication (lead or zinc), or metabolic (hepatopathy, sepsis, pancreatitis). Fecal and esophageal/crop cytology and culture/sensitivity should be performed to reveal primary or secondary pathogens (see discussion under diagnostic testing). CBC count, chemistry panel, heavy metal testing, plasma EPH, and chlamydiophila testing may be useful also. Radiographs may identify foreign body, dilated proventriculus, ileus, or organomegaly, but must be performed with care in birds with GI motility disorders to prevent regurgitation and aspiration. Fluoroscopy or barium series can identify delayed gastric empty time or an obstruction. Ultrasound and biopsy can identify liver disease, masses, or intestinal disease further. Toxin plants can cause serious burns or systemic signs. Contact the poison control center for recommendations for treatment. Treatment for heavy metal intoxication was discussed previously in the neurological disease section. GI obstructions are treated with fluids until stable. Surgical exploratory in recommended. Appropriate antibiotics and/or antifungal medications are indicated. Metoclopramide (Reglan,) or cisapride (compounding pharmacies, 0.5 mg/kg by mouth three times daily) may assist improve crop motility and control regurgitation, but should not be used in cases of GI obstruction. No studies have been performed in birds for dosing, pharmacokinetics, or toxicity for either cisapride or metoclopramide [33].

Delayed emptying of the crop (crop stasis) may occur with any illness that causes debilitation and may not indicate a localized problem. Crop stasis in neonates is common and may be secondary to poor husbandry or improper feedings. A complete blood count, chemistry panel, and electrolyte levels should be performed to assess hydration, leukocyte count, metabolic, and electrolyte abnormalities [46]. Soften impacted material with warm water. Massage material and the fluid; then withdraw the material out into a large bore red rubber tube. This procedure is moderately stressful and must be done with care in debilitated birds. Thickened ingesta may cause proliferation of bacteria and yeast and contribute to dehydration and infection. The birds are treated with fluid therapy and nutritional support with tube feedings. Antibiotics (ie, trimethoprim sulfadiazine at 30 mg/kg by mouth twice daily) and antifungal therapy (nystatin at 100,000 to 300,000 IU/kg every 12 hours by mouth for 7 to 14 days) are given when large numbers of gram-negative bacteria and yeast are seen on crop smears. The owner should be instructed on proper feeding methods [33].

Diarrhea

Differentiation of diarrhea into large and small bowel disease is difficult with the exception that small bowel disease is more likely in the presence of with melena, and large bowel/cloacal disease in the presence of frank blood. Etiology of diarrhea is diet change or indiscretion, infections (avian gastric yeast, chlamydiophila, gram-negative bacteria, yeast, virus), protozoan (Giardia, cryptosporidium) toxins (plants, zinc or lead), systemic disease, GI foreign body, or neoplasia. The clinician must differentiate between true diarrhea and watery stool caused by polyuria. Malnutrition, especially hypovitaminosis A, predisposes a bird to GI disease.

The presence of blood in the stool can have several causes. Cloacal papillomas (primarily South American birds) can cause frank bleeding into the cloaca. Hematuria is seen commonly with zinc and lead toxicity (Amazons and cockatiels). Cloacal trauma and irritation can cause presence of blood in stool.

Medications and stress can cause stool changes. The stool should be evaluated with a Gram's stain, direct cytology, and culture of abnormal findings. Cloacal mucosa is examined for papilloma and trauma. Provide supportive care and treat for suspected infections, yeast, and protozoan parasites as necessary. Radiographs are recommended for toxin, foreign body, and systemic disease. Treat for underlying cause.

Renal disease

Kidney disease is common in avian species. Most studies have been done on chickens or other nonpet birds. Many retrospective studies and case reports support the conclusion that renal diseases are clinically significant in many species of birds (S. Echols and H. Gerlach, personal communication, 2006).

Birds have many of the same kidney functions as is seen in small animals, including renal regulation of water by means of electrolyte balance, endocrine function (production of active form of vitamin D and erythropoietin-like substance production), and osmoregulation (arginine vasotocin, norepinephrine, aldosterone, rennin angiotensin, and prolactin). The kidneys auto-regulate renal blood flow as in small animals between blood pressures of 60 to 110 mm Hg. At mean arterial pressures less than 50 mm Hg, glomerular filtration rate decreases. Avian kidneys are different from small animal kidneys in two significant ways: excretion of uric acid as the end product of nitrogenous waste and the presence of the renal portal system. The renal portal system shifts blood from the legs and coelomic organs directly through the kidneys or into the vena cava through the action of a valve under the control of the sympathetic (SNS) and cholinergic nervous system. Stress, handling, and hypovolemia (any factors stimulating the SNS) cause the valve to close, and blood is shifted directly to the vena cava and central blood flow. For this reason, injection medication into the leg muscles is unlikely to have negative consequences, as stress of restraint and handling will cause blood flow to return to the heart, as is does in mammalian species [53].

The most common clinical signs of renal failure are polyuria and polydipsia. Dehydration, anorexia, and feather picking over the synsacrum also have been noted. As renal failure progresses, oliguria and then anuria will occur. The most diagnostic test is a persistently elevated uric acid in a normally hydrated bird. A pure urine sample is difficult to obtain (see urinalysis in procedures). Other diagnostics are ultrasound, especially for diagnosis of renal enlargement or neoplasia. Calcification of the kidney may be seen in some cases on radiographs. A CBC and chemistry panel and other serology should be done to rule out other diseases. Blood pressure is measured to rule out hypertension. When the bird is stable, an endoscopic kidney biopsy should be performed [53].

In the past, etiologies of renal disease in psittacine birds have been extrapolated on information on renal disease in chickens and other nonpsittacines. More information is forthcoming with the acceptance and increasing frequency of renal biopsy of the psittacine kidney. Gout is reported commonly and may be caused by reduced of the excretion of renal urates or by increased dietary protein. There are two types of gout: visceral gout with uric acid deposition on visceral organs, and articular gout with accumulation of uric acid in the synovial tendon sheaths and joints. Nephritis is a nonspecific inflammation of the kidney and may involve interstitium, tubules, or glomerulus. Glomerulopathies are assumed to be immune-mediated (specific etiologies such as fungal, viral, and bacterial agents), but the exact cause is often unknown. In one retrospective postmortem examination on cockatiels, 67% of the birds had glomerular atherosclerosis [54]. In people, high cholesterol levels clearly are associated with the development of atherosclerosis, but a link between high blood cholesterol levels and atherosclerosis in psittacine birds has not been established [55]. Some common diseases in birds potentially could interfere with cholesterol metabolism, such as hepatopathies, iron storage disease, amyloidosis, goiter, and obesity, and thus contribute to atherosclerosis [56]. One of the authors (Lichtenberger) belies that glomerulonephropathies are common in birds, and changes may be secondary to another disease process and eventual atherosclerosis and hypertension. Future studies are warranted evaluation of cholesterol, low-density lipoproteins, and blood pressure measurements in birds with renal disease.

There is a report on diet-induced renal disease of color variety psittacine birds (S. Echols, unpublished data). The birds affected are color variety cockatiels, lovebirds, budgerigars, and parrotlets that have consumed a predominantly pelleted diet. Lesions seen on kidney biopsy were tubular nephrosis, which theoretically may be related to decreased water consumption when consuming pelleted diets. The disease is reported to be reversible by changing the diet to vegetables, fruit, and a small amount of seeds (S. Echols, personal communication, 2006). More work is needed to confirm this theory.

Other less common renal disease include nutritional, vitamin D toxicosis, congenital, urolithiasis, and trauma. Renal neoplasia is common, especially in the budgerigars. Renal carcinomas most frequently reported are kidney tumor. The birds present after 5 years of age with one-legged lameness and abdominal enlargement. Renal tumors may induce hypertension by activation of the RAAS. Renal tumors are common in psittacine birds, primarily parakeets [11]. An author documented hypertension (systolic blood pressure >300 mm Hg) in two parakeets with renal tumors. The parakeets were treated with benazepril (0.5 mg/kg twice daily by mouth), which lowered the systolic blood pressure to 110 to 130 mm Hg within 1 week. The parakeets lived for 4 months.

Treatment for renal failure regardless of the cause will be to correct dehydration, elevated uric acid, and electrolyte and acid-base imbalances. The bird should be stabilized with heat and fluids as discussed elsewhere in this issue. The bird with an elevated uric acid should be anesthetized and an IO catheter placed. Radiographs, ultrasound, and other diagnostics are performed. Blood pressure is measured. The bird is rehydrated as discussed elsewhere in this issue. Immediately after rehydration, the uric acid is rechecked, and if still elevated, diuresis is initiated. The bird is continued on fluids at thee to four times maintenance (3 to 4 mL/kg/h) for diuresis until uric acid value is normal or near normal. The bird should be tube-fed if not eating as discussed elsewhere in this issue. The tube feeding amounts can be calculated as part of the total diuresis fluid amount to be given. When the bird is eating on its own, fluids and tube feeding should be tapered by 50% per day. Oliguria and anuria are treated when decreased to no urine production occurs after rehydration. Lasix at 1 mg/kg intramuscularly can be given and fluids continued. If there is no urine production within 1 hour, prognosis is poor.

The consequences of glomerulonephropathies in small animals are a result of immune-mediated (secondary to hepatopathies, heartworm disease infections, or chronic skin disease neoplasia) glomerular injury. After the deposition of immune complexes, complement platelet aggregation, neutrophils, and activation of the coagulation system contribute to the glomerular damage. There is reduced renal blood flow, proteinuria, hypertension, and production of thromboxane, which causes vasoconstriction and platelet aggregation. Arterial hypertension is seen in 80% of dogs with glomerular disease. The coagulation system is activated, and pulmonary thromboembolisms are a common sequelae.

In dogs, treatment measures for glomerular disease are prophylactic treatment of a thromboembolism with use of low-dose aspirin (0.5 mg/kg every 24 hours by mouth). The low-dose aspirin selectively inhibits thromboxane (vasoconstrictor, platelet aggregation) without preventing the beneficial effects of prostacyclin formation (eg, vasodilation, inhibition of platelet aggregation). Omega-3 polysaturated fatty acids (as found in fish oil) may suppress glomerular inflammation and coagulation by interfering with the production of proinflammatory prostaglandins. Hypertension is treated with benazepril (0.5 mg/kg). This is also beneficial for decreasing proteinuria. No specific therapy is given for amyloidosis. Colchicine (0.03 mg/kg/d by mouth) may delay or prevent amyloid fibril deposition and may decrease serum amyloid A concentration. The authors recommend that glomerular disease in birds be treated with omega-3 fatty acids, low-dose aspirin, and benazepril (ie, for documented hypertension and/or proteinuria).

All other renal failure diseases must be treated appropriately depending on underlying etiology. Bacterial nephropathy is treated with broad-spectrum antibiotics pending culture of the biopsied kidney tissue. Renal fibrosis and amyloidosis are treated with colchicine. Articular gout is treated with colchicine (0.03 mg/kg) and allopurinol. Articular gout lesions can be opened aseptically to express the uric acid crystals and decrease painful joints [11].

Hypertension

The definition of hypertension in birds is somewhat vague. A study of normal conscious and anesthetized psittacine birds of different species reports mean systolic indirect Doppler arterial pressures of 90 to 180 mmHg and 120 to 180 mmHg, respectively (Fig. 5). In an authors' experience, systolic indirect Doppler blood pressures greater than 200 mm Hg (in conscious and anesthetized birds) are taken to indicate hypertension in birds [57]. In raptors, that value may be higher. One of the authors (Lichtenberger) believes that hypertension in anesthetized raptors is indicated by systolic indirect blood pressure greater than 240 mm Hg.

Pathophysiology and clinical consequences

An increase in systemic vascular resistance (SVR) is the common denominator in most hypertensive crises. This increase is mediated by increased

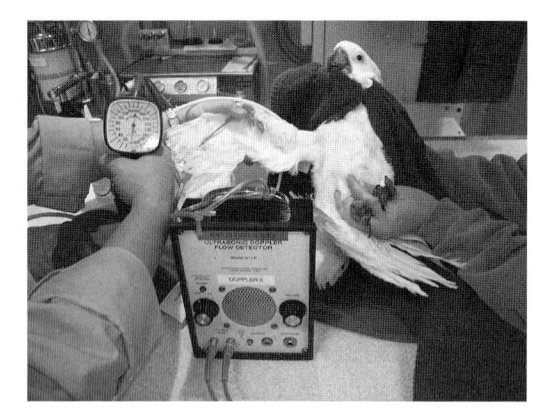

Fig. 5. Indirect blood pressure monitoring. Use of the Doppler indirect blood pressure monitor in a bird.

levels of circulating catecholamines, increased alpha-adrenergic activity, and activation of the renin–angiotensin–aldosterone system. The rise in arterial pressure increases renal perfusion and induces a pressure naturesis. This is important to remember, because most patients presenting with hypertensive crises tend to have a relative hypovolemia. Baroreceptors are stimulated by the resultant decrease in effective arterial circulating volume and produce further increases in the alpha-adrenergic and beta-adrenergic tone. This causes a further increase in blood pressure [58].

Most organs control perfusion by the process of autoregulation. Organ blood flow can be maintained at a relatively constant level over a wide range of perfusion pressures (usually 60 to 150 mm Hg). Target organ damage occurs when systemic pressures exceed the usual autoregulatory range. This may result in endothelial damage, platelet and fibrin deposition, ischemia, fibrinoid necrosis, and/or hemorrhage. The eyes, brain, heart, and kidneys are affected most commonly. Signs of organ damage may be the presenting complaint in some patients with severe hypertension. The patients may present for ocular lesions (ie, retinal hemorrhages, detachments, and/or papilledema), neurological signs (ie, confusion or seizures), cardiovascular signs (ie, ventricular hypertrophy and congestive heart failure), or renal system abnormalities (ie, glomerulonephritis) [58].

Etiology of hypertension

Primary or essential hypertension

Primary hypertension is common in people, and has been documented in dogs, although the prevalence is extremely low. Its presence in other animals and birds is unknown [58,59].

Renal disease. Renal failure is associated relatively commonly with severe hypertension in dogs and cats (ie, 60% of renal failure patients), particularly in patients with protein-losing nephropathy (PLN) [58,59]. The presence of PLN and hypertension in birds is unknown. An author has treated a parakeet with hypertension secondary to a renal tumor.

Atherosclerosis

Atherosclerosis denotes inner arterial wall thickening in association with lipid deposition. Affected large arteries often appear grossly thickened, yellow-white, and have a narrowed lumen. Histological deposits of plaque containing cholesterol, lipid material, focal calcification, and lipophages thicken the inner sections of arterial wall (intima and inner media). There can be widespread involvement of arteries from many organs [60]. The disease in people commonly is associated with extensive plaque formation, arterial calcification, or thrombosis [61].

Clinical diagnosis of atherosclerosis is difficult, and the prognosis for animals with clinical signs related to stenosing atherosclerosis is poor. History of a high-cholesterol diet may be important and may lead to obesity. Obesity in psittacine birds is common and occurs when birds are fed a high-cholesterol and high-fat diet. Physical examination may reveal an extremely obese bird. To an authors' knowledge, no reports of obesity and hypertension have been documented in the avian species. Blood pressure measurement may be used to diagnose hypertension. Future studies need to be performed in birds on high-fat, high-cholesterol diets. Blood tests for cholesterol, low-density lipoproteins, and thyroid testing may be warranted. ECG and echocardiography evaluation may detect primary or secondary heart changes. Hypertension accelerates atherosclerosis because of the high pressure changes in the artery [60].

Atherosclerosis is suspected strongly as being an inflammatory disease developing in response to injury in the vessel wall in humans. Infiltration of the mononuclear lymphocytes into the intima, local expansion of vascular smooth muscle cells, and accumulation of extracellular matrix are believed to be the pathogenesis of the inflammation. Previously determined risk factors including hyperlipidemia and hypercholesterolemia are believed to enhance leukocyte adhesion to damaged endothelium and reduce local immune response. The role of inflammation in the development of psittacine atherosclerosis has yet to be determined [60,61].

Possible risk factors for atherosclerosis include:

Obesity and decreased exercise
High-fat/cholesterol diet
Hypothyroidism
Exposure to stress factors as cold, cigarette smoke
Hypertension

Treatment for atherosclerosis includes reducing fat and cholesterol in the diet, increasing exercise, ruling out hypothyroidism, and decreasing stress factors such as exposure to cold and cigarette smoke. Blood cholesterol reducing agents (eg, statins such as lovastatin) have not been used in birds. Most human lipid-lowering drugs are not licensed for use in small animals or birds. Certain drugs, however, have been used in birds, and there are anecdotal reports of successful treatment. These drugs are to be used with caution, and every effort should be made to monitor blood chemistry, hematology, lipoprotein concentrations, and blood pressure [61].

> Omega-3 fatty acids. These drugs reduce serum cholesterol and triglyceride concentrations by decreasing the synthesis of very low-density lipoprotein (VLDL) and low-density lipoprotein (LDL). There is a liquid human product that can be used at 0.22 mL/kg body weight, by mouth every 24 hours (Optomega). This drug has been used by the authors for hyperlipidemia with hypertension in a parrot [61].
> Chitosan. This is a fiber supplement made from shellfish that reportedly binds lipids in the diet and decreases absorption of them. The drug is given 30 minutes before meals and given separately from the omega fatty acids by several hours. The drug is available in health food stores. This drug has been used with apparent success in an eclectus parrot with hyperlipidemia and hypertension (Lennox and Lichtenberger).
> Niacin. This drug acts primarily to reduce hepatic triglyceride synthesis. There is a new drug that has been used in cats and dogs (acipimox, 5 mg/kg by mouth every 24 hours).
> Statins. These drugs are of less value for lowering triglycerides, but may be effective in reducing cholesterol.

Arterial hdefinition treatment is also a possibility for treating atherosclerosis.

Antihypertensive medications

Unless evidence for hypertension-related organ injury is seen (eg, retinal lesions, neurological signs, renal disease), the decision to initiate antihypertensive therapy is not an emergency. The initial blood pressure should be taken, and every effort should be made to minimize the risk that measured elevations in blood pressure represent a transient white coat or stress effect, rather than a sustained elevation in blood pressure [61].

The optimum endpoint for antihypertensive therapy has not been established for dogs, cats, or birds with hypertension. In the absence of such information, treatment for arterial hypertension should be initiated cautiously with the goal of reducing blood pressure by 25% over weeks in patients without hypertension-related injury [61].

Angiotensin converting enzyme (ACE) inhibitors. Angiotensin converting enzyme (ACE) inhibitors inhibit the conversion of angiotensin I to angiotensin II, and thus attenuate angiotensin-mediated vasoconstriction and aldosterone release. These drugs also decrease glomerular efferent arteriolar vasoconstriction, and help reduce protein loss and inhibit the progression of glomerulosclerosis by lowering glomerular filtration pressure. ACE inhibitors such as benazepril (0.5 mg/kg twice daily) have the potential renoprotective benefits and are therefore appropriate options for renal patients with hypertension [58]. In the authors' experience, ACE inhibitors generally produce a relatively small reduction in blood pressure in dogs and cats. Because of their beneficial role in altering intraglomerular hemodynamics, proteinuria, and profibrotic effects of the intrarenal rennin-angiotensin system, however, ACE inhibitors may have renoprotective effects even in the absence of achieving adequate blood pressure control. Furthermore, in dogs with naturally occurring glomerulopathies, enalapril significantly reduced proteinuria and may have been beneficial in stabilizing renal function.

One of the authors (Lichtenberger) has measured a systolic blood pressure in two parakeets with renal tumors at greater than 300 mmHg. The birds was started on antihypertensive medication (Benazepril or enalapril 0.5 mg/kg twice daily by mouth) and returned weekly for Doppler blood pressure measurements [15]. Because of the stress level of the bird, he was anesthetized under sevoflurane anesthesia for weekly blood pressure measurements. Blood pressure was controlled in both birds for 4 to 6 months. An Amazon bird presented for seizuring at an author's (Lichtenberger) clinic. The indirect systolic blood pressure was greater than 240 mm Hg. The bird was started on benazepril 0.5 mg twice daily, and after 1 week the blood pressure was 150 mm Hg. The bird is doing well 6 months later without seizures and on benazepril. There are several other cases treated by the authors (Lichtenberger and Lennox) for hypertension, with the most common presenting complaint neurologic disease. (eg, seizures, ataxia, weakness, and blindness).

Calcium channel blockers. Calcium channel blockers (CCBs) preferentially antagonize preglomerular vasoconstriction, which theoretically should not reduce glomerular hypertension. CCBs, however, appear to have additional renoprotective properties. They may prevent renal injury by limiting renal growth, by reducing mesangial entrapment of macromolecules, and by attenuating the mitogenic effects of diverse cytokines and growth factors (eg, PDGF, platelet-activating factor). In addition, CCBs inhibit the proliferation of mesangial cells [58]. In the authors' experience, CCBs have been effective antihypertensive agents in dogs and cats with renal and cardiac disease [61]. Because it is usually highly effective, has few adverse effects, and has a rapid onset, the long-acting dihydropyridine calcium antagonist amlodipine is the antihypertensive of choice for most dogs and cats. Future studies are needed in birds for evaluation of amlodipine toxicity and dose recommendations.

Summary

Acute respiratory distress, trauma, reproductive diseases, neurological diseases, GI diseases, renal disease, and hypertension are the most common syndromes affecting the pet bird that presents in an emergency situation. Knowledge of these and other disease processes, indicated diagnostic testing, and immediate treatment protocols are critical to provide efficient and effective care to the pet bird in crisis.

References

[1] Quesenberry KE, Hillyer EV. Supportive care and emergency therapy. In: Ritchie BW, Harrison GJ, Harrison LR, editors. Avian medicine: principles and application. Lake Worth (FL): Wingers Publishing; 1994. p. 382–416.
[2] Jenkins JR, et al. Avian critical care and emergency medicine. In: Altman RB, Clubb SL, Dorrestein GM, editors. Avian medicine and surgery. Philadelphia: WB Saunders; 1997. p. 839–63.
[3] Harrison GJ, Lightfoot TL, Flinchum GB. Emergency and critical care. In: Harrison GJ, Lightfoot TL, editors. Clinical avian medicine. Palm Beach (FL): Spix Publishing; 2005. p. 213–31.
[4] Lichtenberger M, Orcutt C, DeBehnke D, et al. Mortality and response to fluid resuscitation after acute blood loss in Mallard ducks (Anas platyrhynnchos). Proc Annu Conf Assoc Avian Vet 2002;65–70.
[5] Fudge AM. Laboratory medicine avian and exotic pets. Philadelphia: W. B. Saunders Co; 2000. p. 1–26.
[6] Fudge A. Avian liver and gastrointestinal testing. In: Fudge A, editor. Laboratory medicine avian and exotic pets. Philadelphia: WB Saunders Company; 2000.
[7] Reavill DR, Lennox AM. A comparison of serum biochemistry values and liver biopsy histopathology results in psittacines. Proc European Assoc Avian Vet Zurich 2007;P327–42.
[8] Lumeij JT. Hepatology. In: Harrison GJ, Lightfoot TL, editors. Clinical avian medicine. Palm Beach (FL): Spix Publishing; 1994. p. 522–38.
[9] Stanford M. Calcium metabolism. In: Harrison G, Lightfoot T, editors. Clinical avian medicine. Palm Beach (FL): Spix Publishing; 2006. p. 141–51.
[10] Harr KE. Biochemistry. In: Harrison G, Lightfoot T, editors. Clinical avian medicine. Palm Beach (FL): Spix Publishing, Inc.; 2006. p. 612–29.
[11] Echols SM. Evaluating and treating the kidneys. In: Harrison JG, Lightfoot TL, editors. Clinical avian medicine, 2Palm Beach (FL): Spix Publishing, Inc.; 2006. p. 451–92.
[12] Orosz S, Dorrestein GM, Speer BL, et al. Urogenital disorders. In: Altman RB, Clubb SL, Dorrestein GM, editors. Avian medicine and surgery. Philadelphia: W.B. Saunders Company; 1997. p. 614–44.
[13] Harrison GJ, McDonald D. Nutritional considerations section II. In: Harrison JG, Lightfoot TL, editors. Clinical avian medicine, Vol 2Palm Beach, (FL): Spix Publishing; 2006. p. 108–40.
[14] Helmer P. Advances in diagnostic imaging. In: Harrison GJ, Lightfoot TL, editors. Clinical avian medicine. Palm Beach (FL): Spix Publishing; 2005. p. 653–60.
[15] Pees M, Krautwald-Junghanns ME, Straub J. Evaluating and treating the cardiovascular system. In: Harrison GJ, Lightfoot TL, editors. Clinical avian medicine. Palm Beach (FL): Spix Publishing; 2005. p. 379–94.
[16] Berry CR. Physical principles of computerized tomography and magnetic resonance imaging. In: Thrall DE, editor. Textbook of veterinary diagnostic radiology. 4th edition. Philadelphia: WB Saunders Co; 2002. p. 28–35.

[17] Kirk R, Bistner S, Ford R. Nebulization therapy. In: Kirk R, Bistner S, Ford R, editors. Handbook of veterinary procedures and emergency treatment. 5th edition. Philadelphia: WB Saunders; 1990. p. 600–2.
[18] Ruijgrok EJ, Fens MH, Bakker-Woudenberg IA, et al. Nebulization of four commercially available amphotericin B formulations in persistently granulocytopenic rats with invasive pulmonary aspergillosis: evidence for long-term biological activity. J Pharm Pharmacol 2005;57:1289–95.
[19] Schulman RL, Crochik SS, Kneller SK, et al. Investigation of pulmonary deposition of a nebulized radiopharmaceutical agent in awake cats. Am J Vet Res 2004;65:806–9.
[20] Graham JE. Approach to the dyspneic avian patient. Semin Avian Exotic Pet Med 2004; 13(3):154–9.
[21] Bennet RA. Avian respiratory emergencies. Conference proceedings of the Atlantic Coast Veterinary Conference; 2002.
[22] Lichtenberger M. Brochodilator therapy: ways and means. Presented at the International Veterinary Emergency and Critical Care Symposium; 2005.
[23] Oglesbee B. Emergency and acute care of campanion avians. Presented at the Waltham/OSU Symposium for the Treatment of Small Animal Diseases; 1998.
[24] Sinn LC. Anesthesiology. In: Ritchie BW, Harrison GJ, Harrison LR, editors. Avian medicine: principles and application. Lake Worth (FL): Wingers Publishing; 1994. p. 1066–80.
[25] Phalen DN. Respiratory medicine of cage and aviary birds. Vet Clin North Am: Exotic Pet Prac 2000;3(2):423–52.
[26] Burr EW. Intranasal caseous fibrinous plug causing upper respiratory distress in two African grey parrots (Psittacus erithacus). Avian Dis 1981;25(2):542–4.
[27] McDonald DE, Lowenstine LJ, Ardans AA. Avian pox in blue-fronted Amazon parrots. J Am Vet Med Assoc 1981;179(11):1218–22.
[28] Altman RB, et al. Soft tissue surgical procedures. In: Altman RB, Clubb SL, Dorrestein GM, editors. Avian medicine and surgery. Philadelphia: W.B. Saunders Company; 1997. p. 704–32.
[29] Edling TM. Anesthesia and monitoring. In: Harrison JG, Lightfoot TL, editors. Clinical avian medicine, vol 2. Palm Beach (FL): Spix Publishing, Inc.; 2006. p. 447–760.
[30] Gorham SL, Akins M, Carter B. Ectopic egg yolk in the abdominal cavity of a cockatiel. Avian Dis 1992;36(3):816–7.
[31] Bonczynski JJ, Ludwig LL, Barton LJ, et al. Comparison of peritoneal fluid and peripheral blood pH, bicarbonate, glucose and lactate concentration as a tool for septic peritonitis in dogs and cats. Vet Surg 2003;32:161–6.
[32] King AS, McLelland J, editors. Birds: Their Structure and Function. Philadelphia: Bailliere Tindall; 1984.
[33] Marx KL. Therapeutic Agents. In: Harrison GJ, Lightfoot TL, editors. Clinical Avian Medicine. Lake Worth (FL): Spix Publishing Inc.; 2005. p. 242–342.
[34] Paul-Murphy J. Pain management. In: Harrison GJ, Lightfoot TL, editors. Clinical avian medicine. Palm Beach (FL): Spix Publishing; 2005. p. 233–40.
[35] Lichtenberger M. Anesthesia protocols and pain management for exotic animal patients. Proc Western Veterinary Conference; 2006.
[36] Hernandez-Divers SJ, Hernandez-Divers SM. Xenographic grafts using porcine small intestine submucosa in the repair of skin defects in 4 birds. J Avian Med Surg 2003;17(4): 224–124.
[37] Aiken S. New concepts in wound management. Presented at the International Veterinary Emergency and Critical Care Symposium; 2004.
[38] Zaen AL, Rietveld. Inhalation trauma due to overheating in a microwave oven. Thorax 1993;48(3):300–2.
[39] Hillyer H, et al. Clinical manifestations of respiratory disorders. In: Altman R, Clubb S, Dorrestein G, editors. Avian medicine and surgery. Philadelphia: WB Saunders; 1997. p. 419–54.

[40] Poonacha KB, William PD, Stamper RD. Encephalitozoonosis in a parrot. J Am Vet Med Assoc 1985;186(7):700–2.
[41] Andre J-P, Delverdier M. Primary bronchial carcinoma with osseous metastasis in an African grey parrot (Psittacus erithacus). J Avian Med Surg 1999;13(3):180–6.
[42] Bowles HL. Reproductive diseases of pet bird species. Vet Clin North Am Exot Anim Pract 2002;5(3):489–506.
[43] Crosta L, Gerlach H, Burkle M, et al. Physiology, diagnosis, and diseases of the avian reproductive tract.
[44] Joyner KL. Theriogenology. In: Ritchie BW, Harrison GJ, Harrison LR, editors. Avian medicine: principles and application. Lake Worth (FL): Wingers Publishing; 1994. p. 748–88.
[45] Bowles HL. Evaluating and treating the reproductive system. In: Harrison GJ, Lightfoot TL, editors. Clinical avian medicine. Palm Beach (FL): Spix Publishing; 2005. p. 519–39.
[46] Bemnen RA. Neurology. In: Ritchie BW, Harrison GJ, Harrison LR, editors. Avian medicine: principles and application. Lake Worth (FL): Wingers Publishing; 1994. p. 723–47.
[47] Degernes LA. Trauma medicine. In: Ritchie BW, Harrison GJ, Harrison LR, editors. Avian medicine: principles and application. Lake Worth (FL): Wingers Publishing; 1994. p. 418–33.
[48] Bemlen RA, et al. Orthopedic surgery. In: Altman RB, Clubb SL, Dorrestein GM, editors. Avian medicine and surgery. Philadelphia: WB Saunders; 1997. p. 733–66.
[49] Murray MJ. Management of the avian trauma case. Semin Avian Exotic Pet Med 1994;3(4): 200–9.
[50] Rupley A. Critical care of pet birds. Procedures, therapeutics, and patient support. Vet Clin North Am Exot Anim Pract 1998;1:21–2.
[51] Stanford M. Calcium metabolism. In: Harrison GJ, Lightfoot TL, editors. Clinical avian medicine. Palm Beach (FL): Spix Publishing; 2005. p. 1–23.
[52] Gerlach H. Chlamydia. In: Ritchie BW, Harrison GJ, Harrison LR, editors. Avian medicine: principles and application. Lake Worth (FL): Wingers Publishing; 1994. p. 984–93.
[53] Raidal SR, Raidal SL. Comparative renal physiology of exotic species. Vet Clin North Am Exot Anim Pract 2006;9:13–31.
[54] Garner MM. Lipid deposition disorders in cockatiels (Nymphicus hollandicus). Proc of AAV 26th ANN Conf. Monterey (CA) 2005;249–52.
[55] Otten BA, Quesenberry KE, Jones MP. Reference ranges for serum lipid levels in amazon parrots. Proc of AAV 22nd Ann Conf. Orlando (FL): 2001. p. 95–7.
[56] Pilny AA. Retrospective of atherosclerosis in psittacine birds: clinical and histopathologic findings in 31 cases. Proc of AAV. 25th Ann Conf. New Orleans (LA): 2004. p. 349–351.
[57] Lichtenberger M. Determination of indirect blood pressure in the companion bird. Semin Avian Exotic Pet Med 2005;14(2):149–52.
[58] Brovida C. Hypertension in renal diseases and failure: the practical aspect. Proc WSAVA 2002.
[59] Brown S. Pathophysiology of systemic hypertension. In: Ettinger SL, Feldman FC, editors. Textbook of Veterinary Internal Medicine. St Louis (MO): Elsevier/Saunders; 2005. p. 472–6.
[60] Dorrestein GM, Fricke C, Krutwald-Junghanns ME. Atherosclerosis in African Grey Parrots (Psittacus eerithacus) and Amazons (Amazona Species) Proc Assoc Avian Vet 2006.
[61] Lichtenberger M. Emergency case approach to hypotension, hypertension and acute respiratory distress. Proc Assoc Av Vet 2006.

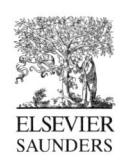

# Emergency Care of Raptors

Jennifer E. Graham, DVM, DABVP-Avian[a,b,*],
J. Jill Heatley, DVM, MS, DABVP-Avian[c,d]

[a]Department of Comparative Medicine, School of Medicine, University of Washington, Box 357910, Seattle, WA 98195, USA
[b]Avian and Exotic Medicine, Angell Animal Medical Center, 350 South Huntington Avenue, Boston, MA 02130, USA
[c]Zoological Medicine Service, Auburn University College of Veterinary Medicine, Auburn, AL 36849, USA
[d]Southeastern Raptor Center, Auburn University College of Veterinary Medicine, Auburn, AL 36849, USA

Emergency presentations of raptors occur based on a variety of debilitating conditions that allow for capture. Important considerations for the veterinarian include origin or use of the bird (eg, wildlife, falconry bird, captive education specimen), duration and nature of illness (acute, chronic, or insidious onset), extent of disease, and potential for recovery. Patient status and temperament help to determine the appropriate range and depth of diagnostic testing. It is vital that the veterinarian is aware of state and federal laws regarding raptorial species; for example, any bird that is completely blind or has sustained injuries that would require amputation of a leg, a foot, or a wing above the cubital joint should be euthanized unless special permission has been granted [1]. Contact local wildlife officials within 24 hours of presentation of any wild raptor and before euthanasia of endangered or threatened raptors or native eagle species to ensure that appropriate guidelines are followed [2]. This article reviews aspects of emergency care for wild and captive raptors, including handling and restraint, short-term hospitalization, triage and patient assessment, sample collection, supportive care procedures, and common emergency presentations.

Handling, restraint, and hospitalization

Raptors vary in their choice of weapons for defense based on species and size. Raptorial species have formidable talons, with the exception of

---

* Corresponding author. Avian and Exotic Medicine, Angell Animal Medical Center, 350 South Huntington Avenue, Boston, MA 02130.
 E-mail address: jennifervet@yahoo.com (J.E. Graham).

vultures, and beaks that can cause significant damage to the handler and bird. The talons, beak, wings, and vomiting may be used singly or in combination, with preference based on species. Vultures have a propensity to bite, especially at the eyes and mouth of the handler, so appropriate precautions should be taken. As a self-defense mechanism, vultures, particularly turkey vultures, are prone to vomit during capture and restraint. Care must be taken to avoid damaging the raptor's feathers during capture and restraint. Additionally, raptors in a poor nutritional plane are prone to fractures with rough handling.

Although trained falconry or educational birds may allow partial examination with minimal restraint if hooded, raptors from the wild must be properly restrained to perform a thorough physical examination (Fig. 1). Choice of equipment should be based on the bird's size, temperament, and planned diagnostics. Nets should be available to capture birds from large aviaries or in the event of an escape. Soft towels or blankets can be used to wrap the bird and avoid damage to the feathers. Goggles for eye protection and varying lengths of leather gloves should be used to protect the hands and arms of the handler (Fig. 2) [2]. Larger raptors, such as eagles, may need two individuals to restrain the bird safely [3]. Varying sizes of hoods or a stockinette is helpful for covering the head of the bird to minimize stress. For wild raptors, a hood that can be adjusted to fit is available [4]. Alternately, covering the raptor's head with a towel can also minimize stress. Good communication and appropriate restraint of the raptor's

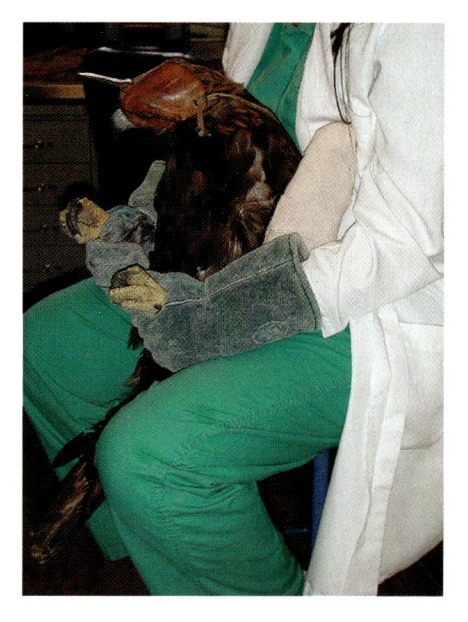

Fig. 1. Restraint of an adult Golden Eagle *(Aquila chrysaetos)* for physical examination.

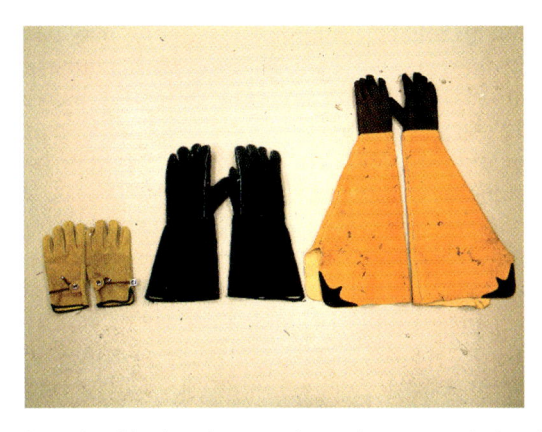

Fig. 2. A variety of lengths of leather gloves can be used to protect the hands and arms of the handler during raptor restraint.

head and feet can avoid injury to the raptor, handler, and examiner. A finger placed between the tarsi of medium-sized raptors can avoid unintentional fractures or self-inflicted damage to the skin [3].

Separate equipment and housing should be used for birds with suspected contagious disease, such as poxvirus, or all equipment and cages should be thoroughly disinfected after use to minimize the risk of disease transmission. Temporary housing must be available for the species in question, with the capability to provide oxygen therapy, nebulization, or heat support as needed. Tail guards, using cardboard or radiology film taped to the tail with masking tape or brown paper tape, may be needed during transport of raptors or when the birds are housed in smaller cages to avoid damage to the tail [3]. The hospitalized raptor should have minimum human or companion animal contact. In particular, wild raptors younger than 6 weeks of age should have minimal human contact to avoid imprinting, especially when they are fed [2]. Even temporary hospitalization of a raptor with barking dogs or free-roaming clinic cats is unacceptable. After stabilization, arrangements for transfer of the raptor to a rehabilitation facility or other suitable housing should be made in a timely manner, usually within 72 hours. Appropriate perching for different species is necessary for even short-term hospitalization to avoid damage to feet and feathers.

Triage and patient assessment

Physical examination is similar to that of other avian species other than capture and restraint. If a raptor is caught out of a flight or even large container or carrier, careful observation of the bird before handling is recommended. The importance of an observational examination cannot be overstated. The observational examination is key in determining the length, depth, and fashion of the physical examination and further diagnostics that the patient is likely to tolerate. Many abnormalities may be obscured by the camouflage of the feathers; however, on observation and examination, these signs can be quite obvious or pronounced. Note any increased respiratory effort or tail bob; posture and awareness of the bird; and any musculoskeletal or neurologic abnormalities, such as a wing droop or head tilt. If a bird is showing extreme respiratory difficulty or weakness, emergency care should be given before performing a complete physical examination.

Weight determination, accurate to the gram, is a necessary part of the raptor physical examination. In diurnal birds of prey, the weight is best obtained when the crop is empty. Although falconry or educational birds may willingly step onto a scale, wild raptors must be appropriately restrained or enclosed to obtain a weight. Medium to large wild raptors can be wrapped in a towel or stockinette, secured in a pet porter or cardboard box, secured on a bird restraint board, or weighed while under anesthesia [3]. Smaller species, such as the screech owl or American kestrel, may be placed in a secured paper bag or small plastic container with ventilation holes.

All equipment for physical examination should be ready before restraint of the raptor. This preparation minimizes handling and examination time, and thus patient stress. If the patient is debilitated, an examination can be performed in a stepwise fashion with small breaks given to the bird between handling, examination, diagnostics, and treatments. Care should be taken to hold the bird upright if the bird is showing signs of respiratory distress or if any fluid or masses are palpated in the coelomic cavity. Any debilitated bird or birds showing signs of shock should be handled as described for psittacine birds (see the article on shock and fluid therapy by Lichtenberger elsewhere in this issue). Oxygen therapy before, during, or after physical examination may be beneficial in the patient with debilitation, shock, or respiratory compromise. If oxygen therapy is needed, an oxygen cage delivering a 50% to 80% humidified oxygen concentration or a facemask with a flow rate of 50 mL/kg/min can be used [5]. Use of an opioid (butorphanol) and midazolam administered intramuscularly can be used for a neuroleptic effect (sedation and to relieve anxiety). Inhalant anesthesia can minimize stress to a fractious or painful patient and allow a complete physical examination, diagnostic sampling, or therapeutic treatment with only a single handler [2].

Raptors with hypovolemic shock need immediate fluid therapy (see section on fluid therapy) after initial stabilization in a warmed and oxygenated incubator for 2 to 4 hours. Signs of the early or compensatory phase of shock in birds include an increased heart rate, normal or increased blood pressure, and normal or increased blood flow as evidenced by bounding pulses and a capillary refill time (CRT) less than 1 second [6]. Birds with continued fluid loss show evidence of the early decompensatory phase of shock with signs that include hypothermia, cool limbs and skin, tachycardia, normal to decreased blood pressure (indirect systolic Doppler blood pressure <90 mm Hg), pale mucous membranes, a prolonged CRT, and mental depression [6]. Birds with decompensatory or terminal shock exhibit bradycardia with low cardiac output, severe hypotension, pale or cyanotic mucous membranes, an absent CRT, weak or absent pulses, hypothermia, oliguria to anuric renal failure, pulmonary edema, and a stupor-to-comatose state; cardiopulmonary arrest commonly occurs at this stage [6].

Replacement of luxations and closure of open wounds may need immediate attention to ensure a positive outcome, but stabilizing the patient may require initiating fluid therapy and shock treatment before in-depth wound care. Initially, a light nonadherent wrap can be placed to minimize bleeding and further trauma to open wounds. When the patient is stable, complete wound care may require analgesia, sedation, or anesthesia. Examine the oral cavity, ears, and nares closely for any signs of blood, which is indicative of head trauma. A complete ophthalmologic examination includes examination of the posterior segment of the eye and should be performed when the bird is stable. Anticonvulsant therapy and steps for prevention of self-inflicted trauma are indicated for seizures. Additional references are available concerning triage and patient assessment [6–20].

Monitoring techniques

Blood pressure, electrocardiography (ECG), pulse quality, CRT, and body temperature are additional physical examination parameters that may be useful in assessing patient status (see the article on monitoring elsewhere in this issue) [7,9,10]. Systolic blood pressure measurements obtained with a Doppler flow detector from the ulnar vessels in awake and isoflurane-anesthetized psittacine birds ranged from 90 to 180 mm Hg [7]. There is limited information regarding published normal blood pressures in raptorial species. One study examining the effects of propofol in Red-Tailed Hawks and Great Horned Owls showed mean direct arterial blood pressure in manually restrained hawks and owls as 187.3 ± 41.7 mm Hg in Red-Tailed Hawks and 203.0 ± 28.4 mm Hg in Great Horned Owls [21]. Guidelines on specific measurements defining hypertension are yet to be determined in raptors. In the authors' experience, inhalant-anesthetized systolic Doppler blood pressure measurements exceeding 240 mm Hg are used as the upper limit value defining hypertension in raptors. Guidelines for fluid therapy for hypovolemia are based on blood pressure measurements as used with mammals and psittacine birds. Raptors should be treated for hypovolemic shock when indirect Doppler blood pressures are less than 90 mm Hg systolic [6].

Pulse quality and CRT help to guide therapy in raptor patients (see previous section). The deep radial artery, which runs alongside the ulnar vein, or the metatarsal artery as it crosses the dorsal surface of the tibiotarsal-tarsometatarsal joint can be used to assess pulse quality [2]. A weak or thready pulse can be a sign of shock, whereas an absent pulse can indicate cardiac asystole, peripheral vasoconstriction attributable to cold, hypovolemia, or hypotension [2]. Oral mucous membrane assessment for CRT can be challenging because of the presence of pigmentation. Vent eversion is an alternative mucous membrane technique for assessment of membrane color. Ulnar vein turgidity is useful for determining vascular perfusion; the vessel should refill immediately when depressed [2].

Body temperature is less often used when assessing the critical awake avian patient. Remote sensing thermometers or conventional digital thermometers can be carefully inserted into the cloaca in unanesthetized birds to measure body temperature. Although cloacal temperature monitoring can be accurate, it depends on body temperature and cloacal activity over time [22]. Remote sensing constant readout thermometers can be used to measure body temperature in anesthetized patients when placed in the esophagus to the level of the heart.

Sample collection

Samples for hematologic and biochemical analysis are preferably obtained before treatment for best diagnostic ability. The patient's needs must be prioritized, however. Raptors in shock must be stabilized before extensive diagnostic sampling. If blood can be safely obtained, it is ideal to collect baseline samples for hematology and chemistry analysis before treatment. A conservative raptor minimum database includes determination of packed cell volume (PCV), total solids, and estimated white blood cell count. Venipuncture sites in raptors include the medial metatarsal vein, jugular vein (the right jugular vein is larger), and cutaneous ulnar or basilic vein. Although total blood volume varies based on the species, in general, 1% of total body weight can be safely collected from the healthy raptor [23]. In the compromised patient, this should be reduced to 0.5% of total body weight. Once the bird is stable, venipuncture for heavy metal testing, aspergillus antigen and antibody testing, additional sample collection, radiographs, respiratory washes, endoscopy with biopsies, and other tests can determine the cause and extent of disease. A fecal parasite examination should be performed on all wild raptors at least once before release [2].

Radiographs are a high-return low-risk diagnostic procedure in stable raptors. Properly positioned radiographs allow visualization of organ size and location; evaluation of the lungs or air sacs; and detection of heavy metal foreign bodies, fractures, and other pathologic findings. Radiographs can be taken without anesthesia in the tractable hooded raptor. Restraint boards and masking or paper tape can be used for positioning of smaller raptors to minimize exposure of personnel to radiation. Inhalant anesthesia may be necessary to obtain properly positioned radiographs when restraint boards are not available or the patient is fractious. Two-view whole-body radiographs are recommended, with additional views taken of extremities if indicated. Additional oblique views of the head are also indicated in cases of skull trauma (Fig. 3). A baseline view of the feet of any raptor affected by pododermatitis can guide prognosis and treatment.

Fluid administration sites

Fluids can be administered orally, subcutaneously, intravenously, or intraosseously. Administration of oral or subcutaneous fluids is reserved for the stable raptor that is less than 5% dehydrated, and standing [2]. Oral fluid administration requires a raptor that can maintain an upright body position and has a functional gastrointestinal tract to avoid regurgitation and aspiration of fluids. The inguinal site, where the inner thigh meets the body wall, is preferred for administration of subcutaneous fluids in raptors [5]. Other potential subcutaneous fluid administration sites include the axillary region, lateral flank, midback, and intrascapular area [11,13]. Subcutaneous fluid administration requires avoidance of fluids entering the coelomic cavity and air sac system.

Intravascular administration of fluids (intravenous or intraosseous) is essential in treatment of the critical raptor patient after initial stabilization in a warmed and oxygenated incubator. Intravenous and intraosseous catheters can be placed under general anesthesia if necessary. Sites for intravenous catheterization include the medial metatarsal vein, the ulnar vein, and the jugular vein. Ulnar vein catheterization is a preferred site, because fluids and drugs can be administered here without regard for the renal portal system. A figure-of-eight bandage can secure the ulnar catheter after it has been glued or sutured in place [5,13]. The catheter site should be checked

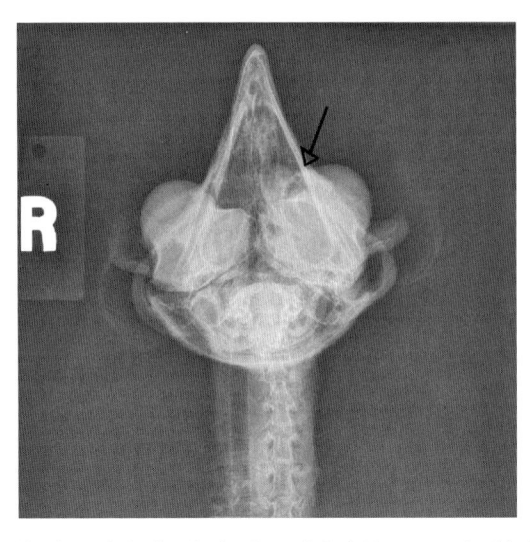

Fig. 3. Radiographic view of the head of a Barred Owl (*Strix varia*) with head trauma. The arrow marks air within the globe of the eye.

daily. Catheterization of the medial metatarsal vein is usually well tolerated by falconry birds [5]. Intravenous catheters can be challenging to maintain in birds because of fragility of vessels, lack of dermal tissues for catheterization, and patient temperament [11,13,14].

Intraosseous catheterization has advantages when compared with intravenous catheterization of the avian patient based on ease of placement and maintenance. Intraosseous catheters usually consist of a small-gauge needle, such as a spinal needle, placed in the distal ulna or proximal tibiotarsus [13]. Pneumatic bones, such as the femur and humerus, should not be used for intraosseous catheters. Intraosseous catheters can be maintained for 3 to 5 days and require the same aseptic technique as intravenous catheters during placement and maintenance [13]. Placement is similar to that of normograde insertion of an intramedullary pin (Fig. 4). For additional information on fluid therapy, see the article by Lichtenberger in this issue.

Transfusion medicine

A transfusion should be considered in critically ill raptors with a PCV less than 20% [5,13,15]. Reasons for anemia in raptors can include trauma; toxin exposure; hemoparasites; and chronic disease of infectious, metabolic, toxic, or neoplastic origin [5,13,15]. Raptors may adapt to anemia of chronic disease, and a transfusion may not be necessary if the underlying cause is treated and the bird does not have severe clinical signs. Factors that should be considered in each case when determining if a transfusion is necessary include severity of clinical signs; patient PCV; cause, severity, and duration of anemia; potential for further blood loss; availability of a donor; and the patient's capacity to tolerate the transfusion procedure [15]. For additional information on transfusion therapy, see the article by Lichtenberger in this issue.

Bandaging and wound management

Open wounds should be cleaned and bandaged until the patient is stable and can tolerate more extensive wound debridement or surgery. Raptors have little subcutaneous fat or other tissue, and immediate wound coverage decreases further tissue damage and desiccation. If immediate wound closure is not possible, packing the wound with moistened sterile gauze sponges or a water-soluble lubricating gel (K-Y Jelly; Johnson and Johnson Products, New Brunswick, New Jersey) limits desiccation [24]. Wounds should be lavaged and debrided when the patient is stable to remove debris before closure or bandaging [24]. Primary wound closure is recommended as soon as possible. When managing wounds by second intention, a variety of topical preparations can be used [24]. Use of water-based preparations is preferred, and topical steroids are avoided in birds. A hydrogel containing acemannan (Carravet Wound Dressing; Carrington Laboratories, Irving,

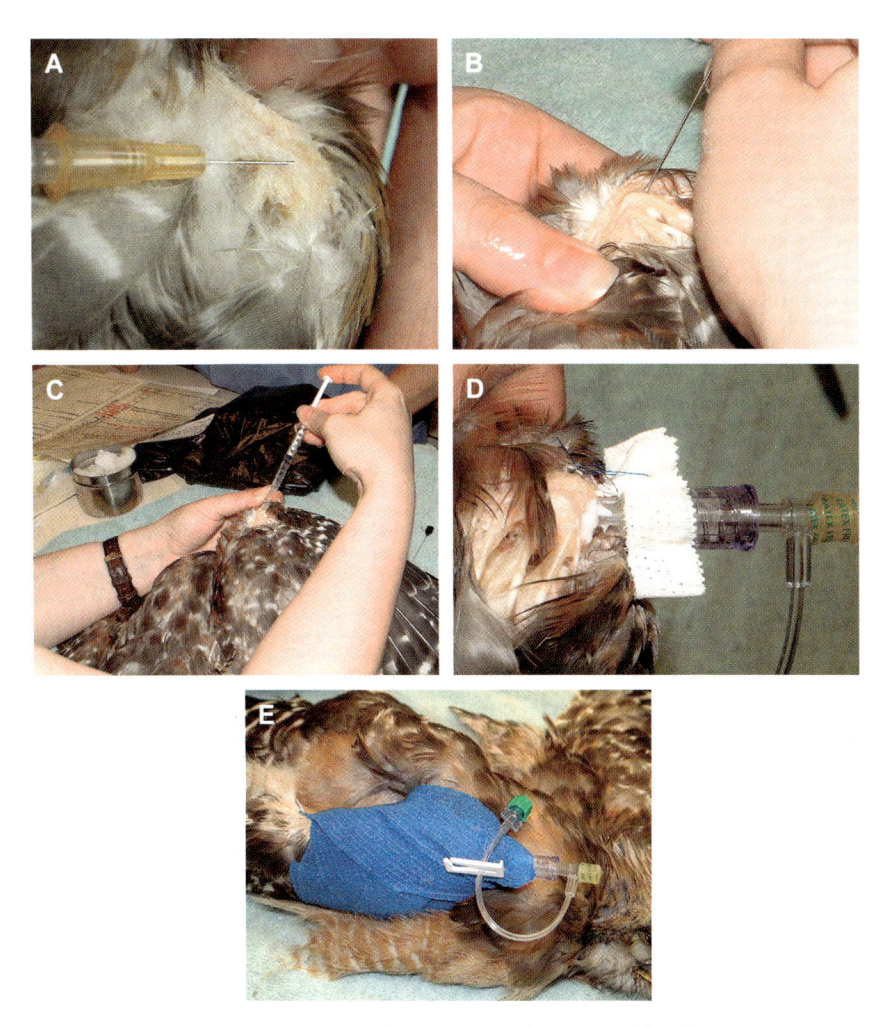

Fig. 4. Placement of a spinal needle in the ulna of a Red-Shouldered hawk (*Buteo lineatus*) cadaver for demonstration of intraosseous catheter placement. Sterile gloves should be worn to ensure aseptic technique. (*A*) Dorsal aspect of the distal radius and ulna is plucked to reveal a landmark for the insertion of the intraosseous catheter, the dorsal ulnar condyle (*Condylus dorsalis ulnaris*). (*B*) After aseptic preparation, the intraosseous catheter (shown here is a 22-gauge spinal needle and stylette) is inserted into the distal ulna with a firm pushing and twisting motion. (*C*) Fluid can sometimes be withdrawn from the intraosseous catheter, and flush should be easily injectable with a tuberculin syringe. Observation of the cutaneous ulnar or basilic vein while flushing the catheter shows clear fluid passing through this vessel with correct catheter placement. (*D*) After placement of the catheter, a catheter cap and extension cap can be added. Antibiotic ointment is lightly applied to the insertion site, and the catheter is fixed to the skin with a tape flange. (*E*) Figure-of-eight bandage is applied to cover the primary catheter portal and lessen wing motion during catheter use.

Texas) stimulates healing in raptor wounds while maintaining moisture. For contaminated wounds, silver sulfadiazine cream (Silvadene Cream; Boots Pharmacueticals, Lincolnshire, Illinois) is a water-based cream with antibacterial and antifungal properties. Nonadherent bandaging materials are recommended to avoid disruption of the healing surface of the wound.

Wing injuries can be stabilized temporarily using figure-of-eight bandages; shoulder and humeral fractures should be further stabilized using a body wrap. Avoid excess pressure across the keel with body wraps that may compromise patient respiration. Cast padding covered with a layer of self-adherent bandage (Vetrap; 3M Health Care, St. Paul, Minnesota) is ideal because it creates a soft padded bandage that is easily held in place and does not damage feathers. Self-adherent bandages can tighten when wet; thus, access of bandaged birds to open containers of water should be limited or monitored [3]. Femoral fractures are managed with cage rest until the bird can withstand surgical fixation. Fractures involving the tibiotarsus can be managed with a Robert-Jones bandage. Tarsometatarsal fractures can be stabilized with a Robert-Jones bandage combined with a ball bandage or incorporated foot cast. Reviews of wound management, bumblefoot treatment, bandage types, and surgical and nonsurgical repair of fractures in raptorial species are available [3,24–31].

Nutritional support

Diets for stable hospitalized raptors should ideally be selected according to the natural diet of the species (eg, fish for bald eagles and osprey). Quail, rats, mice, day-old chicks, ducklings, rabbits, and fish are common items fed to hospitalized raptors [3]. Replacement fluid therapy is critical before nutritional support is instituted. Oral supplementation with isotonic tube-feeding formulas can be initiated in raptors with moderate to severe starvation before feeding prey items if gastrointestinal function is questionable [5]. Raptors naturally eat a diet low in carbohydrates (2%) and high in fat (2%–28%) and protein (17%–20%) [5]. Severely debilitated raptors with a body condition score of 1 cannot readily digest whole-prey items and should be fed items devoid of casting material, such as fur and feathers, to avoid refeeding syndrome. If the debilitated raptor is consistently producing feces while on the liquid diet, Coturnix Quail minus the feet, feathers, and gastrointestinal tract can be ground and fed to the convalescing raptor by the third to fourth day of supportive care [5]. Cut pieces of quail meat soaked in oral electrolyte solution can be offered for a short time (less than 5 days) before instituting whole-prey items once gastrointestinal transit time is normal [5]. Alternatively, the quail (minus feet, feathers or skin, and gastrointestinal tract) can be ground with a meat grinder into patties and fed, with additional frozen for storage, or mixed with ground beef, chicken liver, egg, or electrolyte preparations [3,5]. Other types of meat can be used, but it is important to remove any feathers, fur, or bone when initially feeding the emaciated raptor. Commercially available feeding formulas, such as a formulated critical care diet (Carnivore Care; Oxbow, Murdock, Nebraska), Lafeber's Critical Care diet (Lafeber Company, Cornell, Illinois), Eukanuba Maximum Calorie diet (Maximum-Calorie; Iams Company, Dayton, Ohio), or Hill's a/d diet (a/d Canine/Feline; Hill's Pet Nutrition, Topeka, Kansas) can be used on a short-term basis. Rigorous nutritional requirements for raptors have not been determined; the stomach capacity of raptors is approximately 40 mL/kg of body weight [32]. Several references discuss nutritional care of debilitated raptors and should be consulted for more complete information [3,5,32].

Pain control

Analgesia in raptors is indicated for any procedure or condition that is perceived by the clinician to cause pain [13,33]. Butorphanol is commonly used in raptors [5,13]. Use caution when considering drugs that can cause respiratory depression, such as butorphanol, in the preoperative or debilitated raptor [13]. A variety of anti-inflammatories, such as meloxicam, carprofen, and others, can be used in raptors [34]. The reader is referred to another article in this issue for a discussion on pain control.

Common emergency presentations

Trauma

Fractures, wounds, head trauma, electrocution, gunshot wounds, and other injuries may cause emergent presentation of raptors. A thorough physical examination is essential to determine the extent of trauma and best approach for treatment. Prioritize therapy, cleanse wounds, and stabilize fractures initially until patient stabilization allows surgical repair and more detailed treatment. Fracture stabilization is of paramount importance in raptors. The high mineral content of avian bones results in sharp fracture fragments that can easily damage adjacent vessels, nerves, skin, and muscle. Luxations generally have a poor prognosis but should be reduced as soon as possible to have the best chance for joint mobility.

Head trauma can be associated with physical examination findings of anisocoria, head tilt, depression, or other neurologic signs; skull fractures; retinal detachment; or hemorrhage from the nares, oral cavity, ears, or anterior chamber of the eye. The most important neurologic signs to monitor every 30 minutes are mentation, pupil symmetry and size, and pupillary light reflex. Changes in pupil size to dilated and loss of pupillary light reflex along with mentation progression to stuporous or coma are documentation of neurologic deterioration. The raptor with head trauma may benefit from oxygen support. Intravenous fluid administration using isotonic saline and colloids (ie, hetastarch) is given in limited volumes (saline at 10 mL/kg and hetastarch at 3 mL/kg) to maintain blood pressure at 80 to 90 mm Hg systolic (hypotensive or limited volume resuscitation) to avoid increasing intracranial pressure. Administration of furosemide or mannitol should be considered in the case of minimal response to initial therapy or deterioration of the presenting neurologic signs. The use of steroids with head trauma is not recommended in human beings, and the authors do not recommend its use in raptors. Steroids can cause immunologic suppression and can lead to secondary bacterial and fungal disease in birds [35]. Sedation of a fractious raptor with head trauma is used to prevent further injury. Ophthalmologic examination of anterior and posterior segments should occur on patient stabilization. Posterior segment examination should include evaluation of the pecten for signs of disruption. Retinal detachment and cataract formation are common sequelae to head trauma [5]. Topical or systemic administration of antibiotics is indicated for corneal ulceration or perforation [12]. Topical ophthalmic nonsteroidal anti-inflammatories can be used to treat uveitis in raptors without corneal ulceration. Tissue plasminogen activator can be injected into the globe of the eye in raptors to ameliorate acute ocular inflammation [36,37]. Anesthesia and technical skill are required for the intracameral injection, however.

Electrocution is not uncommon, especially in immature raptors, with a higher incidence in the winter months [5]. Evidence of electrocution may not be evident for several days after injury [5]. Clinical consequences of electrocution in birds include cardiac arrest, pericardial effusion, neurogenic pulmonary edema (causing acute respiratory distress), and thermal burns (particularly of the heat, feet, and carpi) [5,38]. Feather damage of the barbs and barbules without damage to the rachis can be a classic sign of electrocution (Fig. 5). Injury may be so severe from electrocution that humane euthanasia is necessary (Fig. 6). If electrocution is suspected, treat symptoms manifested. Pericardial effusion is diagnosed with the help of

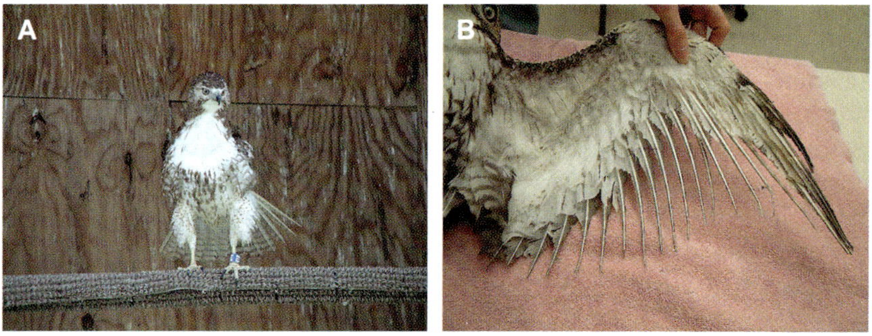

Fig. 5. (*A*) In some cases of electrocution, such as in this immature Red-Tailed Hawk (*Buteo jamaicensis*), feather damage may be the only abnormality found on physical examination. (*B*) Closer view of the damaged feathers of the hawk. A classic sign of electrocution in raptors is feather damage of the barbs and barbules, without damage to the rachis.

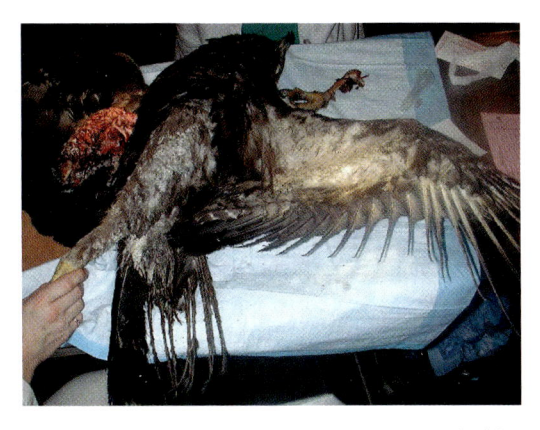

Fig. 6. Electrocution of this Golden Eagle (*Aquila chrysaetos*) resulted in complete traumatic amputation of the right leg, necessitating humane euthanasia.

an echocardiogram and treatment with pericardiocentesis. Neurogenic pulmonary edema causing acute respiratory distress may respond to one dose of furosemide (Lasix; 2 mg/kg) and supportive care with oxygen and sedation. The pulmonary edema resulting from electrocution is secondary to a capillary permeability–induced alveolar injury; therefore, continued administration of the diuretic is not recommended. Systemic administration of antibiotics, antifungals, and nonsteroidal anti-inflammatories as well as topical wound therapy may also be indicated. The prognosis for electrocution varies from fair to grave depending on the extent and severity of the damage. Even if injury is limited to feather damage, this may prevent release of a wild raptor for a molt cycle for up to 1 year.

Respiratory disease

In cases of respiratory distress, the raptor patient should immediately be placed in an oxygen-enriched environment (Fig. 7). Because severely dyspneic birds do not tolerate handling, an oxygen cage with greater than 70% oxygen concentration is recommended. This can be accomplished with commercially available intensive care units with an oxygen flow rate of 5 L. Butorphanol (1 mg/kg) with midazolam (0.25–0.5 mg/kg), administered intramuscularly, may provide mild sedation and reduce anxiety associated with acute respiratory distress in the avian patient. Use terbutaline (Table 1) administered intramuscularly as a bronchodilator initially until localization of the respiratory lesion is accomplished based on breathing pattern, history, and a brief physical examination. Humidification of oxygenated air by bubbling through an isotonic solution is recommended to assist with clearance of respiratory secretions and foreign material in the trachea and bronchi [17]. Commercially manufactured intensive care units for birds can provide oxygen, heat, and humidity and are helpful in

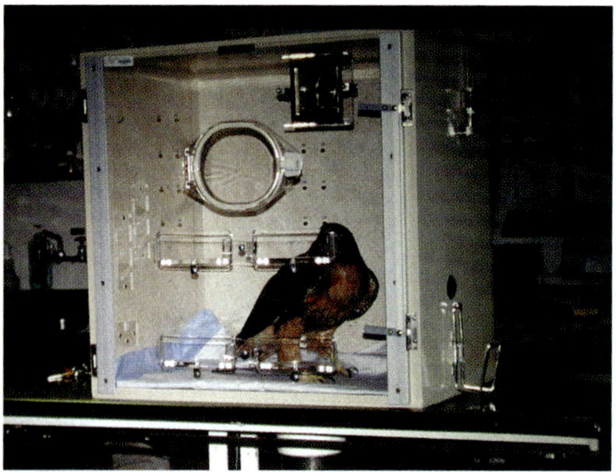

Fig. 7. Use of an oxygenated cage for treatment of respiratory distress in a mature Red-Tailed Hawk *(Buteo jamaicensis)*.

emergency situations. Each incubator unit should be tested for temperature, humidity, and oxygen concentration before use.

Tracheal obstruction in raptors is commonly caused by aspergillosis or inhalation of food. In emergency situations involving occlusion of the upper respiratory tract, such as tracheal granulomas, foreign bodies, or severe head or facial trauma, air sac intubation may be necessary to ensure air flow through the respiratory tract. The existence of the air sac system of the avian respiratory tract allows this means of ventilation, which is not possible in mammals. Sedation with a low dose of midazolam, local lidocaine block, or inhalant anesthesia may be necessary for placement of the air sac cannula. Commercially made avian air sac cannulas (20-French Non-cuffed Tube with Retention Disk; Cook Veterinary Products, Bloomington, Indiana) are available, or various types of tubing or standard endotracheal tubing can be modified for this purpose. Appropriate characteristics of an air sac cannula include material that should be rigid enough not to collapse, be short enough and flexible enough to avoid damage of internal organs on placement, have an internal diameter roughly 10% larger than the patient's trachea, and can be affixed to the body wall. A cuff that can be inflated inside the body wall to stabilize the tube and an external opening that can be easily temporarily occluded to test the necessity of maintaining cannulation are also desirable characteristics. A standard small animal cuffed endotracheal tube 3.0 mm internal diameter can be used in larger birds. Red rubber urethral catheters are also acceptable. In extremely small birds, the authors have used 20- or 22-gauge intravenous catheters to cannulate the air sac. The air sac cannula is placed in the caudal thoracic or abdominal air sac. The point of entry is typically between the last two ribs, caudal to the last rib or just caudal to the thigh muscles. The first two insertion sites usually enter the caudal thoracic air sac, whereas the last site enters the abdominal air sac. The left abdominal air sac is larger than the right; therefore, the bird should be placed in right lateral recumbency if an approach is made caudal to the thigh muscles. In a bird with large ovarian follicles, it may be beneficial to use a right-sided approach to avoid the reproductive tract. It is important to make sure that the placement of the cannula has a minimal impact on movement of the leg.

The bird is placed in right or left lateral recumbency, and the area of cannula insertion is plucked and aseptically prepared. A small skin incision (approximately the diameter of the cannula) is made with a scalpel blade, and small mosquito hemostats are used to dissect bluntly through the abdominal wall musculature. Some force is required to pierce the air sac and overlying peritoneum. Once the air sac is entered, the cannula is passed between the open ends of the hemostats. In the case of a cuffed tube, the cuff should be inflated to keep the cannula in place and the air sac inflated. The cannula can be maintained in place by using a piece of tape in a butterfly fashion or by using the Chinese finger knot technique. The latter method is done by placing a purse-string suture around the skin and cannula (leaving a large tail to the suture) and then wrapping the suture around the cannula, tying a knot after each pass around the circumference of the catheter for approximately 1 cm of the cannula. The patency of the cannula can be tested by holding a microscope slide up to the end of the cannula and watching for condensation on the slide with each respiration. Alternatively, the downy portion of a feather can be used to see if there is airflow in and out of the cannula. The exposed end of the cannula should be positioned so that it does not interfere with movement of the patient's leg.

Aspergillosis is a common mycotic disease in raptors that occurs more frequently in the golden eagle, goshawk, gyrfalcon, snowy owl, and immature red-tailed hawk [3,39]. Ubiquitous spores of *Aspergillus* species can infect immunocompromised raptors, those provided poor sanitation and husbandry, or raptors with other diseases. Disease may be acute, with extensive miliary granulomas throughout the lungs, or chronic, with formation of small to large granulomas in the tracheobronchial syrinx, lungs, pericardium, air sacs, and other organs [40]. Aspergillosis should be a differential diagnosis for any debilitated or emaciated raptor with respiratory abnormalities. Diagnostic tests that can aid in the diagnosis of aspergillosis include hematology, plasma biochemistry, radiography, serology, fungal culture, and polymerase chain reaction (PCR) [39]. Definitive diagnosis is with the use of endoscopy and cytologic fungal identification or culture. Treatment may be prolonged and may include systemic, topical, and nebulized antifungal agents. The prognosis for successful treatment is generally poor to guarded [39]. A complete review of clinical signs, diagnosis, and treatment of aspergillosis is highly recommended for the avian practitioner [3,5,12,39,41–44].

Respiratory difficulty or distress in raptors also occurs as a result of foreign body inhalation, inhaled toxins, and respiratory system trauma. If upper airway obstructive disease (tracheal) is not present, placement of

Table 1
Formulary of common emergency drugs used in raptors

Drug	Route and dosage	Comments
Aminophylline	4 mg/kg PO q 6–12 hours	Can give orally after initial response
	10 mg/kg IV q 3 hours	Use for pulmonary edema
Atropine sulfate	0.2–0.5 mg/kg IM, IV, IO	Bradycardia, CPR, organophosphate toxicity
Butorphanol	0.3–1 mg/kg IM	Opioid agonist-antagonist; doses >1 mg/kg may cause recumbency
Calcium EDTA	10–50 mg/kg IM q 12 hours for 5–10 days	Lead and zinc toxicity; maintain hydration and monitor for polyuria/polydypsea
Calcium gluconate	50–100 mg/kg IM, IV (slow bolus)	Hypocalcemia: dilute 50 mg/mL; hyperkalemia; facilitates potassium movement across cell membranes
Carprofen	2–5 mg/kg PO, SC, IM, IV q 12–24 hours	Analgesic, anti-inflammatory
Cefazolin	50–100 mg/kg PO, IM q 12 hours	First-generation cephalosporin
Charcoal, activated	52 mg/kg PO once	Adsorbs toxins from intestinal tract; component of oiled bird treatment
Dexamethasone sodium phosphate	2–6 mg/kg IM, IV (1 dose)	Shock; see text for contraindications concerning steroid use in avian species
Dextrose (50%)	50–100 mg/kg IV (slow bolus to effect)	Hypoglycemia; can dilute with fluids
	500–1000 mg/kg IV (slow bolus)	Hypoglycemia; can dilute with fluids
Dextran 70	10–20 mL/kg	Hypovolemic shock
Diazepam	0.5–1.0 mg/kg IM, IV prn	Seizures
Dimercaptosuccinic acid (DMSA)	25–35 mg/kg PO q 12 hours for 5 days per week for 3–5 weeks	Lead toxicity; may be effective for zinc and mercury toxicity; can use with calcium EDTA
Dimethylsulfoxide (DMSO) 90%	1 mL/kg topical to affected area q 4–7 days	Analgesic, anti-inflammatory; systemic absorption
Doxapram	5–10 mg/kg IM, IV once	Respiratory depression or arrest
	20 mg/kg IM, IV, IO	CPR; respiratory depression

Drug	Dose	Notes
Enrofloxacin	10–15 mg/kg PO, IM, IV q 12 hours	Broad-spectrum quinolone; IM formulation is alkaline (painful) and should not be given repeatedly; in general, avoid IV use in birds (IV administration in owls may result in weakness, tachycardia, vasoconstriction)
Epinephrine	0.5–1.0 mL/kg IM, IV, IO, IT	CPR; bradycardia
Fluids	10–25 mL/kg IV, IO	Bolus over 5–7 minutes
	50–90 mL/kg fluids SC, IV, IO	
Furosemide	2–5 mg/kg IM	Diuretic; overdose can cause dehydration and electrolyte abnormalities
Hemoglobin glutamer-200 (Oxyglobin)	10 mL/kg IV	Hemoglobin replacement product
Hetastarch	10–15 mL/kg IV (slow) q 8 hours for 1–4 treatments	Hypoproteinemia, hypovolemia
Itraconazole	5–10 mg/kg PO q 12–24 hours	Most species or systemic mycoses
Ketoprofen	2 mg/kg PO, SC, IM	Analgesia, anti-inflammatory
Mannitol	0.2–2.0 g/kg IV (slow) q 24 hours	Cerebral edema; anuric renal failure
Meloxicam	0.1–0.2 mg/kg PO, IM q 24 hours	Analgesia, anti-inflammatory
Metronidazole	50 mg/kg PO q 24 hours	Anaerobic activity; antiprotozoal
Midazolam	0.5–1.0 mg/kg IM, IV q 8 hours	Sedation
Penicillamine	30–55 mg/kg PO q 12 hours for 7–14 days	Lead, zinc toxicity; preferred chelator for copper toxicity; may be used for mercury toxicity
Phenobarbital	—	
Pralidoxime (2-PAM)	10–100 mg/kg IM q 24–48 hours or repeat once in 6 hours	Administer within 24–36 hours of organophosphate intoxication; use lower dose in combination with atropine
Prednisolone sodium succinate	15–30 mg/kg IV	Head trauma; CPR (see text for contraindications concerning steroid use in avian species)
Silver sulfadiazine	Topical q 12–24 hours	Burns, ulcers
Sodium bicarbonate	1 mEq/kg q 15–30 minutes to maximum of 4 mEq/kg total dose	Metabolic acidosis
	5 mEq/kg IV, IO once	CPR

(continued on next page)

Table 1 (*continued*)

Drug	Route and dosage	Comments
Terbinafine	10–15 mg/kg PO q 12–24 hours	Mycotic infections; can be used in combination with itraconazole
Terbutaline	0.01 mg/kg IM q 6–8 hours 0.01 mg/kg with saline, 9 mL, q 6–8 hours nebulization	Inhaled toxin
Ticarcillin/clavulanic acid	200 mg/kg IM, IV q 12 hours	Extended-spectrum penicillin
Vitamin K₁	0.2–2.2 mg/kg IM q 4–8 hours until stable, then q 24 hours PO, IM for 14–28 days	Rodenticide toxicity

Abbreviations: CPR, cardiopulmonary resuscitation; EDTA, ethylenediaminetetraacetic acid; IM, intramuscular; IO, intraosseous; IT, intratracheal; IV, intravenous; PO, by mouth; prn, as needed; q, every; SC, subcutaneous.

Data from Huckabee J. Raptor therapeutics. Vet Clin North Am Exot Anim Pract 2000;3:91–116; and Pollock C, Carpenter J, Antinoff N. Birds. In: Carpenter J, editor. Exotic animal formulary. 3rd edition St. Louis (MO): Elsevier; 2005. p. 135–314.

an air sac cannula may not benefit the bird. The bird should be placed in an incubator with oxygen. A bronchodilator (terbutaline) and sedation (butorphanol and midazolam) to relieve anxiety can be administered intramuscularly. Radiographs and endoscopy may be needed to determine the extent of disease after the bird is stabilized. Respiratory distress associated with inhaled toxic fumes and environmental pollutants occurs in wild and captive raptors [5]. In cases of suspected inhalation toxicosis, immediate oxygen support is ideal and saline nebulization can also be beneficial. Bronchodilators, such as terbutaline (Brethine; Novartis Pharmaceuticals Corporation, East Hanover, New Jersey), are initially given intramuscularly to birds showing signs of respiratory distress from an inhalant toxin exposure (ie, pollen, polytetrafluoroethylene, cigarette smoke, hypersensitivity syndrome) [45]. Repeated use of the bronchodilator can be continued parentally or with use of a nebulizer. The prognosis for respiratory toxicosis may vary from good to grave depending on the extent and severity of the toxins. Tracheal surgery may be necessary in cases of tracheal trauma or rupture causing subcutaneous emphysema. Juvenile and adult raptors may incur tracheal or air sac trauma from predator attack, a fall from the nest, or other trauma. The accumulation of subcutaneous air may result in respiratory compromise. Subcutaneous emphysema can be relieved by fine-needle aspiration or by creation of a small skin incision that is sutured to the body wall and left open to allow healing of the air sac before healing of the skin.

Toxin exposure

Wild and captive raptors are susceptible to the toxic effects of heavy metal, pesticides, oil, and other environmental contaminants. General treatment of toxicity should include removal of the offending agent when feasible, supportive care, and treatment of clinical signs. When the toxicant is known, a specific antidote should also be given if possible. The prognosis for raptor intoxication can vary from good to grave depending on amount and time of toxin exposure and type of intoxication. All raptors with suspected toxicosis should receive a complete necropsy, with results reported to local and regional US Fish and Wildlife Service (FWS) authorities.

Raptors may be shot or ingest metal. Heavy metal poisoning is common in raptors and may result in a variety of signs, including regurgitation, weight loss, neurologic signs, and death [3,5]. Radiographs and determination of blood lead and zinc levels can assist in diagnosis. The clinician is reminded that evidence of metal opacity in radiographs does not ensure the diagnosis of lead or zinc toxicity. Numerous metallic opacities in the gastrointestinal tract on radiographs with clinical signs of metal toxicity make the diagnosis more likely, however. Treatment involves supportive care with fluids to ensure hydration and heavy metal chelators. Surgical removal or endoscopy may be required when metal pieces are not passed in the stool [3,5]. Mercury poisoning occurs in fish-eating raptors, causing weakness, weight loss, and incoordination [5]. Pesticide exposure, including herbicides, rodenticides, and insecticides, causes disease in raptorial species [3,5]. Blood acetylcholinesterase level determination is available for use in determining organophosphate exposure. Atropine and supportive care, including anticonvulsants and pralidoxime (2-PAM), can be used to treat anticholinesterase (organophosphate) toxicity [5]. Vitamin K therapy is indicated in cases of suspected rodenticide ingestion. Venipuncture should be limited in cases of suspected rodenticide intoxication to limit blood loss. Birds with rodenticide ingestion may present with anemia, subcutaneous hemorrhage, or intracavity bleeding.

Oil-contaminated birds may present with respiratory distress, seizures, hypothermia, hypoglycemia, anemia, hypoproteinemia, or lethargy [46,47]. Organ dysfunction is common with petroleum product intoxication; thus, determination of plasma biochemistry or bile acids is followed to assess liver and kidney function. Treatment is based on immediate oil removal and supportive care, including thermal support, fluid therapy, nutritional support, and treatment of secondary disease. Stabilized birds should have oil removed from feathers using dishwashing detergent (Dawn Liquid Dishwashing Detergent; Proctor and Gamble, Cincinnati, Ohio) in warm-water baths (106°F). Water should be softened to 2 to 3 grains of hardness to allow complete removal of oil and prevent crystallization in the feathers, which could result in lack of waterproofing [46]. Thorough rinsing is necessary to ensure complete oil and soap removal [46,47]. Repeat washings because of incomplete removal of soap or oil are associated with increased mortality [46].

Emaciated birds

Emaciation is a common presentation in young raptors that have not learned to hunt prey successfully or in birds facing harsh winter conditions. Emaciated raptors have a body condition score of 1/5 as determined by a near lack of palpable pectoral musculature, and these patients cannot readily digest whole-prey items. Clinical findings can vary in emaciated raptors but commonly include anemia and hypoproteinemia. The emaciated raptor should be fed items devoid of casting material, such as fur and feathers (see section on nutritional support). Replacement fluid therapy is critical in the first 12 to 24 hours before nutritional support is instituted. Intravenous or intraosseous administration of colloid or crystalloid fluid is given; hetastarch or whole-blood transfusions may be necessary in cases of severe hypoproteinemia or anemia. Supplemental heat or oxygen may also be beneficial for the debilitated bird (see the section on nutritional support for more detailed information on feeding debilitated raptors). Because these birds are compromised, supportive care, including antibiotic or antifungal therapy, may be indicated.

Other emergency presentations

Other common causes of emergency presentations of raptors include bacterial, viral, or parasitic infection; hypoglycemia; gastrointestinal stasis or foreign body ingestion; seizures; frostbite; and metabolic bone disease from malnutrition. Raptors are susceptible to *Pasteurella multocida* and sepsis from other gram-negative bacteria from predator bites. Emergency stabilization, supportive care, and broad-spectrum antibiotic therapy (eg, ticarcillin/clavulanic acid and enrofloxacin therapy) are indicated. In case of seizures, intramuscular administration of midazolam or intravenous administration of diazepam can be used. If the seizures cannot be controlled in this manner, phenobarbital (4 mg/kg administered intramuscularly or intravenously) is given every 20 minutes for two doses and then continued orally at a rate of 2 mg/kg every 12 hours. When anticonvulsant therapy is unable to control the seizures, the raptor can be placed under isoflurane or sevoflurane inhalant anesthesia until the phenobarbital takes effect (eg, 15–30 minutes). Appropriate diagnostics (including blood work and radiographs) are indicated once the patient is stable to determine the type and extent of disease. Detailed discussions of diagnosis and therapy for diseases affecting raptorial species are available [2,3,5,12,13,48,49]. Practitioners working with raptors should be aware of the potential for birds of prey to transmit zoonotic diseases, including mycobacteriosis, rabies virus, chlamydophilosis, salmonellosis, and viral encephalitides [50].

Euthanasia

Regional FWS offices are listed on the Internet [51] and must be consulted before euthanasia of any threatened, endangered, or native eagle species. Raptors can be euthanized by administration of intravenous euthanasia solution. Alternatively, raptors can be anesthetized and then given euthanasia solution into the occipital sinus or by means of intracardiac injection. Practitioners should be aware of guidelines regulating captive maintenance of raptors [1]. Any wild bird that is completely blind and any bird that has sustained injuries that would require amputation of a leg, a foot, or a wing above the cubital joint should be euthanized unless special permission has been granted [1]. Veterinarians are permitted to euthanize raptors based on welfare, nonreleasability, or poor prognosis without any additional licensure. Clients bringing in injured raptors should sign a release form that gives the veterinarian permission for any necessary treatment, including euthanasia.

Summary

Raptorial species should be quickly assessed on emergency presentation to determine the best approach for care. Restraint techniques and approach to care may vary depending on whether the bird is used for falconry or presents from the wild. Common causes of emergent raptor presentations include trauma, respiratory disease, toxin exposure, and emaciation. Treatment should be aimed at stabilizing the patient and providing a low-stress environment to help facilitate rapid recovery and rehabilitation. Raptor patients benefit from supportive care, including thermal, fluid, and nutritional support. Administration of cardiopulmonary cerebral resuscitation, antibiotics, antifungals, and analgesics is appropriate for raptors through a variety of routes. Humane euthanasia may be indicated depending on the severity of disease and prognosis for recovery.

References

[1] Code of Federal Regulations 50:21 specific permit provisions: rehabilitation permits. Available at: http://www.fws.gov/permits/ltr/ltr.shtml. Accessed April 24, 2006.
[2] Heatley J, Marks S, Mitchell M, et al. Raptor emergency and critical care: assessment and examination. Compendium. 2001;23(5):442–8.
[3] Samour J. Management of raptors. In: Harrison G, Lightfoot T, editors. Clinical avian medicine, vol. 2. Palm Beach (FL): Spix Publishing; 2006. p. 915–56.
[4] DragonHoods Falconry Products. Available at: http://www.dragonhoods.com/. Accessed May 1, 2006.
[5] Joseph V. Emergency care of raptors. Vet Clin North Am Exot Anim Pract 1998;1(1):77–98.
[6] Lichtenberger M. Principles of shock and fluid therapy in special species. Seminars in Avian and Exotic Pet Medicine 2004;13(3):142–53.
[7] Lichtenberger M. Determination of indirect blood pressure in the companion bird. Seminars in Avian and Exotic Pet Medicine 2005;14(2):149–52.
[8] Quesenberry K, Hillyer E. Supportive care and emergency therapy. In: Ritchie B, Harrison G, Harrison L, editors. Avian medicine: principles and application. Lake Worth (FL): Wingers Publishing; 1994. p. 382–416.
[9] Lumeij J, Ritchie B. Cardiovascular system. In: Ritchie B, Harrison G, Harrison L, editors. Avian medicine: principles and application. Lake Worth (FL): Winger's Publishing, Inc.; 1994. p. 694–722.
[10] Pees M, Krautwald-Junghanns M, Straub J. Evaluating and treating the cardiovascular system. In: Harrison G, Lightfoot T, editors. Clinical avian medicine, vol. 1. Palm Beach (FL): Spix Publishing; 2006. p. 379–94.
[11] Jones M, Pollock C. Supportive care and shock. In: Olsen G, Orosz S, editors. Manual of avian medicine. St. Louis (MO): Mosby, Inc.; 2000. p. 17–46.
[12] Huckabee J. Raptor therapeutics. Vet Clin North Am Exot Anim Pract 2000;3:91–116.
[13] Heatley J, Marks S, Mitchell M, et al. Raptor emergency and critical care: therapy and techniques. Compendium 2001;23(6):561–70.
[14] Ritchie B, Otto C, Latimer K, et al. A technique of intraosseous cannulation for intravenous therapy in birds. Compendium 1990;12:55–9.
[15] Morrisey J. Transfusion medicine in birds: Western Veterinary Conference 2004. Veterinary Information Network Online Proceedings. Available at: http://www.vin.com/Members/Proceedings/Proceedings.plx?CID=wvc2004&PID=pr05739&O=VIN. Accessed May 1, 2006.
[16] Finnegan M, Daniel G, Ramsay E. Evaluation of whole blood transfusions in domestic pigeons (*Columba livia*). J Avian Med Surg 1997;11(1):7–14.
[17] Clippinger T. Diseases of the lower respiratory tract of companion birds. Seminars in Avian and Exotic Pet Medicine. 1997;6(4):201–8.

[18] Graham J. Approach to the dyspneic avian patient. Seminars in Avian and Exotic Pet Medicine. 2004;13(3):154–9.
[19] Harris D. Therapeutic avian techniques. Seminars in Avian and Exotic Pet Medicine 1997; 6(2):55–62.
[20] Costello M. Principles of cardiopulmonary cerebral resuscitation in special species. Seminars in Avian and Exotic Pet Medicine 2004;13(2):132–41.
[21] Hawkins M, Wright B, Pascoe P, et al. Pharmacokinetics and anesthetic and cardiopulmonary effects of propofol in red-tailed hawks (Buteo jamaicensis) and great horned owls (Bubo virginianus). Am J Vet Res 2003;64(6):677–83.
[22] Edling T. Updates in anesthesia and monitoring. In: Harrison G, Lightfoot T, editors. Clinical avian medicine, vol. 2. Palm Beach (FL): Spix Publishing; 2006. p. 747–60.
[23] Campbell T. Hematology. In: Ritchie B, Harrison G, Harrison L, editors. Avian medicine: principles and application. Lake Worth (FL): Wingers Publishing; 1994. p. 176–98.
[24] Burke H, Swaim S, Amalsadvala T. Review of wound management in raptors. J Avian Med Surg 2002;16(3):180–91.
[25] Harcourt-Brown N. Foot and leg problems. In: Beynon P, Forbes N, Harcourt-Brown N, editors. Manual of raptors, pigeons, and waterfowl. Cheltenham (UK): British Small Animal Vet Assoc, Ltd; 1996. p. 147–68.
[26] Harcourt-Brown N. Bumblefoot. In: Samour J, editor. Avian medicine. London: Harcourt Publishers, Ltd; 2000. p. 126–31.
[27] Redig P. Fractures. In: Samour J, editor. Avian medicine. London: Harcourt Publishers, Ltd; 2000. p. 131–65.
[28] Remple J. Raptor bumblefoot: a new treatment technique. In: Redig P, Cooper J, Remple D, et al, editors. Raptor biomedicine. Minneapolis (MN): University of Minnesota Press; 1993. p. 154–60.
[29] Remple J, Forbes N, et al. Antibiotic-impregnated beads in the treatment of bumblefoot in raptors. In: Lumeij J, Remple J, Redig P, et al, editors. Raptor biomedicine III. Lake Worth (FL): Zoological Education Network; 2000. p. 255–63.
[30] Riddle K, Hoolihan J. Form-fitting, composite-casting method for avian appendages. In: Redig P, Cooper J, Remple D, editors. Raptor biomedicine. Minneapolis (MN): University of Minnesota Press; 1993. p. 161–4.
[31] Ferrell S, Graham J, Swaim S. Avian wound healing and management. In: Proceedings of the Annual Conference of the Association of Avian Veterinarians. Monterey; 2002. p. 337–47.
[32] Redig P. Nursing avian patients. In: Beynon P, Forbes N, Harcourt-Brown N, editors. Manual of raptors, pigeons, and waterfowl. Cheltenham (UK): British Small Animal Vet Assoc Ltd; 1996. p. 42–6.
[33] Clubb S, Paul-Murphy J, Fudge A, et al. Pain management in clinical practice. J Avian Med Surg. 1998;12(4):276–8.
[34] Pollock C, Carpenter J, Antinoff N. Birds. In: Carpenter J, editor. Exotic animal formulary. 3rd edition. St. Louis (MO): Elsevier; 2005. p. 135–314.
[35] Westerhof I, Brom Vd, Mol J. Responsiveness of the glucocorticoid-suppressed pituitary-adrenocortical system of pigeons (Columba livia domestica) to stimulation with arginine vasopressin. Avian Dis 1995;40:312–20.
[36] Andrew S, Clippinger T, Brooks D, et al. Penetrating keratoplasty for treatment of corneal protrusion in a great horned owl (Bubo virginianus). Vet Ophthalmol 2002;5(3):201–5.
[37] Korbel R. Investigations into intraocular injection of recombinant tissue plasminogen activator (rTPA) for the treatment of trauma-induced intraocular hemorrhages in birds. In: Proceedings of the Annual Conference of the Association of Avian Veterinarians. Pittsburgh; 2003. p. 97.
[38] Haas D. Clinical signs and treatment of large birds injured by electrocution. In: Redig P, Cooper J, Remple D, editors. Raptor biomedicine. Minneapolis (MN): University of Minnesota Press; 1993. p. 180.
[39] Jones M. Selected infectious diseases of birds of prey. Journal of Exotic Pet Medicine 2006; 15(1):5–17.

[40] Redig P. Fungal diseases. In: Samour J, editor. Avian medicine. London: Harcourt Publishers Ltd; 2000. p. 275–87.
[41] Deem S. Fungal diseases of birds of prey. Vet Clin North Am Exot Anim Pract 2003;6(2): 363–76.
[42] Dahlhausen R. Implications of mycoses in clinical disorders. In: Harrison G, Lightfoot T, editors. Clinical avian medicine, vol. II. Palm Beach(FL): Spix Publishing; 2006. p. 691–704.
[43] Jones M. The diagnosis of aspergillosis in birds. Seminars in Avian and Exotic Pet Medicine 2000;9:52–8.
[44] Langenberg J. Emerging antifungals and the use of voriconazole with amphotericin to treat aspergillosis. In: Proceedings of the Annual Conference of the Association of Avian Veterinarians. New Orleans; 2004. p. 21–4.
[45] Lichtenberger M. Treatment of respiratory inhalant toxins in 4 psittacine birds. In: Proceedings of the Annual Conference of the Association of Avian Veterinarians. Pittsburgh; 2003. p. 39–43.
[46] Mazet J, Newman S, Gilardi K, et al. Advances in oiled bird emergency medicine and management. J Avian Med Surg 2002;16(2):146–9.
[47] Richardson J. Implications of toxic substances in clinical disorders. In: Harrison G, Lightfoot T, editors. Clinical avian medicine volume II. Palm Beach (FL): Spix Publishing; 2006. p. 711–9.
[48] Deem S. Raptor medicine: basic principles and noninfectious conditions. Compendium of Continuing Education for the Practicing Veterinarian 1999;21(4):205–15.
[49] Deem S. Infectious and parasitic diseases of raptors. Compendium of Continuing Education for the Practicing Veterinarian 1999;21(3):329–38.
[50] Carpenter J, Gentz E, et al. Zoonotic disease of avian origin. In: Altman R, Clubb S, Dorrestein G, editors. Avian medicine and surgery. Philadelphia: WB Saunders; 1997. p. 350–63.
[51] US Fish and Wildlife Service Regional Boundaries. Available at: http://www.fws.gov/where/. Accessed May 1, 2006.

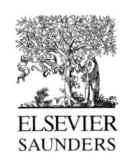

Bandaging, Endoscopy, and Surgery in the Emergency Avian Patient

Will Chavez, DVM[a],
M. Scott Echols, DVM, DABVP-Avian[b],*

[a]*Private Practice, West Hills, CA, USA*
[b]*Westgate Pet and Bird Hospital, 4534 Westgate Boulevard, Suite 100, Austin, TX 78745, USA*

Birds are commonly brought into the hospital with an emergency requiring initial stabilization (see the article by Lichtenberger elsewhere in this issue) and analgesia (see the article by Lichtenberger and Ko elsewhere in this issue). Bandaging includes soft bandage material and splints applied for temporary support or permanent fixation of fractures. The second part of this article describes diagnostic procedures using endoscopy to examine the oral cavity and internal organs. The third part of the article discusses placement of a feeding tube, air sac cannulation, and emergency surgical procedures. Review of special equipment required should enable the veterinarian to perform successful basic surgical procedures.

Bandaging techniques

Bandaging techniques are useful in stabilizing traumatic injuries, fractures, and intravenous and intraosseous catheters. The avian leg is anatomically similar to the mammalian leg, except for the tarsometatarsus of the foot. It is difficult to immobilize femoral fractures with external fixation alone. The cardinal rule of splinting must always be followed: to immobilize the joint above and below the fracture. Bandaging material should be soft and pliable as cast padding for the initial layer, followed by the application of a self-adherent bandage (Vetwrap; 3M Company Animal Care Products, St. Paul, Minnesota) for the outer layer. The bandage can be reinforced, when necessary, with wooden splints, aluminum rods, or human orthopedic products, such as Orthoplast (Johnson & Johnson Products, New

* Corresponding author.
E-mail address: spotdvm@aol.com (M.S. Echols).

Brunswick, New Jersey) or Hexcelite (Hexcel Medical Company, Dublin, California) [1]. At room temperature, Hexcelite and Orthoplast are firm, but after they are placed in hot water, they can be made to conform to the shape of a bird's limb. Water-miscible ointments are applied to the skin over wounds. Oil-based ointments should be avoided because they inhibit normal thermoregulatory function of the feathers. Semiocclusive bandages (Teguderm; 3M Company Animal Care Products) are useful for abrasions and self-induced traumatic lesions [1].The rectangular sheets are cut into strips before removing the opposite backing material. Most simple midshaft fractures heal within 3 weeks in the avian patient [2]. Other fractures may require 4 to 6 weeks to heal. Open fractures and comminuted fractures must be given a guarded prognosis. Open fractures should be treated with antibiotics. The clinician should advise the owner of the bird to use smooth-sided cages without perches (aquarium or plastic carrier) to prevent climbing during the healing period. As a note, joints bound too long with a bandage may develop decreased range of motion. Splinted or otherwise bandaged birds should be regularly evaluated by an avian veterinarian.

Tape splint

Tarsometatarsal fractures are easily diagnosed by palpation and can be supported with the use of a tape splint in birds weighing less than 300 g (Fig. 1). For larger birds, a Thomas splint, a bandage incorporating support material (eg, modified Robert Jones bandage), or surgical fixation is recommended. The tape splint should include a stirrup passing longitudinally down the lateral tarsometatarsus under the foot and back up the medial side [1].Overlapping strips of adhesive tape are placed laterally and medially in a horizontal fashion, with the sticky side toward the limb, beginning just proximal to the stifle and continuing distal to immobilize the hock. The tape is pressed together with a hemostat on each side of the leg. Several layers are necessary to give strength to the splint. Alternatively, a thin band of Vetwrap can be placed over the leg with tape applied as discussed previously. Obviously, care must be taken when removing tape bandages.

"Football" type bandage

The "football" type bandage is used to immobilize toes. A large ball of soft gauze is placed within the grasp of the foot (Fig. 2). The toes are then bound to this ball by wrapping more gauze over and around them. The whole ball may be taped to the foot. The bird may be able to bear weight on it.

Plastic spica bandage

Plastic splints can be used for simple aligned fractures of the femur in birds weighing less than 300 g. A splint can be molded from the human orthopedic

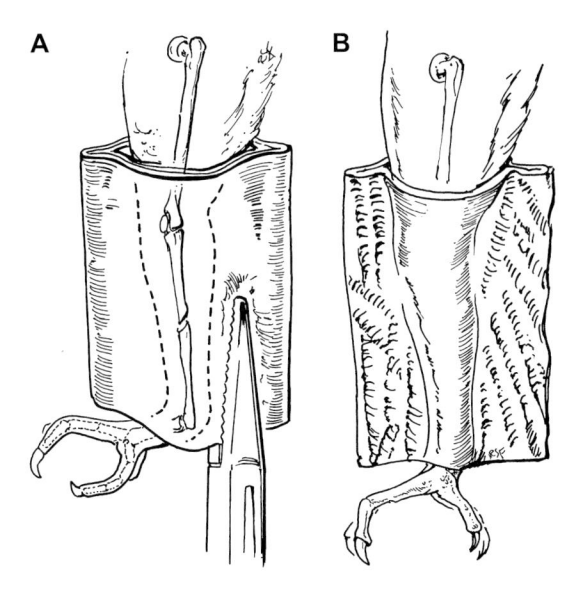

Fig. 1. Tape splint. A tape splint is used for fractures of the tibia and proximal tarsometatarsus. The tape is wrapped around the bird's leg to keep the fractured segments in apposition. (*A*) Tibiotarsal-tarsometatarsal joint is flexed in the normal standing position for the species, and the tape is crimped with a hemostat. (*B*) Tape is crimped as close as possible to the muscles surrounding the tibia. With proper angulation of the tibiotarsal-tarsometatarsal joint, the bird can perch in a normal standing position. Alternatively, a thin band of Vetwrap can be placed over the leg first and tape applied as described previously. The addition of Vetwrap can make later tape removal less traumatic. (*From* Altman RB, Clubb SL, Dorrestine GM, et al, editors. Avian medicine and surgery. Philadelphia: WB Saunders; 1997; with permission.)

products or padded aluminum finger splints (Fig. 3). This splint is a modification of a Robert Jones bandage, except that the padded molded splint extends from the tibiotarsus proximally and over the bird's pelvis in an inverted U-shape to immobilize the femur against the body of the bird.

Modified Robert Jones bandage

The Robert Jones bandage should be limited to any fracture of tibiotarsus or soft tissue injuries of the hock joint or distal. This bandage is used in birds weighing less than 500 g [1,3]. First, cut the Orthoplast in an L-shape. The size of the arms of the "L" need to be adjusted for differently sized birds. Hold the leg in a functional position, and make the vertical portion of the "L" as long as the tibiotarsus. The horizontal portion should be as long as the tarsometatarsus, and the last portion is used to wrap around the foot for stability. Next, place a layer of padding material around the leg from the foot up to just above the stifle. Follow the cast padding with a layer of cling or cotton gauze, tightening gently while wrapping. Then, heat the thermoplastic splint in hot water until it becomes clear and malleable. Position the splint along the lateral aspect of the leg, and wrap the final layer of Vetwrap around the material before the

Step 1 **Step 2**

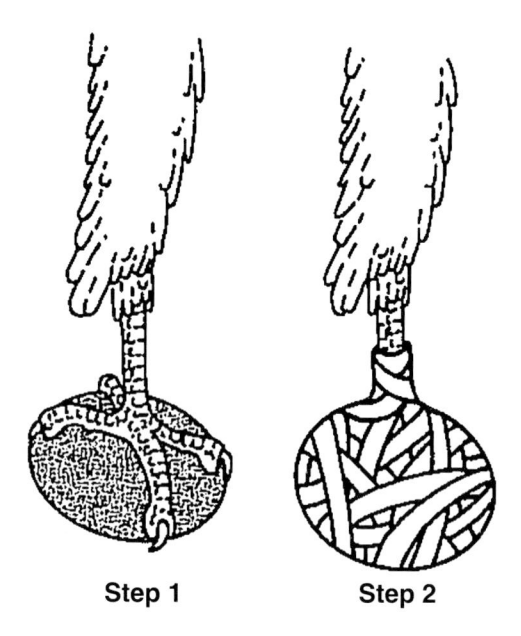

Fig. 2. "Football" splint. This splint is used for immobilization of the toes. (*Step 1*) A large ball of soft gauze is placed within the grasp of the foot. (*Step 2*) The toes are then bound to the ball by wrapping gauze over and around them. Tape is then placed over the gauze. (*From* Kirk RW, editor. Current veterinary therapy VII. Philadelphia; WB Saunders; 1980. p. 664; with permission.)

splint hardens. If the Orthoplast splint does not conform properly, simply replace it in the hot water until it becomes malleable again.

Schroeder-Thomas splint

The use of a Schroeder-Thomas splint is limited to fractures of the tarsometatarsus and distal one third of the tibiotarsus (Fig. 4) [1–3]. Indications for these splints include fractures of the tarsometatarsus in small psittacine birds (bone is too small for any orthopedic repair) and fractures close to the hock. This bandage should not be used in fractures of the femur and proximal two thirds of the tibiotarsus. The wire material used in the splint should be made with two right-angled bends next to the ring at the top so that the splint is parallel to the long axis of the leg. Position the leg so that there is some flexion at the hock joint. A light bandage is applied to the leg with gauze and tape. The leg is suspended within the splint by alternating strips of tape placed cranially and caudally, with the toes extended to the end of the splint. The splint is covered with bandage material. The fracture healing should occur over 4 to 6 weeks, and the bandage should be changed every other week [1–3].

Ehmer type bandage

The leg can be placed in an Ehmer sling like the kind used in a dog or cat. The tarsometatarsus can be folded against the tibia, and gauze can be

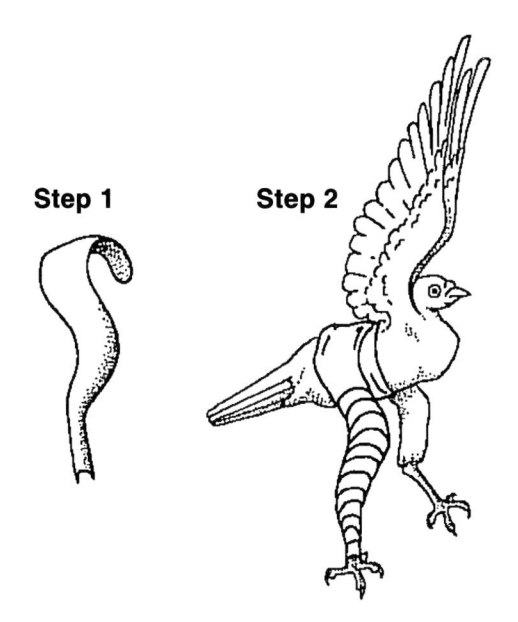

Fig. 3. Plastic leg splint or spica. This splint is used for immobilization of the stifle, femur, and hip. The plastic leg splint is made of Orthoplast or Hexcelite. (*Step 1*) The splint is heated in water and then shaped to fit laterally over the thigh with a curved "tongue" that extends over the back behind the wings. (*Step 2*) The leg is wrapped with cotton padding, and the splint is fit over the cotton. The splint is covered with tape or Vetwrap. (*From* Kirk RW, editor. Current veterinary therapy VII. Philadelphia: WB Saunders; 1980. p. 664; with permission.)

wrapped around both of them. If necessary, they can be bound to the body (Fig. 5). This bandage can be used for a dislocated hip or for temporary stabilization of fractures involving the leg.

Figure-of-eight bandage

The patient with wing fractures commonly presents with a dropped wing. Some fractures heal well after treatment with external coaptation, with return to full function. Bandages can be used for wing fractures in birds not required to return to full flight (aviary and cage birds). The wing is especially amendable to splinting because it can be splinted in the normal physiologic position. A figure-of-eight bandage provides adequate stabilization for fractures of the radius and ulna, carpometacarpus, and digits (Fig. 6) [1–3]. This bandage is also effective for some fractures of the pectoral girdle and humerus when used in conjunction with a body wrap [1–3]. This bandage is easier to place in sedated patients, especially psittacines. You may need to trim the bandage material to 1-inch-wide strips for small patients. Hold the wing in a normal flexed position away from the body, with primary and secondary wing feathers parallel to each other as the carpus is flexed. Incorporate all scapular feathers (those growing from the bird's shoulder) into the bandage. Apply a layer of cast

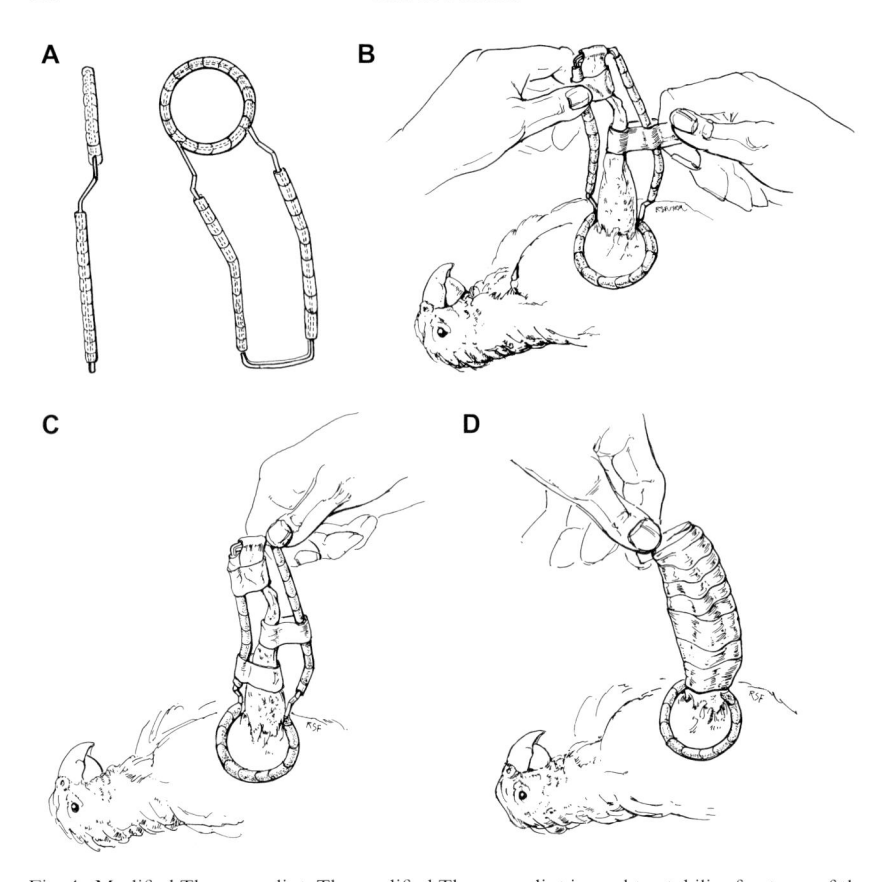

Fig. 4. Modified Thomas splint. The modified Thomas splint is used to stabilize fractures of the tarsometatarsus and distal one third of the tibiotarsus. (*A*) Wire is bent, shaped, and padded to conform to the bird's leg. (*B, C*) Leg is placed through the loop of the splint. (*B*) Distal end of the foot is transfixed to the splint. Gauze or tape is wrapped around the leg to maintain proper alignment of the fracture fragments. (*D*) Tape or Vetwrap is placed around the splint, covering the leg. (*From* Altman RB, Clubb SL, Dorrestine GM, et al, editors. Avian medicine and surgery. Philadelphia: WB Saunders; 1997; with permission.)

padding or light gauze wrap, beginning as high in the axilla as possible on the medial aspect of the humerus. Continue the wrap on the dorsal surface of the wing up to the carpus, and then circle the carpus from a lateral to medial direction, ending on the ventral portion of the carpus. Pass the bandage along the ventral wing surface from the carpus and back to the axillary region. Repeat this cycle until the wing is held lightly but securely in a flexed position. Avoid excessive layering because this causes a bulky and uncomfortable bandage. The gauze or cast padding should be covered with a layer of Vetwrap or similar material. To form a body wrap, use the padding material to hold the wrapped wing next to the body in a natural position. The padding is placed around the body and under the opposite wing at the axillary region. It may

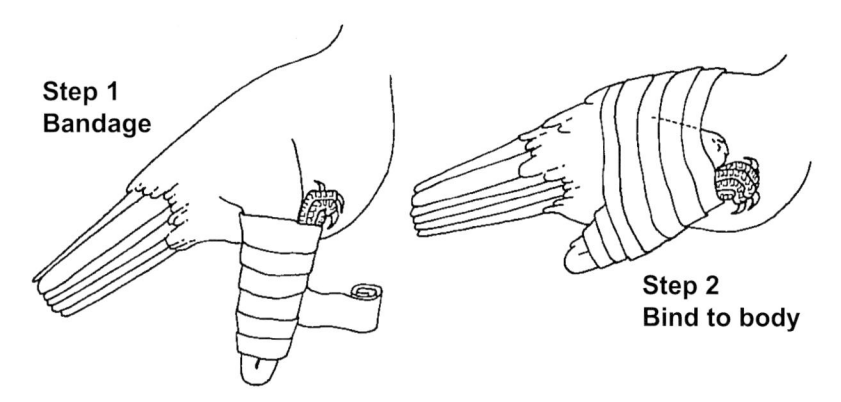

Fig. 5. Ehmer-type sling. This bandage can be used temporarily for fractures of the leg. (*Step 1*) Bind the tarsometatarsus to the tibia. (*Step 2*) Bind the folded leg to the body. (*From* Kirk RW, editor. Current veterinary therapy VII. Philadelphia: WB Saunders; 1980. p. 665; with permission.)

help to place the body wrap bandage material cranial and caudal to the opposite wing, forming a vest. Follow the padding layer with a thin layer of Vetwrap or similar material. Be careful that the caudal extent of the ventral portion of the body wrap does not interfere with leg movement.

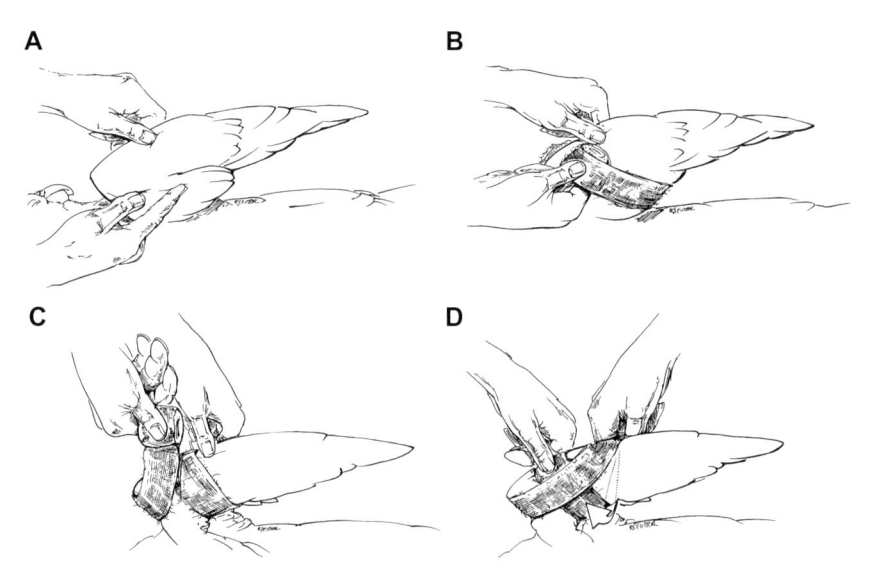

Fig. 6. Figure-of-eight bandage splint. The figure-of-eight bandage can be used for fractures of the wing distal to the humerus. With fractures of the humerus or shoulder girdle, the wing needs to be bandaged to the body. (*A*) Wing is held in its normal flexed position. (*B*) Gauze is wrapped around the ventral aspect of the humerus and brought over the dorsal aspect of the wing. (*C*) Gauze is then wrapped over the humeroradioulnar joint and around the carpus. (*D*) Gauze is then brought under the wing and wrapped back over the dorsum and under the humerus. (*From* Altman RB, Clubb SL, Dorrestine GM, et al, editors. Avian medicine and surgery. Philadelphia: WB Saunders; 1997; with permission.)

Endoscopy

Endoscopy equipment

Endoscopes are fiberoptic probes that use magnification to facilitate visual inspection of the oral cavity, trachea, gastrointestinal tract, and coelomic cavity. The basic equipment for avian endoscopy is a light source, a fiberoptic cable, and a small-diameter endoscope. The 2.7-mm diameter rigid scope can be used for tracheal examination in patients larger than the Amazon bird and for coelomic evaluation of most psittacines and passerines [4–7]. The upper gastrointestinal system of birds as small as cockatiels and as large as macaws may also be explored with this sized scope. The 2.7-mm endoscope has a 5-French instrument channel for placement of 5-French biopsy or grasping forceps [5–7].

Tracheal/upper respiratory endoscopic evaluation

The most common use of emergency endoscopy is for the avian patient presented with upper airway obstruction (see the articles on avian and raptor emergency elsewhere in this issue). The bird with acute respiratory distress attributable to upper airway obstruction requires anesthesia for placement of an air sac tube, as described elsewhere in this article in the section on surgical procedures. Ideally, after placement of the air sac tube, endoscopic examination of the trachea and syrinx for removal of a foreign body (eg, seed in a trachea, diagnostic sampling [eg, aspergillosis granulomas]) is recommended.

Keeping the head and neck straight to accommodate the rigid scope easily, insert the tip of the scope into the glottis. Gently advance the rigid scope, making sure that the trachea can properly accommodate it without causing significant trauma to the tracheal lumen. The trachea often narrows as it approaches the lungs, and this may ultimately make it difficult to reach the tracheal bifurcation. If the scope cannot be advanced the full length of the trachea, keeping the neck straight allows the light to illuminate several centimeters beyond the tip of the scope. If an obstruction is discovered, a decision needs to be made whether there is a possibility of removing it with additional endoscopic instrumentation. The endoscopic sheath increases the diameter size significantly. If the sheathed endoscope can advance to the obstruction site, flexible forceps can be advanced within the lumen of the sheath. Advance 5-French endoscopic grasping forceps to grasp the object and gently extract it. If the obstruction is attributable to an abnormal tissue growth or infectious granuloma, advance 5-French endoscopic biopsy forceps and gently tease or dislodge the obstructive mass. Extreme care must be taken not to lacerate the trachea or damage the surface, which can lead to stricture formation. If a sheathed endoscope cannot be advanced, use of a red rubber tube and suction to remove the foreign material can be attempted. Tracheotomy may be the last consideration.

The choanal/inner nasal area can also be evaluated endoscopically. Seeds and abscesses may obstruct the nasal area.

Upper gastrointestinal endoscopic evaluation

Foreign body ingestion is a common indication for endoscopy. If the foreign body is present in the crop, it is easily removed with the help of an endoscope and graspers or by means of an ingluviotomy. If the foreign body has already traveled to the proventriculus or ventriculus, depending on the bird's length, rigid endoscopy may still be a viable option. In larger birds, such as large macaws, a rigid endoscope does not adequately reach the proventriculus if introducing the scope through the oral cavity. Alternatively, the endoscope can be introduced through an incision made at the base of the crop, bypassing the head and proximal esophagus. A sheathed endoscope with 5-French endoscopic forceps is used to extract the foreign body gently. Care must be taken to position the object to be removed in a fashion that is least likely to result in trauma to the gastric lumen while the object being removed. Irrigation or air insufflation of the proventriculus may be necessary to obtain better visualization of the gastric lumen.

Coelomic endoscopy

Endoscopy of the coelomic cavity may be used to perform diagnostic and surgical techniques that avoid unnecessary surgery. Coelomic endoscopy is recommended for use in the stable patient and should not be performed as an emergency procedure. Coelomic endoscopy should be performed by an experienced avian veterinarian. Coelomic endoscopy is used to examine gonads and follicular development, air sacs, and lungs. Samples may be taken for biopsy and for fungal or bacteriologic culture. Other organs that can be visualized and biopsied are the liver, kidney, adrenals, spleen, and intestines.

Surgical procedures

Thorough patient evaluation is extremely important in the exotic pet prior to surgery. The exotic patient needs to be stabilized before and during anesthesia and surgery (see the article by Lichtenberger elsewhere in this issue). Anesthetic and analgesic protocols are given in the article by Lichtenberger and Ko elsewhere in this issue.

Avian patients are usually fasted for 3 to 4 hours before surgery. Birds commonly aspirate food and fluids that may seep up from the crop through the relatively wide proximal esophagus. Depending on the consistency of the crop contents, the food may be removed with a metal gavage or red rubber or feeding tube.

Ideally, all avian patients should be anesthetized, intubated, and monitored while undergoing preparation for surgery (see the article by Lichtenberger and Ko elsewhere in this issue). Birds need the feathers plucked from the intended surgical site. Feathers in most birds grow in tracts or pterylae, which are separated by featherless areas called apteria. Contour and covert feathers can be easily removed by pulling at the feather individually in the direction of growth. The large wing feathers are anchored in the periosteum with muscle and ligament attachments. These feathers can prove difficult to detach, and care should be taken not to harm the underlying tissues during plucking. The limb should be securely grasped in one hand while the feather is pulled out individually with the other hand in the direction of the feather growth. The surgical site is aseptically prepared.

Because of chlorhexidine's broader spectrum of antimicrobial activity and longer residual effects, it is generally preferred over iodine-based preparations. Chlorhexidine solution is also considered nontoxic and hypoallergenic.

Surgical approach to the coelom

There are many times when an emergency surgical approach to the coelomic, or abdominal, cavity is warranted. Avian species are often presented with conditions that require emergency coelomic surgery. The ventral midline and left lateral incisions are the two most common surgical approaches to the avian coelomic cavity. The ventral midline incision commonly incorporates additional incisions along the keel or pubis to create better visualization and is called the partial flap, full flap, or transabdominal incision (Fig. 7) [8,9]. The left lateral site is the same site used for endoscopy or air sac tube placement. This area is also known as the sternal notch. The ventral midline incision may be best reserved for exploratory procedures, liver biopsy, intestinal surgery, and procedures addressing large masses and eggs and fluid-related problems (eg, yolk peritonitis). The left lateral celiotomy generally provides the best exposure to the female reproductive tract, proventriculus, ventriculus, left kidney, and spleen.

Surgical equipment

Microsurgical pack

A microsurgical instrument pack is ideal for any patient weighing less than 1000 g. An avian microsurgical pack should ideally contain the following instruments:

>Micro-Halstead mosquito hemostatic forceps (2), straight
>Micro-Halstead mosquito hemostatic forceps (2), curved
>Baby-Mixter hemostatic forceps (2), straight
>Baby-Mixter hemostatic forceps (2), curved
>Micro-Adson forceps (1), serrated
>Micro-Adson forceps (1), fine toothed
>Micro-Adson forceps (1), DeBakey
>Jeweler's forceps (1), straight

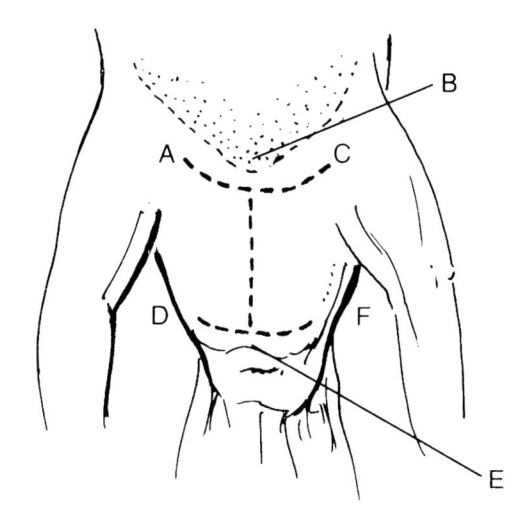

Fig. 7. Ventral approaches to the coelomic cavity. (*B-E*) Ventral midline incision. (*A-B-E*) Partial flap incision. (*A-B-E-D*) Full flap incision. (*A-B-C*) Transabdominal incision. Use caution when incising caudally along B to E, because the ileum is relatively superficial and can easily be accidentally lacerated or transected. (*From* Altman RB, Clubb SL, Dorrestine GM, et al, editors. Avian medicine and surgery. Philadelphia: WB Saunders; 1997. p. 710; with permission.)

Jeweler's forceps (1), curved
Retinal forceps (1)
Iris scissors (1), straight
Iris scissors (1), curved
Adventitia scissors (1)
Spring-handled scissors (1)
Needle holder (1), extra-delicate Hegar or Olsen-Hegar, with 1.2-mm ultrafine serrated or carbide tips
Castroviejo needle holder (1) without a lock (straight or curved)
Scalpel blade handle (1), number 7, with number 15 or number 11 size blades
Thumbscrew eyelid retractor (1) (used as coelomic wall retractors in small patients)
Cotton-tipped applicators
Gauze sponges, 2 × 2 synthetic nonwoven

Specialized surgical equipment
Hemostatic clips. Hemostatic clips (Hemoclip; Weck, Research Triangle Park, North Carolina) should also be readily available because they are the best method for controlling bleeding in the avian patient. Ligating vessels with sutures in the small body cavity of avian species is difficult and can result in excessive traumatic tissue handling, excessive bleeding, and increased surgical time [8,9]. Hemostatic clips are available in multiple sizes, including the applicator (one for each sized clip) and the clip cartridge.

Angled tipped applicators and disposable clip guns that automatically reload are also available from human medical supply distribution companies.

Retractors. The mini-Balfour retractor may be useful in patients within a weight range of 500 to 1200 g. Alm retractors are used for birds weighing 200 to 400 g. For small birds weighing less than 200 g, the small animal eyelid retractor or a Heiss retractor (Heiss Blunt Retractor, number 17011-10; Fine Service Tools, Foster City, California) is recommended. One of the authors' (WC) favorite instruments is a plastic ring retractor that uses hooks attached to elastic cords (Lone Star Medical Products, Houston, Texas). The retractor surrounds the incision site with a plastic ring and multiple small hooks on elastic bands used to retract the tissues. The retractor allows maximum exposure and minimal tissue trauma.

Surgical drapes. Clear adhesive surgical drapes are often the best choice for draping material in the avian patient. They not only keep the patient's surgical area sterile but have monitoring and body heat retention advantages.

Radiosurgery (electrosurgery) equipment. Radiosurgery is a term applied to radiosurgical units that generate waves that can provide a cutting or coagulation effect [8]. These units offer significant advantages in that they reduce blood loss by coagulation and the surgical time spent on providing hemostasis while incising through tissue [8]. Most units provide monopolar and bipolar operating capabilities. Monopolar devices operate by emitting a current from a handheld probe-like electrode that is received by a ground plate, which is placed underneath the patient's body. With the bipolar instrument (Elman International Manufacturing, Hewlett, New York), the electrodes are in close proximity. Additionally, bipolar radiosurgery instruments have a bend of 45°, ultimately transmitting generated wave currents with a greater degree of control and less tissue damage for birds weighing less than 2 kg compared with the monopolar versions [8].

Magnification. Depending on the surgical procedure to be performed, magnification can be considered a useful advantage in the avian patient, especially with those patients weighing less than 1 kg. Binocular magnification loupes are available with several degrees of magnification and can be fitted with a fiberoptic halogen lamp to improve the illumination of the surgical site. Magnification in the range of 2.5 to 8 times is generally considered adequate for most microsurgical procedures.

Surgical procedures

Air sac cannulation

In emergency situations involving occlusion of the upper respiratory tract, such as tracheal granulomas, foreign bodies, or severe head or facial trauma, air sac intubation may be necessary to ensure air flow through the respiratory tract. The air sac cannula is similar to using a tracheostomy in mammals in that both can bypass tracheal obstructions. After tube placement, respiratory distress resolves almost instantaneously in birds with upper airway obstruction. An air sac tube may also improve respiration in birds with tracheal obstructions and lower airway disease, although the improvement in breathing is usually less dramatic. The air sac cannula is placed in the caudal thoracic or abdominal air sac. The point of entry is typically between the last two ribs, caudal to the last rib (sternal notch) or just caudal to the thigh muscles (Fig. 8). The first two insertion sites usually enter the caudal thoracic air sac, whereas the last site enters the abdominal air sac. The left abdominal air sac is larger than the right, and if using the last site, place the bird in right lateral recumbency. In a bird with large ovarian follicles, it may be beneficial to use a right-sided approach to avoid the reproductive tract. It is important to make sure that placement of the cannula has a minimal impact on movement of the leg. The size of the tube depends on the size of the bird (12 French in a 500-g bird, 10 French in a 300-g bird, and 8 French in a 100-g bird); ideally, a cuffed endotracheal tube is used, although sterile red rubber tubes or intravenous tubing can be used in smaller birds. In extremely small birds, one author (WC) uses 20- or 22-gauge intravenous catheters to cannulate the air sac. In general, the internal

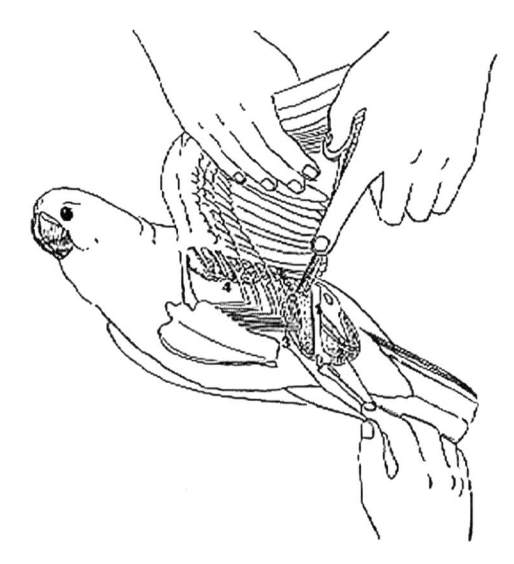

Fig. 8. Placement of a tube in the air sac. The tube inserted into the abdominal air sac can be used to provide oxygen or gas anesthesia. The tube is placed by making a small incision through the skin and muscles in the area of the sternal notch. Femur (*1*), abdominal air sac (*2*), eighth rib (*3*), and lung (*4*). (*From* Ritchie BW, Harrison GJ, Harrison LR, editors. Avian medicine: principles and application. Lake Worth (FL): Wingers Publishing; 1994. p. 397; with permission.)

diameter of the air sac cannula should match or slightly exceed the patient's tracheal diameter.

The area of cannula insertion is plucked and aseptically prepared. A small skin incision (approximately the diameter of the tube being used) is made with a scalpel blade, and small mosquito hemostats are then used to dissect bluntly through the abdominal wall musculature. It may require a bit of force to pierce the air sac and overlying peritoneum. Once the air sac is entered, the cannula is passed between the open ends of the hemostats. If there is a cuff on the tube, it should be inflated; this helps to keep the cannula in place and the air sac inflated (Fig. 9). The cannula can be maintained in place by using a piece of tape in a butterfly fashion or by using the Chinese finger knot technique. The latter method is done by placing a purse-string suture around the skin and cannula (leaving a large tail to the suture) and then wrapping the suture around the cannula, tying a knot after each pass around the circumference of the catheter for approximately 1 cm of the cannula. The patency of the cannula can be tested by holding a microscope slide up to the end of the cannula and watching for condensation on the slide with each respiration. Alternatively, the downy portion of a feather can be used to see if there is air flow in and out of the cannula. The exposed end of the cannula should be positioned so that it does not interfere with movement of the patient's leg. The tube is maintained in place until the respiratory condition is treated and the bird can breathe normally without the

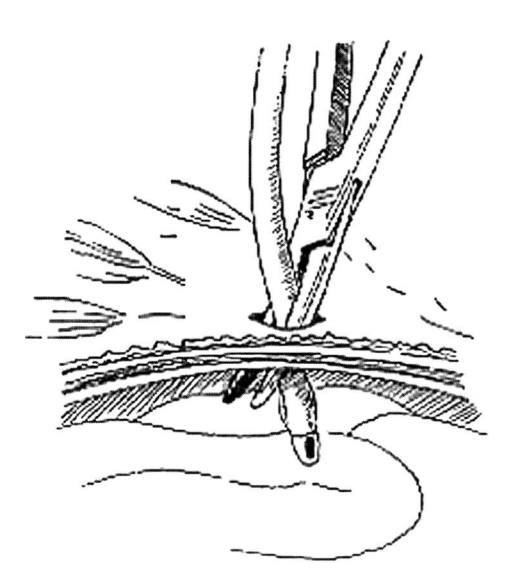

Fig. 9. Placement of a tube in the air sac. The air sac tube is inserted between the jaws of the hemostats into the abdominal air sac and sutured to the skin. (*From* Ritchie BW, Harrison GJ, Harrison LR, editors. Avian medicine: principles and application. Lake Worth (FL): Wingers Publishing; 1994. p. 397; with permission.)

tube. One author (WC) has placed an air sac tube in a bird with aspergillosis and maintained it in place during the initial 8 weeks of antifungal therapy.

Esophagostomy tube placement

Persistently regurgitating birds or those with beak, esophagus, or crop injuries may need to have a feeding tube placed into the proventriculus. The feeding tube is made of polyurethane or silicone. Tubes that are too flexible may be chilled before placement to increase stiffness. The French unit measures the outer lumen diameter of a tube (French unit is equal to 0.33 mm). Polyvinylchloride tubes (Infant Feeding Tube; Argyle Division of Sherwood Medical, St. Louis, Missouri) or red rubber tubes (Sovereign Feeding Tube; Monoject Division of Sherwood Medical) are the least expensive but may harden within 2 weeks and irritate the esophagus. Tubes made of silicone (Cook Nasal Feeding Tube; Cook Veterinary Products, Bloomington, Indiana) are less irritating. The tube size varies according to the size of the patient (12 French for a 500-g bird, 10 French for a 300-g bird, and 8 French for a 100-g bird).

The tube is measured from the midcervix (midneck) to the distal edge of the keel. The tube is cut on the proximal end to the measured point. The midcervix on the right side of the neck is aseptically prepared. A hemostat is inserted orally into the esophagus to aid in identification and to prevent the incision from penetrating the opposite side of the esophagus. An esophagostomy small stab incision is made over the forceps. Guide the tube into the esophagostomy site and into the crop. The crop is held with one hand, and the tube is passed into the thoracic esophagus and then into the proventriculus. The tube is then sutured into place using a Chinese finger knot. Food is given by a slow bolus using a syringe (Fig. 10). The initial amount given should be half of the amount that would be given into the crop. These volumes are slowly increased during the first 24 to 48 hours so that the maximum nutritional requirements (given in milliliters per feeding) are administered every 6 hours (Table 1).

Salpingohysterectomy

Egg binding is probably the most common avian coelomic cavity abnormality. The condition is relatively easy to diagnose and can lead to emergency surgical intervention. Medical intervention is often successful (see the article on avian emergencies elsewhere in this issue) and should always be attempted before considering surgery. Any avian patient that is not completely stable or has an infectious process at time of emergency surgery is a poor candidate and carries a guarded prognosis. Once a decision has been made to remove the reproductive tract or egg surgically, the patient has to be prepared and secured on the surgical table in a position to allow left lateral or midline access. After the skin and muscle layers have been incised, an incision must be made through the air sac to access the oviduct, a long convoluted tubular organ that extends from the left ovary down to

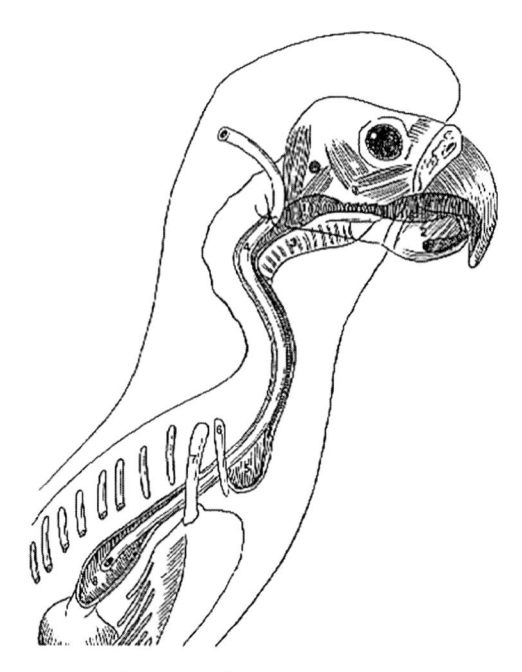

Fig. 10. Esophagostomy tube placement. The esophagostomy tube is used to supply food to the proventriculus and bypass the oral cavity, esophagus, and crop. Esophagus (*1*), tongue (*2*), trachea (*3*), tube in esophagus (*4*), crop (*5*), clavicle (*6*), coracoid (*7*), and proventriculus (*8*). (*From* Ritchie BW, Harrison GJ, Harrison LR, editors. Avian medicine: principles and application. Lake Worth (FL): Wingers Publishing; 1994. p.1112; with permission.)

the left side of the cloaca. The cranial infundibular portion of the oviduct can often be gently elevated away from its dorsal attachments. Radiosurgical bipolar forceps can be used when dissecting out the oviduct, ligaments, and any small arteries or veins. Hemostatic clips can be used to control bleeding as well, and absorbent gelatin sponges can be applied when the origin of bleeding cannot be accurately localized.

The rest of the oviduct can be gently excised out of the coelomic cavity, paying careful attention to additional branches of ovarian and oviductal

Table 1
Suggested esophagostomy tube feeding volumes in various psittacine species

Species of bird	Volumes (mL per feeding)
Budgerigar	1
Lovebird	2
Cockatiel	2–3
Conure	2–6
Amazon Parrot	8–17
Cockatoo	10–20
Large Macaw	17–25

arteries. A larger hemoclip can be placed just proximal to oviduct/cloacal junction, being careful not to include the white tubular ureter that attaches nearby to the cloaca. The hemoclip needs to be large enough to secure the entire width of the uterus to prevent cloacal spillage into the coelomic cavity. Well-developed or cystic follicles should be removed with gentle suction. Gentle manipulation can be used to detach follicles from the ovary but may result in yolk spillage. Any yolk or oviductal fluid that spills into the cavity should be cleaned with sterile cotton-tipped applicators, followed by applicators that have been soaked in warm sterile saline. Saline lavage with significant amounts of fluid is not advised in avian patients that have had air sacs incised. The fluid could seep into the air sac and invade the respiratory system, potentially causing death. All excised tissues should be saved for appropriate diagnostic testing. Muscle and skin layers should be closed individually with a simple continuous pattern using a 3-0 to 6-0 absorbable suture.

Proventriculotomy/ventriculotomy

With the exception of foreign body ingestion, rarely is a proventriculotomy or ventriculotomy considered an emergency surgical procedure. Additionally, less invasive procedures, such as endoscopy, are generally effective in removing foreign bodies from the lumen of either organ. Some foreign bodies can be managed with medical therapy if relatively small and known to be nontoxic. Although it is typically recommended to fast birds for 10 to 12 hours to achieve ventricular emptying, if the procedure is recommended as an emergency procedure, fasting for a long period may not be an option. Because the authors have usually attempted to remove the foreign body with endoscopy plus irrigation before considering surgery, this flushing creates a gastric lavage effect making the patient suitable for surgery sooner. Radiographs assist in guidance on whether to opt for a left lateral or ventral midline celiotomy.

Once the coelomic cavity has been surgically exposed, stay sutures can be placed in the white tendinous portion of the ventriculus and the organ can be exteriorized to create better visualization. The proventriculus is relatively fixed in its position inside the coelomic cavity, and attempts to exteriorize it should not be made. As with any gastrointestinal surgery, packing helps to prevent contamination and exteriorized organs should be kept moist with warm saline-soaked applicators. The relative avascularity, thinness, and location between the proventriculus and ventriculus make the isthmus an ideal site for the incision. The incision can be extended cranially toward a relatively avascular area of the proventriculus or caudally in the direction of the ventriculus. Endoscopy may prove useful in visualizing the interior of both organs. Although irrigation and suction may be of use, the small capacity of both organs could easily lead to contamination of the coelomic cavity. The incised organ can be closed with a fine monofilament absorbable suture using a simple continuous pattern. The sutured area should then be oversewn with a continuous inverting pattern to prevent dehiscence. Alternatively, the ventriculus may be approached by way of the caudoventral sac. This approach requires a meticulous closing technique incorporating a closely placed simple interrupted suture pattern (because a second overlaying inverting pattern is not possible in this area of the ventriculus).

Summary

The emergency clinician may need to perform procedures after initial stabilization of avian patients. Bandaging techniques should be performed as a temporary or permanent method of stabilization of fractures. Endoscopy is becoming a popular technique for emergency evaluation of the trachea and syrinx and gastrointestinal foreign body removal. Avian veterinarians commonly perform endoscopic biopsies of coelomic organs as a less invasive method than surgery. The clinician should be prepared through education of avian anatomy and surgical techniques before attempting surgery on birds. The techniques used in avian surgery often require microsurgery instruments. The actual procedures are too numerous to list here; however, the foundation of emergency avian surgery involves the techniques discussed in this article.

References

[1] McCluggage DM, et al. Bandaging. In: Altman RB, Clubb SL, Dorrestine GM, editors. Avian medicine and surgery. Philadelphia: W.B. Saunders; 1997. p. 828–34.
[2] Degernes LA. Trauma medicine. In: Ritchie BW, Harrison GJ, Harrison LR, editors. Avian medicine: principles and application. Lake Worth (FL): Wingers Publishing Inc; 1994. p. 418–33.
[3] Roush JC. Avian orthopedics. In: Kirk RW, editor. Current veterinary therapy XII small animal practice. Philadelphia: W.B. Saunders; 1996. p. 662–73.
[4] Satterfield WC. Diagnostic laparoscopy in birds. In: Kirk RW, editor. Current veterinary therapy XII small animal practice. Philadelphia: W.B. Saunders; 1996. p. 659–73.
[5] Hochleithner M, et al. Endoscopy. In: Altman RB, Clubb SL, Dorrestine GM, editors. Avian medicine and surgery. Philadelphia: W.B. Saunders; 1997. p. 631–51.
[6] Lierz M. Diagnostic value of endoscopy and biopsy. In: Harrison GJ, Lightfoot TL, editors. Clinical avian medicine. Palm Beach (FL): Spix Publishing Inc; 2006. p. 776–829.
[7] Bowles HL, Odberg E, Harrison GJ, et al. Surgical resolution of soft tissue disorders. In: Harrison GJ, Lightfoot TL, editors. Clinical avian medicine. Palm Beach (FL): Spix Publishing Inc; 2006. p. 776–829.
[8] Altman RD, et al. General surgical considerations. In: Altman RB, Clubb SL, Dorrestine GM, editors. Avian medicine and surgery. Philadelphia: W.B. Saunders; 1997. p. 691–702.
[9] Jenkins JR. Emergency avian surgery. Vet Clin North Am Exot Anim Pract Crit Care 1998;1: 43–58.

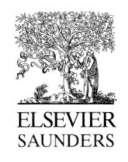

Critical Care of the Rabbit

Joanne Paul-Murphy, DVM, DACZM

Special Species Health, Department of Surgical Sciences, School of Veterinary Medicine, University of Wisconsin, 2015 Linden Drive, Madison, WI 53706, USA

Emergency and critical care principles are similar for all mammals. However, the physiology and natural behaviors of rabbits create an animal that is stressed easily and requires specialized handling techniques. It is important to evaluate rabbits efficiently and stabilize them as quickly as possible before moving into the definitive diagnostic phase of their care. A thorough clinical history, systematic physical examination, and multiple diagnostic tests are ideal, but when a rabbit is in critical condition, emergency stabilization and fluid resuscitation must take priority (see the article by Lichtenberger in this issue). Rabbits are different from traditional companion animals because they have evolved as a prey species, an animal that needs to conceal signs of illness to escape predation. Common emergency presentations include gastrointestinal disorders, prolonged anorexia, respiratory distress, neoplasia, neurologic symptoms, exposure to toxins, trauma, and urinary infections or obstruction.

A few equipment items can make rabbit urgent care procedures more efficient. The examination room should have a digital gram scale with a skid-resistant surface for rapid and accurate weights. Infrared tympanic temperature scanners work well and alleviate the trepidation of rectal thermometer placement. A stainless steel nasal speculum (www.welchallyn.com) provides a rapid but limited dental examination. An essential feature for the care of rabbits in critical condition is a quiet area of the intensive care ward for procedures and hospitalization. Incubators such as the Lyons cage (www.lyonusa.com) are ideal for the critical patient, to provide heat and oxygen support. Equipment items needed for rabbits include small masks that fit easily over the nose for anesthesia or oxygen supplementation. A selection of small endotracheal tubes (2.0-mm and 2.5-mm outside diameter) facilitates endotracheal intubation. Small-diameter pediatric feeding tubes (3.5F to 10.0F) are needed for nasogastric (NG) feeding or oral fluids,

E-mail address: jpmurphy@svm.vetmed.wisc.edu

and low-flow infusion pumps are essential for accurate and safe fluid therapy. Common therapeutics used in rabbit critical care and mentioned in this article are given in Table 1.

Dietary history

A thorough history including standard questions is important when examining any rabbit. In addition, the dietary information for rabbits can vary greatly and may affect diagnosis and treatment. Many rabbit owners are unaware of the nutritional recommendations for their rabbit and may be feeding inappropriate food items, excessive amounts of pellets, or inadequate amounts of hay. Owners may be feeding alfalfa hay or alfalfa pellets rather than the recommended grass hay. The House Rabbit Society (http://www.rabbit.org) provides some of the best client information about appropriate diets for nonreproductive pet rabbits. Rabbits require large amounts of indigestible fiber in their diet. Fiber stimulates cecal-colic motility, and can be protective against enteritis. Excessive amounts of carbohydrates such as cereals or fruits can slow motility and potentiate cecal impaction. Simple carbohydrates can also have a negative impact on gut fermentation, leading to excess production of gas. Heath problems associated with rabbits fed an inappropriate diet are obesity, chronic intermittent soft stools, and episodes of anorexia, often associated with alterations in gastrointestinal motility. Additionally, dystrophic calcification or uroliths can be associated with high-calcium diets.

Diet is a critical component of pet rabbit health and longevity; therefore, dietary recommendations should be discussed with owners before the animal is sent home.

Physical examination

Critically ill rabbits may not tolerate excessive handling and should be observed while in the carrier before handling. The character of feces and urine in the carrier should be noted. Mentation and respiratory rate and character can be assessed. Rabbit respiratory rates are normally rapid, 30 to 60 breaths per minute. The rabbit is an obligate nasal breather; therefore, observation of nasal movements can be used when chest movements are difficult to assess. When respiratory distress is evident, one should briefly auscultate heart and lungs and quickly place the patient in an oxygen cage. Respiratory sounds heard by auscultation of the chest are normally loud or harsh because of referred upper respiratory sounds created as air is pulled through the narrow nasal turbinates.

Rabbits should be examined on a skid-free surface or the body wrapped in a towel if the rabbit is panicky. One should keep a hand on the rabbit at all times, even if the rabbit is recumbent, and obtain heart rate, color of mucous membranes, capillary refill time, blood pressure, and body temperature

Table 1
Selected critical-care drugs for rabbits

Agent	Dose	Route	Indication
Albendazole	8–20 mg/kg q 24 h 14 d	PO	Encephalitozoonosis
Ca-EDTA	27 mg/kg q 6 h for 5 d; dilute to 10 mg/mL with 0.4% NaCl/2.5% dextrose	SC	Heavy metal toxicosis
Cisapride	0.5 mg/kg bid to tid	PO	Motility enhancement; used through nasogastric tube
Doxapram	2 mg/kg respiratory q 15 min	SC, IV	Respiratory stimulant
Enrofloxacin	5–10 mg/kg	SC, PO	Antimicrobial
Fenbendazole	20 mg/kg q 24 h × 28 d	PO	Encephalitozoonosis
Flumazenil	150 mg/kg	IV	Benzodiazepine antagonist
Furosemide	1–4 mg/kg q 6–8 h	IM	Diuretic
Lidocaine w/out Epinephrine	1–2 mg/kg	IV	Antiarrhythmic
	2–4 mg/kg intratracheally		
Marbofloxacin	2 mg/kg q 24 h	IV, IM, PO	Antimicrobial
Meclizine	2–12 mg/kg q 24 h	IM	Torticollis with rolling
Metoclopramide	0.2–1 mg/kg q 6–8 h or 0.2 mg/kg/h CRI	PO, SC	Stimulation of gastrointestinal motility (controversial)
Midazolam	1–2 mg/kg	IM	Sedative
	0.25–0.5 mg/kg	IV, IM	Anticonvulsant
Oxytocin	1–3 units q 2–4 h as needed	IM	Stimulation of uterine contractions
Propofol	2–4 mg/kg; give slowly to effect	IV	Anesthesia induction
Trimethoprim sulfa	15–30 mg/kg q 12 h	PO	

Abbreviations: IM, intramuscular; IV, intravenous; PO, by mouth; SC, subcutaneous.

(www.admon.com) to determine the rabbit's perfusion status. When present, perfusion abnormalities (bradycardia, hypotension, and hypothermia) may be corrected with intravenous (IV) fluid resuscitation and heat (see the article by Lichtenberger in this isssue for shock resuscitation).

Skin tenting and moistness of the mucous membranes determine hydration status. Palpation of the stomach is recommended for all rabbits. Food should be present in the stomach, but a firm, dry mass of material is suspicious of delayed gastric emptying or dehydration. A bloated, tympanic, painful abdomen is serious and requires differentiation between gastric bloat and gaseous distention of the cecum or colon. The dental examination is usually the final procedure because it may be tolerated poorly. A limited examination is possible in the unanesthetized rabbit using a stainless steel nasal speculum placed over each arcade of cheek teeth. If any long dental "points" or gingival ulcers are noted, a complete oral examination must be done. General anesthesia is required but, if dental disease is not the primary cause of the rabbit's critical condition, a complete examination can be delayed until the rabbit is stabilized.

Diagnostic procedures

Intravenous catheterization

Venous access is always recommended when hospitalizing a rabbit in critical condition. Twenty-four–gauge catheters can be placed in most small rabbits, and twenty-two–gauge catheters can be placed easily when rabbits weigh over 3 kg. The cephalic or saphenous veins are well suited for indwelling catheters. Lateral auricular veins tolerate small-gauge indwelling catheters but sloughing of the ear tip has been reported, even with short-term placement. Fluids can be infused using fluid or syringe pumps. The catheter site can be covered with nonadhesive tape when a rabbit chews the catheter. Elizabethan collars are stressful and should be only a last resort when treating rabbits. Cloth Elizabethan collars are tolerated better than plastic ones.

Intraosseous catheterization

When IV catheterization has failed, or the veins are too small, fragile, or hypotensive to place an IV catheter, an intraosseous catheter is extremely beneficial. The proximal tibia is the recommended site to place a 20-gauge, 1-in spinal needle. When spinal needles are not available, a sterilized 18- to 20-gauge needle with appropriately sized cerclage wire (for stylets) can be used. After aseptic preparation of the tibia, local anesthetic is used to block the skin and periosteum, and the spinal needle is passed lateral to the tibial crest, parallel to the long axis of the tibia. A butterfly tape is sutured to the skin and a figure-eight bandage is placed around the knee and over the catheter.

Venipuncture

Several peripheral sites are available for venipuncture: the marginal ear vein, central ear artery, jugular vein, cephalic vein, femoral vein, and lateral saphenous vein. The cephalic vein is usually spared from venipuncture to preserve the site for IV catheter placement. The lateral saphenous vein is visualized easily just above the hock when alcohol is applied to the area. It is the most common site for venipuncture. The rabbit is held with minimal restraint in lateral recumbency. The vein is occluded at the level of the knee, which also aids in preventing withdrawal of the limb. The vessel is located more dorsal on the tibia than in a dog and runs in an upside down "Y" pattern. A 25-gauge needle and 1-mL syringe are used for venipuncture.

Normal reference ranges for hematologic and serum chemistry values are similar to dogs and cats. Normal rabbit lactic acid values have been determined on three different testing devices (Nova Biomedical, Waltham, Massachusetts; Idexx Veterinary Chemistry Analyzer, Westbrook, Maine; Point of Care Portable Lactate, Arkray, Kyoto, Japan) (M. Lichtenberger, personal communication, 2006). The values from 20 clinically healthy rabbits ranged from 2.9 to 10.2 mmol/L. These values are higher than those seen in dogs and cats. Values as high as 23 mmol/L have been seen in rabbits with gastric stasis, and may be related to production of D lactate in the stomach (GA Zell and M. Lichtenberger, personal communication, 2006).

Normal blood glucose is 75 to 155 g/dL in healthy rabbits. Hypoglycemia is common in young rabbits that have been anorexic for several days (M. Lichtenberger, personal communication, 2006). The rabbits often present seizuring. Hyperglycemia is common in critically ill rabbits and likely a response to stress. Glucose levels of 250 to 460 have been seen in critically ill rabbits; these levels return to normal with stabilization and fluid therapy.

Cystocentesis or urethral catheterization

Cystocentesis is done without sedation, but restraint is critical. With the rabbit held in dorsal recumbency, the handler cradles the rabbit between his/her forearms or on his/her lap. A small amount of alcohol in front of the pubis is sufficient to visualize the midline without shaving the fur. A 22-gauge, 1-in needle and a 6-mL syringe should be used for collection. Ultrasound needle guidance is recommended when available. Catheterization is possible in the conscious rabbit and is easier to perform with males than with females. Sedation with midazolam, with or without the addition of an opioid, is recommended by this author. The procedure is similar to that described for small animals.

Normal reference ranges for a urinalysis are similar to small animals, with a pH of 8.2, calcium carbonate crystals, and inactive sediment. The urine should be centrifuged and interpretation of specific gravity performed on the supernatant. Specific gravity of normal rabbit urine (n = 100) has a broad range, 1.002 to 1.040 (mean of 1.027) (M. Lichtenberger, personal communication, 2006). The rabbit has a low collecting duct permeability to urea which could explain the absence of a marked enhancement of concentrating ability [1]. The rabbit's specific gravity values differ from those of carnivorous animals or the omnivorous rat, which ingest large quantities of meat over short periods in the wild state. Herbivores more commonly graze over lengthy periods of the day. It has been suggested that an evolutionary development of the renal concentrating mechanism has arisen to accommodate differences in temporal generation of urea [2].

Diagnostic imaging

Critically ill rabbits should not be restrained for diagnostic radiographs until after stabilization and fluid resuscitation. Some rabbits allow lateral views without struggling. Rabbits may need to be sedated for the best radiographic positioning, which can be accomplished using a combination of tranquilizer and opioid. A high dose of meloxicam, 1 mg/kg intramuscularly (which can be reversed with flumazenil following the procedure), can provide sufficient sedation for helical CT of the skull. Helical CT has numerous advantages, but is especially useful for rabbit skull diagnostic imaging (Fig. 1).

Interpreting radiographs of the abdomen and chest of the rabbit follows guidelines similar to those for small animals. Knowledge of the normal anatomy is required because of the anatomic differences of the gastrointestinal tract in the rabbit. Rabbits have a large amount of retroperitoneal fat. A mat of hair in the stomach is a normal finding in a healthy rabbit. Rabbits have potential for a large cecal volume. A large, gas-distended cecum and clinical signs of shock are consistent with enterotoxemia [3,4].

Ultrasound examination is useful for rabbits with liver, kidney, urinary, reproductive, and cardiac disease. Reference resources for normal measurements are limited but the clinician should perform ultrasonic and echocardiogram examinations similar to those for dogs and cats. Ultrasound is especially helpful in evaluating the female rabbit reproductive tract and the kidneys.

Therapeutic techniques

Enteral feeding and nasogastric tubes

Early enteral feeding decreases pain, helps with motility of the gastrointestinal tract, and decreases bacterial translocation. Hepatic lipidosis develops quickly in the rabbit and can be averted with enteral feeding. Critically ill rabbits often are too weak or too nauseous to eat from a syringe. An NG tube can be less stressful in the critical patient than force feeding with a syringe. The primary disadvantage of NG tubes for enteral alimentation occurs when the small diameter precludes administration of the insoluble fiber that is required for the rabbit's gastrointestinal motility.

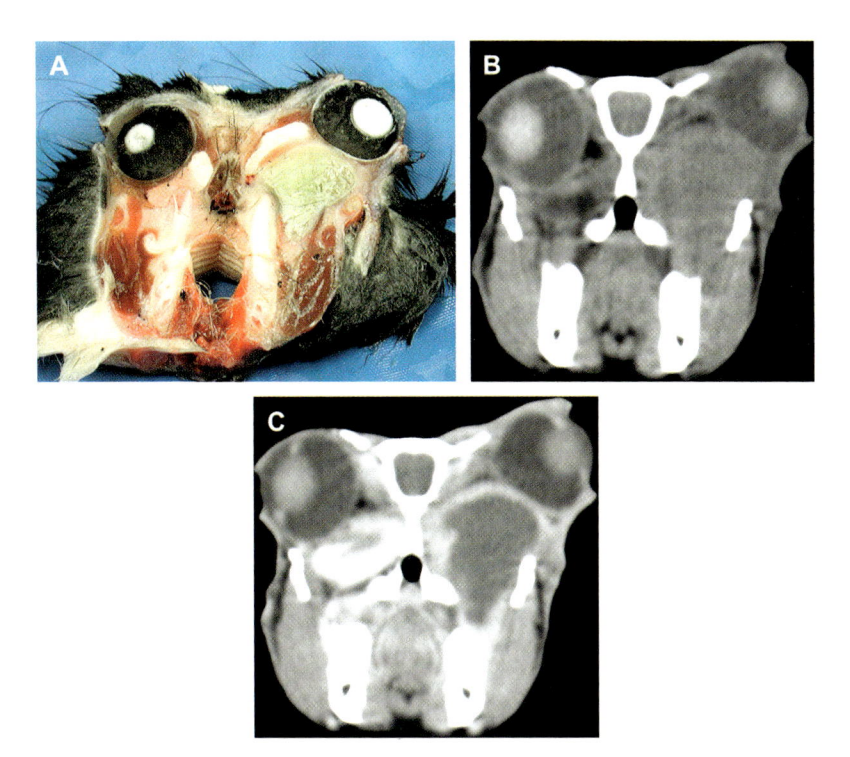

Fig. 1. Transverse section of the rabbit head viewed from rostral (*A*) at the level of the orbits defines a well-delineated area of suppurative inflammation in the left orbit that indents the posterior sclera and fills the dependent orbital structures adjacent to the maxilla and mandible. (*Courtesy of* Richard Dubielzig, DVM, Madison, WI). CT study of the head before (*B*) and after (*C*) application of IV contrast medium. Left retrobulbar mass extending to the medial aspect of the mandible, displacing the globe rostrolaterally (1.9 × 2.4 cm).

Most commercial veterinary enteral diets are produced for carnivores and are completely unsuitable for the herbivorous rabbit. Human enteral diets (eg, Ensure [www.ensure.org/entrust] or Sustacal [www.drugs.com/cons/Sustacal.html]) provide calories with high fat content and are low in fiber. The fiber in human enteral products is a digestible cellulose fiber. Nondigestible fiber is essential for the rabbit hind-gut production of short-chain fatty acids and for stimulation of gastrointestinal motility. Crude fiber of less than 12% has been associated with diarrhea in rabbits [5]. The percentage of crude fiber in commercial enteral products is usually less than 2%. Liquid canine or feline products are completely inappropriate because of the high fat and carbohydrate concentrations.

The most suitable enteral diets for syringe feeding rabbits have a high percentage of nondigestible fiber, low fat, and relatively low carbohydrates. Herbivore enteral diets are available commercially from Oxbow Pet Products (www.oxbowhay.com). The Oxbow products have been specifically formulated for nutritional support of herbivorous small mammals. The kcal is given on a dry-matter basis, with 2.69 kcal/gram of dry weight of the powder. When mixed as directed, Critical Care Enteral powder/water (1:1.5 v/v) provides approximately 1.9 kcal/mL and the slurry can be used for syringe feeding of stable patients in hospital or for home feeding by the owner. The syringe is placed into the diastema, the large space between the incisors and premolars. Syringe feeding needs to be done slowly, to avoid aspiration. Unfortunately, this formulation will clog a 5F or 8F NG tube even when blenderized, and is not suitable for NG tube feeding.

When a rabbit has had anorexia for more than 24 hours and is weak and dehydrated, an NG tube is part of the treatment plan to deliver calories and rehydrate the stomach contents (Fig. 2). A 5F or 8F soft, flexible pediatric feeding tube is used (Argyle tube, Kendall Company, Mansfield, Massachusetts [http://www.imed.com/shop/detail.cfm/sku/K1185]) because these are softer than a red rubber tube, and a stylet is not necessary. The length necessary to reach the stomach is determined by measuring from the nose to the last rib. A local anesthetic (2% lidocaine gel) is placed into the rabbit's nostril 5 to 10 minutes before passing the tube. The rabbit must be restrained properly and its back protected, and the head is ventrally flexed but with the neck straight (to avoid compression of the trachea) by an assistant. The tube is passed ventrally and medially into the ventral nasal meatus. The end of the tube is advanced until it reaches the stomach. Verification of placement is determined with a radiograph or by aspiration of gastric contents.

The Advanced Nutrition Support Enterals for Herbivores from Rock-Solid Herpetoculture (www.rocksolidherpetoculture.com) is an enteral diet for herbivorous reptiles. The powder diet has 8% fiber concentration and, although this is lower than rabbits require, it is suitable for temporary NG tube nutrition for 2 to 3 days (Susan Donagnue, personal communication,

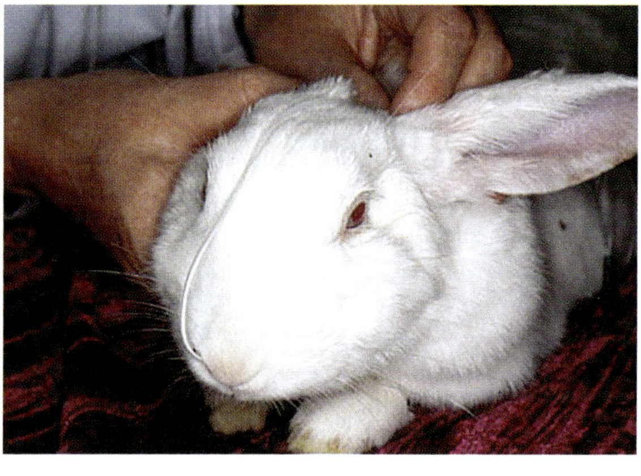

Fig. 2. An NG tube has been passed through the ventral nasal meatus of the rabbit and extends into the stomach. The tube can be secured to the hair or skin between the ears.

2003). The NG formulation using the RockSolid enteral herbivore diet is prepared by mixing 13 mL/kg of powder with 20 mL/kg of water to provide approximately 1.2 kcal/mL when mixed. The slurry is delivered by syringe into the NG tube every 6 hours, and it is followed by 5 to 6 mL of water after each feeding to keep the tube patent and provide additional fluid. Most rabbits with uncomplicated gastric stasis will start to eat and produce slightly soft stools after 12 to 36 hours. The tube can remain in place until the rabbit eats on its own and starts to produce stool. A complication that has been observed is nasal discharge from tube irritation. The tube should be removed and antibiotics included in the treatment protocol (M. Lichtenberger, personal communication, 2006).

Percutaneous placement of gastrostomy tubes has been adapted to the rabbit using a technique similar to that for other companion animals [6]. Complications of abscessed subcutaneous space and peritonitis are common. Most rabbits do not tolerate the tubes so the procedure must be performed under general anesthesia. This procedure is not recommended.

Surgical placement and chronic maintenance of a pharyngostomy tube has been described for the healthy rabbit [7], but it is not a common critical care procedure. Abscesses can develop along the subcutaneous path of the catheter, and the anatomic placement should be practiced in less critical patients or cadavers before patient use. The tube sometimes may be required in long-term feeding or in fractures of the jaw.

Regardless of the level of enteral support selected for a critical rabbit, food should be available at all times for voluntary consumption. The rabbit's customary diet should be provided: same brand, same bowl, same amount, and so forth. Timothy hay should be part of the rabbit's normal diet. Placing fresh grass, timothy hay, or alfalfa hay in front of the rabbit may stimulate the appetite. Fresh greens, such as dandelion greens, broccoli flowers and stem, cilantro, dark leaf lettuce, watercress, Brussels sprouts, celery leaves, cabbage, and endive may entice a rabbit to eat and can to be offered ad libitum until the rabbit returns to a normal appetite.

Nutritional requirements

Correction of fluid and electrolyte imbalances should be initiated before nutritional support. The goal is to restore nitrogen balance by providing protein and sufficient energy for maintenance and illness. Protein should be 26% of the total calories and fiber should be 13.6% dry matter [6]. Amounts to feed vary with the disease, the method of feeding, and the diet selected. Calculation of the rabbit's kcal requirement per day is the most accurate method of determining adequate nutrition, rather than relying on charts of recipes. The approximate basal energy requirement should be calculated using the following formula:

$70(\text{Body weight in kg})^{0.75} = \text{BMR in kcal/d}$,

where *BMR* is basal metabolic rate

The BMR is adjusted for each patient; it is increased if the rabbit is hypermetabolic and reduced if hypometabolic. The BMR is multiplied by an illness factor between 1.2 and 2.0 to account for metabolic needs above resting. Starvation actually decreases the metabolic rate and these rabbits require fewer calories than usual.

$$\text{Illness factor} \times \text{BMR in kcal/d} = \text{Illness energy requirement in kcal/d}$$

The illness energy requirement in kcal/day is matched to the weight of dry enteral powder (in grams), which varies with the product used. When using Oxbow Critical Care, the illness energy requirement should be divided by 2.69 because this is the kcal/gram of dry powder. Rock Solid Herpetoculture enteral product is approximately 3 kcal/gram dry powder; therefore, the illness energy requirement is divided by 3. One should weigh out the total daily grams of dry powder and divide this into several small meals spaced evenly over 24 hours. Weighing and feeding based on dry product is more accurate because it is independent of the amount of water being added, which can vary, depending on the accuracy of the person mixing the food. More or less water can be added to facilitate passage through a feeding tube and to meet the fluid needs of the patient.

Nutritional support is started gradually. Patients in good condition can receive 75% to 100% of their daily energy need over the first 24 to 48 hours, whereas debilitated patients receive 40% to 70% of their daily energy requirement, gradually increased over a 3- to 5-day period.

An example might be a 2-kg adult rabbit with a 2-day history of anorexia and gastrointestinal stasis caused by chronic malocclusive dental disease. The rabbit is alert and responsive, and has been rehydrated with fluids. The treatment plan includes syringe feeding of Oxbow Critical Care for 2 days of hospitalization.

1. Calculate BMR: $70(2)^{0.75} = 117.6$ kcal
2. Determine an illness factor based on rabbit's condition: use 1.6
3. Multiply BMR by illness factor: $1.6 \times 117.6 = 188.2$ kcal
4. Use Oxbow Critical Care: 2.7 kcal per gram dry powder
5. $188.2/2.7 = 69.7$ g of dry powder per day
6. Mix 23 g dry powder with 34 mL warm water every 8 hours for the first 24 hours

Anesthesia/analgesia

Signs of pain may be subtle, such as a change in respiration, a reluctance to move, apprehension, sudden aggression, persistently squinting of the eyes or a worried or anxious expression, and an inability to rest or sleep normally. A rabbit with abdominal pain or sore feet may lie stretched out or sit in a hunched position. Bruxism is a sign of severe pain, often gastrointestinal in origin; however, rabbits normally can exhibit quieter, infrequent tooth grinding as a sign of contentment (although this is a much softer noise than that heard with pain). It is unusual for rabbits to vocalize, but when they experience sudden pain or anxiety, they may give a high-pitched squeal. Pain in rabbits is underdiagnosed and when it is recognized, it is often underestimated. It is difficult to differentiate pain from anxiety in rabbits, especially because often they are combined and can be manifested by similar changes in behavior. For the most commonly used drugs for analgesia and anesthesia, see the article by Lichtenberger and Ko in this issue.

Anorexia

Anorexia is a common, nonspecific sign of stress in rabbits. Stress may be caused by pain, systemic disease, gastrointestinal stasis, or even "anxiety." Any period of anorexia lasting more than 1 to 2 days is a potential emergency. Anorexic rabbits become dehydrated, which slows gastrointestinal motility and eventually leads to hypovolemia. A complete physical examination, including an oral examination for dental disease, is indicated. If a minimum amount of blood is obtained for diagnostic testing, the packed cell volume (PCV), total solids, blood glucose, and azostix are determined. The PCV, total solids, and azostix values become elevated with hypovolemia. Anorexia can induce hypoglycemia but, in some emergency presentations, a stress-induced hyperglycemia may be evident. When evaluating a serum chemistry profile, lactic acid concentrations become elevated because of poor perfusion, but the degree of elevation may also be caused by gastric production of D lactate (M. Lichtenberger, personal communication, 2006). Rabbits with an infectious disease rarely have an elevated white blood cell count, but rather, show a shift in the percentages of the various leukocytes to a heterophil-dominated differential. Commonly, rabbits with an acute infection present with 60% or more heterophils, and 30% or less lymphocytes. Occasionally, rabbits with an acute infectious process have a normal differential and a decrease in total white blood cell numbers. Stress, or endogenous corticosteroid release, results in a marked lymphocytopenia [8]. A fecal occult-blood test is recommended to determine if the condition has progressed to gastrointestinal bleeding. Anorexia can progress quickly to hepatic lipidosis in rabbits, and elevated liver enzymes occur in these cases [9].

Gastrointestinal stasis

Gastrointestinal stasis is a common cause of anorexia in the rabbit, but anorexia or decreased fiber intake also causes gastrointestinal stasis. The underlying causes of gastrointestinal stasis can be varied and sometimes vague. Rabbits with gastrointestinal stasis often have a history of inappropriate diet, or stress in the household. The primary clinical signs are decreased appetite, abdominal discomfort, and reduction in stool pellet size and amount to absence of stool production. Low-fiber diets lead to decreased intestinal motility and abnormal cecal fermentation changes in the pH and microbial dysbiosis. A firm, doughy mass palpable in the cranial abdomen (the stomach containing food, hair, and decreased fluid) is consistent with gastrointestinal stasis [10,11]. Complete blood count, chemistry profile, and urinalysis are performed to rule out an underlying cause (ie, renal disease).

Gastric obstruction is rare in rabbits, but must be ruled out before treatment with prokinetics is initiated. If the rabbit is still defecating, obstruction is less likely. Aggressive rehydration treatment improves gastrointestinal motility and greatly decreases the potential for gastric hair mats to obstruct outflow at the pylorus or duodenum. Obstruction of the upper gastrointestinal tract presents with severe gas distension of the stomach to the degree of typany, pain, tachypnea, and septic shock. Decompression of the stomach can be accomplished by passing an NG tube. Surgery is required in cases of obstruction, although, after stabilization and treatment for shock, prognosis is still guarded [10–16].

The cecum can be the site of gaseous distension caused by ileus and may be secondary to overgrowth of *Clostridium* spp within the cecum. This condition can be differentiated from gastric distention by palpation, radiographs, and a lack of improvement after passing an NG tube. Radiographs can be useful to differentiate a tympanic abdomen caused by gastrointestinal stasis from gastric obstruction, because in ileus, gas accumulates in the cecum and frequently the stomach is filled with ingesta (Fig. 3). Primary enterotoxemia can have gaseous distension throughout the gastrointestinal tract.

Rabbits with gastrointestinal stasis (including nonobstructive mats of hair) are best managed with systemic and enteric rehydration and increasing fiber in the diet. If the rabbit is still eating and drinking, syringe feeding is an effective method for rehydration and caloric support. Grass hay and high-fiber vegetables should also be offered. If the rabbit is not eating, hospitalization with NG tube placement for oral rehydration and feeding is

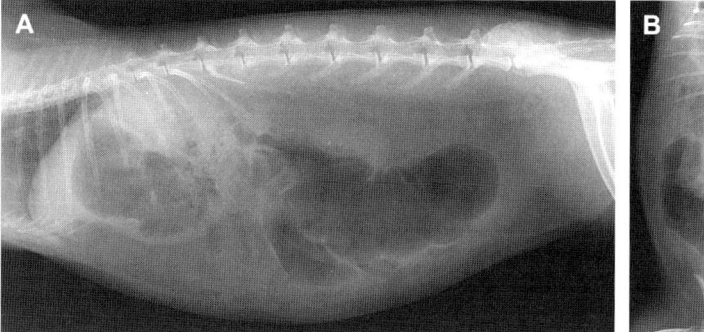

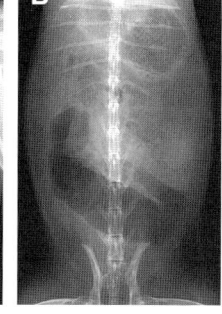

Fig. 3. Lateral (*A*) and ventrodorsal (*B*) radiographs of a rabbit. Roentgen signs include gas distention of the cecum. Mixed soft tissue, and mineral and gas opacities, are present within the stomach. Feces are present within the rectum and there is minimal dilatation of the small intestines. These findings are consistent with cecal tympany associated with gastrointestinal stasis.

necessary. In severe cases, IV or intraosseous fluid therapy may be indicated. A thorough oral examination to check for malocclusion, enamel points, and oral abscesses should be performed (see later discussion).

Prokinetics may be of benefit to promote motility of the stomach and intestines of rabbits. The use of metoclopramide as a motility agent, either subcutaneously or as a constant rate infusion, is anecdotal. Cisapride may be available through compounding pharmaceutic agencies. Oral cisapride in rabbits is absorbed rapidly from the gastrointestinal tract, with a plasma half-life similar to that in dogs [17]. Other data show that cisapride may modify the contractile responses of the isolated rabbit intestine to ranitidine, having a potentiating effect up to a certain concentration. The conclusion is that coadministration of the two drugs may lead to enhanced motility [18].

Malocclusion of incisors-premolars and molar teeth

Malocclusion of the incisors and cheek teeth (premolars and molars) frequently causes anorexia and may be accompanied by drooling. Rabbits may present with saliva-matted fur or even dermatitis under the chin. Malocclusion of incisors is determined easily by visual inspection and corrected by trimming the incisors evenly. When a rabbit is in critical condition because of dental disease, it is rarely malocclusion of the incisors alone causing the problem. Incisor-premolar-molar malocclusion with periodontal and endodontal disease is a serious dental disease complex that may include one or more of the following: incisor malocclusion; distortion of the premolar-molar occlusal plane; sharp points or spikes; periodontal disease; periapic changes; apical elongation; oral soft tissue lesions; and maxillofacial abscess formation [19]. Initial stabilization may require supportive care, including fluid therapy and nutritional support. Following stabilization, a thorough visual examination of the teeth requires general anesthesia and the use of oral speculums specifically designed for rabbits and rodents to open the mouth vertically, and a pouch dilator to open the mouth horizontally (Fig. 4). Alternatively, a specialized dentistry board can be used to elevate and open the mouth (Sontec Instruments Incorporated Englewood, CO, [www.sontecinstruments.com]). Skull radiographs or helical CT should be included in a complete dental examination to identify any areas of osteomyelitis or abscessation. For rabbits in critical condition, it is recommended that dental disease be approached in stages, with the first procedure being removal of points and reduction of tooth height using a straight hand-piece with a round diamond burr. Extractions can be very time consuming and are best delayed until the patient is no longer in critical condition.

Uterine disorders

If the female rabbit is intact, reproductive disorders must be considered in the differential diagnoses for anorexia. Uterine adenocarcinoma is the most

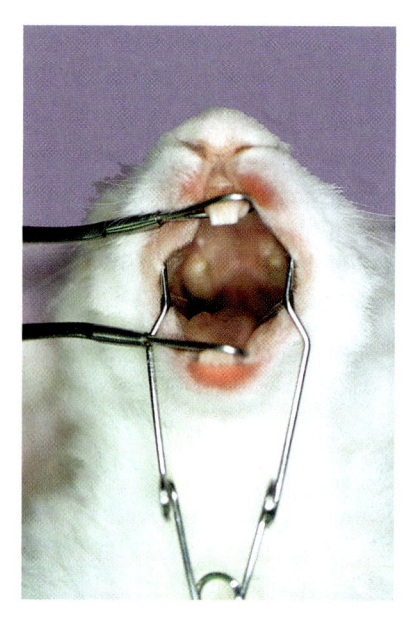

Fig. 4. Oral examination of the anesthetized rabbit is facilitated by using an oral speculum to open the mouth vertically and a pouch dilator to open the mouth horizontally.

prevalent disorder, but pyometra, uterine torsion, and endometrial venous aneurysm all palpate similarly, as fluctuant or doughy masses in the caudal abdomen. Radiographically, an enlarged uterine mass will be identified. The rabbit typically presents for red urine, and urinary bladder disease can be differentiated by a urine sample collected by cystocentesis and abdominal ultrasound. Abdominal ultrasound can distinguish fluid in the uterus and multiple nodules, and can identify local invasion of neoplasia. If uterine adenocarcinoma is suspected, thoracic radiographs are indicated to rule out pulmonary metastasis. All conditions require surgical intervention following stabilization of the rabbit. The most serious condition is multiple endometrial venous aneurysms, which cause episodic bleeding in the lumen of the uterus. Typically, cylindrical blood clots molded within the uterine horns are passed with the urine, and are highly suggestive of this condition, which is seen more commonly in younger does of larger breeds. Although the cause has not been elucidated, venous aneurysms in other animals occur secondary to trauma or congenital defects of the uterine wall. Rabbits with endometrial venous aneurysms may become severely anemic and may require transfusion (PCV < 10). Affected does are at a high risk for fatal exsanguinations from uterine hemorrhage. The rabbit should be stabilized with fluids and transfusion (see the article by Lichtenberger in this issue), and an oophorohysterectomy should be performed.

Dystocia or retained fetuses are uncommon in rabbits and usually this is accompanied by breeding within the past 28 days or delivery of one or more rabbits in the past 24 hours. Signs of dystocia include persistent contractions, straining, and bloody or greenish-brown vaginal discharge. Fetuses are usually palpable, although radiography or abdominal ultrasound will confirm the diagnosis. Abnormalities in the fetuses or in the width of the pelvic canal can be determined with radiographs. Assistance usually requires gentle manual removal of the fetuses and rapid removal of fetal membranes if the neonate is alive. Oxytocin can assist uterine contractions. If the rabbit has a history of prolonged delivery with uterine inertia, a serum chemistry profile is obtained primarily for a calcium and glucose evaluation. Treatment of hypocalcemia is 1 mL/kg of 10% calcium gluconate IV 30 minutes before administering the oxytocin. Heart rate should be observed for bradycardia during bolus administration. The doe should be placed in a quiet dark room for 30 to 60 minutes after administration. Cesarean section is indicated if the injection of oxytocin gets no response.

Renal disease

Acute renal failure is a syndrome characterized by the sudden onset of filtration failure by the kidneys, accumulation of uremic toxins, and dysregulation of fluid, electrolytes, and acid-base balance. It is potentially reversible, if diagnosed quickly and treated aggressively. Azotemia is defined as an elevation in blood urea nitrogen and creatinine. Usually, the serum urea nitrogen is elevated severely in an azotemic rabbit, whereas the creatinine may only be mildly elevated. One reason for this is thought to be the decreased muscle mass, compared with dogs and cats.

The three common causes of acute renal failure in rabbits are

1. Prenal (eg, shock, hypovolemia, as in gastric stasis): The presence of mild to moderate azotemia, clinical dehydration, hypovolemia or hypotension, in conjunction with a urine-specific gravity (USG) that is not isosthenuric (USG > 1030) confirms a diagnosis of prerenal azotemia.
2. Postrenal: The most common causes of postrenal disease include partial or complete obstruction of the urethra or bladder by uroliths, blood clots, or sand, and mucous plugs.
3. Intrinsic renal disease (eg, glomerular nephritis, tubular damage or interstitial renal disease, as with *Encephalitozoon cuniculi*): Intrinsic renal disease is usually an acute onset of chronic renal failure.

Acute renal failure is potentially reversible, whereas chronic renal failure is not completely reversible; therefore, these conditions need to be differentiated. Both acute and chronic renal failures have elevations in blood urea nitrogen and creatinine. In chronic renal failure, the rabbit has a history of chronic loss of body condition, anemia, polydipsia, polyuria, and isosthenuria (eg, 1.010 to 1.015). Kidneys in chronic renal failure appear small ultrasonographically (measuring less than 3 cm in length × 2 cm in width), with abnormal architecture. In acute renal failure, the rabbit has a normal body condition, normal hematocrit value, and no history of polyuria or polydipsia. A urinalysis (± culture and sensitivity) is used to rule out infection, and *E cuniculi* serology should be done in suspected cases. Serology is of limited use in rabbits because it does not indicate that this parasite is the cause of the clinical signs. Many rabbits have been exposed to *E cuniculi* and are infected, but do not show clinical signs of renal disease. A positive test only means that the rabbit has had previous exposure to the parasite; it is not an indication that the parasite is responsible for any of the clinical signs. A negative titer will reliably rule out *E cuniculi* from the differential.

Treatment of acute renal failure involves fluid therapy divided into three parts: (1) correction of perfusion (2) correction of dehydration deficits (3) diuresis to correct azotemia, electrolyte, and acid base status (see the article by Lichtenberger in this issue). Correction of the primary cause needs to be addressed (ie, treatment of gastric stasis, removal of offending drug, or treatment for *E cuniculi*). Once the animal is normotensive and rehydrated, one should record the volume of urine produced every 4 hours. This phase is the polyuric or diuresis phase of acute renal failure. Measurement of urine volume can be accomplished by continuous urinary bladder catheterization or by placing preweighed diapers under the vulva or penis. The volume of urine voided on the diaper can be estimated by assuming 1 mL equals 1 g. The volume of fluid to be administered in each 4-hour period is the sum of calculated maintenance requirements (2 mL/kg/hr) and urine volume from the previous interval. Weighing the rabbit twice a day can provide insight into how effective (or ineffective) the fluid therapy is. If the rabbit has lost weight, then the replacement fluid therapy is ineffective. Ongoing losses (eg, diarrhea) also must be estimated and added to the volume of fluids administered; it is safe to assume that most patients with acute renal failure become 3% to 5% dehydrated each day as a result of ongoing losses. Therefore, the final calculated volume of fluids administered should be increased by 3% to 5%.

In many instances, once the polyuric phase of acute renal failure (ARF) occurs, such large volumes of urine are produced that only aggressive fluid administration allows one to keep up with the patient's fluid requirements. The urine production may be as high as 5 to 10 mL/kg/hr, which is added to maintenance fluid requirements and ongoing losses (ie, 5–10 × maintenance requirements may be required during the diuresis phase). Rule-of-thumb replacement using 2 to 2.5 times maintenance fluids for diuresis is ineffective and will lead to dehydration and ineffective urine production.

Fluids are discontinued gradually when hydration and urine production are restored (fluids in and urine out are matched), serum urea and creatinine are normal (stabilized), and the patient is eating and drinking. The fluids should be tapered by 50% per day. The taper of fluids prevents medullary washout.

Urolithiasis

Urolithiasis refers to the presence of calculi in the urinary system. Rabbits can have any combination of cystic, urethral, renal, and ureteral calculi. The cause of urolithiasis in rabbits is not understood fully, but several factors are involved, including anatomy, nutrition, body condition, and, rarely, infection. Hypercalciuria or crystalluria is a clinical condition seen frequently in pet rabbits. Affected rabbits have a large amount of amorphous, pasty-to-slightly-gritty, calcium-based "sand" or "sludge" in a distended bladder, which can be seen radiographically (Fig. 5). Frequently, a doughlike mass is palpated in the caudal abdomen. Rabbits have an unusual calcium metabolism in that the intestinal absorption of calcium does not directly depend on vitamin D. Increases in dietary calcium directly increase urinary excretion of calcium. The fractional urinary excretion of calcium is less than 2% in most mammals, whereas the range for rabbits is 45% to 60% [20,21]. Voided urine may appear only slightly turbid; however, with manual bladder expression, copious amounts of pasty urine are passed. Expressing urine is painful because of the abrasive material passing along the urethra. Urine can be obtained for analysis by cystocentesis or catheterization. Analysis yields crystalluria; numerous calcium oxalate crystals are common, but ammonium phosphate, calcium carbonate, and monohydrate crystals are also observed frequently. Proteinuria and hematuria are common additional findings. If bacteria are found on cytology, urine obtained on cystocentesis should be submitted for culture. *Pseudomonas* species and *Escherichia coli* are bacteria known to cause cystitis. Results of a complete blood count and serum biochemistry assay assist in assessing renal function and developing a prognosis.

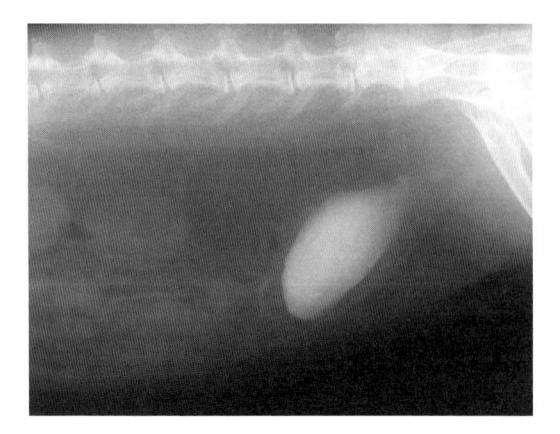

Fig. 5. Lateral radiograph of a rabbit abdomen. Roentgen signs include the urinary bladder with mineral material. A linear mineral opacity is outlining the ventral bladder wall. These findings are consistent with crystalluria.

The rabbit can be started on IV or subcutaneous fluids for diuresis and flushing of the bladder. The bladder should be manually expressed daily for 2 to 4 days to encourage passage of crystals and residual calcium "sand" that may not be voided during normal micturition. A technique similar to voiding, urohydropropulsion, which is used in dogs and cats [22], can be used in rabbits for the nonsurgical removal of fine, granular or small, smooth cystic calculi. Midazolam can be administered to help relax the urethralis muscle, in addition to an opioid for analgesia. The rabbit should be held in an upright position so that the vertebral column is vertical, and steady pressure applied to the bladder. Hematuria is expected to occur for 1 to 2 days following urohydropropulsion [22]. Diet change to reduce weight by giving timothy hay and green vegetables and increasing exercise may help to reduce bladder sand production and accumulation.

Urethral obstruction

A history of strangury or dysuria and a full, firm urinary bladder is consistent with urethral obstruction. The urethra can be obstructed with a single discreet stone, but more commonly the material is an accumulation of "sludge" material. The diagnosis of urolithiasis should be confirmed radiographically. Midazolam relaxes the urethral sphincter muscles, assisting in passage of a urinary catheter. Catheterization of the urethra should be performed carefully with a 3.5F or 5.0F soft catheter of sufficient length to pass the length of the vagina or penile urethra. The catheter tip should be lubricated with sterile lidocaine gel for local analgesia. Indwelling urinary catheters usually are not necessary. Following catheterization and unblocking of the urethra, the critical supportive treatment, with fluid therapy for correction of perfusion and dehydration and diuresis for the hypercalciuria, is given as described earlier for renal failure. Rarely is the urolith firmly lodged in the urethra, but in those cases, surgery is required. Bacterial cystitis is common and is thought to be one of the predisposing causes for urolithiasis in rabbits; therefore, a urine culture should be submitted. Initial treatment should include broad-spectrum antibiotics until culture results can be used to select the most appropriate antimicrobial when indicated.

Diarrhea

Inappropriate diet

Rabbits with intermittent soft stool often have a history of low-fiber diet, high-carbohydrate diet, change in diet, or parasites. When coccidian of the genus *Eimeria* are identified on fecal examination, these can be treated with sulfa drugs but may not be the primary cause of the diarrhea. Inappropriate diet may result in changes in cecal pH or intestinal dysbiosis. Rabbits on an inappropriate diet respond well to correction of the diet [8,11,14]. A high-carbohydrate, low-fiber diet and can result in severe dysbiosis and diarrhea, sometimes accompanied by gas-distended loops of bowel and a painful abdomen. These rabbits need the supportive care described earlier for gastrointestinal stasis.

Inappropriate antibiotic therapy

Normal adult rabbit small intestine, cecum, and colon are inhabited predominantly by the strict anaerobe *Bacteroides*. Studies have identified the facultative anerobic flora in rabbit gastrointestinal content to be primarily staphylococci, whereas coliforms and lactobacilli are rarely detected [23]. Inappropriate antibiotic therapy may result in gastrointestinal dysbiosis and watery, and sometimes bloody, diarrhea. Antibiotics such as amoxicillin, penicillin, ampicillin, clindamycin, lincomycin, erythromycin, and cephalosporins have been reported to cause enteritis. Narrow-spectrum antimicrobials suppress normal gastrointestinal flora, allowing other flora to proliferate, leading to changes in intestinal pH and sometimes progressing to enterotoxemia caused by iota-like toxins from an overgrowth of *Clostridium spiroforme* [8,11,13–15]. These animals are very ill and require hospitalization and treatment as given for gastric stasis. The antibiotic in question should be stopped. Metronidazole (20 mg/kg every 2 hours) can be administered to decrease the growth of clostridium. Several therapies have been recommended for antibiotic-associated enteritis, including *Lactobacillus*, cholestyramine and transfaunation (oral administration of a fecal slurry from a healthy rabbit) and are all anecdotal [19]. *Lactobacillus* may be inhibitory to pathogenic *E coli* [24] because, although it is not thought to be present in healthy rabbit gastrointestinal flora, it does provide some improvement when used therapeutically. Cholestyramine is anion exchange resin that binds bacterial toxins associated with antibiotic-induced enterotoxemia [25].

Mucoid enteritis

Mucoid enteritis has been described as an increase in cecal mucous production of unknown cause, generally in young rabbits. A high morbidity and mortality is associated with this disease syndrome. As described for diarrheas with other causes, rabbits with mucoid enteritis may be dehydrated and anorexic. Supportive care as for gastric stasis is followed.

Red urine

Red urine is perceived frequently by new rabbit owners as an emergency because of blood in the urine. Nonpathologic porphyrin pigments often cause red color in the urine, and a urine dipstick test or urine sediment cytology is a useful, quick assessment to distinguish blood from porphyrins [26,27]. Cystocentesis for urine examination and ultrasound of the caudal abdomen differentiate urinary tract from reproductive tract disorders (see discussion of reproductive disorders). Urinary tract disorders, such as cystitis, pyelonephritis, and urolithiasis (see earlier discussion), can also result in hematuria, treated using typical small animal methods [15,26].

Acute respiratory distress

Rabbits are obligate nasal breathers, and nasal infection is the most common respiratory disease seen in domestic rabbits, usually caused by a polybacterial infection, primarily *Pasteurella multocida* or *Bordetella bronchiseptica*, although other causes such as aspergillosis are possible [28]. The rabbit may have a history of intermittent nasal or ocular discharge, or the presentation may be acute. Physical examination findings may include mucopurulent discharge from the nose or eyes, or uveitis. Thoracic auscultation may consist of referred upper respiratory sounds, or crackles and wheezes in affected lung fields if pneumonia is also present. Animals with severe upper airway disease may be dyspneic because of mucopurulent plugs in the nares and are immediately more comfortable once the nares are cleared. Pneumonia may be unapparent to the owners until late in the course of the disease [10]. Bacterial pneumonia is characterized by dyspnea, tachypnea, and hyperthermia. Radiographs provide critical information in the diagnosis of pneumonia. Ideally, diagnosis is also based on culture and sensitivity. Rhinoscopic evaluation of the nares, or bronchoscopy of the lungs, is recommended for culture sampling [29].

Rabbits with bacterial upper respiratory disease or may benefit from oxygen therapy and nebulization with bronchodilators, as used in small animals.

Neoplasia

Primary mediastinal neoplasia, such as thymoma or lymphoma, or generalized metastatic lung neoplasia, such as uterine adenocarcinoma, are common in rabbits. Radiographs and thoracic ultrasound with fine-needle aspirates of the mass are useful in the diagnosis. Mediastinal masses in the rabbit have been associated with exophthalmos or respiratory distress because of increased pressure on the venous return to the heart, causing engorgement of the large orbital sinus, or pressure on the trachea, respectively [30]. Thoracotomy and surgical removal of the mediastinal mass is the treatment of choice, although radiation therapy can be palliative and can extend the life of the rabbit significantly.

Cardiac disease

As in other mammals, left-sided cardiac disease in rabbits can result in pulmonary edema (ie, dilated cardiomyopathy, mitral regurgitation) and right-sided cardiac disease can cause pleural effusion. The rabbit may have a history of exercise intolerance. A murmur may or may not be auscultated during the physical examination. Radiographs and echocardiography are essential for the diagnosis. Furosemide is useful in relieving pulmonary edema, and thoracocentesis is useful for pleural effusion. Other cardiac medications used in the treatment of dogs and cats are useful in the treatment of cardiac disease in rabbits.

Neurologic signs

Seizures are uncommon in rabbits, but can be the result of a serious condition. If the animal is seizuring at presentation, midazolam may be administered IV [16]. Hypoglycemia is seen in young, anorexic rabbits and may lead to seizures. Blood glucose should be checked and treated with 50% glucose IV (0.25mL/kg) mixed with an equal volume of 0.9% saline.

Lead poisoning may be seen in rabbits allowed free roam of a house in which chewing of lead material is possible. Neurologic signs seen with lead toxicosis are subtle, and include anorexia, progressive depression, and lethargy. Rabbits are often anemic with chronic heavy metal toxicity. Metallic opacities may be apparent radiographically in the stomach and blood lead levels greater than 10 g/dL are diagnostic. Lead toxicosis can be treated as in other small mammals. The treatment of choice is chelation with Ca-EDTA (versenate) for 5 days. The Ca-EDTA can be given subcutaneously, but because it is irritating to tissues, needs to be diluted to 10 mg/mL, using 0.4% sodium chloride (NaCl) and 2.5% dextrose. Two courses of treatment, 1 week apart, may be required.

Posterior paresis/paralysis

Vertebral fracture/subluxation

Fracture of the lumbar vertebrae at L6-L7 is a frequent cause of acute posterior paresis/paralysis in a rabbit. Vertebral fracture or subluxation is commonly the result of improper handling or injury to a startled rabbit that jumps from a chair or table. Additional clinical signs may include loss of skin sensation over the lumbar regions and a flaccid, full urinary bladder. Diagnosis with CT (myelograms are poorly tolerated in rabbits) and treatment protocols are similar to those for small animals. Steroids are controversial in small animals and they are not recommended in rabbits. Nonsteroidal anti-inflammatory drugs (NSAIDs) can be used to decrease inflammation and pain (see the article by Lichtenberger and Ko in this issue).

Encephalitozoon cuniculi

E cuniculi can cause posterior paresis, vestibular disease, uveitis, or renal failure. Unfortunately, the subtle signs may be overlooked until the clinical signs are severe enough to prompt the owner to seek veterinary care. Positive antibody titers to *E cuniculi* only confirm exposure to the organism, but, when combined with compatible clinical signs, are suggestive of infection. A negative antibody titer is reliable to rule out *E cuniculi*. Definitive diagnosis of *E cuniculi* can only be made by histopathologic identification of the organism. Treatments for *E cuniculi* are aimed at elimination of the parasite and supportive care. Treatments include albendazole or fenbendazole. Fenbendazole given orally for 28 days has been reported to eliminate the organism, although the drug is only parasitostatic and does not reverse the tissue damage created by the organism [31]. NSAIDS may be useful in rabbits with normal perfusion, hydration, and renal function.

Head tilt

Head tilt ("wry neck" or torticollis) is a common emergency presentation of the pet rabbit. The most common causes are otitis media (*P multocida*) and *E cuniculi,* but other causes of head tilt in rabbits include otitis externa, *Baylisascaris*, listeriosis, toxoplasmosis, rabies, or other diseases affecting the nervous system, such as trauma or neoplasia. Only one report exists of rabies in a pet rabbit, which had a history of an encounter with a wild skunk [32]. Rabbits with *Baylisascaris* have a history of contact with raccoon or skunk feces, often through hay or bedding. The signs of disease called visceral larval migrans depend on the amount of damage from the migrating larvae and the organ or organs affected. Treatment with high doses of ivermectin may reduce the load of migrating parasites. NSAIDs may assist in decreasing inflammation associated with the larval tracts.

Otitis media

Pasteurella multocida

Otitis media is the most common cause of head tilt in the rabbit [8]. With pasteurellosis, the rabbit may have a history of upper respiratory disease or the presentation may be acute. Infection may progress from the nasal cavity to the middle or inner ear by way of the eustachian tube. At physical examination, mucopurulent material may be observed behind the tympanic membrane, or the membrane may be ruptured. Cultures of the aural discharge are diagnostic in the event of tympanic membrane rupture. Nystagmus is rarely noted. Helical CT images or skull radiographs are useful in evaluating middle ear and bullae disease. Measurement of antibody titers to *P multocida* and *E cuniculi* is of questionable diagnostic value because most rabbits have been exposed to both organisms and will have measurable antibody titers, although negative titers prompt the clinician to look for other causes. Pasteurellosis can be treated with enrofloxacin or other antibiotics such as trimethoprim sulfa or injectable procaine penicillin (for a short period of time), but torticollis may persist. Meclizine has been useful in reducing disorientation in rabbits with head tilt, but is anecdotal [12]. *E cuniculi* is treated as indicated earlier. Nutritional support, with food placed directly in front of the rabbit, is important.

Heat stress

Rabbits are very susceptible to heat stress and generally have a history of exposure to elevated temperatures. Heat-stressed rabbits are dehydrated, weak, and disoriented, and may seizure. Body temperature may be higher than 106°F. These animals must be cooled slowly with IV fluids and a tepid bath [26]. Following recovery, rabbits should be monitored closely for 3 to 5 days for renal failure or additional metabolic abnormalities.

Myiasis

Larvae of the *Cuterebra* sp may infect rabbits housed or allowed to roam outdoors. These opportunistic, large, nonfeeding flies lay eggs near animals, and when an animal wanders past, the eggs attach and hatch in response to the host's body heat. Larvae pupate in the subcutis, causing one or more swellings, especially in the neck, dorsum, and axillary regions. Each swelling encapsulates a larva and has a visible breathing hole on the skin. An advanced-stage larva is about 2.5 cm in length and width. About a month after infestation, the *Cuterebra* larvae fall out of the skin on the ground and pupate. Treatment includes supportive care, removal of the larvae, and treatment of the wound site.

Pregnancy toxemia

Rabbits with pregnancy toxemia generally are overweight and near the end of pregnancy, although this disease can also occur in the postparturient and pseudopregnant rabbit. These rabbits are weak, ataxic, and depressed, and they can progress quickly to coma or death. They are ketonuric, which can be detected using a quick urine dipstick. Treatment is supportive, with IV or intraosseous balanced electrolyte solutions with additional 5% dextrose [32].

References

[1] Gunther RA, Rabinowitz L. Urea and renal concentrating ability in the rabbit. Kidney Int 1980;17:205–22.
[2] Marsh DJ. Solute and water flows in thin limbs of Henles' loop in the hamster kidney. Am J Physiol 1970;218:824–31.
[3] Silverman S, Tell L. Radiology of rodents, rabbits & ferrets: an atlas of normal anatomy and positioning. St. Louis (MO): Elsevier Saunders; 2005.
[4] Rubel GA, Isenbugel E, Wolvekamp P. Atlas of diagnostic radiology of exotic pets: small mammals, birds, reptiles and amphibians. [International edition issued by Schlutersche,

Hannover, Wolfe Publishing Limited, London]. Philadelphia: W.B. Saunders Company; 1991. [London Wolfe Pub].
[5] Cheeke PR. Rabbit feeding and nutrition. Orlando (FL): Academic Press; 1987.
[6] Smith DA, Olson PO, Mathews KA. Nutritional support for rabbits using the percutaneously placed gastrostomy tube: a preliminary study. J Am Anim Hosp Assoc 1997;33(1): 48–54.
[7] Rogers G, Taylor C, Austin JC, et al. A pharyngostomy technique for chronic oral dosing of rabbits. Lab Anim Sci 1988;38:619–20.
[8] Harkness JE, Wagner JE. The biology and medicine of rabbits and rodents. Baltimore (MD): Williams & Wilkins; 1995.
[9] Brown SA, Rosenthal KL. The anorexic rabbit. Proceedings of the North American Veterinary Conference. Orlando (FL): January 1997. p. 788.
[10] Eisele PH. Analgesia in small mammals. Proceedings of the North American Veterinary Conference. Orlando (FL): January 1997. p. 796–9.
[11] Hillyer EV. Pet rabbits. Vet Clin North Am Small Anim Pract 1994;24(1):25–65.
[12] Carpenter JW. Exotic animal formulary. 3rd edition. St. Louis (MO): Turtleback; 2004.
[13] Harrenstein L. Critical care of ferrets, rabbits and rodents. Seminars in Avian and Exotic Pet Medicine 1994;3(4):217–28.
[14] Jenkins JR. Rabbits. In: Jenkins JR, Brown SA, editors. A practitioner's guide to rabbits and ferrets. Lakewood (CO): The American Animal Hospital Association; 1993.
[15] Gentz EJ, Harrenstien LA, Carpenter JW. Dealing with gastrointestinal, genitourinary, and musculoskeletal problems in rabbits. Vet Med 1995;90(4):365–72.
[16] Stein S, Walshaw S. Rabbits. In: Laber-Laird K, Swindle M, Flecknell P, editors. Handbook of rodent and rabbit medicine. Oxford (UK): Pergamon; 1996. p. 183–218.
[17] Michiels M, Monbalie J, Hendriks R, et al. Pharmacokinetics and tissue distribution of the new gastrokinetic agent cisapride in rat, rabbit and dog [abstract]. Arzneimittelforschung 1987;37(10):59–67.
[18] Langer JC, Bramlett G. Effect of prokinetic agents on ileal contractility in a rabbit model of gastroschisis. J Pediatr Surg 1997;32(4):605–8.
[19] Fann MK, O'Rourke D. Normal bacterial flora of the rabbit gastrointestinal tract: a clinical approach. Seminars in Avian & Exotic Pet Medicine: Bacterial Disease 2001;10(1):45–7.
[20] Buss SL, Bourdeau JE. Calcium balance in laboratory rabbits. Miner Electrolyte Metab 1984;10:127–32.
[21] Cheeke PR, Amberg JW. Comparative calcium excretion by rats and rabbits. J Anim Sci 1973;37:450–4.
[22] Lulich JP, Osborne CA, Carson M. Nonsurgical removal of urocystoliths in dogs and cats by voiding urohydropropulsion. J Am Vet Med Assoc 1993;203:660–3.
[23] Linaje R, Coloma MD, Perez-Martinez G, et al. Characterization of faecal enterococci from rabbits for the selection of probiotic strains. J Appl Microbiol 2004;96:761–71.
[24] Abo-El-Khair IAA, Awny N. Influence of feeding Lactobacillus acidophilus cells on serum cholesterol levels of rabbits. Egypt Journal of Microbiology 1993;28:259–69.
[25] Lipman NS, Weischedel AK, Connors MJ, et al. Utilization of cholestyramine resin as a preventive treatment for antibiotic (clindamycin) induced enterotoxaemia in the rabbit. Lab Anim 1992;26(11):1–8.
[26] Paul-Murphy J. Reproductive and urogenital disorders. In: Hillyer EV, Quesenberry KE, editors. Ferrets, rabbits and rodents clinical medicine and surgery. Philadelphia: WB Saunders Co; 1997. p. 202–11.
[27] Samman S, Fussell SH, Rose CI. Prophyria in a New Zealand white rabbit. Can Vet J 1991; 32:622–3.
[28] Rougier S, Galland D, Boucher S, et al. Epidemiology and susceptibility of pathogenic bacteria responsible for upper respiratory tract infections in pet rabbits. Vet Microbiol 2006; 115(1–3):192–8.

[29] Hernandez-Divers SJ. Endoscopic evaluation of the respiratory system of rabbits. Exotic DVM 2002;4(3):55–8.
[30] Vernau KM, Clarke-Scott HA, Sullivan N. Thymoma in a geriatric rabbit with hypercalcemia and periodic exophthalmos. J Am Vet Med Assoc 1995;206:802–22.
[31] Suter C, Muller-Doblies UU, Hatt JM, et al. Prevention and treatment of Encephalitozoon cuniculi infection in rabbits with fenbendazole. Vet Rec 2001;148(15):478–80.
[32] CDC Veterinary Public Health Notes. Rabbit rabies. J Am Vet Med Assoc 1981;179:84.

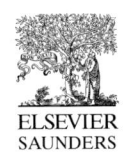

Emergency Medicine of the Ferret
Christal Pollock, DVM, DABVP-Avian

30 Severance Circle, Apartment 206, Cleveland Heights, OH 44118, USA

Ferrets most commonly require supportive and critical care for gastrointestinal disease, cardiac disease, neoplasia, or endocrinopathy. The emergency veterinarian must be familiar with anatomy and husbandry that differs from cats and dogs. Various emergency procedures and diagnostics are discussed here, along with diseases most commonly encountered in emergency situations.

The average small animal veterinarian may easily become comfortable with ferrets. Ferrets are hardy and relatively stoic, and as members of the order Carnivora, ferrets are predator species that approach the world in a manner similar to cats and dogs. A small number of medical problems are seen very commonly in ferrets. Careful study of these conditions and attention to the unique aspects of ferret anatomy and behavior prepare the small animal veterinarian for basic emergency care of the ferret.

"Ferret-centric" information

Taxonomy

Ferrets are members of the order Carnivora and family Mustelidae, making them close relatives to the mink, skunk, weasel, and otter. The scientific name of the ferret *Mustela putorius furo* literally translates as "stinky thief." This name reflects the curious, sometimes mischievous, nature of the ferret and their distinctive musky odor. Most ferrets seen in clinical practice have been de-scented and neutered, which reduces but does not totally eliminate this musky scent. This scent is much more pungent in the intact ferret, particularly the intact male.

The pet ferret is not an exotic animal whose natural environment must be duplicated in captivity [1]. Ferrets have been domesticated for more than 2000 years. In the United Kingdom and Canada, ferrets are generally

---

E-mail address: christal7@mac.com

outdoor pets used for hunting rabbits, groundhogs, and other small mammals. Their long, skinny shape allows ferrets to follow prey down into burrows and flush them out so they may be captured with nets or snares. Ferrets are popular indoor pets in the United States. Most American ferrets come from large ferret farms or ranches where they are neutered and de-scented at an early age. Despite their domesticity and popularity, ferrets are poorly understood. There are many state, county, or city laws that describe them as "wild," "non-domestic," or "dangerous" animals [2].

Vocabulary terms and physiologic values

A female ferret is a "jill," and a male ferret is a "hob." Probably the most common term used by pet owners is "kit," which designates a neonatal or juvenile ferret. Less commonly used by pet owners are terms such as "gib" (neutered male) and "sprite" (neutered female) [2]. Selected physiologic values for the domestic ferret are given in Table 1.

Anatomy

Knowledge of basic carnivore anatomy is an excellent starting point for dealing with the ferret; however, there are some unique anatomic characteristics of the ferret. First, the ferret spine is extremely flexible, allowing 180° turns within narrow passageways. The vertebral formula is C7 T15 L5 (6 or 7) S3 Cd18 [2].

As strict carnivores designed to eat small, whole prey, ferrets possess a short, simple gastrointestinal tract with no cecum or ileocolic valve.

Table 1
Basic biologic characteristics of the ferret [36]

Life stage	
Achieve adult size	3–4 months
Puberty	4–5 months
Sexual maturity	6–12 months
Lifespan	6–8 years (maximum, 10–12 years)
Adult body weight	0.6–1.2 kg*
Temperature	100°F–103°F
Pulse	170–250 bpm
Respiratory rate	32–36 bpm
Litter size	1–18 kits (average, 8)
Gestation	41–43 days
Birth weight	6–12 g
Eyes and ears open	32 and 24 days
Weaning age	6–8 weeks
Body weight	Males 0.8–1.2 kg; females 0.6–1.0 kg
Dental formula	2 (I 3/3 C1/1 P3/3 M1/2 = 34
Urine volume	26–28 mL/24 h
Vertebral formula	C7 T15 L5 (6 or 7) S3 Cd18

* Males are larger, weighing 0.8 to 1.2 kg, while females are smaller and more petite.

Transit time is rapid and may be as brief as 3 hours. The presence of only minimal microbial flora means the ferret gut handles most antibiotics well. This same lack of microbial flora means that carbohydrates are digested poorly and fiber not at all. The dental formula of the ferret is 2 (I 3/3 C1/1 P3/3 M1/2) = 34 [2,3].

Husbandry

Nutrition

Ferrets require high quality, animal-based dietary protein. Diets should contain 30% to 35% crude protein and 15% to 20% fat. Typical diets fed to pet ferrets in the United States include commercial ferret foods and good quality cat foods.

When feeding the hospitalized ferret, always learn about the home diet, because some individuals may resist sudden dietary changes. Also ask if the ferret drinks from a water bottle or bowl. Dishes should be heavy enough to prevent the curious ferret from overturning them. Unless drastically overfilled, a large bowl makes it difficult for the ferret to access the food, so small or shallow dishes work best. Food should be available at all times unless the ferret is being fasted, because the normal ferret eats small amounts of food frequently [4].

Good choices for feeding the anorectic ferret include Prescription Diet a/d (Hill's Pet Nutrition; Topeka, KS), Carnivore Care (Oxbow Pet Product; Murdock, NE), and Eukanuba Maximum-Calorie (The Iams Company; Dayton, OH). Chicken baby food is readily accepted and may be fed on a short-term basis [2,4]. Warming food may increase acceptability. Nutri-Cal (Tomyln; EVSCO Pharmaceuticals; Buena, NJ), Ferrotone (8-in-1 Pet Products; Hauppauge, NY) and other sugar-containing formulations can cause rebound hypoglycemia in ferrets with insulinoma and should be avoided in those animals.

Illness quickly leads to minimal body fat stores and then cachexia. Hepatic lipidosis develops quickly in the ferret, and therefore enteral nutrition is recommended after initial stabilization with fluids. The ferret is easily force-fed by holding the ferret by the "scruff" in one hand and force-feeding with the other hand. When syringe feeding a ferret, begin with 5 to 10 mL per feeding at least three to four times daily. Small, extremely weak, or highly resistant ferrets should be offered a minimum of 2 to 3 mL more frequently. Large ferrets with good appetites may take up to 20 mL per meal. Try offering water to debilitated ferrets in a shallow crock, even if the individual normally drinks from a water bottle.

For long-term management, esophagostomy or pharyngostomy tubes may be considered in rare instances. Place an 8- to 10-Fr feeding tube using the same method described for cats. Apply a butterfly tape piece to the tube, suture it into place, and add a light wrap around neck [5,6]. Gastric feeding tubes have been placed experimentally in the ferret, but not in clinical patients [7]. When the gut must be bypassed, partial or total parenteral nutrition may also be used [6].

Housing the pet ferret

Ferrets are often kept in large, multilevel cages at home. They also require supervised exercise outside of the cage within "ferret-proofed" rooms. Ferret proofing includes all measures taken to keep the pet ferret safe. Holes to the outside or to areas from which ferrets cannot be retrieved are blocked. The bottoms of all couches, chairs, and mattresses are covered with a thin piece of wood or hardware cloth to prevent burrowing and chewing in soft foam rubber. Access to foam or latex rubber should also be avoided, because ferrets often chew such items, including athletic shoe soles, rubber bands, stereo speakers, and headphones. Reclining chairs have been implicated in the death of many ferrets and should be removed from any ferret-proofed environment [2,6].

In the hospital, maintain ferrets in escape-proof enclosures, because they can squeeze through openings as small as 1 inch in diameter if there is any give to the material. Probably the best choice for ferret housing is a standard stainless steel cage with small spacing between vertical bars. Cages with larger bar spacing may be adapted by attaching a piece of Plexiglas to the cage front at least half the height of the door or taller. This Plexiglas cover prevents escape and is easily removed for cleaning. Hospitalized ferrets may also be maintained in plastic rabbit cages, avian hospital cages, or incubators. Monitor ferrets closely in avian cages or incubators, because they may easily overheat [4,6].

Always provide burrowing material, such as a large towel or pillowcase, unless the patient requires an intravenous or urinary catheter. In these cases, remove burrowing material or provide something small like a surgical towel, otherwise the line will invariably become entangled as the ferret burrows.

Ferrets often use a back corner of the cage as a latrine; therefore, place the litter box in the back of the cage. Offer a pan with one very low side for weak or ataxic ferrets [4].

Handling and restraint

Except for their natural, exuberant wiggliness, most ferrets are easily handled using minimal restraint. Gently grasp the ferret around the chest with one hand while lightly supporting the rump with the other hand. Most ferrets also relax when held snugly but gently against the body with a flexed arm. With the exception of kits, most ferrets rarely bite when handled gently [4].

Manual restraint is required for uncomfortable procedures such as checking body temperature. There are two main methods of physical restraint of the ferret: scruffing and stretching. To scruff, gently yet firmly grasp the ferret by the loose skin at the nape of the neck (Fig. 1). Then allow the ferret to hang from its scruff with all four feet suspended off the ground. In many

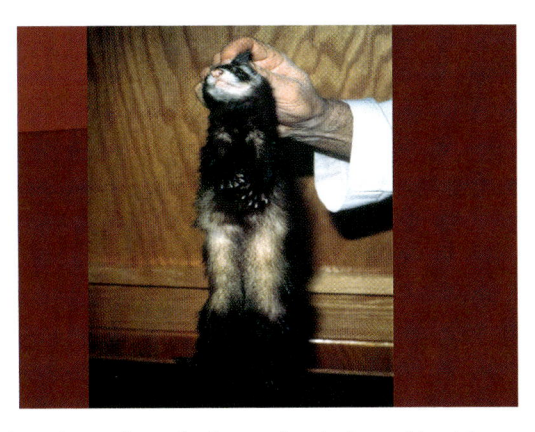

Fig. 1. Scruff the ferret by gently yet firmly grasping the loose skin at the nape of the neck, then suspend all four feet off the ground.

ferrets, this causes total and complete relaxation, including a jaw-popping yawn.

To stretch, hold the ferret in lateral recumbency while grasping the scruff in one hand and placing the other hand securely around the pelvis. Do not hold the rear limbs, as one would in a cat, because this always makes ferrets struggle. A distraction, like Nutri-Cal or meat baby food, may also prove helpful as long as the ferret is not being restrained to check blood glucose levels.

Hospital personnel with influenza should avoid contact with ferrets [6].

Anamnesis

Signalment and history are crucial in developing an initial differential diagnosis list (Tables 2 and 3) [6]. After discussing the reason for presentation, including onset and progression of clinical signs, obtain a detailed general history. What diet is fed at home, including treats? Low quality cat food containing plant-based protein promotes development of struvite crystalluria. Does the ferret drink from a water bottle or bowl? What is the housing set-up? Is the ferret usually caged? Anecdotally, lack of time outside the cage for exercise and play has been correlated with increased incidence of *Helicobacter* gastritis. This is most likely related to increased boredom and stress when playtime is not offered. When out of the cage, is the ferret supervised and is the environment ferret-proofed? Is the pet a chewer? Have any toys or household items been recently destroyed? Younger ferrets commonly chew rubber and sponge material with increased risk for foreign body ingestion. And who is the primary caretaker? Whenever a young child is in the household, the risk for trauma increases greatly.

Discuss details of the ferret's medical history, including appetite, activity level, and eliminations. Has there been any vomiting or diarrhea? What is the vaccination status? Although the incidence of disease is

Table 2
Important differentials in the ferret based on clinical signs

Clinical sign	Differential diagnoses	Comments
Alopecia		
Metabolic	**Adrenal disease**	
	Ovarian remnant disease	
	Seasonal alopecia	(Tail); hair typically regrows in several weeks, may be more common in males
Anorexia		
Metabolic	Cardiomyopathy	
	Ovarian remnant disease	
	Urethral obstruction	
Neoplasia	Lymphosarcoma	
Idiopathic	Myofasciitis	
Infectious, inflammatory	Epizootic catarrhal enteritis	
	Proliferative bowel disease	
Trauma	**Gastrointestinal foreign body**	
Ascites		
Metabolic	Cardiomyopathy	
Neoplasia	Lymphosarcoma	
Ataxia		
Metabolic	**Insulinoma**	
	Cardiomyopathy	
Idiopathic	Myofasciitis	
Collapse	See *Weakness*	
Constipation		Rare in the ferret, more likely stranguria or dysuria
Depression		
Metabolic	**Insulinoma**	
	Cardiomyopathy	
	Urethral obstruction	
Neoplasia	**Lymphosarcoma**	
Idiopathic	Myofasciitis	
Infectious, inflammatory	Epizootic catarrhal enteritis	
Trauma	Gastrointestinal foreign body	
	Traumatic household injury	
	Heat stroke	
Diarrhea		
Metabolic	(Ovarian remnant disease)	(Melena)
	(Renal disease)	
	(Liver disease)	
Nutritional	Dietary indiscretion	
Infectious, inflammatory	***Helicobacter* gastritis**	
	Proliferative bowel disease	(Large bowel)
	Lymphocytic-plasmacytic gastroenteritis	
	Eosinophilic gastroenteritis	

(*continued on next page*)

Table 2 (continued)

Clinical sign	Differential diagnoses	Comments
	Epizootic catarrhal enteritis	(Green, mucoid; "bird seed" appearance)
	Influenza	(Transient diarrhea sometimes occurs)
	Campylobacter	Hematochezia, fever
	Salmonella	Hematochezia, fever
	(*Giardia*)	
	(Coccidiosis)	
Trauma	Gastrointestinal foreign body	
	Trichobezoar	
	Heat stroke	Melena, bloody diarrhea
Toxin	(Toxin exposure)	
Dyspnea		
Metabolic	Cardiomyopathy	
Neoplasia	Lymphosarcoma	Cranial mediastinal mass or pulmonary involvement
Infectious, inflammatory	Influenza virus	
Trauma	Traumatic household injury	
	Heat stroke	Associated with tachypnea
Dysuria	See *Stranguria*	
Ecchymosis	See *Petechia*	
Fever		
Idiopathic	Myofasciitis	
Infectious, inflammatory	**Influenza virus**	
	Canine distemper virus	
Trauma	**Overheating, including heat stroke or exhaustion**	
Lethargy	See *Depression*	
Lymphadenopathy		
Neoplasia	**Lymphosarcoma**	
Nausea, vomiting		
Metabolic	**Insulinoma**	
	Renal disease[a]	
	Hepatic disease[a]	
Inflammatory, infectious	***Helicobacter* gastritis**	
	Lymphocytic-plasmacytic gastroenteritis	
	Eosinophilic gastroenteritis	
	Epizootic catarrhal enteritis	
Trauma	Gastrointestinal foreign body[a]	
	Heat stroke	
Petechia		
Metabolic	Ovarian remnant disease	
Pruritus		
Metabolic	Adrenal disease	
Inflammatory, infectious	(Ectoparasites)	
	Cardiomyopathy	

(*continued on next page*)

Table 2 (*continued*)

Clinical sign	Differential diagnoses	Comments
Rear limb weakness[b]		
Metabolic	**Insulinoma**	
	Cardiomyopathy	
Idiopathic	Myofasciitis	
Trauma	Traumatic household injury	
Rectal prolapse		
Inflammatory, infectious	**Proliferative bowel disease** (Coccidiosis) (Neoplasia)	
Respiratory signs		
Metabolic	Cardiomyopathy	
Inflammatory, infectious	Influenza	
Seizure activity		
Metabolic	Insulinoma	
Trauma	Heat stroke	
Skin mass	Mast cell tumor	
Stranguria		
Nutritional	Struvite crystalluria	
Metabolic	**Prostatomegaly secondary to adrenal disease**	
Inflammatory, infectious	(Cystitis) (Prostatic abscess)	
Vulvar swelling		
Metabolic	**Adrenal disease**	
	Ovarian remnant disease	
	Intact female	
Weakness		
Metabolic	Insulinoma	
	Ovarian remnant disease	
Neoplasia	Lymphosarcoma	
Idiopathic	Myofasciitis	

The most important or common differentials are **bolded**.
[a] Vomiting is rare, but may occur intermittently.
[b] Anything that causes generalized weakness may initially manifest as rear limb weakness in the ferret.

rare, ferrets are exquisitely sensitive to canine distemper virus. Ferrets are also prone to vaccination reactions. Has there been exposure to a new animal recently, or has the ferret visited a show or pet store? Epizootic catarrhal enteritis may develop after exposure with a young, newly acquired ferret.

Know ferret-specific signs of disease. Signs of nausea in the ferret may include copious drooling (ptyalism) and pawing vigorously at the mouth, in addition to retching and gagging. Signs of abdominal pain may include bruxism or teeth grinding.

Table 3
Important differentials in the ferret based on clinical pathologic findings

Test result	Differential diagnoses	Comments
Hypoglycemia		
Metabolic	Insulinoma	
	(Liver disease)	
	Heat stroke	
Inflammatory, infectious	Sepsis	
Anemia		
Metabolic	Ovarian remnant disease	Pancytopenia
	Adrenal disease	Mild to moderate nonregenerative
Neoplasia	Lymphosarcoma	Nonregenerative
Inflammatory, infectious	*Helicobacter* gastritis	Regenerative anemia
Trauma	Gastrointestinal foreign body	Regenerative anemia
	Flea bite infestation	
Azotemia		
Metabolic	Urethral obstruction	
	Heat stroke	
Hyperkalemia		
Metabolic	Urethral obstruction	
	Heat stroke	
Elevated ALT		
Metabolic	Hepatic lipidosis secondary to insulinoma	
	Cardiomyopathy	
Creatine kinase, elevated		
Metabolic	Heat stroke	
Idiopathic	Myofasciitis	

Physical examination

Cardiopulmonary arrest requires immediate treatment (see the article on shock and fluid resuscitation elsewhere in this issue).

Modify the length of the physical examination based on the ferret's cardiopulmonary status. Place any ferret showing signs of respiratory distress in an oxygen-rich environment. Carefully observe the ferret's breathing pattern and auscult respiratory sounds. The long, thin chest of the ferret places the apex heart beat more caudally than in the cat or dog. The heart sits between the sixth and eighth ribs, usually three to four ribs caudal to the elbow. Auscult the entire length of the thoracic cavity, ideally with the use of a pediatric or infant stethoscope. A common finding in the ferret is a prominent respiratory sinus arrhythmia. There are five different breathing patterns associated with audible or auscultated sounds that help to localize the cause of respiratory distress.

Breathing patterns

An upper airway lesion creates a normal breathing pattern with a loud inspiratory wheeze [8–10]. Referred upper airway sounds are heard on auscultation of the chest. Potential causes of laryngeal obstruction include foreign body, neoplasia, or abscess of the upper airway. Laryngeal paralysis has not been reported in the ferret. Perform an oral examination to identify the obstruction for biopsy, culture and sensitivity, or removal of the foreign body.

Lower airway lesions such as tracheal obstruction also create a normal breathing pattern, but this is associated with soft expiratory stridor, pronounced gagging, and swallowing. Upper airway sounds are present on auscultation.

Small airway disease creates a soft expiratory wheeze with synchronous movement of the chest and abdomen. There is a wheezing sound on auscultation of the chest. The lesion is located within the small bronchi and is usually secondary to a small airway inhalant toxin or asthma. This is very rare in the ferret.

There are no audible respiratory sounds in parenchymal disease; however, there is synchronous movement of the chest and abdomen. Respiratory wheezes are heard on auscultation of the chest. Differentials include pulmonary edema secondary to heart disease (see Cardiovascular disease) and pneumonia (see Respiratory disease).

Pleural space disease creates no audible respiratory sounds, but a dyssynchronous breathing pattern is observed with the chest and abdomen moving opposite to each other. Dull lung sounds are heard on auscultation of the chest. The pleural space is filled with air (pneumothorax) or blood (hemothorax) in cases of trauma, or pleural effusion in cases of cardiac disease or lymphosarcoma (see Cardiac disease and Neoplasia).

When the cardiovascular and pulmonary systems are normal, physical examination may be continued in a systematic fashion. Normal physiologic parameters are given in Table 1. Evaluate the moistness of the mucous membranes for evidence of dehydration and treat with fluids as described in the article on shock and fluid therapy by Lichtenberger elsewhere in this issue. Ferrets derived from a ferret farm have two small dots tattooed in the pinna of the right ear. This tattoo signifies that the ferret has been de-scented and neutered. Within the ears, it is common to find dark brown, waxy discharge. Excessive wax or more commonly granular ear discharge may be associated with *Otodectes cyanotis* mite infestation [11]. Broken canines are a common finding in older ferrets.

Lymph nodes may feel enlarged in big male or overweight ferrets because of the presence of surrounding fat, but the nodes still feel soft and pliable. Firmness or asymmetry of the lymph nodes suggests lymphadenopathy and warrants fine-needle aspiration. Enlargement of two or more nodes justifies a full diagnostic workup.

Palpate the abdomen while lifting the front half of the ferret off the table. Ferrets normally have relaxed abdomens that are easy to palpate. The normal ferret spleen is large for the size of the animal, measuring approximately 5 cm long, 2 cm wide, and 1 cm thick [6]. Palpate the spleen gently for clean edges and homogenous consistency. Splenomegaly is a common incidental finding in ferrets older than 1 year of age, most frequently caused by extramedullary hematopoiesis. Even a spleen so big and pendulous that the animal has difficulty lifting its abdomen off the ground may not be pathologic in origin. Ultrasonography and fine-needle aspirate cytology may be indicated for evaluation of the enlarged spleen [2,6,11].

Examine the hair coat for evidence of alopecia, particularly over the flanks, shoulders, and tail base. Seasonal alopecia is a common finding in which fur falls out, typically along the tail, and then regrows within several weeks. Also check for evidence of skin excoriations, which may be created in the pruritic ferret.

Ferrets are easy to sex. The prepuce is on the ventral abdomen just caudal to the umbilicus, and the os penis is readily palpable. Check the prepuce for redness, which may be seen with excessive licking when urogenital disease leads to discomfort. The female urogenital opening is a slit in the perineal region just ventral to the anus. Always check for vulvar swelling, which may be observed with estrus, ovarian remnant syndrome, or adrenal disease (Fig. 2).

Allow the ferret to walk around the room at the end of the examination. Signs of generalized weakness may include a loss of the normal hump in the back while in motion and rear limb weakness or ataxia. A ferret allowed to explore an examination room often eliminates in one corner. Normal stool is slightly soft and formed.

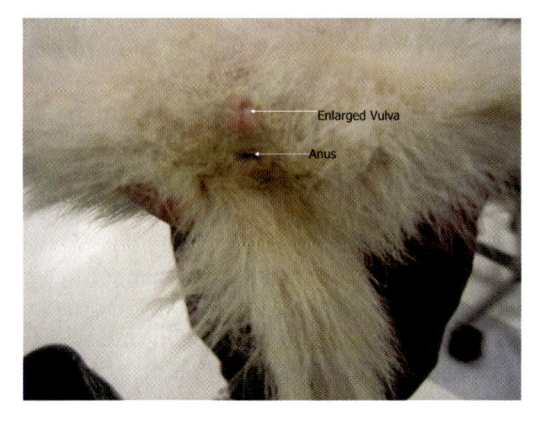

Fig. 2. This figure shows vulvar swelling in the female ferret. Female ferrets should always be evaluated for vulvar swelling on physical examination. Vulvar swelling may develop with estrus, ovarian remnant syndrome, or adrenal disease.

Diagnostics and therapeutics

Clinical pathology

Ideally one should obtain a biochemistry panel and complete blood count, including reticulocyte count, in the debilitated ferret. Minimum stat blood work should include hematocrit, total protein, blood glucose level, and blood urea nitrogen (BUN).

Normal hematocrit is higher in the ferret (46%–61%), and erythrocyte counts may be as high as 17.4×10^6 cells/µL. The normal mean reticulocyte count for female albino ferrets is 5.3% and 4% for male albino ferrets. Reticulocyte counts may be as high as 10% or even exceed 12% with regenerative anemia. The white cell count in ferrets normally ranges from 2500 to 8000 cells/cm. Typically neutrophils predominate, with lymphocyte counts usually less than 50%. Normal total protein is 5.1 to 7.4 g/dL [12].

Isoflurane and sevoflurane significantly decrease hematocrit, hemoglobin, plasma protein, red blood cell count, and white cell count. Maximum effects occur 15 minutes after induction. Values should return to their original state 45 minutes after anesthesia [13–15].

Biochemistry panel

Ferret biochemistry values are similar to those found in other mammals with few exceptions. For instance, liver enzyme values and serum bile acids are similar to those of dogs and cats. Alanine aminotransferase (ALT), serum alkaline phosphatase (ALP), total bilirubin levels, and serum bile acids increase with liver disease and liver dysfunction.

Blood glucose levels normally range from 90 to 120 mg/dL in the fasting ferret. Insulinoma is a very common disease of middle-aged to older ferrets, leading to hypoglycemia. Blood glucose levels less than 90 mg/dL are suspicious for insulinoma in the fasting ferret, whereas levels less than 70 mg/dL are strongly suggestive of insulinoma. Ferrets suspected of having insulinoma do not necessarily need to be fasted. When fasting is performed, it should last for no more than 2 to 3 hours, and the patient should be carefully monitored during that time.

Normal serum creatinine in the ferret is usually half that seen in the dog and cat. Creatinine often ranges from 0.1 to 0.3 mg/dL and is almost always less than 0.5 mg/dL. Elevations in creatinine may be incremental, if they occur at all [16]. Creatinine levels between 0.7 to 1.0 mg/dL signify azotemia in the ferret. Always be sure to evaluate serum phosphorus and urine specific gravity (USG) in any ferret suspected of having renal disease. Elevations in BUN and phosphorus are common with renal disease. Ferret urine is usually isosthenuric with a USG between 1.010 and 1.115 in chronic renal failure [2].

Normal electrolyte values are similar to those in a cat. Lactate measurements are normally between 1 and 3 mmol/dL. Electrolyte values are elevated in the poorly perfused ferret and decrease with fluid resuscitation as in the dog and cat (M. Lichtenberger, personal communication, 2007).

Venipuncture

Restraint for venipuncture is challenging in the conscious ferret. Practice venipuncture on healthy anesthetized patients or cadavers. Inhalant anesthesia lowers hematocrit and white blood cell count and is not recommended for the purpose of collecting a blood sample in the critically ill patient.

Use a 1- to 3-mL syringe paired with a 25- to 27-gauge needle in most ferrets. In large males, a 22- or 23-gauge needle may also be used for jugular venipuncture. A small 0.3- to 0.5-mL insulin syringe with a 28- to 30-gauge needle may be used for small vessels. The thick skin of the ferret necessitates use of a new, sharp needle with every venipuncture attempt. The maximum volume of blood that may be collected in healthy ferrets is 1% of body weight in grams. Place samples in microtainers (Calgary Laboratory Services; Calgary, AB, Canada) [2,12].

There are several options for venipuncture sites. The jugular vein and cranial vena cava are the most popular sites for collection of large blood volumes. The jugular vein lies in a more lateral position than in the cat and dog. The thick skin over the neck can sometimes make it difficult to find the vessel.

Blood collection from the cranial vena cava is easily done on the conscious ferret with practice. The heart is located caudal in the chest, making caval venipuncture safe. Lay the ferret on its back with its forelimbs extended straight down toward its tail. Palpate a slight depression or notch between the manubrium and first rib. Slowly insert a 25-gauge needle attached to a 1- or 3-mL syringe at a 45° angle to the skin. Aim the needle at the opposite hip and slowly insert the needle to the level of the hub while gently applying negative pressure. Then slowly withdraw the needle until the syringe begins to fill with blood (Fig. 3). If the patient moves, remove the needle quickly to avoid lacerating the vessel. Avoid caval sticks in patients in which pancytopenia is suspected [11].

The lateral saphenous is a good alternative, especially for collection of smaller blood volumes. This vessel may be easiest to access when using the straight segment of the vessel, which lies proximal to the tarsus, as in the dog.

Venous catheterization

The cephalic vein is the best site for intravenous catheter placement. This vessel is usually visible, but the overlying skin may be thick. A 22-gauge needle with the bevel side up may be used to make a small nick in the skin to prevent burring of the catheter. Ferrets rarely chew at catheter sites. Alternative sites for catheter placement include the lateral saphenous vein and the jugular vein [6,11].

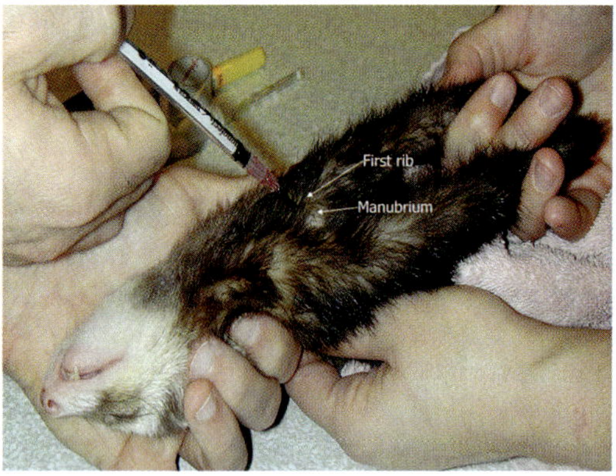

Fig. 3. The cranial vena cava is an alternate site for collection of large blood volumes. The ferret is wrapped in a towel and both forelegs are pulled back. The second person extends the neck and inserts a 25-gauge needle with an attached 1 mL syringe between the manubrium and first rib at a 45° angle and directed toward the opposite back leg. Insert the needle to the hub and pull back on plunger as the needle is slowly withdrawn until blood begins to fill the syringe.

An intraosseous catheter can be placed when intravenous catheterization fails. The lateral tibia and proximal femur are the most common sites for placement. Use a 22- gauge spinal needle with a stylet or a 20- or 18-gauge hypodermic needle. Use sterilized orthopedic wire within the hypodermic needle as a stylet to prevent occlusion with bone marrow. Aseptically prepare the skin and inject 0.1 mL of lidocaine 2% with 0.1 mL bupivacaine 0.5% into the periosteum, subcutaneous tissue, and skin.

Urinalysis

As in dogs and cats, there are multiple options for urine collection. Cystocentesis, when indicated, may be performed by palpation or guided by ultrasound. Insert the needle through the lateral body wall as in the cat. Use a 3- to 6-mL syringe attached to a 1-inch, 22- to 25-gauge needle. Some ferrets may be manually restrained, whereas others may require sedation with buprenorphine or butorphanol (see the article on analgesia/anesthesia elsewhere in this issue). Repeated cystocentesis is not recommended because of the thin bladder wall.

Radiology

Whole body radiographs are generally taken in ferrets using tabletop technique, high-speed film, and fine screen cassettes. The appearance of the normal ferret radiograph is similar to that of other carnivorous species [11].

The long, lean body shape of the ferret means that the heart is positioned more caudally within the thoracic cavity. The normal ferret heart may seem slightly more globoid on survey radiographs. On lateral films, the right ventricle may seem slightly elevated from the sternum because of the accumulation of fat around the ligament, which extends from heart to sternum. This normal finding should not be confused with the presence of pneumothorax. When evaluating the thoracic cavity, be sure to include the cranial thorax [6,11]. The size of the cardiac silhouette can be quantified by use of the modified vertebral heart score (VHS), which measures heart length and width on the right lateral radiograph. These measurements are added together and expressed in centimeters. Normal mean VHS value in the ferret is 4.00 cm (range, 3.75–4.07 cm) (Fig. 4) [17].

There is normally a large amount of fat outlining abdominal organs in the ferret. Splenomegaly is a common finding. The stomach is normally devoid of gas, whereas there is little to no gas in the intestinal tract [16,18].

Contrast radiography

Give barium at 8 to 15 mL/kg by mouth or by stomach tube for upper gastrointestinal evaluation. Strawberry flavored barium is readily accepted by ferrets. When a gastrointestinal perforation is suspected, use iohexol mixed with tap water at a 1:1 ratio at the same dose. Take radiographs immediately and then at 5, 10, 20, 40, 60, 90, 120, and 150 minutes after the barium is administered. Gastric emptying usually begins immediately, although total emptying of the stomach takes longer in sedated ferrets than in awake ferrets (130 ± 40 minutes and 75 ± 54 minutes, respectively). The barium-filled small intestines are best visualized at 20 and 40 minutes. The width of the small bowel does not normally exceed 5 to 7 mm [11,16].

When performing an excretory urogram, the recommended intravenous dosage is 2 mL/kg of iodinated contrast agent [2].

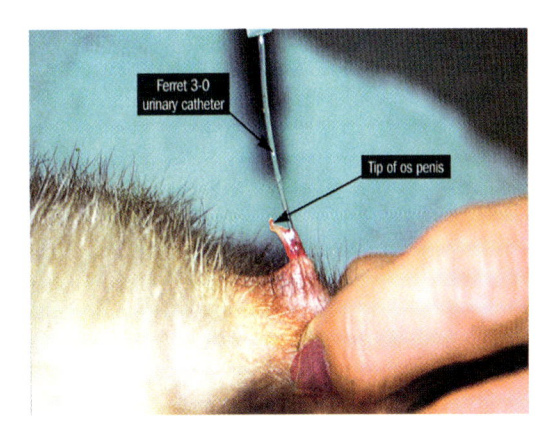

Fig. 4. Urethral catheterization of a male ferret using a 3-French urinary catheter. The S shape of the tip of the penis is shown.

Ultrasonography

Ultrasound is commonly performed to evaluate abdominal organs as in cats and dogs. Measurements that differ from those in cats are kidneys measuring 3 × 3 cm and adrenal gland width less than 3 mm [2].

Normal echocardiographic measurements have also been evaluated in the ferret (Table 4) [19,20]. The most common heart disease in the ferret is dilated cardiomyopathy, although hypertrophic cardiomyopathy, mitral valvular disease, and heartworm disease have been described.

Electrocardiogram

Apply flattened ECG clips to these small patients. Also use ECG coupling gel for awake ferrets, because they often object strongly to the use of alcohol. It may help to distract the ferret by slowly giving Nutri-Cal or chicken baby food by syringe. The most common ECG results include sinus arrhythmia and sinus tachycardia. For more information on monitoring, see the article by Lichtenberger elsewhere in this issue.

Lymph node aspiration

A good, representative lymph node aspirate may be difficult to obtain because of the large amount of fat that often surrounds peripheral lymph nodes in the ferret. Carefully palpate the enlarged, firm node to distinguish it from the surrounding fat. Use a 25- to 22-gauge needle and stab the gland multiple times [11]. Attach an air-filled 6-mL syringe to the needle and push the sample onto the slide, then spread the sample gently and evenly across the slide.

Although a lymph node biopsy is not an emergency procedure, popliteal nodectomy may be indicated if lymph node aspiration cannot be used to

Table 4
Echocardiographic variables in the normal, anesthetized, male ferret [26]

Parameter	Mean value ± SD	Range
Age (months)	10–20	—
Gender	—	—
Body weight (kg)	1.4 ± 0.2	—
Heart rate (bpm)	196.0 ± 26.5	140–240
Mean electrical axis, frontal plane (degrees)	+86.13 ± 2.50	79.6–90.0
Lead II measurements		
P amplitude (mV)	n/a	n/a
P duration (sec)	n/a	n/a
PR interval (sec)	0.0560 ± 0.0086	0.04–0.08
QRS duration (sec)	0.0440 ± 0.0079	0.035–0.060
R amplitude (mV)	2.21 ± 0.42	1.4–3.0
QT interval (sec)	0.109 ± 0.018	0.08–0.14

Abbreviation: n/a, not available.

achieve a representative cytologic sample. Popliteal nodectomy is generally associated with minimal, if any, bleeding [2].

Splenic aspiration

Clip a small region of fur, aseptically clean the site, then palpate and immobilize the spleen. Splenic aspiration may be performed on awake ferrets with good restraint, although anesthesia or sedation may be indicated for ultrasound-guided aspiration of a focal lesion. Use a 22- to 25-gauge needle and a 3-mL syringe [11].

Bone marrow aspiration

Bone marrow aspiration is performed as in cats and dogs under anesthesia. Potential sites include the iliac crest, humerus, and the proximal femur, with the proximal femur being the most popular site. Clip a small area of overlying fur, aseptically prepare the site, and make a small skin incision using a 15 blade. Use an 18- to 20-gauge, 1.5-in spinal needle or a Jamshidi biopsy needle attached to a 6-mL syringe [11].

Tracheal wash

Tracheal wash is best performed as in the cat, through a sterile endotracheal tube with a red rubber catheter. Infuse at least 2 to 3 mL of sterile saline [11].

Urinary catheter placement

Urinary catheter placement may be challenging in the male ferret because of its small size and a J-shaped os penis. Anesthesia is required for adequate muscle relaxation and restraint in the form of gas anesthesia or parenteral combinations (see the article by Lichtenberger and Ko on analgesia/anesthesia elsewhere in this issue). Avoid high-dose ketamine in ferrets that have urethral obstruction. Most ferrets should be intubated and maintained on isoflurane or sevoflurane when anesthetized for extended periods. Using a 24-gauge catheter with the needle removed may be helpful in finding and dilating the urethral opening. Afterward, a 3-Fr 11-in ferret urinary catheter (Slippery Sam, Global Veterinary Products; New Buffalo, MI) or a 22- or 20-gauge jugular catheter may be placed in most ferrets (Fig. 5). Use a 3.5-Fr red rubber catheter in larger males. Pre-measure the length of red rubber or jugular catheters. Keeping red rubber catheters in the freezer until time of placement may enhance ease of insertion. Leaving the jugular catheter stylet in place may also facilitate careful passage. Resistance most often occurs as the catheter is passed around the pelvic flexure. Gently flush the urethra with sterile saline solution to help the catheter pass.

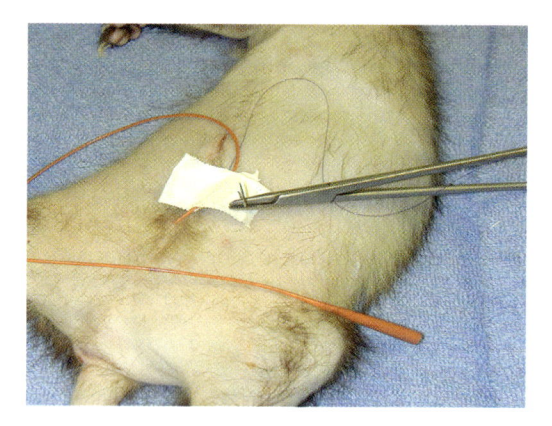

Fig. 5. Urethral catheterization using a 3.5-French red rubber catheter and suturing in place using a tape butterfly.

When urinary catheterization proves difficult, removing a small amount of urine once by way of cystocentesis can reduce pressure and allow passage of the urinary catheter. Repeated cystocentesis is not recommended because of the thin and possibly necrotic bladder wall, which may easily rupture. When catheter placement fails, a percutaneous cystostomy may be performed (see later discussion on urethral obstruction).

Suture butterfly tape strips near the prepuce to secure the catheter, then fasten the catheter or attached tubing to the tail base to minimize tension on the line (Fig. 6). Bandaging the ferret's abdomen may also minimize risk for rotation. Attach a closed collection system using a small intravenous bag

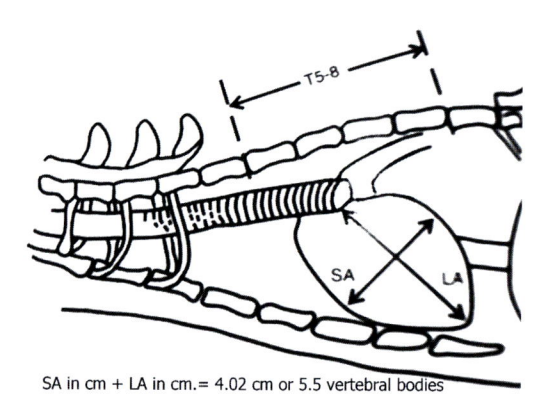

Fig. 6. Drawings of lateral (*right*) views of the thorax indicating measurements of the cardiac silhouette in long axis (*LA*) and short axis (*SA*). The sum of the LA and SA measurements is expressed in centimeters or in vertebrae length, beginning at the cranial edge of the fifth thoracic vertebrae (T5) and estimated to the nearest 0.25 vertebrae. The vertebrae width and length measurements are added to obtain a vertebrae heart score. (*Adapted from* Stepien RL, Benson KG, Forrest LJ. Radiographic measurement of cardiac size in normal ferrets. Vet Radiol Ultrasound 1999;40:606–10).

and monitor urine production. The normal ferret produces 26 to 28 mL of urine over a 24-hour period (range, 8–48 mL) [11,21].

Female ferret

Place the female ferret in ventral recumbency and elevate the rear quarters with a rolled towel. Aseptically prepare the vulva and perivulvar region, and then insert a vaginal speculum or otoscope. Locate the urethral opening on the floor of the vestibule 1 cm cranial to the clitoral fossa. Introduce a 3.5-Fr red rubber catheter, which may be fitted with a wire stylet [6].

Thoracocentesis

Use a 21- to 23-gauge butterfly catheter attached to a 12-mL syringe and stopcock to remove air or fluid for cytologic evaluation and culture. Ultrasonography may be helpful in guiding needle insertion. Ferrets rarely allow thoracocentesis with manual restraint alone, and needle laceration of the lung may occur when the ferret struggles. Consider chemical restraint using isoflurane, sevoflurane, or etomidate (2 mg/kg intravenously) with midazolam (0.25–0.50 mg/kg intravenously) before this procedure (M. Lichtenberger, personal communication, 2006). Repeat survey radiographs and echocardiogram afterward for more detailed evaluation of the thoracic cavity.

Pain management

As a general rule, ferrets are stoic animals. Anticipate procedures and conditions that should be painful and provide preemptive analgesia. Signs of pain in the ferret may include anorexia, lethargy, crying, stiff movements, inability to sleep in a natural, curled position, and squinting (see the article by Lichtenberger and Ko on analgesia and anesthesia elsewhere in this issue) [11].

Drug therapy

Dosages for medications administered to ferrets are often extrapolated from small animal medicine (Table 5). Ferrets are difficult to pill, and the recommended form of oral drug administration is liquid, especially sweet pediatric suspensions or syrups. Avoid fish flavors. Many drugs available only in tablet form may be compounded with the help of a pharmacist or crushed and mixed with a small amount of Nutri-Cal or baby food. Even when the formulation should be palatable, the ferret may still need to be scruffed for successful drug administration. It is common for ferrets to drool or paw violently at the mouth after bitter medications such as metronidazole are given [11].

Metabolism of acetaminophen is slow in ferrets. Activity of the hepatic enzyme, glucuronosyltransferase, is similar to that of cats [22].

Table 5
Drug dosages for ferrets [7,5,15,24]

Drug	Dosage	Route	Frequency	Comments
Amoxicillin	10–20 mg/kg	PO	Every 12 h	Give with metronidazole and for management of *Helicobacter* gastritis
Amoxicillin/clavulanate	22 mg/kg	PO	Every 8 h	Respiratory or UTI
Cephalexin	15 mg/kg	PO	Every 12 h	Antibiotic well suited for respiratory or urinary tract infections
Chloramphenicol	50 mg/kg	PO, SC, IM	Every 12 h	Careful to warn owners of aplastic anemia (see text on PBD)
Chlorpheniramine	1–2 mg/kg	PO	Every 8–12 h	Antihistamine that may relieve some symptoms of upper respiratory tract disease
Cisapride	0.5 mg/kg	PO	Every 8–24 h	
Dexamethasone sodium phosphate	0.2 mg/kg	IV		Slow bolus with insulinoma
Diazoxide	5–30 mg/kg	PO	Every 12 h	
Digoxin	0.01 mg/kg	PO	Every 12–24 h	
Diphenhydramine	0.5–2.0 mg/kg	IM, IV	Every 8–12 h	Hypersensitivity reaction
	2–4 mg/kg	PO		Upper respiratory disease
Enalapril	0.5 mg/kg	PO	Every 48 h	
Enrofloxacin	5 mg/kg	PO	Every 12 h	
Etomidate	1–2 mg/kg	IV		Always combined midazolam/diazepam
Famotidine	0.25–0.50 mg/kg	PO, IM, IV	Every 24 h	Histamine blocker
Fipronil (Frontline)	1 pump of spray or 1/5th of cat tube	Topical	Every 30–60 d	
Furosemide	1–4 mg/kg	PO, SC, IM	Every 8–12 h	
Human chorionic gonadotropin	100 IU	IM		Repeat in 7d if vulvar swelling has not resolved with estrogen toxicity
Imidacloprid (Advantage)	1 cat dose	Topical	Every 30 d	

Drug	Dose	Route	Frequency	Notes
Ivermectin	0.2–0.4 mg/kg	PO, SC	Once	Repeat in 14 d for anthelmintic treatment
	0.05 mg/kg	PO, SC	Every 30 d	Heartworm prevention
Leuprolide acetate	125 ug/kg	IM		Adrenal disease
	250–400 ug/kg	IM		Urethral obstruction secondary to adrenal disease
Lufenuron	30–45 mg/kg	PO	Every 30 d	
Metoclopramide	0.2–1.0 mg/kg	PO, SC	Every 6–8 h	
Metronidazole	20 mg/kg	PO	Every 12 h	Give with amoxicillin and bismuth in the management of *Helicobacter* gastritis
Prednisolone sodium succinate	22 mg/kg	IV		Slow bolus
Prednisone, prednisolone	0.5–2.0 mg/kg	PO, SC	Every 12–24 h	Insulinoma (be sure to use an alcohol-free formulation such as Pediapred)
Ranitidine	0.25–1.00 mg/kg	PO, SC	Every 12 h	Inflammatory bowel disease
	2–4 mg/kg	PO	Every 8 h	Histamine blocker
Selamectin	6 mg/kg	Topical		
Sucralfate	25–100 mg/kg	PO	Every 6–8 h	Stagger administration of sucralfate with other drugs and feedings that must be absorbed orally and so sucralfate is given on an empty stomach
Terbutaline	0.01 mg/kg	SC, IM		
Trimethoprim/sulfa	30 mg/kg	PO	Every 12 h	

Abbreviations: IM, intramuscular; IV, intravenous; IT, intratracheal; PO, per os; SC, subcutaneous.

Acetaminophen ingestion leads to methemoglobinemia and seizure activity. Treatment for intoxication is similar to that in a cat.

Care must be given when administrating any nonsteroidal anti-inflammatory drug (NSAID) to the debilitated ferret. NSAIDs promote a reduction in renal blood flow, gastrointestinal ulceration, and platelet dysfunction. Because of the salicylate present in the preparation, use of bismuth subsalicylate (Pepto-Bismol, Proctor & Gamble; Cincinnati, OH) is not recommended in the treatment of *Helicobacter* gastritis (M. Lichtenberger, personal communication, 2007).

Common diseases of the ferret

Gastrointestinal diseases

In addition to gagging and retching, signs of nausea in the ferret may include heavy drooling and clawing vigorously at the mouth. A unique sign of abdominal pain in the ferret is bruxism or teeth grinding.

Gastrointestinal foreign body

Gastrointestinal (GI) foreign bodies are common in young ferrets younger than 1 to 2 years of age. Ferrets enjoy chewing foam, sponge, or soft rubber items, such as shoe soles or latex rubber toys. Linear foreign bodies are rare. When outside of the cage, affected ferrets may go unsupervised in a home that is not ferret-proofed (see earlier section on housing the pet ferret).

The most consistent clinical signs of GI foreign body are anorexia and subsequent weight loss and lethargy. Depending on the location of the foreign body, the poor appetite may wax and wane. Signs of nausea and abdominal pain and diarrhea, potentially including melena, are variably seen. Vomiting is rare.

Some foreign bodies may be palpable on physical examination, especially intestinal foreign bodies. A foreign body may be associated with variable amounts of gas within the gut and evidence of segmental ileus on survey radiographs. Obstruction is typically associated with gaseous distension of the stomach or a pronounced intestinal gas pattern [16]. A barium series may also help to identify complete obstruction; however, the soft, spongy materials usually eaten by the ferret are rarely identified directly on films.

Treatment of GI foreign body depends on the location of the object and the clinical signs of the patient. Initially the patient should be rehydrated (see the article by Lichtenberger elsewhere in this issue). Some partial obstructions may pass after fluid therapy, but many foreign body obstructions require surgical removal.

Helicobacter *gastritis*

One of the reasons ferrets are kept as laboratory animals is for the study of the commensal microbe, *Helicobacter mustelae*. In many individuals, *Helicobacter* is not associated with disease; however, this organism may overgrow with stress or concurrent disease leading to gastritis and ulcers. *Helicobacter* gastritis may be reported in any age ferret. There may have been a recent change in the ferret's environment, such as introduction of a new ferret or moving to a new home. The incidence of disease may also be higher in ferrets that are caged continuously. Ferrets require at least a couple of hours of exercise daily.

Onset of clinical signs of *Helicobacter* gastritis may be acute or chronic. Nonspecific signs of illness, such as anorexia, lethargy, and weight loss, as well as vomiting, ptyalism, pawing at the mouth, bruxism, and diarrhea, including melena, may be observed.

Diagnosis of *Helicobacter* gastritis is often presumptive. Complete blood count results may include regenerative anemia and microcytosis. Radiographic findings may be similar to those seen with gastrointestinal foreign body (variable amounts of gas, segmental ileus).

Specific treatment for *Helicobacter* gastritis in the ferret is based on amoxicillin and metronidazole paired with sucralfate and the histamine (H2) blocker, ranitidine or famotidine. Combination of metronidazole and amoxicillin is much more effective than any one of these drugs alone, and in fact, use of a single drug may promote microbial resistance. Because of the presence of salicylate, bismuth subsalicylate is not recommended (M. Licthenberger, personal communication, 2007). The newer generation macrolide, clarithromycin, may be used in ferrets nonresponsive to antibiotics, H2 blockers, and sucralfate. Supportive care should include fluid therapy and force-feeding (see earlier discussion on nutritional support).

Epizootic catarrhal enteritis

First recognized in the early 1990s, epizootic catarrhal enteritis or ECE is strongly believed to be caused by coronavirus [23]. Although all ages may be affected, clinical disease is generally mild in young ferrets and most severe in middle-aged to older ferrets. History with ECE may involve exposure to a new, young ferret that may have had mild, transient diarrhea.

Clinical signs of ECE include nonspecific signs of illness (anorexia, lethargy), vomiting, and diarrhea. Diarrhea may be variable in appearance; however, stool may be profuse, green, and mucoid or brown with many mucosal shreds (also known as "bird seed stool"). Diagnosis is usually one of exclusion, although definitive diagnosis requires biopsy and histopathology. Radiographic evidence of profound gastrointestinal ileus may be observed.

Treatment focuses on aggressive fluid therapy and kaolin-pectin or sucralfate. Antibiotics are a reasonable part of empiric treatment, because bacteria such as *Campylobacter* may also cause enteritis. Isolate all ferrets that are suspected to have ECE [2].

Proliferative bowel disease

The obligate intracellular bacteria, *Lawsonia intracellularis*, cause proliferative bowel disease or PBD. Although prevalence of disease is low, PBD is most commonly seen in young ferrets, particularly those ranging from 10 to 16 weeks of age. Improvement in ferret nutrition is believed to be responsible for the decreasing incidence of PBD.

Clinical signs include anorexia, weight loss, and large bowel diarrhea (blood, mucus, excessive straining, and increased frequency of defecation). Severe tenesmus may lead to rectal prolapse in some kits. Thickened loops of bowel may be palpated on physical examination. Perform fecal parasite testing to exclude the presence of coccidia. Survey radiographs and baseline blood work may also be indicated.

Rehydrate ferrets and administer antibiotics, such as metronidazole, amoxicillin, or chloramphenicol, if diarrhea is present. Provide latex gloves for the owner administering chloramphenicol, and warn of the potential for rare, idiosyncratic aplastic anemia in humans. In rare instances, a dose-related, reversible anemia has also been reported in other species [20]. Mild rectal prolapse may resolve with antibiotic treatment alone, while the delicate tissue is protected with a gentle, topical zinc oxide preparation. In rare instances, purse-string sutures are required for more severe prolapses. Stay sutures may be left in place up to 3 days [2].

Lymphocytic-plasmacytic gastroenteritis and eosinophilic gastroenteritis

Infiltrative or inflammatory bowel diseases are generally seen in middle-aged to older ferrets. Although no clinical studies have been performed, eosinophilic gastroenteritis is theorized to be associated with parasite infestation or food allergy. Clinical signs may include anorexia, chronic weight loss, chronic diarrhea, and vomiting, as well as signs of nausea and abdominal pain. Some ferrets treated for presumptive ECE, *Helicobacter* gastritis, or PBD may develop chronic gastrointestinal signs caused by inflammatory bowel disease. Physical examination may reveal thickened intestinal loops and enlarged mesenteric lymph nodes. Stabilize ferrets with fluids before obtaining a definitive diagnosis through pediatric endoscopy or surgical gastric and intestinal biopsies. Although the anthelmintic, ivermectin, may be administered to ferrets with eosinophilic gastroenteritis, prednisone seems to be the mainstay of treatment for both conditions. Other medications that have been tried include azathioprine and metronidazole [2,3].

Endocrine diseases of ferrets

Insulinoma

Insulinoma or pancreatic beta cell tumor is commonly seen in middle-aged to older pet ferrets in the United States. Presentation of clinical signs varies. Affected ferrets may exhibit acute onset, intermittent episodes of hypoglycemia, or clinical signs that may develop slowly and insidiously. Signs of hypoglycemia frequently include depression, a dazed or glazed appearance in the eyes (star-gazing), posterior paresis and ataxia, and signs of nausea (copious drooling, pawing at the mouth, retching, and gagging).

Affected ferrets may begin to sleep longer and harder. If hypoglycemia becomes severe enough the ferret may collapse. Seizure activity may be seen with severe hypoglycemia.

Physical examination is often unremarkable except for evidence of generalized weakness, such as posterior paresis, ataxia, or collapse, and possible weight loss. Signs of concurrent illness are common in middle-aged to older ferrets, particularly signs of adrenal disease discussed later.

Diagnosis of insulinoma generally relies on history, clinical findings, and persistent hypoglycemia. Normal fasting blood glucose levels range from 90 to 120 mg/dL. Fasting blood glucose less than 90 mg/dL is suspicious for insulinoma; blood glucose less than 70 mg/dL is strongly suggestive. If insulinoma is suspected, it is not necessary to fast the ferret; however, if fasting is performed, do so for no more than 2 to 3 hours while monitoring the ferret closely and carefully. Until proven otherwise, a ferret with persistent hypoglycemia almost invariably has insulinoma. Insulin/glucose ratios are not useful for diagnosing insulinomas in ferrets. Starvation may also lead to hypoglycemia. Other, rare causes of hypoglycemia in the ferret include liver disease, neoplasia, sepsis, starvation, and heatstroke.

The remainder of the biochemistry panel is usually normal in ferrets with insulinoma. Liver enzyme elevation may occur with secondary hepatic lipidosis, or much less commonly, metastasis of the beta cell tumor to the liver.

Survey whole-body radiographs are usually unremarkable, although incidental splenomegaly may be observed. Abdominal ultrasonography may reveal nodular enlargements near the stomach that can, in rare instances, be large beta cell tumor nodules. More commonly these nodules represent lymphadenopathy of the prominent lymph nodes that lie along the lesser curvature of the stomach.

Mild to moderate hypoglycemic episodes may be managed on an outpatient basis. If the ferret is alert enough to swallow, feed an easily digestible, animal protein-based food such as Oxbow Carnivore Care or Hill's prescription diet a/d. Avoid sugar-based products such as Nutri-Cal, because they may promote rebound hypoglycemia.

Hospitalization is recommended for severe hypoglycemic episodes that do not respond to oral treatments or that include profound signs of hypoglycemia, such as collapse or seizure activity. Administer 0.25 to 0.50 mL of 50% dextrose slow bolus intravenously over at least 10 to 15 minutes. Dilute 50% dextrose in a 1:1 concentration with saline or sterile water. If dextrose is administered alone, the functional beta cell tumor may be stimulated to secrete more insulin. This can lead to an ever-worsening cycle of hypoglycemia, dextrose administration, and subsequent insulin secretion; therefore, also administer dexamethasone sodium phosphate (0.1 mg/kg intravenously) to facilitate entry of glucose into the cells (M. Lichtenberger, personal communication, 2007).

Depending on clinical response to intravenous dextrose bolus, the ferret may then be fed a high-protein meal or the patient may require constant rate infusion containing 2.5% to 5% dextrose. When a ferret with insulinoma is maintained on intravenous fluids, it is essential that infusion truly be continuous. Starting and stopping fluids containing dextrose only stimulates insulin secretion and potentially worsens the patient's condition.

Concurrent administration of prednisolone solution or syrup (1 mg/kg orally every 12 hours) also promotes uptake of glucose by cells. Use an alcohol-free formulation (Pediapred Oral Liquid, Celltech Pharmaceuticals; Rochester, NY), because alcohol lowers blood glucose. Diazoxide is a secondary drug used for the treatment of insulinoma. Diazoxide is frequently ineffective in ferrets that have not already responded to medical management. It is rarely used in emergency situations unless the ferret continues to be unresponsive. Adverse effects of diazoxide may include nausea and vomiting.

When a ferret presents with hypoglycemic seizures nonresponsive to dextrose administration, give midazolam (0.2–0.5 mg/kg intravenously) or diazepam (1–2 mg intravenously to effect). If additional anticonvulsant therapy is needed, administer phenobarbital (4 mg/kg intravenously every 20 minutes for two doses), and continue the patient on oral phenobarbital (2 mg/kg every 12 hours) if need be. Oral phenobarbital may be given for up to 6 weeks and then slowly tapered off over a 2-week period (M. Lichtenberger, personal communication, 2007).

If the ferret continues to suffer from persistent and severe hypoglycemia, then constant rate infusion dexamethasone (0.5–1.0 mg/kg slow bolus intravenously over 6 hours, repeat every 12–24 hours as needed) may prove helpful [24]. The rare ferret suffering from severe signs of insulinoma does not respond to medical management and requires surgical debulkment of the pancreas for clinical signs to resolve. Although only a palliative measure, surgical debulkment of the beta cell tumor is the treatment of choice. Exploratory laparotomy should always be performed at this time, because many ferrets have concurrent adrenal gland disease.

Client education is crucial for owners of affected ferrets. Teach owners to recognize signs of hypoglycemia and to prevent hypoglycemic episodes from occurring. Owners (and clinicians) should recognize situations that may use blood glucose and may precipitate a hypoglycemic crisis, such as stress, travel, and exercise. Minimize stressors whenever possible and ensure that the ferret eats afterward. Other important preventive measures include feeding high-protein, meat-based foods frequently and avoiding foods containing simple sugars and carbohydrates.

Ovarian remnant syndrome

Ferrets are induced ovulators. Approximately half of estrous females remain in heat until bred or artificially stimulated to ovulate. Persistent estrus leads to estrogen toxicity of hematopoietic tissue and subsequent severe, potentially fatal, pancytopenia. Persistent estrus used to be a common problem; however, now that ferret farms routinely spay ferrets before they are purchased, this condition is much less common. Today, persistent estrus is most commonly observed in spayed female ferrets less than 2 years of age when a portion of the ovary is accidentally left at the time of the early spay procedure.

Clinical signs include lethargy, weakness, pallor, vulvar swelling, and possibly vulvar discharge. Severe disease is also associated with evidence of bleeding (melena, petechia, ecchymoses) secondary to thrombocytopenia and endocrine alopecia.

Diagnosis relies on physical examination, complete blood count, and reticulocyte count. Abdominal ultrasound and bone marrow aspirate cytology are also recommended. Affected ferrets require aggressive supportive care. Ferrets with severe anemia benefit from oxygen administration and intravenous Oxyglobin (Biopure; Cambridge, MA) (11–15 mL/kg over 4 hours) until a blood transfusion is available (see article by Lichtenberger elsewhere in this issue) [25,26]. Leuprolide acetate or human chorionic gonadotropin may prove effective in reducing estrogen levels. Definitive treatment is exploratory surgery to excise the ovarian remnant.

Adrenal disease

Adrenal disease of the ferret involves hyperplasia, benign neoplasia, or malignant neoplasia of the zona reticularis. Disease of this adrenal tissue leads to an increase in sex hormones (estrogens, progestins, and androgens) and not glucocorticoids. Adrenal disease is extremely common in middle-aged to older neutered ferrets in the United States. Adrenal disease is common in ferrets in the United States. Pathogenesis of disease in the United States is likely multifactorial and is theorized to include early sterilization, consumption of processed diets, and exposure to artificial photoperiods [2].

The most consistent clinical sign of adrenal disease is dorsally symmetric endocrine alopecia, which typically begins over the tail base and flanks or less commonly over the shoulders. Approximately one third of affected ferrets also display intense pruritus. Approximately 75% of affected females have vulvar swelling. Affected males occasionally develop dysuria or stranguria secondary to androgen-induced prostatomegaly. Adrenomegaly may be palpable on physical examination in some cases [2].

Minimum database findings are frequently unremarkable. Ferrets with long-standing adrenal disease may have mild to moderate nonregenerative anemia. Survey whole-body radiographs are usually not helpful. Calcification is rare, and only profoundly enlarged adrenals may be seen on survey films [2].

Ultrasonography is a diagnostic test of choice. The width of the normal adrenal gland is usually 3 mm or less. Adrenal gland disease is associated with widening of the adrenal gland from a classic lentil bean shape to a football shape that often measures at least 3.5 mm across. Diagnosis of adrenal disease in the ferret may also be based on the University of Tennessee's adrenal hormone panel, which measures three sex hormones, including estradiol, 17-hydroxyprogesterone, and androstenedione. Levels that exceed normal are highly suggestive of adrenal disease, although false negatives are possible [2].

The treatment of choice for adrenal disease is surgery. When surgery is not an option because of poor condition, extreme old age, or financial concerns, medical management involves use of hormonal manipulation, such as leuprolide acetate or melatonin [2,27].

Diabetes

Diabetes mellitus is uncommon in the ferret. The condition is most commonly a transient sequela to surgical pancreatic debulkment for insulinoma. Treatment is rarely necessary in this scenario, but when initiated it is extrapolated directly from care of cats and dogs [28].

Neoplasia

The most common neoplasms of the ferret are adrenal disease and insulinoma (see section on endocrinology).

Lymphosarcoma

Lymphosarcoma or lymphoma is the third most common neoplasm of the ferret. Neoplasia involving mature, well-differentiated lymphocytes or lymphocytic lymphoma is most common in older ferrets. Disease most commonly affects lymph nodes, followed by spread to parenchyma. Affected ferrets may be presented for chronic or intermittent lethargy, anorexia, and subsequent weight loss. The most common physical examination finding is generalized lymphadenopathy in which lymph nodes feel firm or asymmetric instead of soft and pliable.

Young ferrets younger than 2 years of age are more commonly afflicted with lymphoblastic lymphosarcoma. Cranial mediastinal masses frequently lead to pleural effusion and dyspnea. On physical examination, the chest is noncompressible, and no heart murmurs or arrhythmias are detected. Although uncommon, pulmonary metastasis may occur with lymphocytic or lymphoblastic lymphosarcoma [2].

Diagnosis of lymphosarcoma relies on cytologic or histologic evaluation of lymph nodes or pleural fluid. Because splenic lymphoma is uncommon in the ferret, splenic aspirates generally reveal extramedullary hematopoiesis. White blood counts are variable, and lymphocyte counts may be markedly elevated. Nonregenerative anemia may be mild to marked. Biochemistry panel results may reflect neoplastic infiltration of organs or concurrent illness.

Chemotherapy protocols in the ferret have been extrapolated from the care of cats and dogs. Ferrets tolerate chemotherapy well; however, only approximately 10% experience remission. If traditional multiagent chemotherapy is not an option, palliative treatment with prednisone (2.2 mg/kg orally every 24 hours) may reduce tumor burden for several months (M. Lichtenberger, personal communication, 2007).

Dermatologic neoplasia

The most common skin tumor of middle-aged to older ferrets is the basal cell tumor. Basal tumors often appear as small, white or pink growths that may have a depressed center. Mast cell tumors are the second most common skin neoplasm. Mast cell tumors are typically small, round, and slightly raised; lesions often bleed and scab over. Both of these tumors are typically benign in ferrets; surgical excision and biopsy is recommended and considered curative [2,29].

Hematopoietic

Anemia

After confirming the presence of anemia, examine the peripheral blood smear for microcytosis or polychromasia, evaluate red blood cell indices, such as mean corpuscular volume (MCV) and mean corpuscular hemoglobin concentration (MCHC), and perform a reticulocyte count. Changes observed with regenerative anemia may include microcytosis or microcytosis and an elevated reticulocyte count. Nonregenerative anemia is associated with normocytic–normochromic red blood cells.

Regenerative anemia in the ferret is most commonly caused by gastrointestinal bleeding secondary to *Helicobacter* gastritis. Heavy flea infestation may also cause regenerative anemia, particularly in juvenile ferrets. Immune-mediated hemolytic anemia has not been identified in ferrets.

The most common cause of nonregenerative anemia in the ferret is anemia of chronic disease caused by adrenal disease. Anemia is generally mild to moderate in adrenal disease. Although incidence is uncommon, estrogen toxicity secondary to ovarian remnant syndrome is the most important cause of profound pancytopenia, including nonregenerative anemia (see section on endocrine disease). Neoplastic infiltration of bone marrow by lymphoma (see section on neoplasia) is another potential cause of pancytopenia.

Thrombocytopenia

Primary immune-mediated thrombocytopenia has not been reported in the ferret. Thrombocytopenia has been reported with estrous-induced pancytopenia.

Coagulopathies

Coagulopathies are rarely reported in the ferret, perhaps because normal coagulation parameters are rarely available (see earlier discussion on blood work for coagulation normals). Coagulopathy secondary to warfarin ingestion has been seen (M. Lichtenberger, personal communication, 2007).

Cardiovascular disease

Heart disease is frequently reported in middle-aged to older ferrets. The most common cardiac disease is dilated cardiomyopathy (DCM). Other heart conditions reported in the ferret include valvular heart disease, hypertrophic cardiomyopathy, and heartworm disease. Because of the small size of the ferret heart, even the presence of one *Dirofilaria immitis* worm can lead to heart failure.

Clinical signs of heart disease in the ferret are similar to those observed in cats and dogs. Nonspecific signs of illness often predominate, such as lethargy, anorexia, weight loss, pallor, and weakness. These signs may not be appreciated until disease is advanced. Additional signs of heart disease may include evidence of generalized weakness, such as posterior paresis or ataxia, and dyspnea or tachypnea.

On physical examination, ascites may be detected in addition to the aforementioned clinical signs. Auscultation may identify a heart murmur, tachycardia, or arrhythmia. Muffled heart sounds may be recognized with pleural effusion, whereas pulmonary edema may lead to harsh lung sounds. Coughing is usually absent.

Stabilize any ferret that presents in distress before performing diagnostic tests. Provide cage rest in an oxygen-rich environment. Low-dose butorphanol (0.4 mg/kg subcutaneously, intramuscularly, intravenously) may help to relieve stress and anxiety.

When heart failure results in a parenchymal disease breathing pattern (see earlier discussion on respiratory distress) and harsh lung sounds, treat for pulmonary edema with furosemide (2–3 mg/kg intravenously, intramuscularly, subcutaneously). Repeat furosemide in 30 minutes if there is no improvement. Nitroglycerine paste (NitroBID, Hoechst Marion Roussel, Kansas City, Missouri) $1/8^{th}$ inch is placed on the gums or tongue. Continue the ferret on continuous rate infusion furosemide (0.2 mg/kg/h intravenously) for 12 hours.

If respiratory distress is present with a dyssynchronous breathing pattern (see earlier discussion on respiratory distress) and muffled breath sounds, pleural disease is most likely. Perform thoracocentesis under anesthesia. Induce with midazolam (0.5 mg/kg intravenously) and etomidate (1–2 mg/kg intravenously) and then intubate the patient. During the brief anesthesia, other additional diagnostics may be performed (M. Lichtenberger, personal communication, 2006).

Obtain radiographs, echocardiography, electrocardiography, and blood pressure readings when the ferret is stable. Complete blood count and biochemistry panel should also be obtained. If only a limited amount of blood is available, be sure to evaluate electrolytes, BUN, creatinine, blood glucose, and hematocrit.

Although there are several tests to diagnose heartworm disease in small animals, none of these tests are validated for use in ferrets. Microfilarias are identified on blood smears in only 25% to 50% of cases. Antigen and antibody testing used in cats may be met with false negative results. Echocardiography is currently the most reliable test in the ferret to confirm the presence of adult worms within the heart [10,19].

Base treatment protocols for heart disease on diagnostic test results. Enalapril, digoxin, and furosemide dosages have all been extrapolated from cats and dogs. Treatment of heartworm disease includes ivermectin (0.05 mg/kg orally, subcutaneously monthly) and prednisone (1 mg/kg orally every 24 hours) until disease has been cleared. Melarsomine (Immiticide, Merial; Duluth, GA) (2.5–3.25 mg/kg deep intramuscularly once under isoflurane sedation, followed 30 days later by two doses at 2.5–3.25 mg/kg 24 hours apart) also seems to be effective and its use may hasten recovery [30,31]. Some ferrets develop complications including anaphylaxis, however, so premedicate with diphenhydramine (0.5–2.0 mg/kg). Heartworm preventive medication (such as once-monthly ivermectin) is recommended for ferrets in climates where such medication is also recommended for the pet cat.

Respiratory disease

Human influenza virus

Several strains of human influenza virus can infect ferrets. Flu may be transmitted from people to ferrets, from ferrets to people, and from ferret to ferret. Disease can appear within 48 hours of exposure, so always ask if anyone in the household has been ill.

Clinical disease most consistently includes signs of upper respiratory infection: nasal discharge, sneezing, severe congestion, fever, and profound lethargy and anorexia. Lower respiratory involvement is less common and often leads to secondary bacterial pneumonia. Ferrets with the flu often seem moribund; however, the death rate in adults is fortunately low. Course of disease typically lasts 7 to 14 days. Treatment frequently includes intensive supportive care (feeding and fluid therapy) and antihistamines such as diphenhydramine (2–4 mg/kg orally every 8–12 hours) to help relieve severe congestion [2].

Bacterial pneumonia

Although bacterial pneumonia may occur secondary to influenza virus infection, primary bacterial pneumonia is uncommon in the ferret.

Anterior mediastinal masses

Cranial mediastinal masses caused by lymphosarcoma are often associated with pleural effusion and dyspnea in young ferrets (as seen earlier in the discussion on lymphosarcoma). Definitive diagnosis is with ultrasound or computer tomography-guided aspiration of the mass, laparoscopy, or surgical biopsy.

Canine distemper virus

Ferrets are exquisitely sensitive to canine distemper virus (CDV). Although the incidence of CDV is rare in pet ferrets in the United States, this disease should always be considered in any unvaccinated individual with consistent signs. Clinical signs include fever, anorexia, oculonasal discharge, coughing, hyperkeratosis of footpads, and a rash involving the lips and chin. Vomiting and diarrhea are uncommon in the ferret with CDV, whereas neurologic signs may be seen with advanced infection. The mortality rate is 100% [2].

Urogenital disease

The two most important causes of urinary tract disease in the male ferret are prostatomegaly secondary to adrenal disease. Struvite uroliths used to be common problems before commercial ferret diets were improved. Urolithiasis was most commonly seen in adult males on a plant-based protein diet such as poor quality cat food. Plant-based protein promotes the development of alkaline urine and the precipitation of magnesium ammonium phosphate or struvite crystals [2].

Currently the most important cause of urethral obstruction is prostatomegaly secondary to adrenal disease. An increase in androgens leads to squamous metaplasia of prostatic glandular epithelium and the development of thick-walled prostatic cysts. In some cases the cysts become infected. Prostatic disease unrelated to adrenal disease, such as abscesses and neoplasia, is rare in the ferret [2].

Clinical signs associated with urolithiasis or prostatic disease may include pollakiuria, stranguria, or dysuria. Owners may misinterpret the straining observed as "constipation." Frequent dribbling may create a wet, urine-stained perineum, and the prepuce may be red from frequent licking. Ferrets are frequently depressed, weak, and very painful. In some instances, these nonspecific signs of illness may be observed without noticeable signs of dysuria [2,6,11].

Diagnosis of urogenital disease relies on signalment, history, and clinical findings. With urethral obstruction, a distended bladder is readily palpable on physical examination.

In the case of urethral obstruction, urinary catheterization is an emergency procedure (see earlier discussion on urethral catheterization and anesthesia). When catheter placement fails, temporary percutaneous cystostomy may be performed to provide cutaneous urinary diversion until definitive treatment may be performed. Temporary cystostomy tube placement is performed as in the dog and cat (Fig. 7). The cystostomy tube may be maintained for 1 to 3 days with use of sedation such as continuous rate infusion fentanyl-ketamine (see the article by Lichtenberger and Ko on analgesia and anesthesia elsewhere in this issue) (Fig. 8). Surgery for the treatment of prostatomegaly is performed only when the ferret is stable. The

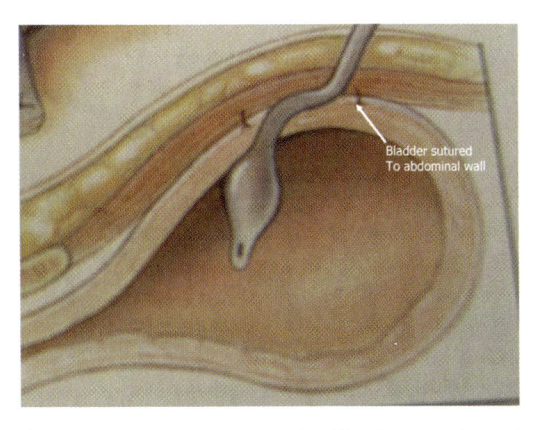

Fig. 7. Placement of a percutaneous cystostomy tube. The diagram shows the Foley catheter in place within the bladder. The bladder wall is sutured to the abdominal wall.

cystostomy catheter is removed following medical or surgical treatment and after the ferret is urinating on its own. Remove the catheter by simply removing skin sutures and deflating the Foley catheter. Allow the wound to heal by secondary intention [32,33].

While placing the urinary catheter under anesthesia, carefully monitor the electrocardiogram for evidence of hyperkalemia. Signs of hyperkalemia include loss of the P wave, widening of the QRS complex, peaked T waves, and a short QY interval. Relief of obstruction and forced diuresis is usually sufficient in the management of hyperkalemia. Medical treatment of hyperkalemia is indicated if an arrhythmia is present in addition to poor perfusion or altered mentation. Give calcium gluconate (50–100 mg/kg slowly bolus intravenously) while carefully monitoring the ECG to temporarily stabilize myocardium, or administer regular insulin (0.2 U/kg intravenously) followed by glucose (1–2 g intravenously for every unit of insulin) to prevent

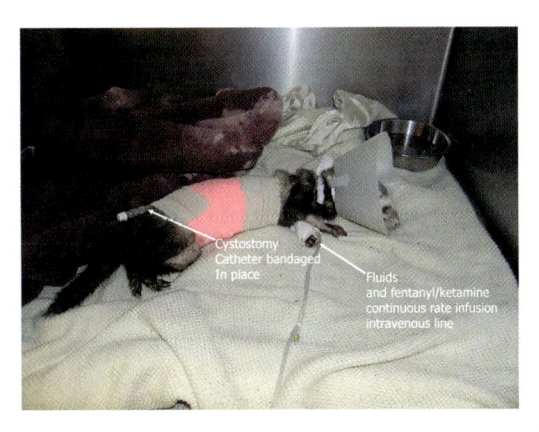

Fig. 8. The ferret is shown with a percutaneous catheter bandaged in place. The ferret is maintained on fluids for support and on a continuous rate infusion (CRI) of fentanyl/ketamine.

hypoglycemia. A patient given insulin/dextrose should initially receive 2.5% dextrose when forced diuresis is begun [2,32].

Blood and urine samples should be collected at the same time as urinary and intravenous catheter placement. Perform urinalysis, urine culture and sensitivity, complete blood count (CBC), and biochemistry panel. If the amount of blood collected is limited, at least evaluate BUN, creatinine, electrolytes, blood glucose, and packed cell volume/total protein. Hyperkalemia and metabolic acidosis are common [2].

On survey radiographs, evaluate the entire length of the urinary tract for radiodense uroliths. Calculi lodged at the os penis may be particularly difficult to detect. Prostatomegaly may appear as a mass lesion dorsal to the urinary bladder, ventrally displacing the bladder [2].

Abdominal ultrasound can be used to identify cystic prostatic hyperplasia or struvite calculi. At the same time, perform ultrasonographic evaluation of the kidneys, bladder, and adrenal glands.

Use crystalloids and colloids to first correct perfusion abnormalities, such as hypotension, and then to rehydrate the patient (see the article by Lichtenberger elsewhere in this issue). Surgical management of adrenal gland disease is performed only after hydration and urine production are restored and laboratory values are normal. Adrenalectomy is the treatment of choice for adrenal disease and associated prostatic cysts. Stabilization before surgery generally requires approximately 24 to 36 hours.

Ferrets with adrenal disease and prostatic cysts should receive high-dose leuprolide acetate (250 µg/kg intramuscularly). Administration of this synthetic gonadotropin-releasing hormone analog may lead to a subsequent reduction in prostatic tissue within 12 to 48 hours of drug administration. This allows better flow of urine through, and even voluntary micturition around, the urinary catheter [2]. Although leuprolide acetate may temporarily or permanently mask clinical signs, growth of the adrenal gland is not affected.

In the treatment of struvite crystalluria, dietary conversion is ineffective in ferrets, because they will not eat a struvite-dissolving diet like Prescription Diet Feline s/d. Begin forced diuresis and schedule surgical removal of urinary calculi as needed.

Trauma

Traumatic injury is a common problem in ferrets because of their curious nature and their propensity for burrowing. Reclining chairs are a common cause of traumatic injury, while household accidents like being stepped on, run over by a wheeled object, falling, or being dropped are additional common complaints. Ferrets may also fight with larger species leading to serious bite or crush injuries [12].

Sequelae to traumatic injury may include conditions that are not particularly common in the ferret, such as pneumothorax and fractures. When fractures do occur, the appendicular skeleton is usually affected. Spinal and pelvic fractures are uncommon. Treatment of fractures and other traumatic injuries may be extrapolated from emergency care of the kitten [2].

Immune-mediated disease

Vaccine reactions
There are many anecdotal reports of vaccine reaction in the ferret. These reactions are usually immediate (within 30 minutes of injection). Less severe reactions can be seen up to several hours after vaccine administration. Reactions are most common when more than one vaccine is given at the same time.

Clinical signs may include vomiting and retching, diarrhea, fever, and red, itchy skin. Some ferrets may also become hyperactive although this behavior is quickly followed by collapse. Diphenhydramine and fluid therapy may be sufficient for the treatment of vaccine reaction. Additional medications that may be used include epinephrine and corticosteroids.

Idiopathic myofasciitis
Idiopathic myofasciitis is a ferret disease first recognized in 2003. Although the pathogenesis is not understood, administration of a specific canine distemper vaccine may be a common factor (see later discussion for additional information) [34].

Immune-mediated hemolytic anemia
Immune-mediated hemolytic anemia has not been identified in ferrets.

Musculoskeletal disease

Idiopathic myofasciitis
Idiopathic myofasciitis or spontaneous inflammatory polymyopathy of the ferret was first recognized in 2003. The cause of this condition is unknown, although it may be immune-mediated. Young ferrets are most commonly affected, although there has been one report in a middle-aged individual [34].

Clinical signs include high fever, lethargy, recumbency, anorexia, posterior paresis and ataxia, pain with movement, and abnormal stools. Minimum database results include leukocytosis with a mature neutrophilia, mild to moderate nonregenerative anemia, mild to moderate elevation in ALT, mild hyperglycemia, and hypoalbuminemia [34].

Although a wide variety of drugs have been tried, including antibiotics, anti-inflammatory agents, glucocorticoids, analgesics, interferon, and cyclophosphamide, all regimens have thus far led to treatment failure. All patients have died or been euthanized [34].

Heat stroke

Because of their long, thin bodies and lack of sweat glands, ferrets are very susceptible to temperature extremes. They may easily develop heat exhaustion or heat stroke when environmental temperature exceeds 80°F. This is particularly true with high humidity in geriatric ferrets or in ferrets with concurrent illness.

The first signs of heat exhaustion in the ferret may include open-mouth breathing and lying prone. Affected ferrets are often profoundly lethargic, and the footpads and mucous membranes may be bright red at first. Signs of nausea, diarrhea, and vomiting, sometimes with blood, may also be seen. Additional clinical findings may include tachycardia, arrhythmia, and tachypnea, but not necessarily an elevated body temperature by the time of presentation. The more severe form of heat illness, heat stroke, may also be associated with signs of central nervous system dysfunction, such as opisthotonus, fixed and dilated pupils, seizure activity, collapse, and even coma, as well as evidence of disseminated intravascular coagulation, such as purpura, conjunctival hemorrhage, melena, bloody diarrhea, hemoptysis, and hematuria. Ferrets may also become oliguric or anuric [2,35].

CBC and coagulation testing may provide evidence of coagulation disorders and hemoconcentration. Biochemistry panel abnormalities may occur with organ damage. The most consistent finding includes elevations in creatine kinase (CK), aspartate aminotransferase (AST), and ALT levels. Azotemia, hyperkalemia, and acid–base imbalance may also be seen. Hypoglycemia may occur secondary to increased use of glucose or hepatic damage. Urinalysis may reveal proteinuria, hematuria, myoglobinuria, or granular casts [2,35].

Immediate cooling is essential. Apply tepid or cool, not cold, water to the patient until temperature is 103°F–104°F. Begin aggressive fluid therapy for perfusion resuscitation and rehydration and to correct and maintain blood pressure. These measures may prevent serious sequelae, such as disseminated intravascular coagulation and renal failure (see the article by Lichtenberger elsewhere in this issue).

Ophthalmologic disease

Ophthalmologic disease is uncommon in the ferret. *Staphylococcus* sp. and *Corynebacterium* sp. are normally isolated from conjunctival and eyelid margins in adult ferrets. Healthy ferrets have a normal mean intraocular pressure of 14.50 ± 3.27 mm Hg, normal mean Schirmer tear test of 5.31 ± 1.32 mm/min, and a mean central corneal thickness of 0.337 ± 0.020 mm [36].

Summary

Ferrets are delightful animals that approach the world in a friendly, often fearless, manner. Even when ill, ferrets are often still very wiggly. The clinician able to use scruffing and stretching techniques is at a distinct advantage for completing important diagnostic or therapeutic procedures. When clinical condition allows, however, also consider chemical restraint in the form of inhalant anesthesia or short-term parenteral anesthesia to collect diagnostic samples or perform procedures. Common emergency conditions seen in the ferret include insulinoma, cardiomyopathy, and urethral obstruction. When developing a diagnostic and therapeutic plan, the ferret veterinarian must seek a balance between species-specific information discussed in this article and information extrapolated from cat and dog medicine. The therapeutic plan must always include close and careful monitoring. Significant changes in the status of these small patients can occur extremely quickly in the course of providing basic supportive care such as intravenous fluids or supplemental heat.

References

[1] Boyce SW, Zingg BM, Lightfoot TL. Behavior of *Mustela putorius furo*. Vet Clin North Am Exot Anim Pract 2001;4:697–712.
[2] Quesenberry KE, Carpenter JW, editors. Ferrets, rabbits, and rodents: clinical medicine and surgery. 2nd edition. St. Louis (MO): WB Saunders Co.; 2003. p. 2–134.
[3] Johnson-Delaney CA. Anatomy and physiology of the gastrointestinal system of the ferret and selected exotic carnivores. In: Proc Annu Meet Assoc Ex Mammal Vet 2006;29–38.
[4] Ball RS. Husbandry and management of the domestic ferret. Lab Anim 2002;31:37–42.
[5] Fisher PG. Esophagostomy tube placement in the ferret. Exotic DVM 2001;2:23–5.
[6] Orcutt CJ. Emergency and critical care of ferrets. Vet Clin North Am Exot Anim Pract 1998; 1:99–126.
[7] Benson KG, Paul-Murphy J, Carr A. Percutaneous placement of a gastric feeding tube in the ferret. Lab Anim 2000;29:44–6.
[8] Atkins LB. Respiratory patterns (ST7A). In: Proc Annu West Vet Conf 2006.
[9] Rudloff E. The first 5 minutes: assessment of the emergency patient. Proceedings, Western Veterinary Conference; 2006.
[10] Vastenburg MH, Boroffka SA, Schoemaker NJ. Echocardiographic measurements in clinically healthy ferrets anesthetized with isoflurane. Veterinary Radiology and Ultrasound 2004;45:228–32.
[11] Castanheira de Matos RE, Morrisey JK. Common procedures in the pet ferret. Vet Clin North Am Exot Anim Pract 2006;9:347–65.
[12] Fudge AM. Ferret hematology. In: Fudge AM, editor. Laboratory medicine: avian and exotic pets. Philadelphia: WB Saunders Co.; 2000. p. 269–72.
[13] Lawson AK, Lichtenberger M, Day T, et al. Comparison of sevoflurane and isoflurane in domestic ferrets (*Mustela putorius furo*). Vet Ther 2006;7:207–12.
[14] Marini RP, Callahan RJ, Jackson LR, et al. Distribution of technetium 99m-labeled red blood cells during isoflurane anesthesia in ferrets. Am J Vet Res 1997;58:781–5.
[15] Marini RP, Jackson LR, Esteves MI, et al. Effect of isoflurane on hematologic variables in ferrets. Am J Vet Res 1994;55:1479–83.
[16] Schwarz LA, Solano M, Manning A, et al. The normal upper gastrointestinal examination in the ferret. Vet Radiol Ultrasound 2003;44:165–72.
[17] Stepien RI, Benson KG, Forrest LJ. Radiographic measurement of cardiac size in normal ferrets. Vet Radiol Ultrasound 1999;40:606–10.
[18] Sirois M. Advances in clinical chemistry. Proceedings, American College of Veterinary Internal Medicine; 2002.

[19] Stepien RI, Benson KG, Wenholz LJ. M-mode and Doppler echocardiographic findings in normal ferrets sedated with ketamine hydrochloride and midazolam. Vet Radiol Ultrasound 2000;41:452–6.
[20] Turton JA, Fagg R, Sones WR, et al. Characterization of the myelotoxicity of chloramphenicol succinate in the B6C3F1 mouse. Int J Exp Pathol 2006;87(2):101–12.
[21] Esteves MI, Marini RP, Ryden EB, et al. Estimation of glomerular filtration rate and evaluation of renal function in ferrets (*Mustela putorius furo*). Am J Vet Res 1994;55:166–72.
[22] Court MH. Acetaminophen UDP-glucuronosyltransferase in ferrets: species and gender differences, and sequence analysis of ferret UGTIA6. Journal of Veterinary Pharmacology and Therapeutics 2001;24:415–22.
[23] Williams BH, Kiupel M, West KH, et al. Coronavirus-associated epizootic catarrhal enteritis in ferrets. J Am Vet Med Assoc 2000;217:526–30.
[24] Nelson RW. Disorders of the endocrine pancreas. In: Nelson RW, Couto CG, editors. Small animal internal medicine. 3rd edition. St. Louis (MO): Mosby; 2003. p. 769–75.
[25] Manning DD, Bell JA. Lack of detectable blood groups in the domestic ferrets: implications for transfusion. J Am Vet Med Assoc 1990;197:84–6.
[26] Orcutt C. Update on oxyglobin use in ferrets. Exotic DVM 2001;3(3):29–30.
[27] Ramer JC, Benson KG, Morrisey JK, et al. Effects of melatonin administration on the clinical course of adrenocortical disease in domestic ferrets. J Am Vet Med Assoc 2006;229(11):1743–8.
[28] Benoit-Biancamano MO, Morin M, Langlois I. Histopathologic lesions of diabetes mellitus in a domestic ferret. Can Vet J 2005;46:895–7.
[29] Parker GA, Picut CA. Histopathologic features and post-surgical sequelae of 57 cutaneous neoplasms in ferrets (*Mustela putorius furo*). Vet Pathol 1993;30(6):499–504.
[30] Antinoff N. Clinical observations in ferrets with naturally occurring heartworm disease, and preliminary evaluation of treatment with ivermectin with and without melarsomine. In: Proceedings Symposium American Heartworm Society: Recent Advances in Heartworm Disease. 2002;45–7.
[31] Supakorndej P, McCall JW, Supakorndej, et al. Evaluation of melarsomine dihydrochloride as a heartworm adulticide for ferrets. Proceedings Symposium American Heartworm Society: Recent Advances in Heartworm Disease. 2002;49–55.
[32] Lichtenberger M. Treatment of urinary obstruction in the male ferret. Proceedings of the Annual Meet International Conf Ex, 2006.
[33] Nolte DM, Carberry CA, Gannon KM, et al. Temporary tube cystostomy as treatment for urinary obstruction secondary to adrenal disease in four ferrets. J Am Anim Hosp Assoc 2003;38:527–32.
[34] Garner MM, Ramsel K, Sidor I, et al. Idiopathic myofasciitis in the domestic ferret. In: Proceedings Annual Meet Assoc Ex Mammal Vet 2006; 65–6.
[35] Wingfield WE. Veterinary emergency medicine secrets. Fort Collins (CO): Hanley & Belfus; 2000.
[36] Montiani-Ferreira F, Mattos BC, Russ HH. Reference values for selected ophthalmic diagnostic tests of the ferret (*Mustela putorius furo*). Vet Ophthalmol 2006;9:209–13.

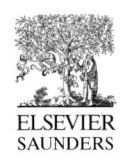

Emergency and Critical Care of Rodents

Michelle G. Hawkins, VMD, DABVP-Avian[a],*,
Jennifer E. Graham, DVM, DABVP-Avian[b,c]

[a]Department of Medicine and Epidemiology, School of Veterinary Medicine, 2108 Tupper Hall, University of California, Davis, Davis, CA 95616, USA
[b]Avian and Exotic Medicine, Angell Animal Medical Center, 350 South Huntington Avenue, Boston, MA 02130, USA
[c]Department of Comparative Medicine, School of Medicine, University of Washington, Box 357910, Seattle, WA 98195, USA

In recent years, the number of rodent species kept as pets has grown considerably and the demand for appropriate veterinary care for these species has also increased. Unfortunately, because rodents are prey species, clinical signs often are masked until the course of the disease is far advanced and the pet is presented on an emergency basis for veterinary care. Today, the rodent species that are presented most commonly in veterinary practice include the guinea pig (*Cavia porcellus*), chinchilla (*Chinchilla laniger*), prairie dog (*Cynomys* sp), rat (*Rattus norvegicus*), mouse (*Mus musculus*), gerbil (*Meriones unguiculatus*), Syrian or golden hamster (*Mesocricetus auratus*), Siberian or dwarf hamster (*Phodopus sungorus*), Chinese hamster (*Cricetus griseus*), and degu (*Octodon* sp). The normal physiologic parameters for some common rodent species are shown in Table 1. However, little data regarding unique medical conditions and their appropriate care are available for some of these species. All mammals within the order Rodentia possess four continuously growing incisors, lack canine teeth, and have an interdental space located between the incisors and cheek teeth. Most rodents are also obligate or dependent nasal breathers. Guinea pigs and chinchillas also have continuously growing premolars and molars. Guinea pigs are unique among rodents in having an absolute requirement for exogenous vitamin C. The principles of emergency and critical care apply equally to rodents; however, the anatomic, physiologic, and behavioral differences among these species require careful consideration when developing an initial plan of emergency therapy. Many

* Corresponding author.
E-mail address: mghawkins@ucdavis.edu (M.G. Hawkins).

Table 1
Normal physiologic parameters for common rodent species

Species	Average weight (g)	Rectal temperature C°/(F°)	Heart rate (beats/min)	Respiratory rate (breaths/min)
Chinchilla	400–800	37.0–38.0 (98.6–100.5)	200–350	40–80
Guinea pig	700–1000	37.0–39.5 (98.6–103.1)	250–380	40–100
Rat	250–520	36.0–37.5 (96.8–99.5)	250–500	70–120
Mouse	20–63	36.5–38.0 (97.7–100.5)	350–700	90–220
Hamster	85–150	37.0–38.0 (98.6–100.5)	250–500	30–140
Gerbil	45–85	37.0–39.0 (98.6–102.2)	250–500	80–160

rodents are predisposed highly to stress, so rapid evaluation and patient stabilization often is required before complete evaluation for a definitive diagnosis can be performed.

Patient handling and restraint

In an emergency situation, the stability of the animal dictates the type of restraint allowable to minimize patient stress. General anesthesia or deep sedation can minimize stress for a fractious or painful patient and can allow for complete physical examination, diagnostic sampling, intravenous (IV) catheter placement, and initiation of therapy, but the risk of adverse effects under anesthesia must be weighed carefully before anesthesia for restraint is considered. The animal may need to be placed in a warm and oxygenated cage before initiation of any restraint. Preoxygenation should be performed whenever possible and always when signs of respiratory distress are present. Sometimes, the benefits of preoxygenation may take 5 minutes or longer in a rodent with a compromised respiratory system.

Handling and restraint of rodents varies with the species. In general, guinea pigs require minimal restraint, but care should be taken to avoid injury from a fall when examining on a table. It is best to support chinchillas with one hand under the thorax and a second hand around the rump. The examiner must avoid holding the chinchilla by the scruff of the neck, because fur slip is common in chinchillas when exuberant restraint is used [1,2]. Prairie dogs can inflict deep and painful bites if not tame, or when stressed. If tame and calm, prairie dogs also can be supported around the chest with one hand and under the hindquarters with the other. Prairie dogs are difficult to scruff, and leather gloves or a towel may be necessary to facilitate handling in some cases [3].

The smaller rodents can be challenging to handle in a way that minimizes patient stress. Wearing examination gloves during restraint of some small rodents may decrease the chances of a bite if the animal bites the glove rather than the hand; however, all rodents are capable of inflicting serious bites. Although gerbils can be very docile and held in a cupped hand, they may require a scruff-of-the-neck or over-the-back technique for complete restraint, taking care not to damage their delicate skin [4,5]. Hamsters are prone to bite, especially if startled; the abundant loose skin over the back and shoulders can be grasped in a full-handed grip for complete immobilization, if needed [4]. Mice can be captured by gently grasping the base of the tail with one hand and then using a scruff-of-the-neck technique with the other hand [4]. Most pet rats are friendly and amenable to handling; if needed, whole-body restraint can be achieved by placing a forefinger below the mandible on one side of the head, and a thumb on the opposite side, above or below the forelimb, with the tail and hind limbs held with the opposite hand [4,6].

Restraint devices are available commercially for all sizes of rodents but are used mainly in the laboratory setting. Small towels are used most commonly as restraint devices to partially "burrito" the companion animal, allowing for examination of individual limbs. Paper towels, syringe cases, and polyethylene or plastic bags with a corner removed have all been reported to facilitate restraint of the small rodent [4]. Any restraint device used with emergency rodent patients should allow for quick release in the event that the rodent becomes severely stressed.

History and physical examination

A comprehensive history is critical in the determination of the disease process and often may help determine the exact cause of the presenting complaint. Often, the history can be obtained while the patient is being stabilized. Dietary history is of utmost concern in the rodent patient. High fiber is necessary for proper hindgut fermentation. Patients that receive diets containing seeds and dried fruits, should be assumed to be consuming large amounts of carbohydrates, which can result in overall malnutrition and gastrointestinal (GI) abnormalities, including diarrhea and dental disease.

The rodent physical examination is similar to that of other mammalian species. If the rodent is debilitated, the examination should proceed in a stepwise fashion, with the most important sections of the examination prioritized in advance, and small breaks from handling given between examination sections. Oxygen supplementation during physical examination may be required.

All equipment needed for the physical examination should be prepared before handling the patient, and all efforts should be made toward minimizing stress for the patient by limiting the time the animal is handled. In addition to the respiratory rate and effort, a significant amount of physical examination information can be obtained before any handling or physical restraint. Symmetry of the eyes, ears, and limbs, and posture and awareness can be evaluated. Ocular or nasal discharge may alert the emergency clinician to diseases of the eyes or upper respiratory tract. In healthy rodents, porphyrin ocular discharge is a normal physiologic finding, but the discharge usually is not seen if the animal is healthy and grooming properly. In some cases, rats are presented on emergency for "bleeding from the eyes" when, in fact, the "porphyrin tears" are simply a sign of other underlying diseases or stress [6,7]. Musculoskeletal or neurologic abnormalities also should be evaluated before handling. If the animal's caging is present, take note of the diet provided and the water containers. It is also important to evaluate the substrate provided in the cage and to note the volume and consistency of urine or feces and whether any odors are present.

The body weight should be obtained as soon as possible, using a gram scale to obtain the most accurate weight of small rodents. The body temperature should be obtained at the onset of examination. Many clinicians avoid taking the body temperatures of small rodents, but the temperature of these animals can be taken if the procedure is performed carefully. It is preferable to use a plastic, flexible thermometer, instead of glass, to avoid injury to the patient [8]. The eyes, oral cavity, ears, nostrils, and integument should be examined closely for any evidence of blood, which may indicate trauma. Because of the pronounced globes of many rodents, trauma of any sort may cause secondary ophthalmic injury, so a thorough ocular examination should always be performed. Also, ocular abnormalities and nasal discharge can be seen secondary to dental disease of the maxillary teeth in guinea pigs and chinchillas. The hair, coat, and skin should also be examined closely because emergency presentation for dermatologic conditions is surprisingly common. Neoplasia and abscesses associated with the integument are also seen frequently in rodents. Abdominal palpation should be performed in all rodents to evaluate for masses, excessive gas ("bloat"), organomegaly, or other abnormalities. The oral examination should be performed last because it is often the most stressful part. However, a complete oral examination is vital, especially in rodents with continuously growing premolars and molars, such as the guinea pig and chinchilla, because dental disease can be the underlying cause of various abnormal clinical signs and emergency presentations.

The external oral examination involves visualization of the incisors in all species and thorough palpation of the ventral mandibles of guinea pigs and chinchillas, because apical elongation of the cheek teeth is common with dental disease in these species. The examination of the oral cavity requires illumination and magnification, which can be accomplished by using a transilluminator and nasal speculum. Alternatively, an otoscope can be used; however, complete examination with this instrument is limited. Ideally, the rodent should be anesthetized, and an endoscopic oral evaluation performed. Intraoral dental disease usually involves buccal elongation of the maxillary cheek teeth and lingual elongation of the mandibular teeth. Tongue entrapment due to lingual points is common with dental disease in guinea pigs and chinchillas.

Sample collection

Stabilization of the patient is mandatory before extensive diagnostic sampling. If blood can be obtained safely, it is ideal to collect baseline samples for hematology and biochemistry analysis before institution of any treatment. Venipuncture can be stressful, even in healthy rodents, because significant restraint is often required to obtain access to appropriate sampling sites. Possible venipuncture sites vary, depending on the species and patient stability. Anesthesia or sedation may be required to facilitate blood collection from any site, but the risk of this must be weighed carefully in the critically ill rodent.

Many techniques have been described for blood sampling in rodents [3–6, 9–13]. Although total blood volume varies according to species, in general, total blood volume is approximately 6% to 8% of body weight; no more than 7% to 10% of the blood volume, or approximately 1% of total body weight, can be collected safely in healthy rodent patients [4,10]. In sick patients presenting on emergency, the general rule of thumb is that no more than 0.5% of total body weight should be collected for blood sampling. The lateral saphenous and cephalic veins are often the most accessible vessels in rodents, and restraint often can be minimized to facilitate collection from these sites. These vessels may yield minimal blood volumes and collapse, even with minimal aspiration pressure, in very small patients. Alternatively, a 0.3-mL insulin syringe, with a swedged-on small-gauge (27-gauge or 29-gauge) needle with the plunger removed, can be introduced into the vein and the blood collected from the hub of the needle inside the syringe barrel into heparinized hematocrit tubes (Fig. 1). A small-gauge hypodermic needle can also be introduced into the vessel, and blood collected in the same manner; however, the use of the syringe barrel technique often provides greater stability of the needle in the vessel during blood collection (see Fig. 1).

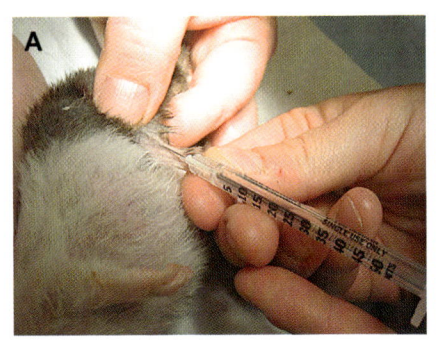

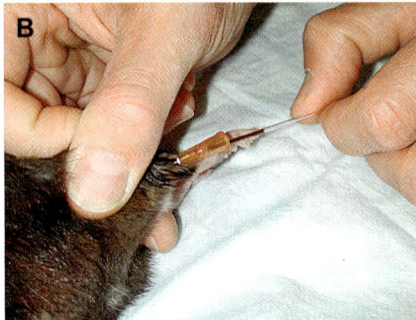

Fig. 1. (*A*) A small-gauge hypodermic needle can be introduced into the vessel and blood collected. (*B*) The use of the syringe barrel technique often provides greater stability of the needle in the vessel during blood collection.

The lateral tail veins can be used to collect small to moderate amounts of blood in gerbils, mice, and rats. The rat has a ventral tail artery that can yield an adequate blood sample, but this technique requires practice [13]. Jugular venipuncture can be challenging because many rodents have short, thick necks with large, fat bodies covering the jugular groove. Restraint for this procedure can be very stressful; often, anesthesia is necessary to facilitate sample collection from this site.

Cranial vena cava venipuncture under anesthesia is also possible in some rodents. The potential risks of this technique include hemorrhage into the thoracic cavity or pericardial sac and penetration of the heart. To minimize these potential complications, use of a 25- to 27-gauge hypodermic needle and a 0.5- to 1-mL syringe is recommended. The angle of the needle and syringe used during cranial vena cava venipuncture is slightly different in some rodents than in other species. For example, in the guinea pig and chinchilla (which have an underdeveloped clavicle), a 25-gauge, five-eighths-inch–length needle is inserted cranial to the manubrium and first rib (Fig. 2). In all other rodents (rat, mouse, hamster, gerbil), a 27-gauge, 0.5-in–length needle is inserted cranial to the clavicle (these rodents have a well-developed clavicle) and at a 45° angle (Fig. 3). The femoral vein is used frequently for venipuncture in anesthetized rodents in the authors' practice and often yields an adequate blood sample (Fig. 4). With the rodent in dorsal recumbency, the femoral artery is palpated deep in the inguinal region, and the needle is inserted parallel to this site. The venipuncture site should be held off for several minutes after collection if the femoral artery is sampled inadvertently (see Fig. 4). Orbital venous plexus collection and cardiac venipuncture are recommended only as terminal procedures in the anesthetized companion rodent patient.

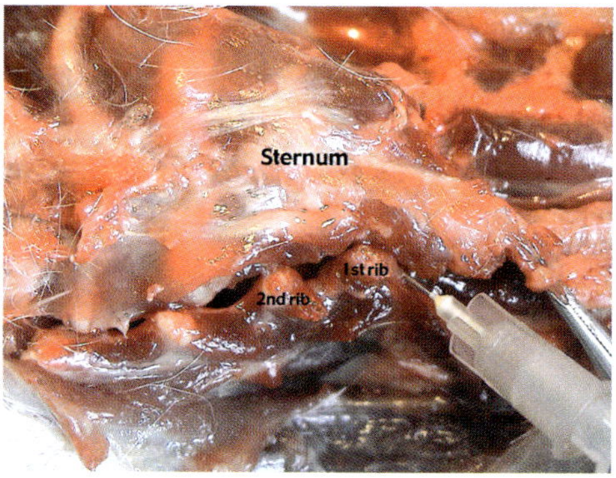

Fig. 2. Correct positioning of the needle for vena cava puncture in a guinea pig cadaver. The guinea pig and chinchilla have underdeveloped clavicles. A 25-gauge, five-eighths–inch needle is inserted cranial to the first rib lateral to the notch of the sternum and directed at a 45° angle toward the opposite hip. (*Courtesy of* Vittorio Capello, DVM, Milano, Italy.)

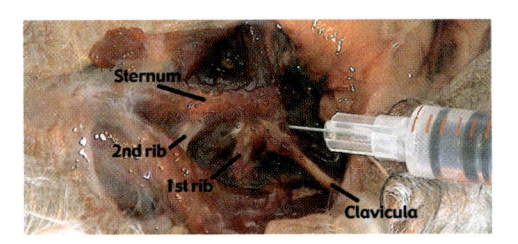

Fig. 3. Correct positioning of the needle for vena cava puncture in a golden hamster cadaver. The needle should be placed between the clavicle and the first rib by inserting the needle cranial to the clavicle. Puncture between the clavicle and the first rib changes the angulation, forcing the needle more laterally, making venipuncture more difficult. (*Courtesy of* Vittorio Capello, Milano, Italy.)

Radiographs may be obtained with or without anesthesia, also depending on patient stability. Restraint boards and masking tape can be used for positioning rodents, to minimize exposure of personnel to radiation [14]. Two-view, whole-body radiographs are recommended, with additional views taken of the skull, thorax, abdomen, and extremities, if indicated. In general, four-view radiographs (dorsoventral (DV), lateral, left and right obliques) should be taken to assess dental disease. In some of the smaller rodents, dental radiographic equipment may be better for radiographic evaluation of the abdomen or distal extremities (Fig. 5). Ultrasound can be a very useful tool for evaluating the small thorax of rodents. Ultrasound is also used widely for abdominal evaluation in rodents, but it can be hindered by the presence of gas in the GI tract. Systematic evaluation of all organs is performed in the same fashion as in other mammals. Ultrasound provides greater imaging detail of abdominal neoplasms and urogenital abnormalities in rodents.

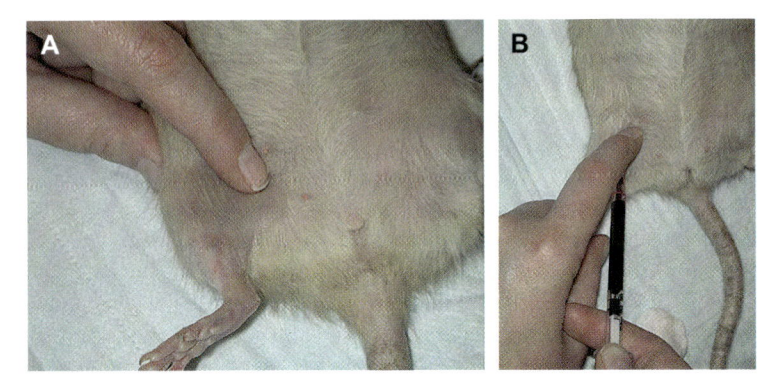

Fig. 4. The femoral vein site for venipuncture is identified by palpation of the femoral artery (*A*) and the needle inserted and directed parallel to the site (*B*).

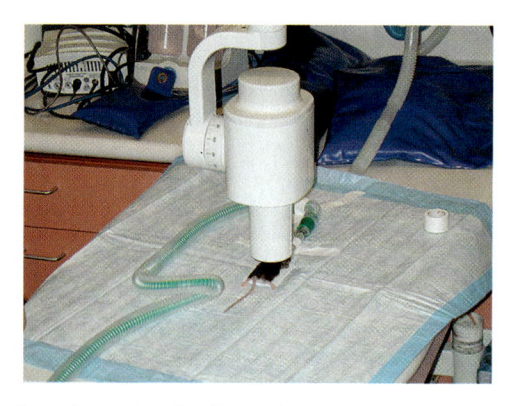

Fig. 5. In some smaller rodents, dental radiography may provide for better radiographic detail of the distal extremities, abdomen, and thorax.

Respiratory washes and cultures, urine collection, and other diagnostic tests may be useful to determine the cause and extent of disease. A direct fecal examination and flotation are advisable, especially in patients showing GI signs.

Triage of the emergency rodent patient

The ABCs (airway, breathing, circulation) of small-animal emergency medicine and the principles of cardiopulmonary-cerebral resuscitation are universal, and apply equally to the small rodent patient. If a rodent is showing extreme respiratory difficulty or open-mouthed breathing, or if the rodent is collapsed or exhibiting weakness, emergency supportive care should be provided before undertaking a complete physical examination.

Respiratory evaluation and support

The respiratory rate and effort should always be evaluated in rodents before handling, and immediate assessment of a patent airway is critical. When an airway obstruction is present, or if the patient is in respiratory arrest, tracheal intubation is a necessity. Tracheal intubation can be challenging in rodents because most are obligate or dependent nasal breathers with limited oral access, so the clinician should be prepared to perform an emergency tracheostomy procedure to provide ventilation, if necessary. In the guinea pig, orotracheal intubation is complicated also by the fusion of the soft palate to the base of the tongue, creating only a small opening called the palatal ostium (Fig. 6) [15,16]. Small endotracheal tubes of 1.0- to 2.5-mm internal diameter are needed most often for small rodent species; the smallest commercially available tubes have an internal diameter of 1 mm. However, tubes less than 2-mm internal diameter often are highly flexible, and kink

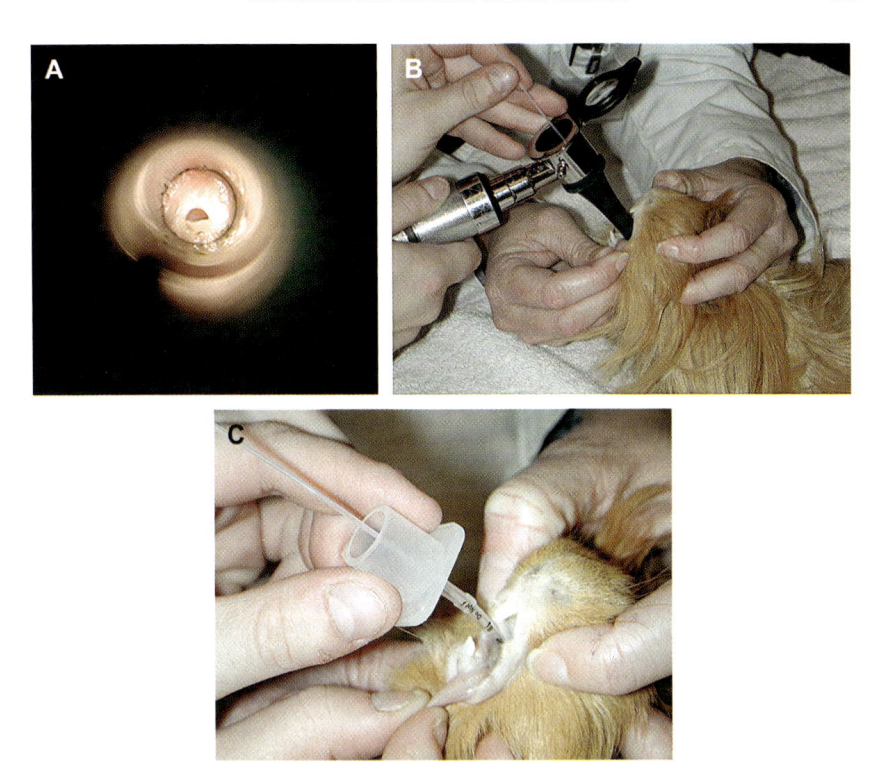

Fig. 6. Guinea pigs have a palatal ostium that can be traumatized easily during intubation. To minimize trauma, an otoscopic cone or endoscope can enhance visualization of the larynx (*A*). A stylet is then placed into the larynx (*B*), allowing the endotracheal tube to be manipulated gently past the palatal ostium (*C*).

easily during use. Very small rodents may be intubated with Teflon IV (14 gauge, 16 gauge), red rubber, or urinary catheters, but occlusion with mucous plugs occurs frequently because of the small internal diameter of these tubes. Care must be taken to ensure that no sharp edges are present on the end of these tubes. Cole tubes are uncuffed endotracheal tubes with a narrow distal insertion tip to allow facilitation of placement into the airway, and a broader shoulder to fit snugly at the larynx. In the authors' experience, these tubes tend to slip from the airway easily. The smallest diameter cuffed tube is 3 mm, which is too large for many rodents. Noncuffed tubes do not provide a sealed airway, so airway protection from aspiration of secretions or GI contents is reduced; therefore, it is imperative that the oral cavity is clean before performing intubation because many rodents store food in their cheek pouches. Elevating the head and neck of the patient may reduce the potential for regurgitation of GI contents into the oral cavity.

An otoscopic cone, modified pediatric blade, or endoscope can help facilitate intubation [17–22]. Otoscopic cones that have been modified by removing a section laterally can facilitate visualization of the epiglottis and direct placement of the endotracheal tube. In smaller rodents and guinea pigs, a stylet may be placed first, to help facilitate endotracheal tube placement and to minimize trauma to the palatal ostium. Endoscopy may provide the best visualization of the epiglottis and may minimize trauma during tube placement. One drop of a 2% lidocaine solution applied directly to the larynx usually reduces laryngospasm and eases tube placement.

If an endotracheal tube cannot be placed, a temporary tracheostomy can be performed. A 2- to 3-cm skin incision is made on the ventral midline parallel to the trachea, just caudal to the larynx. The SC fat and fascia are dissected bluntly, which minimizes the potential to cut through blood vessels imbedded in the fat that can bleed excessively. Blunt dissection is continued through the paired strap muscles to isolate the trachea. A transverse incision is made between the tracheal rings that should not exceed 50% of the circumference of the trachea. Stay sutures are placed in the trachea cranial and caudal to the tracheostomy site. An endotracheal tube is inserted into the trachea and secured in place.

Intermittent positive-pressure ventilation should be administered with 100% oxygen at a rate of 20 to 30 breaths/min at 8 to 10 cm H_2O airway pressure, if respiratory arrest is present [23]. If the patient is not intubated, positive pressure ventilation by way of a tight-fitting mask can provide indirect ventilation; however, this method must be monitored carefully because aerophagia can occur and may lead to severe GI dilatation and tympany. Generally, nasal intubation is not practical in rodents because of the small size of the nasal cavity.

If a rodent is showing signs of respiratory distress but does not require intubation, the patient should be placed immediately into a quiet, oxygen-enriched environment. If a commercial oxygen cage is not available, one can be fashioned from an induction chamber or a small pet carrier covered with a plastic bag, or, if the patient is small enough, the rodent can be placed inside a large anesthetic facemask (Fig. 7). The use of oxygen delivered through an anesthetic mask over the nose or by nasal insufflation is feasible, but can be very stressful for the rodent patient. The authors recommend the use of sedation and oxygen delivery in a quiet environment to minimize stress, if this technique for oxygen delivery is to be used. Humidification of oxygenated air by bubbling through an isotonic fluid solution is recommended, to assist with clearance of respiratory secretions and foreign material within the trachea and bronchi. Commercially manufactured intensive care units can provide oxygen, heat, and humidity.

Nebulization can be useful for delivering moisture or topical medications to the mucous membranes of the respiratory system [24]. Inhalant delivery of aerosolized medication offers a number of theoretic benefits, including a large absorptive surface area across a permeable membrane, a low-enzyme environment potentially resulting in reduced drug degradation, avoidance of hepatic first-pass metabolism, potential for high drug concentrations

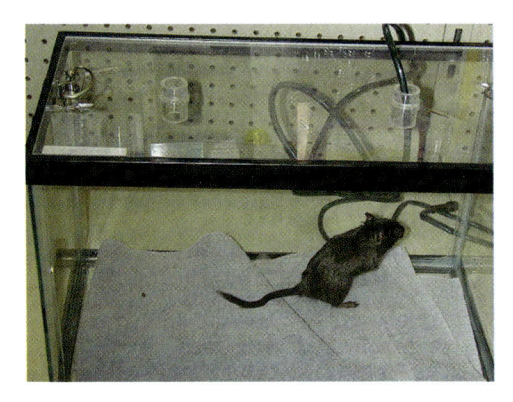

Fig. 7. If a rodent is showing signs of respiratory distress but does not require intubation, the patient should be placed immediately into a quiet, oxygen-enriched environment. (*Courtesy of* Marla Lichtenberger, DVM, Mequon, WI.)

directly at the site of disease [25], and reduced potential for systemic toxicity. In veterinary medicine, the literature on inhalant therapy is extremely sparse and what does exist focuses more on aerosol drug delivery to horses than to small pet animal species. Only two published studies in conscious, unsedated cats and rats have demonstrated the ability to deliver particles to the lower airways by way of nebulization [25,26]. Regardless, aerosol delivery of medication has become popular for the treatment of dogs, cats, small mammals, and birds with respiratory disease. Administering nebulized particles using positive-pressure ventilation through an endotracheal tube is the most efficient method for lower airway particle delivery, but this procedure usually is not practical in a clinical setting. Nebulization has been administered to small mammals in a closed cage, induction chamber, or aquarium or by way of a face mask. Typically, the systemic drug dose has been diluted empirically in saline and delivered over a single 15- to 30-minute nebulization session.

The most frequently used antibiotic medications for nebulization are the aminoglycoside antibiotics, but no guidelines have been established for administering these drugs by this route. Amphotericin B has been used effectively by way of nebulization for lower airway fungal disease in rats [25]. Parental bronchodilators, such as terbutaline, have also been used empirically by way of nebulization, in small exotic mammals with lower airway disease. In rats, terbutaline (0.01 mg/kg) often is given intramuscularly (IM) initially or subcutaneous (SC) while the rat is placed into an oxygen environment, and then terbutaline is nebulized for subsequent treatment.

Mucolytic therapy with N-acetylcysteine by way of nebulization also has been used by some clinicians to facilitate the clearance of respiratory secretions. Because of its potential irritation to the airways, a bronchodilator should precede therapy with N-acetylcysteine, and therefore, nebulization with this drug should be considered with caution in small exotic animals.

During the physical examination, care should be taken to hold the patient upright, and oxygen support should be provided if there are signs of respiratory distress or if any fluid or masses are palpated in the abdominal cavity. Clinical signs of respiratory disease may be subtle, but can include discharge from the eyes or nares, tachypnea, abnormal respiratory sounds, and open-mouthed breathing. Because of the small size of the rodent thorax, it is sometimes difficult to auscultate the normal breathing patterns; the use of a neonatal or pediatric stethoscope often facilitates this part of the examination.

Circulatory evaluation and support

The heart should be auscultated, and the heart rate and any abnormalities in rhythm should be recorded. An ECG can also be used to evaluate cardiac rhythm, but, because of the rapid heart rate of many small rodents, the ECG complexes can be difficult to assess at standard speeds of 25 mm/sec. A number of ECG devices are now available that can provide speeds of 100 and 200 mm/sec, allowing accurate evaluation of the small complexes. Needle ECG leads are ideal for small rodents because they provide excellent conduction without the use of gels or alcohol that can cool the body temperature of the patient. Alternatively, metal alligator clips attached to a hypodermic needle or to an alcohol-soaked cotton ball can be used (Fig. 8). It is important not to saturate the patient with alcohol because it can cause rapid reduction in body temperature.

Perfusion is assessed by evaluating the color and capillary refill time of the oral, rectal, or vaginal mucous membranes, the femoral pulse quality, the heart rate, and the blood pressure. Indirect blood pressure monitoring can be performed using a Doppler ultrasonic probe to detect the arterial flow, a pressure cuff to occlude arterial blood flow, and a sphygmomanometer to measure pressures. An oscillometric device can be used that measures pressures automatically by detecting the pressure changes in the cuff as it is deflated, but these devices can be unreliable in the small hypotensive or hypothermic patient. The general rule for size of blood pressure cuffs is the same as for other mammals, in that the size of the cuff should approximate 40% of the circumference of the limb on which it is used. Cuffs that are too large can give falsely decreased pressures. The cuff can be placed above the carpus or tarsus, or a tail cuff designed specifically for rodents can be placed over the base of the tail. The Doppler ultrasonic probe can then be placed between the carpal/tarsal pad and the pads of the feet over the digital arterial branches, or on the ventral surface of the tail over the ventral tail artery; shaving of these areas is sometimes necessary (Fig. 9). The pressures determined with use of a sphygmomanometer are thought to correlate with systolic pressures, whereas the oscillometric devices can provide systolic, diastolic, and mean arterial pressures. The clinician should evaluate the

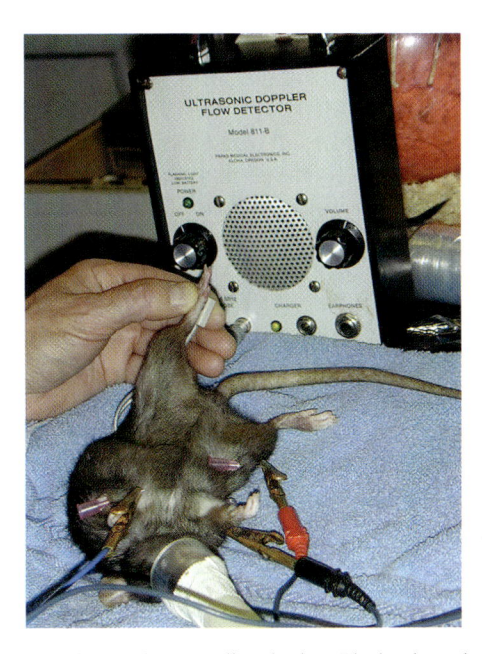

Fig. 8. An ECG can be used to evaluate cardiac rhythm. Placing hypodermic needles through the skin and attaching alligator clips to the hypodermic needle can provide appropriate signal conduction while minimizing trauma. (*Courtesy of* Marla Lichtenberger, DVM, Mequon, WI.)

patient carefully and respond to trends in the oscillometric measurements, rather than rely on the absolute number generated. Normal systolic blood pressure measurements obtained with Doppler flow detection in small mammal patients range from 90 to 120 mm Hg [27].

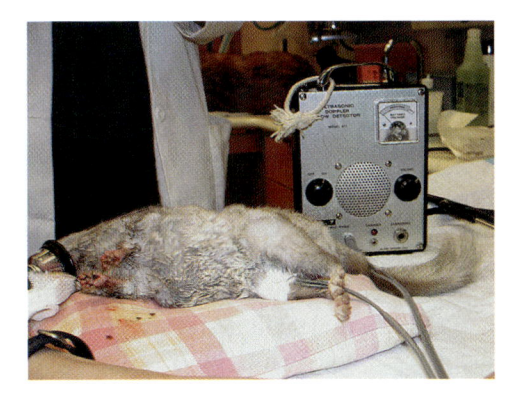

Fig. 9. Pulse rate and subjective changes in pulse quality by evaluating loudness of signal can be assessed using a Doppler ultrasonic probe placed over an artery. Indirect blood pressure monitoring can be performed using a Doppler ultrasonic probe to detect the arterial flow, a pneumatic pressure cuff to occlude arterial blood flow, and a sphygmomanometer to measure pressures.

General supportive care

Environmental support

Rodents should always be hospitalized away from noise and any predator species (ferrets, cats, and so forth) to minimize stress. Noise also should be minimized during the physical examination and diagnostic procedures.

Thermal support is often necessary for the emergency rodent patient. The exception to this rule is head trauma, where heat support may cause vasodilation of intracranial vessels and exacerbate hemorrhage. The clinician should realize that normal body temperatures of rodents vary and can be as low as 95.7°F in prairie dogs [3]. Caution should be exercised when providing thermal support because many small rodents are susceptible to heat stress; chinchillas are particularly prone to temperatures higher than 75°F [1,2]. An obtunded patient may be unable to move away from a heat source when becoming overheated. Careful monitoring is essential when supplemental heat is being provided, and body temperatures should be taken frequently.

Fluid therapy

Fluid therapy for hypovolemic resuscitation is described in the article by Lichtenberger in this issue. The percentage of dehydration can be estimated subjectively, based on body weight, mucous membrane dryness, decreased skin turgor, sunken eyes, and altered mentation, but these parameters can also be affected by decreased body fat and increased age. Dehydration deficits greater than 5% ideally require IV fluid replacement; a constant-rate infusion of a crystalloid fluid is necessary to support patients that are dehydrated and have ongoing losses. Fluid requirements for dehydration are calculated as

$$\%\text{dehydration} \times \text{kg} \times 1000 \text{ mL/L} = \text{fluid deficit (L)}$$

Dehydration requirements should be added to those fluids provided for daily maintenance fluid requirements and ongoing losses. Fifty to seventy-five percent of the calculated fluid deficit can be replaced in the first 24 hours. An objective way to assess whether the fluid volume is adequate is to evaluate body weight regularly throughout the day. Acute weight loss may sometimes be associated with fluid loss, and can be used to determine the patient at risk of becoming dehydrated.

All fluids should be warmed to the body temperature of the patient, regardless of the route of administration. Fluids can be warmed to 38° to 39°C without affecting their composition [28]. Fluid-line warmers are available commercially; alternatively, the fluid line may be passed though a bowl of warm water to maintain the fluid temperature. The protocol for fluid therapy should be based on packed cell volume (PCV), total protein, urine output, and, ideally, blood pressure and acid-base status. Although urinary catheterization of rodents can be used to determine urinary output objectively, it usually is not practical in small rodents. Alternatively, urine output can be evaluated subjectively by weighing dry bedding before placing it into the rodent's cage and then weighing the bedding after removal. Hospital pads are often preweighed and placed into the cage for urine collection.

Oral fluids should be given only if the rodent is stable, less than 5% dehydrated, and standing. Care must be taken when administering oral fluids to ensure that the GI tract is functioning properly and that fluid is not aspirated. SC fluids are used only when venous access cannot be obtained. An ideal site for administration of SC fluids in most rodents is the SC space over the neck or back. Intraperitoneal fluids can be given in the lower left quadrant, with the head of the patient lower than the abdomen, to allow the viscera to slide forward [4,29].

In an emergency situation, IV or intraosseous (IO) fluids may be required to provide replacement fluids. Sedation or inhalant anesthesia may be necessary for IV catheter placement in the stressed rodent patient. IV catheters can be placed in the cephalic, lateral saphenous, or femoral veins in larger rodents such as chinchillas, guinea pigs, and rats (Fig. 10). The author prefers the cephalic vein for IV catheterization in most cases. The superficial lateral tail vein can also be used for short-term catheter placement in the rat. Peripheral catheterization is difficult in prairie dogs because of fat surrounding the vessels, and in very small rodents because of small vessel size [3,30]. Although jugular catheterization can be performed in rodents, a surgical cut-down procedure under anesthesia is necessary. Most often, small-bore, over-the-needle catheters (24-gauge or smaller) are necessary for small

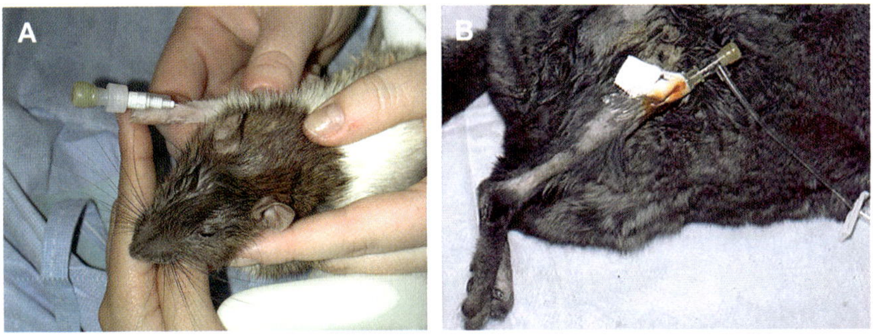

Fig. 10. In an emergency situation, IV or IO fluids may be required to provide replacement fluids. (*A*) IV catheters can be placed in the cephalic, lateral saphenous, or femoral veins in larger rodents such as chinchillas, guinea pigs, and rats. Catheters should be secured with a bandage tape butterfly and sutured in place, and careful monitoring is essential. (*B*) Common sites for IO catheter placement in the rodent include the femur, through the trochanteric fossa, or the tibia, through the tibial crest. Placement is similar to that of a normograde insertion of an intramedullary pin and requires strict aseptic technique during placement and maintenance.

rodent patients. However, catheter maintenance may be hindered by vessel fragility and patient temperament. The catheter site should be prepared aseptically. Catheters should be secured with a bandage-tape butterfly and sutured in place. Jugular catheters, if left in-dwelling, require 24-hour monitoring because fatal hemorrhage can occur if the rodent pulls or chews on the catheter and damages the vessel. Generally, rats, mice, and hamsters are intolerant of bandaging material and other equipment such as indwelling catheters, and will attempt to chew and remove the materials, even when they are severely compromised, so careful monitoring of the IV catheter is essential.

IO catheterization can be useful in smaller patients or during cardiovascular collapse (see Fig. 10) [31]. IO catheter maintenance is easier to achieve because of stability in the medullary cavity. Products that can be used as IO catheters include 18- to 24-gauge, 1- to 1.5-in spinal needles or 18- to 25-gauge 1-in hypodermic needles, depending on the size of the species. The length of the catheter should be long enough to extend one third to one half of the length of the medullary cavity. A wire stylet may be necessary to reduce the potential for a bone core plugging the catheter during placement. The authors prepare several hypodermic needles (25- to 18-gauge needles) with wire stylets (stainless steel sutures) and sterilizes them for use in rodent IO catheterization. Common sites for IO catheter placement in the rodent include the femur, through the trochanteric fossa, or the tibia, through the tibial crest. Placement is similar to that of a normograde insertion of an intramedullary pin, and requires strict aseptic technique during placement and maintenance. Once the cortex is penetrated, the catheter should advance easily with little resistance. Further resistance indicates most likely that the opposite cortex has been penetrated. The cannula should be flushed with heparinized saline immediately because the bone marrow quickly clots. The insertion site should be covered with an antibiotic ointment, and the cannula secured with a bandage-tape butterfly and suture. A bandage can be placed over the cannula site for additional security, and to prevent possible trauma, or damage to the catheter. IO catheters have been reported to remain patent for 72 hours without flushing; however, if fluid therapy is not continuous, it is recommended that the catheter be flushed gently with heparinized saline twice daily. Complications associated with IO catheterization include penetration of both cortices, failure to enter the medullary cavity properly, and extravasation of fluids with associated pain. IO catheterization is contraindicated in patients that are septic or have metabolic bone disease. Administration of alkaline or hypertonic solutions can cause pain, so these solutions should be diluted before delivery thorough an IO catheter, and the catheter flushed with heparinized saline after any drug injection. IO catheters should be used primarily for short-term vascular volume expansion, until an IV catheter site can be obtained. Many rodents appear to become uncomfortable on limbs supporting IO catheters, even after short-term placement.

Dextrose solutions may be added to crystalloid solutions for the treatment of hypoglycemia only when hypoglycemia has been documented by a blood glucose measurement. An initial bolus of 50% dextrose at 0.25 mL/kg can be given as a 1:1 dilution with saline IV. The parenteral use of dextrose should be conservative because it may induce compartmental shifts in electrolytes and water, which ultimately could lead to further dehydration.

A whole blood transfusion may be indicated in critically ill rodents when blood loss is severe (>30% blood volume) or the PCV is less than 20%. As in other species, continued blood loss, nonregenerative anemia with PCV 12% to 15% or below, and clotting disorders (such as seen with anticoagulant rodenticides) are indicators used to determine the potential need for a whole blood transfusion [32]. Considerations for performing a blood transfusion include the degree of clinical signs, the patient's hematocrit, the cause and degree of anemia (acute blood loss versus chronic conditions), potential for further blood loss, availability of a donor, and the patient's capacity for handling the stress of catheter placement. For blood transfusion specifics, see the article by Lichtenberger in this issue.

Nutritional support

Nutritional support is a crucial component of treatment, and is vital to resolve or prevent gastric stasis and ileus in rodents. Replacement-fluid therapy also must play a role in nutritional support because the GI tract must be hydrated to facilitate motility and function during nutritional therapy. In general, sick rodents tolerate hand feeding by syringe extremely well; a nasogastric tube is rarely required for enteral nutrition. Nasogastric tube placement is more difficult in the small rodent patient and no nutritionally complete fiber diet will pass through these small lumen tubes. Attempts can be made to mix these formulations with other formulas, such as isotonic feeding formulas or baby food, to reduce the particle size; however, the nutritional value of the food will also be reduced. Often, patience is required to feed small boluses of food with a 1-mL syringe directed into the interdental space, with breaks given to the patient as needed. In the author's experience, rodent patients respond positively with minimal stress to this type of enteral support. Currently, a timothy hay–based critical care feeding formula for herbivores (Oxbow Critical Care, Oxbow Pet Products, Murdock, Nebraska) is available commercially; when mixed with water, it provides a high-fiber, homogeneous, palatable mixture for anorectic herbivores. Although blending pellets and greens with water is an alternative to the commercial diet, it is more time consuming and generally results in a less homogenous mixture. Total parenteral nutrition and partial enteral nutrition are not used commonly in small exotic animal medicine because of catheter-related complications, patient tolerance, and the lack of appropriate formulations for herbivorous species.

Guinea pigs require an exogenous source of vitamin C [33] and in some cases will present on emergency with clinical signs of hypovitaminosis C (scurvy), such as hindlimb weakness or lameness, anorexia, and diarrhea [34]. Vitamin C supplementation is provided routinely to the hospitalized, critically ill guinea pig at 50 to100 mg/kg/day [34].

Pain management

Information on pain management for rodents is included in the article by Lichtenberger and Ko in this issue.

Antibiotics

Antibiotics are commonly used empirically in rodent emergency medicine, often before obtaining culture and sensitivity results. However, specific antibiotic use always must be considered carefully in rodents. Some rodents, such as the guinea pig and hamster, have a predominately gram-positive GI flora and are very sensitive to dysbiosis associated with antibiotic use [35]. Antibiotics, including oral penicillins, macrolides, and lincosamides, can destroy normal gut flora in some rodents, and permit fatal dysbiosis [34–36]. Before results from culture and sensitivity, first-line antibiotics commonly used in rodents include the fluoroquinolones (enrofloxacin, ciprofloxacin), trimethoprim-sulfa, and chloramphenicol. Even these antibiotics may cause GI disruption in some individuals, so patients should be monitored closely at all times when on antibiotics. Chloramphenicol can be hematotoxic in humans and animals [37], so appropriate precautions must be considered before prescribing this antibiotic.

Emergency presentations

Trauma

Wounds, fractures, head trauma, ocular trauma, electrocution, and other traumatic injuries are often primary causes for emergency presentation of rodents. The patient should be assessed for internal trauma, such as pulmonary contusions, fractures, and organ trauma, and these concerns addressed immediately. Fractures and wounds should be cleaned and stabilized initially, and pain management should be provided accordingly, until the rodent is stable enough to undergo surgical repair or more aggressive treatment.

Wounds commonly occur in the rodent patient from predator bites, attacks from conspecifics, accidental falls or trauma from owners, and injury from sharp corners or other items within the cage. Severe wounds, such as tail slip in the gerbil, may require surgical intervention when the patient is stable [1,5]. Bite wounds, specifically from dogs and cats, can result in fatal septicemia. Wounds should be cleansed thoroughly and antibacterial therapy should be instituted immediately. Generally, bite wounds and punctures should be left open to heal by second intention, whenever possible. Sulfa antibiotics generally provide a good spectrum for cat-bite wounds and most are usually safe for use in the sensitive rodent GI tract.

Fractures can be challenging to manage in the rodent patient because of the small size of the extremities. In an emergency situation, modified Robert-Jones bandages and splints can be applied to fractures distal to the humerus or femur. Adaptations to the bandage, such as abdominal taping or wrapping, may be necessary to prevent bandage slipping in the small rodent patient [30]. Many small rodent species are intolerant of bandages, so external coaptation may not provide the best option for long-term fracture repair in these species. Small Elizabethan collars are available commercially, or can be made out of radiology film, to prevent chewing of the bandage, but some rodents will not tolerate collars. In some cases, sedation may allow for Elizabethan collar placement and better tolerance. External fixators are often the stabilization of choice in small rodents because they are often tolerated better, and can be applied once the patient is stable. When external fixators or external coaptation are not tolerated, maintaining the rodent soley on soft bedding may be attempted, but there is a risk of mal-union or non-union of the fracture with this method.

Head trauma can be associated with physical examination findings of anisocoria; head tilt; depression; skull fractures; retinal detachment; or hemorrhage from the nostrils, oral cavity, ears, or into the anterior chamber of the eye. Oxygen support is usually prudent in the rodent with evidence of head trauma. Care should be taken to avoid hypothermia or hyperthermia. The rodent should be maintained on soft bedding; excessive movement may require sedation. The neurologic status, including mentation, pupil symmetry, position, and papillary light reflex should be assessed often, every 30 minutes at a minimum. Dilated and nonresponsive pupils may suggest a brainstem lesion, which carries a poor prognosis. Diuretic use should be considered only with deterioration of mentation or with pupillary assessment. The use of steroids in humans is no longer recommended in head trauma and therefore not recommended by the author.

Globe proptosis is a common emergency presentation in rodents, especially in hamsters, and can be secondary to improper restraint, trauma, molar abscessation, sialodacryoadenitis, and infection [7,30]. The lid margins around the globe should be retracted gently following cleansing and lubrication of the eye, with gentle pressure applied to the intact globe to reduce the prolapse. Ophthalmic lubricants and antibiotics can be used to treat the eye for 7 to 10 days after replacement. Topical steroid use should be avoided, but nonsteroidal anti-inflammatory drug (NSAID) ophthalmic preparations may be used with caution. The total dose used of an NSAID ophthalmic in a rodent patient should not exceed the maximum calculated systemic dose for that (NSAID) medication. If NSAIDs are also given orally for pain relief, either the ophthalmic or the systemic dose may need to be adjusted accordingly. Tarsorrhaphy may be necessary to prevent recurrence of the proptosis. Enucleation may be necessary if the trauma is severe, or if the proptosed globe cannot be replaced [7]. Topical or systemic antibiotics are indicated in the event of corneal ulceration or perforation. Topical NSAIDs, such as 0.03% flurbiprofen (Flurbiprofen sodium ophthalmic solution, Bausch & Lomb, Rochester, New York) can be used for treatment of uveitis.

Rodents naturally gnaw on many substrates; if not supervised carefully, the small exotic mammal may gnaw or chew on furniture, carpet, and electrical wires, leading to foreign body ingestion or electrocution. Evidence of electrocution may not be evident for 24 to 48 hours after electrocution injury. Electrocution may be associated with thermal burns in the oral cavity and on the limbs; cardiac arrest; pericardial effusion; central nervous system damage; neurogenic pulmonary edema; and muscle or generalized convulsions (Fig. 11). If electrocution is suspected, aggressive therapy may be necessary to save the injured rodent. Treatment of pulmonary edema with a diuretic is controversial because it is thought that the pulmonary edema is caused by a permeability injury. The author recommends one dose of furosemide IM when respiratory distress accompanies electrocution. Often,

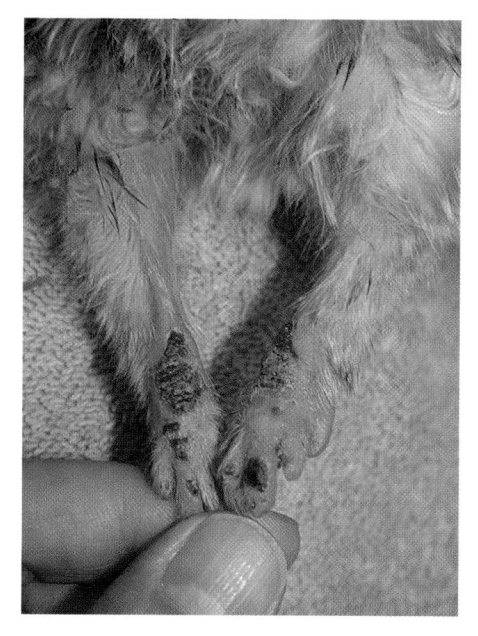

Fig. 11. Electrocution may be associated with thermal burns in the oral cavity and on the limbs, which may not be evident for several days after injury.

antibiotics, NSAIDs and sedation are required. Additionally, topical therapy for wounds may be needed.

Respiratory disease

Pneumonia, foreign body inhalation, and thoracic trauma are some of the common respiratory emergencies seen in rodents. Infectious pneumonias are also common. Bacterial organisms are implicated most commonly in pet rodents, but viral disease is also possible and, in some cases, a complex of viral and bacterial causes can be present [7]. Inappropriate husbandry conditions and stress often predispose to secondary infection. Antibiotics, fluid therapy, oxygen support, bronchodilators, nebulization, and minimal patient handling can help stabilize the patient with pneumonia. Radiographs and cultures are beneficial, once the patient is stable, to best direct therapy. Cultures of material collected from tracheal or bronchoalveolar lavage are ideal in cases of pneumonia, but it may not be possible to collect them safely in the distressed patient. Viral screening can be performed on patients who are refractory to antibiotic therapy. In many cases, especially in rats, respiratory disease can be a chronic recurring problem, necessitating the frequent use of antibiotics.

Neoplasia is a very common condition in small rodents, and often the first clinical signs of the disease are respiratory signs from metastatic disease to the lungs. Other underlying conditions, such as cardiac disease and pleural effusion, should be ruled out in the dyspneic rodent patient. Cardiac disease is very common in the hamster and prairie dog [3,7].

Foreign-body inhalation/aspiration and esophageal foreign body, or choke, are causes for emergency presentations of rodents with respiratory distress. If a patient was clinically normal before a sudden onset of respiratory distress, foreign-body aspiration or an esophageal foreign body should be ruled out. These patients often present with green fluid around the nostrils, or drooling. Immediate oxygen support is beneficial, to stabilize the patient. A low dose of a sedative often helps calm the patient and may even allow for the passage of the foreign material. Saline nebulization is helpful to deliver moisture to the upper respiratory passages, which helps dissolve food material that may be partially obstructing the upper airway. In some cases, anesthesia and attempts to remove the lodged material by way of endoscopy may be necessary. It is prudent to treat recovered patients with antibiotics and, potentially, antifungal medications to prevent secondary bacterial or fungal pneumonia in the case of foreign-body aspiration.

Thoracic trauma due to falling or crushing injuries is common in small rodents and can result in pneumothorax or hemothorax. Radiographs are necessary to assess the degree of thoracic trauma. Thoracocentesis, ideally ultrasound-guided, can be performed using a 25-gauge butterfly catheter and 3- or 6-mL syringe to aspirate fluid or air. Hospitalization and oxygen therapy are recommended, with repeat thoracic radiographs, ultrasound, or thoracocentesis to ensure resolution of the problem.

Cardiac disease

Although not as common as primary respiratory disease, cardiac disease does occur in rodent patients. Cardiac disease should be ruled out in any patient presenting with signs of dyspnea, tachypnea, rales, tachycardia, arrhythmia, poor peripheral pulses, cyanosis, or ascites. Radiographs, cardiac ultrasound, and electrocardiogram are used to assess cardiac disease in rodent patients. Diuretics, angiotensin-converting enzyme, and digoxin have been used in the rodent patient [7,30,38,39]. Dilated cardiomyopathy is seen commonly in prairie dogs older than 3 years [3]. Cardiomyopathy and atrial thrombosis are common in older hamsters [7,40].

Neurologic emergencies/toxins

Seizuring can have various causes in rodents. In gerbils, approximately 20% to 40% develop seizure-like activity beginning at 2 months of age, which most outgrow with time. The seizures usually pass within a few minutes and appear to have no lasting effect. No successful treatment is known at this time [5,41]. Pruritis associated with ectoparasites, such as with *Trixacarus caviae*, are other possible causes of seizures or seizure-like behavior, especially in the guinea pig [42–44]. Thiamine deficiency, *Listeria monocytogenes*, and cerebral nematodiasis are reported causes of seizures in chinchillas [45–48]. Lymphocytic choriomeningitis is an important zoonotic disease that can cause neurologic disease in rodents, including guinea pigs and chinchillas [1,2,7,49]. Hypoglycemia can occur in any rodent unable to access food and may be seen more commonly in young rodents.

Any seizuring rodent should be treated initially with a benzodiazepine, such as diazepam or midazolam, IV, IO, or rectally for seizure control. The author has attempted to control seizure activity in rodents that are unresponsive to benzodiazepines with phenobarbital, using two doses of 4 mg/kg IM approximately 20 minutes apart as a loading dose. Phenobarbital can be continued 12 hours later at 2 mg/kg by mouth twice daily. Dextrose and calcium gluconate may be needed if hypoglycemia or hypocalcemia are present. Diagnostics should be directed at determining an underlying cause for the seizures. Additional supportive care, including supplemental heat, fluid therapy, and oxygen support, may be indicated.

Spontaneous radiculoneuropathy occurs commonly in aged rats and may manifest with hindlimb paresis or weakness [50–52]. This degenerative disease of the spinal nerve roots, with concurrent atrophy of the skeletal muscles in the epaxial and hindlimb region, may not be noticed initially by the owner. The clinical signs may appear acutely, so trauma is the most common presenting complaint in the emergency setting. Usually, the rat will be alert and still eating. Often, analgesia using NSAIDs is prescribed, with little effect.

Ingested toxins, including heavy metals and anticoagulant rodenticides, may result in various clinical signs, including neurologic signs, hemorrhage, and death. Exposure to pesticides, including herbicides, rodenticides, and insecticides, may cause disease when ingested or absorbed cutaneously. Vitamin K therapy at standard mammalian dosages is indicated in cases of suspected rodenticide ingestion. Venipuncture should be avoided in cases of suspected rodenticide ingestion, to avoid excessive blood loss. Gastric lavage and administration of activated charcoal can be performed in the case of toxin ingestion. Additional treatment involves supportive care, including thermal support, fluid therapy, nutritional support, decontamination, and treatment of secondary disease. In the case of heavy metal toxicosis, heavy metal chelators and potential removal of the toxic material when present may be indicated.

Gastrointestinal emergencies

Emergency presentations for GI conditions are quite common in rodents. Underlying dental disease with secondary anorexia and ileus is undoubtedly the most common reason for emergency presentations of chinchillas and guinea pigs of all ages. Aged hamsters and gerbils often present with these signs secondary to incisor elongation. Clinical signs may be nonspecific and may include anorexia and bruxism, or the patient may be painful on abdominal palpation, or may exhibit GI stasis, diarrhea, or rectal or intestinal prolapse. A thorough oral examination is important to confirm intraoral disease. However, radiographs are often necessary to confirm apical changes, especially of the maxillary cheek teeth.

GI stasis can result from any abnormality causing pain or anorexia in the rodent. Inadequate fiber in the diet is often a predisposing factor. The GI contents may become dehydrated during stasis, exacerbating GI pain and possibly leading to partial or complete GI obstruction. Clinical signs of GI stasis include decreased size or absence of fecal material, anorexia, bruxism, pain on abdominal palpation, decreased GI sounds, and respiratory or cardiovascular compromise. GI stasis can also result in the accumulation of gas within the intestinal tract that can become life threatening. Chinchillas appear quite prone to gastric "bloat" [1,2]. Diagnostics, including abdominal radiographs, are necessary to determine the extent of disease. Gastric decompression is needed in cases of gastric tympany and can be accomplished by passing a large red rubber tube into the stomach through the oral cavity or, alternatively, a needle used as a trocar can be passed percutaneously. Trocarization is not without the risk of gastric or cecal rupture or peritonitis. Simethicone has also been suggested for absorbing gas from the GI tract; care must be taken to ensure that the GI contents are well hydrated because simethicone can also dehydrate and act as a foreign body in the face of dehydrated GI contents. In situations of GI stasis without secondary gas accumulation, medical therapy, including aggressive fluid therapy and analgesics to minimize pain associated with GI stasis, should be instituted. Antibiotics should not be considered an empiric therapy in rodents with GI disease because of the sensitive nature of the rodent GI tract to some antibiotics. Bacterial culture results or suspicions that the GI disease is caused by specific bacteria should be weighed carefully in the decision for antibiotic use.

Chinchillas and guinea pigs are presented most commonly on emergency for dental disease because their incisors and cheek teeth are growing continuously. The clinical signs of dental disease in rodents are often nonspecific, and include anorexia, weight loss, and GI stasis. Other signs can include excessive salivation, diarrhea, dysphagia, ocular or nasal discharge, and swellings on the lower mandible and upper maxilla due to tooth root elongation. The animal may not be able to close its mouth completely or may be uncomfortable when the jaw is manipulated. Protrusion of the globe can be seen if there is an abscess or bony changes caudal to the globe. In severely affected animals, systemic signs of disease may be evident, with death seen in severe cases. Treatment for the emergency patient with dental disorders is targeted initially at nutritional, fluid, and analgesic support. Once the patient is stabilized, dental therapy can be performed, including crown-height adjustment of the affected teeth. The prognosis depends on the extent of the disease at the time of presentation; often, multiple visits for tooth crown-height adjustment under anesthesia are necessary [53–55].

Diarrhea can be a serious problem in small rodents because hypoglycemia, dehydration, hypothermia, and electrolyte imbalances can occur quickly. Diarrhea is often described in rodents, especially in hamsters, as "wet tail." This term is general, and should not be confused with a specific type of bacteria. Warmed fluids with or without dextrose should be administered, and supplemental thermal support should be initiated. When hypoalbuminemia is present, colloids may be necessary to maintain oncotic pressure. Antibiotic therapy is initiated if a bacterial cause for the diarrhea is suspected. Protozoal parasites are a common cause of diarrhea in young rodents, particularly hamsters and chinchillas [2,56], so fecal examinations, including a wet mount for direct examination and fecal flotation, should be performed. Dietary correction with adequate fiber provision is important in treating diarrhea.

Intestinal torsion, intussusception, impaction, or ingested foreign bodies can result in partial or complete GI obstruction [57]. Supportive care, including fluids and analgesia, are important while initiating diagnostics. Radiographs, ultrasound, and GI contrast studies may be necessary to determine if surgery is required. Although medical management alone may be sufficient to resolve some cases of impaction, rapid surgical intervention may be necessary if the patient is in shock and deteriorating. Intestinal torsion and intussusception require immediate surgical intervention.

Rectal or intestinal prolapse occurs in rodents, particularly in hamsters [7]. Although a simple rectal prolapse can be resolved with a purse-string suture, intestinal prolapse carries a grave prognosis [30]. The underlying cause of the prolapse must be determined and corrected.

Fecal impaction is identified occasionally in older guinea pigs, but the cause has not yet been identified. This syndrome is seen most commonly in older intact guinea pigs. Some clinicians believe that it may be related to increased testosterone, as seen in older male dogs with perineal hernias (Tom Donnelly, personal communication, 2006). The guinea pig usually is presented for straining to defecate or for constipation. Commonly, the only physical examination abnormalities detected will be an enlarged rectum impacted with normal, soft feces. Suggested therapy has included a diet change to increase fiber, along with daily manual expression of stools. Neutering at a later age does not seem to correct the problem.

Reproductive emergencies

Dystocia, pregnancy toxemia, vaginal or uterine prolapse, and paraphimosis are reproductive emergencies often seen in rodent patients. Dystocia is common in guinea pigs that have not been bred for the first time before 7 to 8 months of age because of fusion of the pubic symphysis [34]. Dystocia should be suspected in gravid sows that are depressed, have failed to complete parturition, are straining, or have a bloody or discolored vaginal discharge [10]. Radiographs can help differentiate between oversized fetuses and uterine inertia. Oxytocin and calcium gluconate can be attempted in the case of uterine inertia, but usually cesarean section or en-bloc oophorohysterectomy are required for fetal–maternal relation abnormalities [10,34]. Oxytocin should never be given to a sow that has been bred for the first time after 8 months of age.

Pregnancy toxemia is seen usually in obese guinea pigs within the last 2 weeks of gestation. Affected animals may be anorectic, dyspneic, and may die acutely. Ketonuria, proteinuria, aciduria, ketonemia, hypoglycemia, and hyperlipidemia can be seen, followed by hyperkalemia, hyponatremia, hypochloremia, and anemia [10,34,58]. The guinea pig with pregnancy toxemia should be resuscitated with aggressive fluid therapy (ie, crystalloids and colloids) as discussed in the article by Lichtenberger in this issue. Perfusion should be corrected first, followed by rehydration therapy over 4 to 6 hours. Hypoglycemia and hypocalcemia should be corrected, and analgesics given as needed. Blood work should be monitored, with the goal being to correct the ketosis and acidosis. As soon as the guinea pig is stabilized, enteral nutritional support should be initiated because excellent nutritional support is vital. An ultrasound should be performed to check for fetal viability; a caesarian section should be considered if the pups are dead. The prognosis of pregnancy toxemia is usually guarded to grave.

Vaginal or uterine prolapse can be seen in rodents associated with parturition or straining from some underlying abnormality such as uterine neoplasia or urinary obstruction. The patient should be stabilized with fluid and analgesic therapy and antibiotics and other treatment as needed, before surgical intervention is attempted. If viable, the prolapsed tissue may be reduced under anesthesia, but ovariohysterectomy should be recommended in most situations [59].

Paraphimosis typically occurs in chinchillas, but can be seen in other rodents [2,7]. A "fur ring" collects around the penis and prevents retraction into the prepuce. This condition can be associated with swelling, urinary obstruction, and vascular compromise of the distal penis [7]. General anesthesia may be required to facilitate removal of the fur ring, along with lubrication and rolling or cutting off the fur.

Urinary obstruction

Urinary obstruction in small rodents is associated most commonly with urinary calculi and is identified most often in guinea pigs, chinchillas, and rats [60–64]. The most common types of calculi identified in these species are calcium based and struvite. In general, guinea pigs with urinary calculi are overrepresented among small mammals. These patients are generally middle-aged or older guinea pigs (>2.5 years old). To date, the etiopathogenesis of urinary calculi development in guinea pigs is not known. The composition of the urinary calculi in guinea pigs is predominately calcium-based, with calcium carbonate calculi most commonly reported through the Urinary Stone Laboratory at the University of California, Davis School of Veterinary Medicine. Clinical signs are associated commonly with the size and location of the calculi. Bladder or urethral calculi can present with signs of acute obstruction, such as anuria, but often are associated also with micturition abnormalities such as hematuria, strangury, or dysuria, and vague clinical signs, such as lethargy and anorexia. If the calculus is located higher in the urinary tract, such as in the ureters or kidneys, micturition abnormalities may be present, along with lethargy, anorexia, and weight loss, which are often the only clinical signs reported. Diagnosis of urinary obstruction or urolithiasis is based on clinical signs; physical examination findings; imaging studies, including radiographs, ultrasonography, excretory IV pyelograms (IVPs; only if azotemia is not present), and CT; urinalysis, and urine culture, if indicated. Urinary calculi in guinea pigs are generally radio-opaque, allowing for ease of identification using survey radiography, but if multiple calculi are present, it may be difficult to determine the anatomic locations of the calculi using survey radiography alone. A complete blood cell count and biochemistry panel should be evaluated to assess kidney function and electrolyte abnormalities.

Medical treatment of urolithiasis in guinea pigs is focused on fluid therapy because the typical calcium-based composition of the common urinary calculi in guinea pigs does not lend itself to dissolution therapy. In some cases, particularly in sows, small calculi may be voided once aggressive fluid therapy has been introduced. However, in many cases, surgical treatment is required.

If the patient is obstructed, therapy should be initiated immediately to relieve the obstruction and correct any metabolic abnormalities. Urinary catheterization should always be attempted under general anesthesia or heavy sedation, but placement can often be difficult because of the small size of the patient. Cystocentesis can be performed to relieve the immediate pressure on the bladder, but rupture can be a potential complication if the bladder wall is compromised severely. Plasma electrolyte concentrations should be evaluated for abnormalities. An ECG should be evaluated if hyperkalemia is present, and fluid therapy to correct the hyperkalemia should be instituted if abnormalities are identified. Elevated blood urea nitrogen with normal to mildly elevated creatinine is often seen in the azotemic guinea pig and should be corrected before surgery.

The prognosis for urinary calculi is guarded because recurrence of calculi is very common, regardless of therapy. Determining the composition of the urinary calculi present in the guinea pig patient is extremely important in establishing the etiopathogenesis, which, in turn, may provide information to improve future treatment options.

Renal failure

Renal failure in small mammals has been reported infrequently. The most common reports of acute renal failure have been in guinea pigs and chinchillas associated with either calcium-based nephrolithiasis or oxalate-containing plant ingestion [65]. Terminal renal amyloidosis is commonly associated with chronic renal failure in geriatric hamsters.

The clinician must differentiate chronic renal failure from acute renal failure, because acute renal failure is potentially reversible. Elevations in blood urea nitrogen and creatinine may be identified with either acute or chronic renal failure. Chronic renal failure usually involves a history of chronic loss of body condition, polydipsia, and polyuria; anemia may be evident on the hemogram.

Treatment of acute renal failure involves aggressive fluid therapy, involving three fluid therapy phases, as is recommended in small animals:

1. Correct perfusion abnormalities when hypotension is present (ie, systolic blood pressure less than 90 mmHg) (see the article by Lichtenberger in this issue on fluid therapy)
2. Rehydration (see the article by Lichtenberger in this issue on fluid therapy)
3. Diuresis

Once the animal is normotensive and rehydrated, the volume of urine produced should be recorded every 4 hours. This phase is the polyuric or diuresis phase of acute renal failure. Measurement of urine volume can be accomplished by placing preweighed diapers under the vulva or penis. The volume of urine voided on the diaper can be estimated by assuming 1 mL equals 1 g. The volume of fluid to be administered in each 4-hour period is the sum of calculated maintenance requirements (3-4 mL/kg/hr) and urine volume for the previous interval. Even weighing the animal twice a day can provide insight into the effectiveness of the fluid therapy protocol. If the animal has lost weight, then the replacement fluid volume may be ineffective.

Fluids should be discontinued gradually when hydration and urine production are restored (ie, when fluids in and urine out are matched), when blood urea nitrogen and creatinine are stabilized, and when the patient is eating and drinking. Fluids should be tapered by approximately 50% per day to minimize medullary washout.

Oral phosphate-binding agents can be used, although no studies have been performed in small mammals on their effectiveness in lowering elevated serum phosphorus.

Miscellaneous emergency conditions

Heat stroke can occur in all rodents with elevations in normal environmental temperature. Heat stroke most commonly occurs in chinchillas at environmental temperatures higher than 75°F [1,2], but it has been reported also in other rodent species when environmental temperatures exceed 80° to 85°F. Animals generally are presented with a history of exposure to elevated environmental temperatures and with clinical signs of hyperthermia and shock. The patient's core body temperature should be reduced to approximately 103°F with cool crystalloid fluids and cool towels, and perfusion deficits should be treated with appropriate fluid therapy. The prognosis for heat stroke is guarded to grave because most animals are affected severely by the time clinical signs are observed.

Summary

Rodent species should be assessed quickly on emergency presentation to determine the best approach for care. Common causes of emergent presentations include trauma, respiratory disease, dental disease, GI disease, reproductive disorders, and urinary tract obstruction. Treatment should be aimed at stabilizing the patient and providing a low-stress environment to help facilitate rapid recovery. Rodent patients benefit from supportive care, including thermal, fluid, and nutritional support. Administration of cardiopulmonary-cerebral resuscitation, antibiotics, and analgesics are appropriate for rodents through various routes.

References

[1] Donnelly T. Disease problems of chinchillas. In: Quesenberry K, Carpenter J, editors. Ferrets, rabbits, and rodents: clinical medicine and surgery. St. Louis (MO): WB Saunders; 2004. p. 255–65.

[2] Strake J, Davis L, LaRegina M, et al. Chinchillas. In: Laber-Laird K, Swindle M, Flecknell PA, editors. Handbook of rodent and rabbit medicine. Exeter (UK): BPC Wheaton Ltd.; 1996. p. 151–81.
[3] Funk R. Medical management of prairie dogs. In: Quesenberry K, Carpenter J, editors. Ferrets, rabbits, and rodents: clinical medicine and surgery. 2nd edition. St. Louis (MO): WB Saunders; 2004. p. 266–73.
[4] Bihun C, Bauck L. Basic anatomy, physiology, husbandry, and clinical techniques. In: Quesenberry K, Carpenter J, editors. Ferrets, rabbits, and rodents: clinical medicine and surgery. 2nd edition. St. Louis (MO): WB Saunders; 2004. p. 286–98.
[5] Laber-Laird K. Gerbils. In: Laber-Laird K, Swindle M, Flecknell PA, editors. Handbook of rodent and rabbit medicine. Exeter (RI): BPC Wheatons; 1996. p. 39–58.
[6] Fallon M. Rats and mice. In: Laber-Laird K, Swindle M, Flecknell PA, editors. Handbook of rodent and rabbit medicine. Exeter (RI): BPC Wheatons; 1996. p. 1–38.
[7] Donnelly T. Disease problems of small rodents. In: Quesenberry K, Carpenter J, editors. Ferrets, rabbits, and rodents: clinical medicine and surgery. St. Louis (MO): WB Saunders; 2004. p. 299–315.
[8] Daviau J. Clinical evaluation of rodents. Vet Clin North Am Exot Anim Pract 1999;2: 429–45.
[9] Adams R, et al. Techniques of experimentation. In: Fox J, Anderson L, Loew F, editors. Laboratory animal medicine. 2nd edition. San Diego (CA): Elsevier; 2002. p. 1005–45.
[10] Quesenberry K, Donnelly T, Hillyer E. Biology, husbandry, and clinical techniques of guinea pigs and chinchillas. In: Quesenberry K, Carpenter J, editors. Ferrets, rabbits, and rodents: clinical medicine and surgery. 2nd edition. St. Louis (MO): WB Saunders; 2004. p. 232–44.
[11] Reuter R. Venipuncture in the guinea pig. Lab Anim Sci 1987;37:245–6.
[12] Hem A, Smith A, Solberg P. Saphenous vein puncture for blood sampling of the mouse, rat, hamster, gerbil, guinea pig, ferret, and mink. Lab Anim 1998;32:364–8.
[13] Bober R. Technical review: drawing blood from the tail artery of a rat. Lab Anim 1988;17: 33–4.
[14] Silverman S, Tell LA. Radiology of rodents, rabbits, and ferrets: an atlas of normal anatomy and positioning. St. Louis (MO): Elsevier; 2005.
[15] Blouin A, Cormier Y. Endotracheal intubation in guinea pigs by direct laryngoscopy. Lab Anim Sci 1987;37:244–5.
[16] Timm KI, Jahn SE, Sedgwick CJ. The palatal ostium of the guinea pig. Lab Anim Sci 1987; 37:801–2.
[17] Heard D. Anesthesia, analgesia, and sedation of small mammals. In: Quesenberry K, Carpenter J, editors. Ferrets, rabbits, and rodents: clinical medicine and surgery. St Louis (MO): WB Saunders; 2004. p. 356–69.
[18] Kujime K, Natelson B. A method for endotracheal intubation of guinea pigs (*Cavis porcellus*). Lab Anim Sci 1981;31:715–6.
[19] Yasaki S, Dyck P. A simple method for rat endotracheal intubation. Lab Anim Sci 1991;35: 596–9.
[20] Tran D, Lawson D. Endotracheal intubation and manual ventilation of the rat. Lab Anim Sci 1986;36:540–1.
[21] Stark R, Nahrwold M, Cohen P. Blind oral tracheal intubation of rats. J Appl Physiol 1981; 51:1355–6.
[22] Cambron H, Latulippe JF, Nguyen T, et al. Orotracheal intubation of rats by transillumination. Lab Anim Sci 1995;45:303–4.
[23] Costello M. Principles of cardiopulmonary cerebral resuscitation in special species. Seminars in Avian and Exotic Pet Medicine 2004;13:132–41.
[24] Kirk R, Bistner S, Ford R. Nebulization therapy. In: Kirk R, Bistner S, Ford R, editors. Handbook of veterinary procedures and emergency treatment. 5th edition. Philadelphia: WB Saunders; 1990. p. 600–2.

[25] Ruijgrok EJ, Fens MH, Bakker-Woudenberg IA, et al. Nebulization of four commercially available amphotericin B formulations in persistently granulocytopenic rats with invasive pulmonary aspergillosis: evidence for long-term biological activity. J Pharm Pharmacol 2005;57:1289–95.
[26] Schulman RL, Crochik SS, Kneller SK, et al. Investigation of pulmonary deposition of a nebulized radiopharmaceutical agent in awake cats. Am J Vet Res 2004;65:806–9.
[27] Lichtenberger M. Principles of shock and fluid therapy in special species. Seminars in Avian and Exotic Pet Medicine 2004;13:142–53.
[28] Curro TG. Anesthesia of pet birds. Seminars in Avian and Exotic Pet Medicine 1998;7: 10–21.
[29] Harkness J. Small rodents. Vet Clin North Am Small Anim Pract 1994;24:89–102.
[30] Antinoff N. Small mammal critical care. Vet Clin North Am Exot Anim Pract 1998;1: 153–75.
[31] Otto C, Crowe D. Intraosseous resuscitation techniques and applications. In: Kirk R, Bonagura J, editors. Current veterinary therapy XI: small animal practice. Philadelphia: WB Saunders; 1992. p. 107–12.
[32] Haskins S. Fluid therapy. In: Kirk R, Bistner S, Ford R, editors. Handbook of veterinary procedures and emergency treatment. Philadelphia: WB Saunders; 1990. p. 574–600.
[33] Nishikimi M, Kawai T, Yagi K. Guinea pigs possess a highly mutated gene for L-gulono-gamma-lactone oxidase, the key enzyme for L-ascorbic acid biosynthesis missing in this species. J Biol Chem 1992;267:21967–72.
[34] O'Rourke D. Disease problems of guinea pigs. In: Quesenberry K, Carpenter J, editors. Ferrets, rabbits, and rodents: clinical medicine and surgery. St. Louis (MO): WB Saunders; 2004. p. 245–54.
[35] Morris TH. Antibiotic therapeutics in laboratory animals. Lab Anim 1995;29:16–36.
[36] Young JD, Hurst WJ, White WJ, et al. An evaluation of ampicillin pharmacokinetics and toxicity in guinea pigs. Lab Anim Sci 1987;37:652–6.
[37] Turton JA, Fagg R, Sones WR, et al. Characterization of the myelotoxicity of chloramphenicol succinate in the B6C3F1 mouse. Int J Exp Pathol 2006;87:101–12.
[38] Ness R. Rodents. In: Carpenter J, editor. Exotic animal formulary. St. Louis (MO): Elsevier; 2005. p. 377–408.
[39] Morrisey J, Carpenter J. Formulary. In: Quesenberry K, Carpenter J, editors. Ferrets, rabbits, and rodents: clinical medicine and surgery. 2nd edition. St. Louis (MO): WB Saunders; 2004. p. 436–44.
[40] Sichuk G, Bettigole RE, Der BK, et al. Influence of sex hormones on thrombosis of left atrium in Syrian (Golden) hamsters. Am J Physiol 1965;208:465–70.
[41] Laming PR, Cosby SL, O'Neill JK. Seizures in the Mongolian gerbil are related to a deficiency in cerebral glutamine synthetase. Comp Biochem Physiol C 1989;94:399–404.
[42] Ellis C, Mori M. Skin diseases of rodents and small exotic mammals. Vet Clin North Am Exot Anim Pract 2001;4:493–542.
[43] Richardson V. The skin. Diseases of domestic guineas pigs. 2nd edition. Malden (MA): Blackwell Science; 2000. p. 1–13.
[44] Timm KI. Pruritus in rabbits, rodents, and ferrets. Vet Clin North Am Small Anim Pract 1988;18:1077–91.
[45] Gray ML, Killinger AH. Listeria monocytogenes and listeric infections. Bacteriol Rev 1966; 30:309–82.
[46] Leader RW, Holte RJ. Studies on three outbreaks of listeriosis in chinchillas. Cornell Vet 1955;45:78–84.
[47] Sanford SE. Cerebrospinal nematodiasis caused by Baylisascaris procyonis in chinchillas. J Vet Diagn Invest 1991;3:77–9.
[48] Wilkerson MJ, Melendy A, Stauber E. An outbreak of listeriosis in a breeding colony of chinchillas. J Vet Diagn Invest 1997;9:320–3.
[49] Hoefer H. Chinchillas. Vet Clin North Am Small Anim Pract 1994;24:103–11.

[50] Anver M, Cohen B, et al. Lesions associated with aging. In: Baker H, editor. The laboratory rat I biology and diseases. New York: Academic; 1979. p. 377–99.
[51] Berg BN, Wolf A, Simms HS, et al. Degenerative lesions of spinal roots and peripheral nerves of aging rats. Gerontologia 1962;6:72–80.
[52] Krinke G, et al. Spontaneous radioneuropathology, aged rats. In: Jones T, editor. Monographs on pathology of laboratory animals: nervous system. New York: Springer-Verlag; 1988. p. 203–8.
[53] Osofsky A, Verstraete F. Dentistry in pet rodents. Compendium on Continuing Education for the Practicing Veterinarian 2006; January: 61–73.
[54] Capello V, Gracis M. Dental instruments and equipment. In: Lennox A, editor. Rabbit and rodent dentistry handbook. Lake Worth (FL): Zoological Education Network, Inc., 2005. p. 193–212.
[55] Crossley D. Treatment of dental disease in rabbits and rodents. Proceedings of the North American Veterinary Conference 2000;995–7.
[56] Shelton GC. Giardiasis in the chinchilla. II. Incidence of the disease and results of experimental infections. Am J Vet Res 1954;15:75–8.
[57] Cunnane SC, Bloom SR. Intussusception in the Syrian golden hamster. Br J Nutr 1990;63: 231–7.
[58] Harrenstein L. Critical care of ferrets, rabbits, and rodents. Sem Avian Exotic Pet Med 1994; 3:217–28.
[59] Bennett R, Mullen H. Soft tissue surgery. In: Quesenberry K, Carpenter J, editors. Ferrets, rabbits, and rodents: clinical medicine and surgery. St. Louis (MO): WB Saunders; 2004. p. 274–84.
[60] Jones RJ, Stephenson R, Fountain D, et al. Urolithiasis in a chinchilla. Vet Rec 1995; 136:400.
[61] Spence S, Skae K. Urolithiasis in a chinchilla. Vet Rec 1995;136:524.
[62] Gaschen L, Ketz C, Lang J, et al. Ultrasonographic detection of adrenal gland tumor and ureterolithiasis in a guinea pig. Vet Radiol Ultrasound 1998;39:43–6.
[63] Stieger SM, Wenker C, Ziegler-Gohm D, et al. Ureterolithiasis and papilloma formation in the ureter of a guinea pig. Vet Radiol Ultrasound 2003;44:326–9.
[64] Fehr M, Rappold S. Urolithiasis in 20 guinea pigs (Cavia porcellus). Tieraerztliche Praxis 1997;25:543–7.
[65] Holowaychuk MK. Renal failure in a guinea pig (Cavia porcellus) following ingestion of oxalate containing plants. Can Vet J 2006;47:787–9.

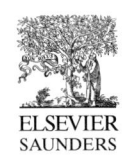

Emergency and Critical Care Procedures in Sugar Gliders (*Petaurus breviceps*), African Hedgehogs (*Atelerix albiventris*), and Prairie Dogs (*Cynomys spp*)

Angela M. Lennox, DVM, DABVP-Avian

Avian and Exotic Animal Clinic of Indianapolis, 9330 Waldemar Road, Indianapolis, IN 46268, USA

The past decade has seen an increase in pet ownership of exotic mammals, especially ferrets and rabbits. Pet stores now commonly feature unusual species, such as the sugar glider, the African Hedgehog, and, until a recent federal ban, the prairie dog. These animals are occasionally seen for routine care and elective surgical neutering, but the most common indication for presentation is treatment of illness.

A common scenario for all exotic pets is chronic disease presenting as an acute onset of illness. These three species fall into the category of prey species, with inherent instincts to hide illness until unable to do so. Therefore, any of these species presented in acute crisis must be carefully evaluated for long-term chronic underlying illness, because any debilitating condition can ultimately result in presentation for emergency care. Table 1 lists selected diseases reported in the literature for each species. More common reasons for presentation for critical care are listed in this article under each species.

Common reasons for emergency presentation

Although all exotic species are susceptible to a wide variety of disease processes, including infectious, traumatic, metabolic, and neoplastic conditions, some of the more commonly encountered in these three species are discussed in more detail in this section. It should be kept in mind that the most common underlying factors in diseases affecting these species are malnutrition and improper husbandry. All efforts at diagnosis and treatment must include careful

E-mail address: birddr@aol.com

Table 1
Disease affecting pet prairie dogs, hedgehogs, and sugar gliders presented in the literature

Prairie dogs	Hedgehogs	Sugar gliders
Cardiomyopathy	Parasitic dermatitis	Metabolic bone disease
Monkeypox	Intervertebral disc disease	Trauma
Pneumonia	Neoplasia	Self-mutilation
Pseudo-odontoma	Digit/limb constriction secondary to sting/fiber	Pneumonia
Trauma	Bacterial enteritis	Urinary tract infection
	Trauma	Neoplasia
	Cardiomyopathy	Pouch infections
	Pneumonia	Enteritis
	Wobbly hedgehog syndrome	

examination of husbandry and explicit recommendations for correction based on the most recent understanding of the needs of these species.

Sugar gliders

Improper husbandry and malnutrition are the most common underlying factors leading to illness in sugar gliders. Hypocalcemia and metabolic bone disease are common and are the result of imbalance of calcium, vitamin D, and phosphorus. Hypoproteinemia is also a common feature of an improper diet [1,2]. The typical diet of the sugar glider with nutritional illness is often fruit and meat, and it may even include commercial pelleted glider diets. The most common presentation of nutritional disease is apparent acute collapse, with the glider typically found on the cage bottom (Fig. 1). Owners often report that the glider seemed completely normal the day before collapse. Hypoglycemic or hypocalcemic sugar gliders may seizure or present with other more subtle central nervous system (CNS) abnormalities [1,2]. Although gliders with metabolic bone disease commonly exhibit hind limb weakness, the author has not commonly noted fractures in these patients. Other less common consequences of improper diet reported in the literature include

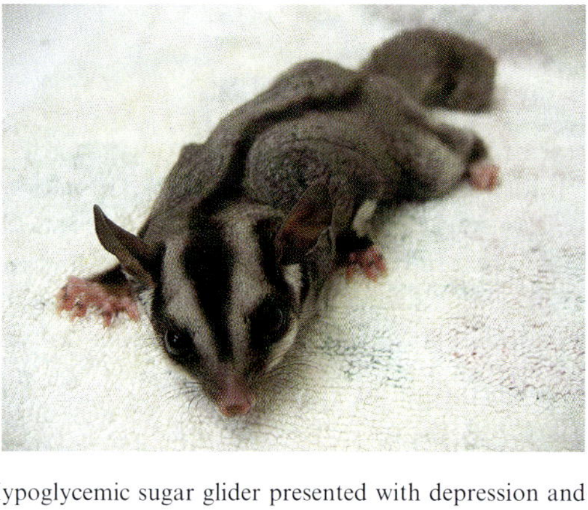

Fig. 1. Hypoglycemic sugar glider presented with depression and lethargy.

encephalomalacia, myonecrosis, cardiac failure, and cataracts [2]. Obesity is also common, especially in gliders fed such items as cat food or in those with a lack of exercise [1]. Pneumonia, enteritis, urinary tract infection, pouch infection, and dental disease have also been reported, as has neoplasia, (primarily hepatic or lymphatic), in older animals [1,2]. Baylisascaris, toxoplasmosis, and listeriosis have produced CNS disease with self-mutilation in glider colonies [2]. An outbreak of histoplasmosis was reported in a zoo colony [3].

Gliders kept as single pets without adequate socialization are prone to self-mutilation of the extremities and genitals. The sugar glider is a laboratory model for serotonin deficiency depression, which can be produced in these animals simply by housing them singly [2]. Predator trauma is occasionally seen as well.

Hedgehogs

Neoplasia is common in African Hedgehogs, and represents most hedgehog disease case reports in the literature. Clinical experience has shown that many cases of neoplasia are diagnosed in chronically debilitated animals presented for urgent care. A review of 14 postmortem submissions found neoplasia to represent 29% of cases [4]. Neoplasms include skeletal sarcoma; oral squamous cell carcinoma; intestinal lymphosarcoma; mammary gland tumors, including adenocarcinoma; thyroid C-cell carcinoma; subcutaneous malignant mast cell tumor; uterine neoplasia; granulosa cell tumor; retrobulbar carcinoma; and intestinal plasmacytoma [5–14]. Gastrointestinal neoplasia usually results in chronic weight loss and anemia. Uterine neoplasia is among the more commonly reported neoplasms and includes adenosarcoma, leiomyosarcoma, and adenoleiomyoma [15]. Other proliferative lesions include endometrial polyps. In a retrospective study of 15 cases of uterine proliferative disease or neoplasia, all cases were associated with vaginal bleeding [16].

Cardiomyopathy has been reported in the literature and anecdotally [17]. Another study of 42 hedgehog necropsy cases revealed cardiomyopathy in 16, or 38% of submissions [18]. Fourteen of 16 hedgehogs with cardiomyopathy were male animals older than 1 year of age. Nine of 16 hedgehogs with cardiomyopathy exhibited one or more clinical signs, including heart murmur, lethargy, icterus, moist rales, anorexia, dyspnea, dehydration, and weight loss. Histopathologic lesions were mainly associated with the left ventricle and included myodegeneration, myonecrosis, atrophy, hypertrophy, and myofiber disarray [18].

Hedgehogs commonly harbor mites, which are thought to be a normal inhabitant of animals in the wild but can become severe in ill or immunocompromised individuals [17]. Predator trauma is uncommon in hedgehogs because of their formidable protective spines. Trauma secondary to falls and other injuries can occur, however. Prolapsed intervertebral disk disease has been reported in the literature [17]. Enteritis and primary respiratory disease are also seen infrequently in hedgehogs, including cases of fatal intestinal cryptosporidiosis and corynebacterial pneumonia [17–20].

Several unusual neurologic abnormalities have been reported in African Hedgehogs, including so-called "wobbly hedgehog syndrome" (WHS), which produces mild ataxia progressing to severe neurologic disease and complete paralysis [21]. Most affected animals are younger than 2 years of age, but older animals can be affected as well. WHS produces vacuolization of the white matter of the brain and spinal cord, with associated neurogenic muscle atrophy without inflammation. Several etiologies have been proposed, but genetics seem to play a role. Treatment is generally unrewarding and has included vitamins E and B, selenium, calcium, prednisone, antibiotics, homeopathic remedies, acupuncture, and physical therapy. In some cases, treatment has seemed to halt the progression of disease temporarily; however, because the disease can be relapsing with variable progression, it is unclear if therapy was actually effective. No treatment has been shown to halt the progression of paralysis [21].

Hedgehogs may be predisposed to ocular proptosis because of shallow orbits. Eight cases of unilateral proptosis revealed histopathologic lesions, including orbital cellulitis, panophthalmitis, and corneal ulceration [22].

Several zoonotic diseases have occasionally been associated with hedgehogs, including *Salmonella* spp, *Yersinia pseudotuberculosis*, *Mycobacterium marinum*, rabies virus, herpesvirus (human herpes simplex), mites, dermatophytosis, and cryptosporidiosis [23,24].

Prairie dogs

The outbreak of monkeypox in pet prairie dogs, certain rodent species, and human contacts in 2003 prompted the Centers for Disease Control and Prevention (CDC) to issue a joint order "prohibiting the transportation, offering for transportation in interstate commerce, or the sale or offering for sale, or offering for any other type of commercial or public distribution, including release in the environment." This order does not apply to transportation of these animals to the veterinarian, nor does it prohibit the veterinarian from providing necessary medical care [25]. Although no new cases have been diagnosed since the original 2003 outbreak, the CDC order was still in effect as of print time of this article. Unless the order is lifted, medical care for prairie dogs in the United States is likely to consist primarily of treatment of adult and geriatric disorders as the current population ages.

Typical causes of presentation for emergency care include trauma from falls or other blunt forces; encounters with other pets, particularly dogs and cats; and electrical injuries from chewing on cords. Older prairie dogs (older than 3–4 years of age) may present with dilated cardiomyopathy. Respiratory distress is common and has a variety of causes. Infectious causes include bacterial, fungal, and viral agents [26]. Most animals diagnosed with monkeypox virus were presented in respiratory distress, often with oral ulcers (Fig. 2) [25]. The author encountered a case of fatal parasitic pneumonia in a prairie dog caused by a pulmonary mite. Respiratory distress can also be secondary to cardiac disease, extreme obesity, or pseudo-odontoma [26].

Pseudo-odontoma is common in prairie dogs and is characterized by root deformation of the maxillary incisor tooth roots, resulting in a space-occupying nasal mass (Fig. 3) [27]. Damage to incisor roots occurs after repeated trauma, typically from constant chewing on cage bars. Because prairie dogs (as well as many rodents) are obligate nasal breathers, affected animals are presented in varying degrees of respiratory distress. In typical severe cases, animals are emaciated and depressed and exhibit increased respiratory effort with mouth breathing. The incisors of these animals may be abnormally short, discolored, misshapen, or fractured.

Neoplasia is not commonly reported in the prairie dog, but reports include multicentric lymphoma, maxillary osteosarcoma, and hepatocellular carcinoma [28–31]. Diseases of zoonotic concern in addition to monkeypox include tularemia and plague. Before the federal ban, epizootics of both occurred in recently captured animals intended for the pet trade [32].

Although of uncertain clinical significance, the prairie dog is a laboratory model for spontaneous gallbladder stone formation. The incidence can be experimentally increased by feeding diets high in cholesterol [33].

General nutrition and husbandry

Although this article does not attempt to delve deeply into nutrition and husbandry, it is apparent that many serious medical illnesses in these species are primarily or indirectly a result of improper care.

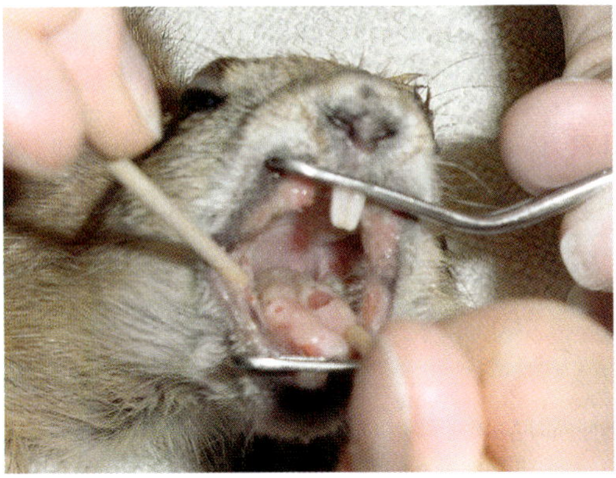

Fig. 2. Oral ulceration is commonly reported in confirmed cases of monkeypox in prairie dogs. Although the owner of this animal was hospitalized with confirmed monkeypox, veterinary personnel were luckily unaffected. Note the ungloved hands of the examiners.

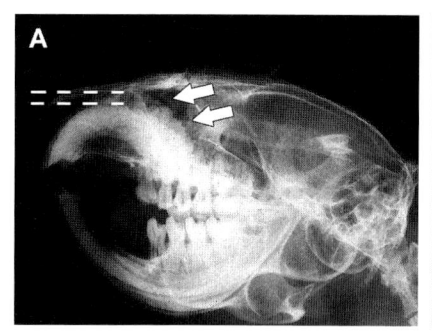

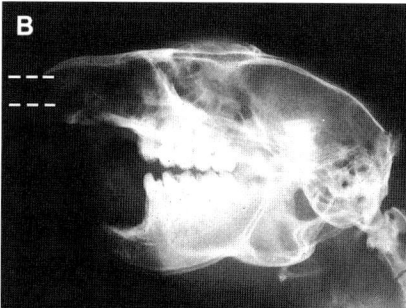

Fig. 3. (*A*) Pseudodontoma in a prairie dog. Note the decreased nasal sinus space (*lines*) and marked tooth root deformities (*arrows*). This animal was presented in severe dyspnea. (*B*) Same patient after extraction of the maxillary incisors, which helped to relieve the space-occupying mass and greatly improved the clinical condition.

Several manufacturers offer complete diets for these three species. Practitioners and owners should be aware that many, if not most, exotic pet diets are offered to the public without benefit of dietary trials, and many manufacturers do not perform quality control or guarantee analysis of the contents. Before recommending a particular commercial diet, veterinarians must be willing to research the diet carefully, which includes directly querying the manufacturer. Characteristics of adequate versus inadequate commercial diets are listed in Table 2.

The natural diet of prairie dogs is native grass. A practical diet for captive prairie dogs is unlimited grass hay and limited quantities of rabbit pellets with or without an occasional rodent block [26]. Animals should be "fed to condition," with adjustments in food volume made based on the individual animal's condition. Obesity is common in animals denied exercise or fed inappropriate items, such as fruits, table foods, and cat and dog food. Prairie dogs require a large enclosure with artificial burrows or tunnels constructed from wood or plastic materials, such as polyvinyl chloride (PVC) pipes. Smooth-sided enclosures rather than metal cage bars are recommended, because prairie dogs

Table 2
Characteristics of adequate versus inadequate commercial diets for exotic pets

Adequate diet	Inadequate diet
Manufactured based on current understanding of composition of natural diet by a nutritional scientist	
Dietary trials performed with adequate numbers of animals raised successfully over multiple generations, with objective measurement of gross parameters	Anecdotal reports of successful use only
Quality control: regular batch testing for guaranteed analysis	No guaranteed analysis

frequently chew on metal cage bars, resulting in potentially catastrophic incisor root disease [27].

African Hedgehogs are insectivores, and the author recommends commercial insectivore diets from reputable companies with experience in manufacturing zoo diets, with the addition of live insects. Before the ready availability of insectivore diet, hedgehogs commonly survived on cat food and insects, and obesity was a common physical examination finding. Hedgehogs are relatively easy to house in flat-bottom cages with commercial bedding material (not cedar), a hide box or shelter for security, and a secure top, because they are actually good climbers.

Of these three species, the most difficult to keep properly is the sugar glider. Native to Australia, the sugar glider is nocturnal and arboreal and lives in a social group [2]. Its natural diet includes insects, arachnids, small vertebrates, blossom nectar, and sap of trees (specifically eucalyptus). Obesity, failure to thrive, and metabolic bone disease are common disorders in captivity [2]. Commercial complete pelleted sugar glider diets currently available do not come close to replicating the sugar glider's natural diet, and the author is unaware of any manufacturers that have completed dietary trials on their products. Several recommended homemade captive diets are presented in Table 3 and have the benefit of some limited dietary research [34]. Gliders require large enclosures with branches to encourage exercise and a nesting box secured in a high position in the cage. Gliders require an ambient temperature greater than 75°F, which usually necessitates a radiant heat source, especially in winter months [1,2].

All three species readily adapt to accepting water in standard commercial water bottles.

Principles of emergency stabilization

The principles of emergency care and stabilization are the same as those established in human and more traditional pet medicine: airway and cardiac support, control of hemorrhage, correction of underlying fluid and electrolyte abnormalities, and restoration of normothermia. This subject is discussed in detail in another article in this issue.

Table 3
Practical homemade diet for sugar gliders

Leadbeater's mixture for nectar-eating opossums (50%)	Commercial insectivore diet (50%)	Treats (less than 5%)
150 mL water 150 mL honey 1 shelled hard-boiled egg 25 g high protein baby cereal 1 tsp zoo/avian vitamin/mineral	Mazuri Brand (St. Louis, MO) Available at: www.mazuri.com	Fruit Insects Lean meat

Data from Ness R, Booth R. Sugar gliders. In: Quesenberry K, Carpenter J, editors. Ferrets, rabbits and rodents, clinical medicine and surgery. St. Louis (MO): WB Saunders; 2004. p. 330–8.

Airway support

Intubation of these species for direct establishment of an airway is difficult and may require an endoscope or other specialized equipment and considerable time not available in case of respiratory collapse. Tracheal intubation by means of tracheotomy can be accomplished quickly in extremely small animals using a standard tracheotomy approach and small endotracheal tubes (1.0–2.5 mm) or smaller diameter red rubber catheters [35].

In less severe cases, oxygen can be delivered by means of a face mask or while the animal is resting quietly in an oxygen chamber. Cardiopulmonary-cerebral resuscitation and airway support are discussed in detail in another article in this issue.

Fluid and vascular support

Optimal fluid therapy is critical for treatment of hypovolemic shock and correction of dehydration. Although little information exists on specific guidelines for treatment of hypovolemic shock in these species, information can be extrapolated from work with other species, including the guinea pig, rabbit, and ferret. For these species, Lichtenberger [36] recommends rapid intravenous infusion of warmed isotonic crystalloids at a rate of 10 to 15 mL/kg, followed by colloids (6% hetastarch; B Braun Medical, Irvine, California) at a rate of 5 mL/kg over 5 to 10 minutes. After achieving a systolic Doppler blood pressure greater than 40 mm Hg, aggressive external heat support is initiated until rectal body temperature reads at least 98°F. Boluses of isotonic crystalloids (10–15 mg/kg) and colloids (5 mL/kg) are continued until the systolic Doppler blood pressure reads greater than 90 mm Hg. At this point, dehydration deficits are calculated and corrected using isotonic crystalloids over a 6-hour period in cases of acute disease and over 12 to 24 hours in cases of more chronic disease [36].

The principles of fluid administration for correction of hypovolemia and dehydration are as follows [31]:

Establish vascular access.
Establish intravenous or intraosseous catheterization.
Begin rewarming in case of hypothermia.
Measure indirect systolic Doppler blood pressure.
Administer warmed isotonic crystalloids at 10 to 15 mg/kg and hetastarch (6%) at 5 mL/kg over 5 to 10 minutes until systolic Doppler blood pressure reads greater than 40 mm Hg
Continue external heat support until rectal body temperature is greater than 90°F.
Administer bolus crystalloids (10–15 mL/kg) and colloids (5 mL/kg) until systolic Doppler blood pressure reads greater than 90 mm Hg.
Calculate dehydration deficit and administer over 6 hours (acute disease processes) or over 12 to 24 hours (more chronic disease processes).

These guidelines are practical and extremely useful for use in prairie dogs, hedgehogs, and sugar gliders. Although measurement of systolic Doppler blood pressure has been reported in these species and has been found to be similar to that in other small mammals, practitioners may find this more challenging in smaller individuals, particularly hedgehogs and sugar gliders. It may be more feasible to monitor blood pressure trends with the aid of anesthesia or sedation. Measurement of indirect systolic blood pressure is accomplished with pediatric blood pressure cuffs and a Doppler vascular monitor (Fig. 4). In most exotic mammals, the cuff is placed at the humerus and the Doppler monitor is placed in a shaved area just above the ventral forelimb footpad [36].

When blood pressure measurement is unsuccessful, practitioners may be forced to make judgment calls regarding perfusion status based on patient response and such parameters as capillary refill time, turgor of visible surface vessels, temperature, and heart rate. When correcting hypothermia, normal body temperatures of these species should be kept in mind, particularly in sugar gliders and African Hedgehogs (Table 4).

Intravenous catheterization is extremely difficult in smaller species and is challenging in prairie dogs because of the presence of subcutaneous fat. The cephalic vein is often the most accessible vein in these species, but intravenous catheterization may require brief sedation in all but the most debilitated patients. The practitioner must make a judgment call regarding the risk of sedation for the purpose of catheterization versus the risk of withholding intravenous therapy in critical cases. Intraosseous administration is another extremely valuable option and has been accomplished by the author and many other exotic practitioners in mammals as small as hamsters. Sedation may not be required in extremely debilitated patients but may be useful in cases in which restraint is stressful or handling is difficult, such as the hedgehog. The most accessible sites for intraosseous administration are the

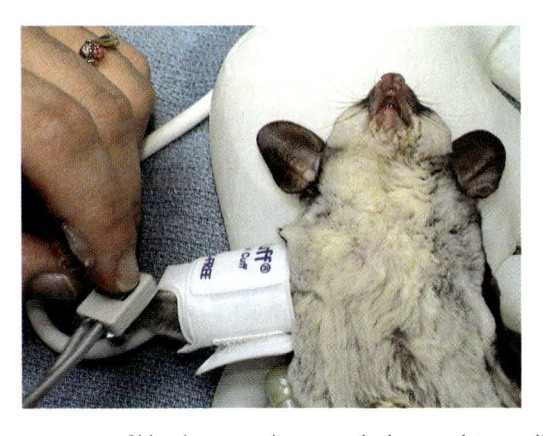

Fig. 4. Indirect measurement of blood pressure in a severely depressed sugar glider using a small pediatric cuff.

Table 4
Physiologic data for prairie dogs, African Hedgehogs, and sugar gliders

	Prairie dog	African Hedgehog	Sugar glider
Rectal temperature (°F)	95.7°F–102.3°F	95.7°F–98.6°F	97.3°F
Heart rate (beats per minute)	83–318	180–280	200–300
Respiratory rate (breaths per minute)		25–50	16–40
Average weight (g)	700–2300	Male: 400–600 Female: 300–600	Male: 100–160 Female: 80–130
Life span (years)	8–10	4–6; reports of up to 8 years	12–14 years (optimal diet only)
Sexual maturity	2–3 years	Male: 12–15 months Female: 8–12 months	Female: 8 months–1 year Male: 12–14 months

Data from Ivey E, Carpenter J. African Hedgehogs; Ness R, Booth R. Sugar gliders; and Funk R. Medical management of prairie dogs. In: Quesenberry K, Carpenter J, editors. Ferrets, rabbits and rodents, clinical medicine and surgery. St. Louis (MO): WB Saunders; 2004. p. 334, 330–2, 267.

proximal tibia by way of the tibial crest (Figs. 5 and 6) or the proximal femur through the trochanteric fossa. The site should be infiltrated with lidocaine before placement of the catheter. Depending on patient size, standard needles for injection are easy to place and maintain. In the prairie dog, a smaller spinal needle with a stylette may be useful to prevent a core of bone from obstructing the catheter lumen. Properly placed intraosseous catheters can also obstruct over time, and sterilized cerclage wire is ideal for use as a stylette to relieve the obstruction. Suggested needle sizes for intraosseous catheters are 25-gauge for sugar gliders, 25- to 22-gauge for hedgehogs, and 22- to 18-gauge for prairie dogs. Standard catheter caps are attached to the properly placed needle and

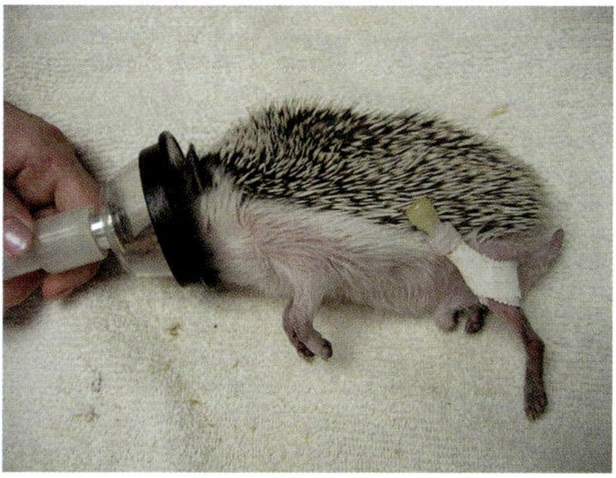

Fig. 5. Placement of an intraosseous catheter in the tibia of a hedgehog. The catheter has been secured with tape and fitted with a standard catheter cap.

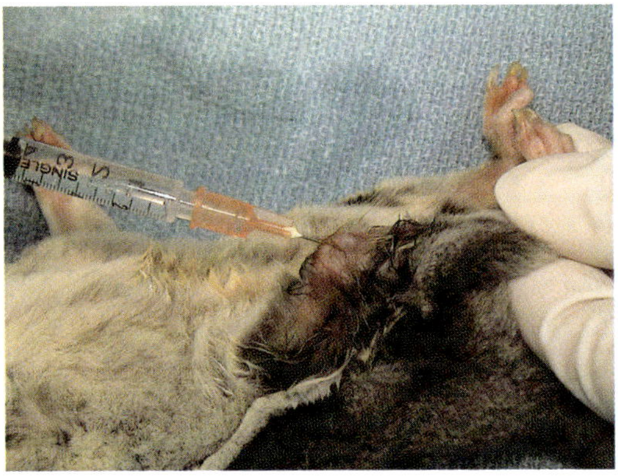

Fig. 6. Injection of lactated Ringer's solution into the tibia of a sugar glider.

securely taped (or sutured) to the leg (see Fig. 6). Postprocedure radiographs in two views must be obtained to ensure proper placement and prevent inadvertent administration of fluids into soft tissues (Figs. 7–9). Relatively soft bones in smaller species make perforation of the opposite cortex and improper placement a common complication, especially in the presence of underlying bone disorders, such as metabolic bone disease (primarily sugar gliders on calcium-deficient diets.)

Note that a tibial intraosseous catheter can be accessed in hedgehogs even when the animal is rolled tightly into a defensive ball (Fig. 10).

Intravenous infusion can be accomplished with a standard fluid administration set, with or without a small animal infusion pump in prairie dogs. In smaller species, a small-volume infusion syringe pump is a safer and more practical option. Syringe pumps are designed for human pediatric use, and many can be set to deliver extremely small volumes over a set period (Fig. 11).

Subcutaneous fluid administration is easy in all three species, although it may be inadequate in cases of marked hypovolemia, dehydration, or other fluid imbalance. Administration of intraperitoneal fluids into the lower left quadrant of the abdomen, with the patient's head held lower than the abdomen to displace the viscera cranially, has also been described [35]. Absorption may be inadequate by method in hypovolemic patients.

Control of hemorrhage

As in other species, wound care can be delayed while patient stabilization is accomplished, but hemorrhage must be controlled immediately. The blood volume of mammals is estimated at 7% to 10% of body weight, and normal healthy individuals can tolerate the loss of approximately 10% of blood volume. Losses in excess of 10% or losses in debilitated patients may lead to vascular collapse. Acute hemorrhage is most commonly controlled with direct

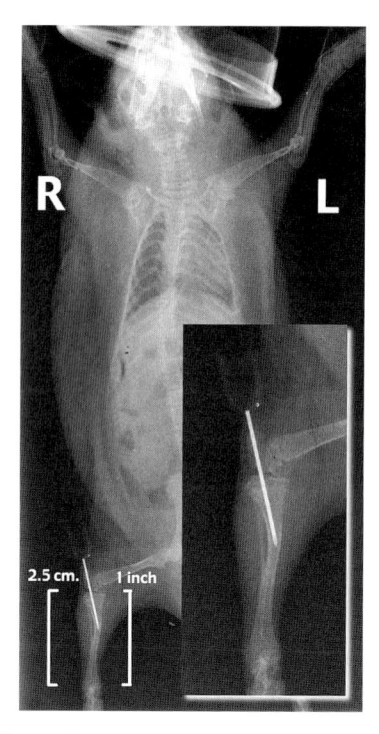

Fig. 7. Ventral/dorsal radiographs demonstrating corrected placement of a 22-gauge needle into the tibia of a hedgehog.

pressure. Silver nitrate or quick-stop products may be used for nail hemorrhage. More severe bleeding may require ligation of the compromised vessel.

Treatment for blood loss includes blood transfusion or the use of colloids with oxygen-carrying ability such as Oxyglobin (Biopure Corporation, Cambridge, MA), and is discussed in detail in another article in this issue.

Rough guidelines for the indication for blood transfusion are similar to those used in other species and include acute blood loss resulting in a packed cell volume (PCV) less than 20% or chronic blood loss with a PCV less than

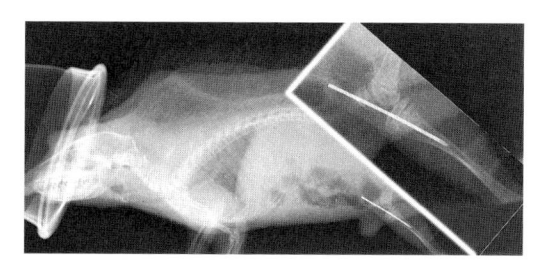

Fig. 8. Lateral radiographs demonstrating corrected placement of a 22-gauge needle into the tibia of a hedgehog.

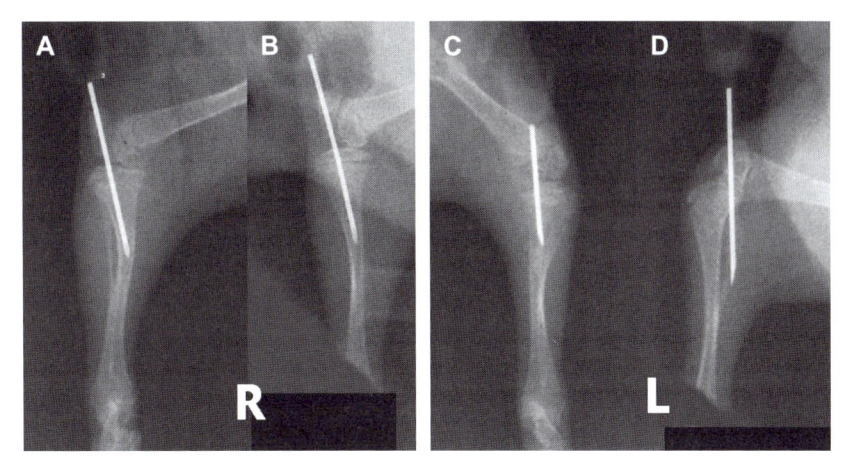

Fig. 9. Demonstration of the importance of radiographs in two views to confirm placement of an intraosseous catheter. The image on the left shows adequate placement. The image on the left shows that the needle has perforated cortical bone and the tip of the needle is entering soft tissue of the leg.

12% to 15% [35]. Overall patient condition (bright and alert versus pale and depressed) is also important when considering transfusion.

Sources of blood donors include the ill pet's house mates or pet stores. The author keeps a list of owners willing to provide blood donors in exchange for clinic credit. Blood is collected from healthy donors under sedation with acid citrate dextrose (ACD), 1 mL per 10 mL of blood, to a maximum 10% of blood volume based on calculated body weight [35]. Blood is administered by means of an intravenous or intraosseous catheter.

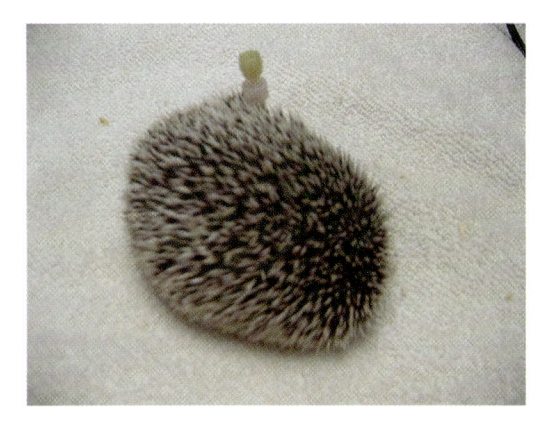

Fig. 10. Intraosseous catheter placed in the tibia of this hedgehog is still accessible even when the animal is rolled into a defensive ball.

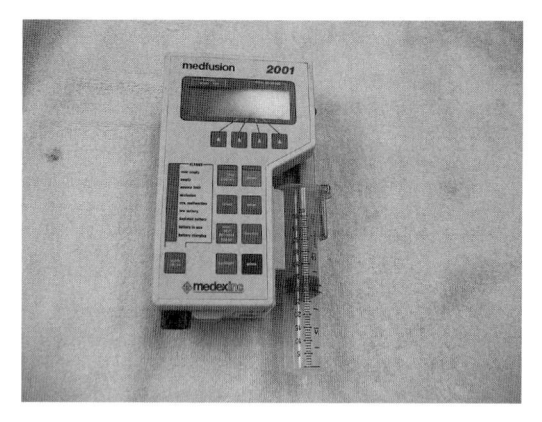

Fig. 11. Pediatric syringe pump capable of infusing small volumes of fluid over a selected length of time.

Establishment of normothermia

Normal body temperatures of prairie dogs, hedgehogs, and sugar gliders are reported in Table 2. Measurement of body temperature is not difficult in debilitated animals. A constant readout flexible temperature probe can be inserted rectally and taped into position and allows monitoring until restoration of the animal's normal temperature is achieved (Fig. 12). Methods for rewarming include the use of heating pads, warm-water bags or bottles, forced air warming devices, radiant heat sources, and commercial small mammal incubators (Fig. 13). Internal (core body temperature) rewarming methods include infusion of warmed intravenous fluids, which has been shown in another article in this issue to be extremely important for the prevention of an afterdrop effect, or the return of cool fluids to the body core

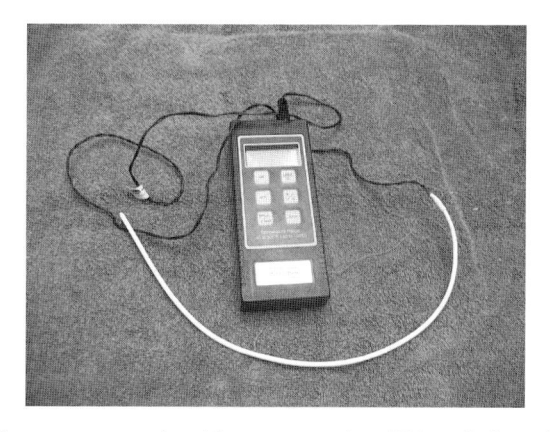

Fig. 12. A flexible temperature probe with constant readout. This probe is small enough for rectal use in prairie dogs and hedgehogs but may be too large for use in smaller sugar gliders.

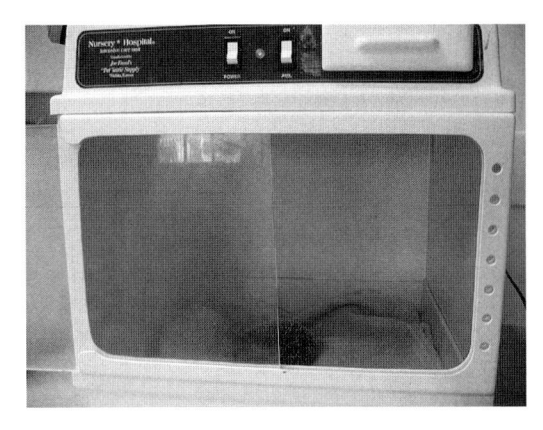

Fig. 13. Variable temperature small animal incubator. Active patients, such as alert sugar gliders, must be put into secure containers before placement into the incubator, because this model has heating coils and mechanical parts in the top of the unit.

and worsening of the animal's condition when external warming alone is used.

Nutritional support

Debilitated animals must be encouraged to eat as quickly as possible. Hand feeding with a syringe is a common procedure and is easily accomplished in prairie dogs and sugar gliders. Prairie dogs are fed commercial powdered hay reconstituted with water and administered by means of a spoon or syringe (Critical Care; Oxbow Hay Company, Murdock, Nebraska; www.oxbowhay.com). A hand-feeding formula for sugar gliders can be prepared in advance and frozen into an ice cube tray for easy access. Formula is made based on the recipe for Leadbeater's solution (see Table 1), with the addition of commercial insectivore diet soaked until soft or powdered in a coffee grinder.

Of the three species, hedgehogs remain the most difficult to hand feed or administer oral medication. Debilitated or tame hedgehogs may lap food from a spoon or accept syringe feeding. Most, however, resist efforts to force feed. Some ill hedgehogs accept live insects when all other food items are refused (Fig. 14). Acceptable hand feeding products for hedgehogs are Carnivore Critical Care (Oxbow Hay CompanyMurdock NE) [37], commercial insectivore diet soaked or ground in a coffee grinder and reconstituted with water, or strained meat baby food.

Animals in need of enteral support that are extremely debilitated or difficult to feed may require an esophagostomy tube. Esophagostomy is well described in small animal literature and is associated with fewer complications than pharyngostomy or nasogastric feeding tubes in dogs and cats [38]. Soft red rubber feeding tubes are selected based on patient size. The tube is implanted in the animal under anesthesia and secured with tape

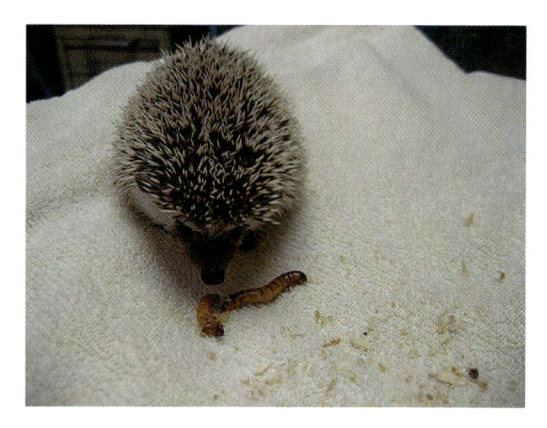

Fig. 14. Ill hedgehogs are often tempted to eat live food, such as mealworms.

sutured to the skin base of the neck. The tube must be long enough to accommodate the animal in a normal position and, in the case of the hedgehog, rolled completely into a defensive position. Feeding formulas for tube feeding are the same as those described previously for hand feeding, depending on species. It should be noted that Oxbow Herbivore Care (Oxbow Hay Company) used as manufactured frequently obstructs smaller bore feeding tubes. This can be overcome by thoroughly grinding the food in a food processor or coffee grinder for 15 minutes (Dawn Hromanik, Oxbow Hay Company, personal communication, 2004).

An alternative product is Herbivore Enteral formula by Rock Solid Herpetoculture [39]. Although marked for and tested on herbivorous reptiles, practitioners have used this product at a rate of 15 mL mixed with 15 mL of water per kilogram of body weight. In rabbits, this amount fed four times daily provides 88 Kcal/kg/day, which meets the suggested energy requirements for a stressed ill rabbit (Marla Lichtenberger, personal communication, 2006.) At a 1:1 volume to liquid ratio, this product provides 1.4 Kcal/mL.

Anesthesia and analgesia in the critical patient

Decisions on anesthesia and analgesia must be made carefully in the critical patient. In many cases, the practitioner must judge between the risk produced by the anesthetic or analgesic agent and the risk produced by pain and accompanying stress. Many exotic animal practitioners are familiar with the simple use of isoflurane or sevoflurane by face mask. An emergency specialty practice with a high volume of exotic mammal patients prefers the following protocol to reduce the stress associated with the application of a face mask further, particularly in those larger species for which some degree of stressful physical restraint may be necessary: buprenorphine, 0.01 to

0.03 mg/kg, or butorphanol, 0.4 mg/kg, and midazolam, 0.25 to 0.05 mg/kg, administered intramuscularly, followed in 10 to 15 minutes by mask anesthesia for the duration of the painful or stressful procedure (Marla Lichtenberger, personal communication, 2006).

Diagnosis and treatment of specific common emergency conditions

Initial treatment of shock and vascular collapse has been described previously. Diagnosis of specific conditions is often delayed until the patient is stable and collection of diagnostic samples and data is feasible.

Blood collection in small mammalian species can be challenging, especially in obese patients. Recently, the vena cava collection technique has been described and is currently the author's choice in nearly all small exotic mammals (Fig. 15) [40]. With practice, blood collection at this site is usually successful even in extremely small, obese, or severely compromised patients. Collection is usually performed with sedation, except in extremely cooperative or debilitated individuals. Other alternatives include any peripheral vein that can be visualized or accessed, including the jugular vein and sometimes cephalic veins in prairie dogs and hedgehogs. (It should be noted that if sedation is chosen for any reason, diagnostic or therapeutic, the practitioner should plan to accomplish as many steps as are safe and feasible in the single procedure rather than subject the patient to multiple attempts at sedation.)

Even a single drop of blood can be of great value when larger volumes are not possible. One drop collected into a hematocrit tube can be used to prepare a blood slide for a differential, a manual white blood cell count by hemocytometer, and determination of hematocrit and total serum solids. Larger volumes are useful for a complete blood cell count, chemistry panels, and even more specialized testing. Normal hematologic data for these three species are presented in Table 5.

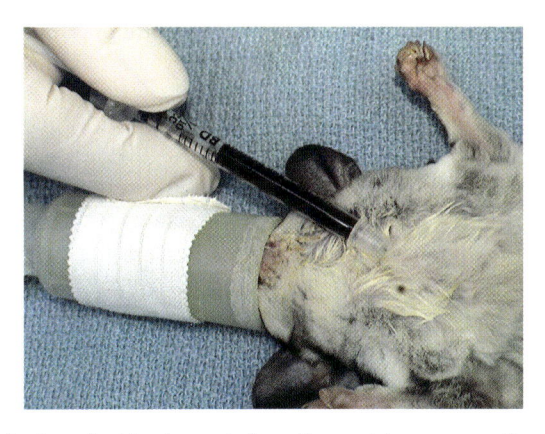

Fig. 15. Collection of a blood sample from the cranial vena cava of a sugar glider.

Table 5
Hematologic and blood chemistry date for prairie dogs, African Hedgehogs, and sugar gliders

	Prairie dog	African Hedgehog	Sugar glider
Hematocrit (%)	36–54	36 (22–64)	45–53
White blood cell count ($\times 10^3$ µL)	1.9–10.0	11 (3–43)	5.0–12.2
Neutrophils	0.9–7.1	5.1 (0.6–37.4)	1.5–3.0
Lymphocytes	0.3–3.5	4.0 (0.9–13.1)	2.8–9.2
Monocytes	0.0–0.7	0.3 (0.0–1.6)	0.1–0.2
Eosinophils	0.0–06	1.2 (0.0–5.1)	0.0–0.1
Basophils	0.0–0.13	0.4 (0.0–1.5)	0
Alkaline phosphatase (IU/L)	25–64	51 (8–92)	—
Alanine aminotransferase (IU/L)	26–91	53 (16–134)	50–106
Amylase (IU/L)	—	510 (244–858)	—
Aspartate aminotransferase (IU/L)	16–53	34 (8–137)	46–179
Bilirubin (mg/dL)	0.1–0.3	0.3 (0.0–1.3)	0.4–0.8
Blood urea nitrogen (mg/dL)	21–44	27 (13–54)	18–24
Calcium (mg/dL)	8.3–10.8	8.8 (5.2–11.3)	6.9–8.4
Chloride (mEq/L)	—	109 (92–128)	—
Cholesterol (mg/dL)	—	131 (86–189)	—
Creatinine kinase (IU/L)	—	863 (333–1964)	210–589
Creatinine (mg/dL)	0.8–2.3	0.4 (0.0–0.8)	0.3–0.5
γ-glutamyl transferase (IU/L)	—	4 (0–12)	—
Glucose (mg/dL)	120–209	89	130–183
Lactate dehydrogenase (IU/L)	—	441 (57–820)	—
Phosphorus (mg/dL)	3.6–10.0	5.3 (2.4–12)	3.8–4.4
Potassium (mEq/L)	4.0–5.7	4.9 (3.2–7.2)	3.3–5.9
Protein (g/dL)	5.8–8.1	5.8 (4.0–7.7)	5.1–6.1
Albumin (g/dL)	2.4–3.9	2.9 (1.8–4.2)	3.5–4.3
Globulin (g/dL)	—	2.7 (1.6–3.9)	—
Sodium (mEq/L)	144–175	141 (120–165)	135–145
Triglycerides (mg/dL)	—	38 (10–96)	—

Data from Ivey E, Carpenter J. African Hedgehogs; Ness R, Booth R. Sugar gliders; and Funk R. Medical management of prairie dogs. In: Quesenberry K, Carpenter J, editors. Ferrets, rabbits and rodents, clinical medicine and surgery. St. Louis (MO): WB Saunders; 2004. p. 345, 335, 269.

Collection of diagnostic-quality radiographs might be possible without sedation in severely debilitated prairie dogs, hedgehogs, and sugar gliders and is possible with difficulty using tape or gauze to restrain an alert sugar glider. In most cases, however, brief sedation greatly reduces patient stress and improves radiographic quality by enhancing proper positioning (Figs. 16 and 17). Sedation for radiography must be delayed in severely debilitated patients.

Other diagnostic tests for these species are similar to those in any other pet species and include urinalysis, sample collection for cytology or culture, bone marrow collection, fecal analysis, and biopsy.

Seizures in sugar gliders

Sugar gliders presenting with CNS signs, including tremors and seizures, may be experiencing hypocalcemia or hypoglycemia. Blood for chemistry

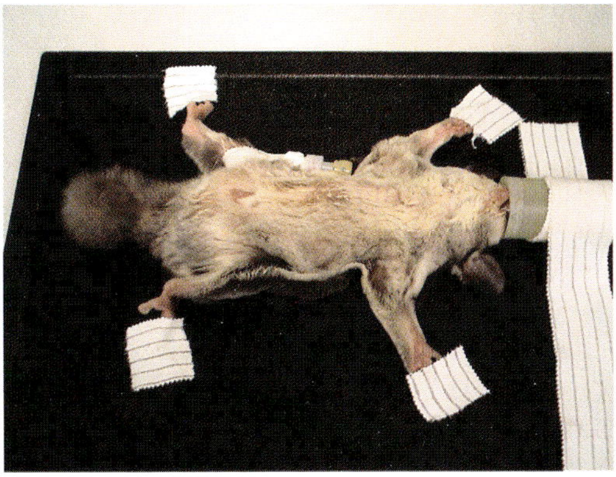

Fig. 16. Brief sedation with isoflurane or sevoflurane facilitates performance of radiographs and should be considered in all but extremely debilitated patients.

analysis should be drawn before beginning therapy if possible. Treatment of hypocalcemia includes calcium gluconate at a rate of 0.2 to 1 mL/kg administered intravenously, intramuscularly, or subcutaneously. Dogs administered rapid intravenous calcium may experience bradycardia, which may be of concern in exotic species as well. The author prefers to monitor patients receiving intravenous calcium with an electrocardiogram (ECG) or by cardiac auscultation. Treatment of hypoglycemia requires the addition of glucose to intravenous resuscitation fluids. Intravenous boluses of 50% dextrose can be administered at a rate of 0.5 mL/kg mixed with equal parts of lactated Ringer's solution. Animals that do not respond to therapy, especially those that have been seizuring for longer periods, may require anticonvulsion medication. Hyperthermia may occur in animals with prolonged seizure activity.

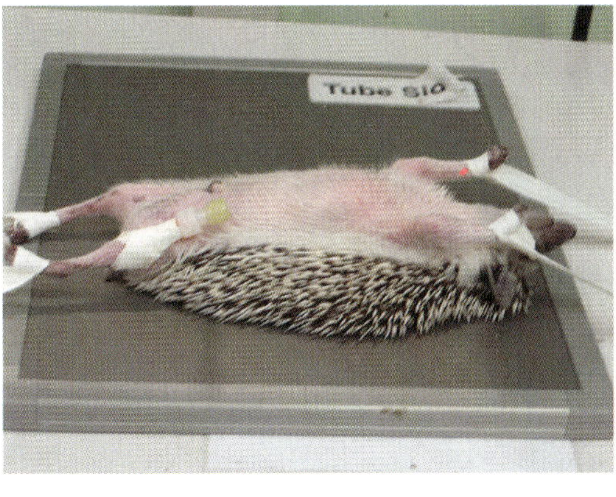

Fig. 17. Brief sedation with isoflurane or sevoflurane for performance of radiographs in a hedgehog. Most procedures, including complete physical examination and sample collection, require sedation in all but extremely debilitated patients.

Pseudo-odontoma of prairie dogs

As mentioned previously, pseudo-odontoma of prairie dogs is progressively debilitating and results in worsening respiratory distress because of impedance of airflow in the nasal cavity by damaged roots of the maxillary incisors. Diagnosis is based on clinical signs and demonstration of root deformation and a nasal mass on skull radiographs (see Fig. 3). Immediate care may include administration of oxygen by means of a face mask or chamber and correction of secondary disorders, such as dehydration and emaciation. In more severely affected animals, general anesthesia for endoscopic-guided endotracheal intubation is possible but difficult because of the unique anatomy of the pharynx and larynx. Other considerations include tracheotomy and retrograde placement of an endotracheal tube or temporary tracheostomy.

Resolution is technically difficult and requires reduction of the nasal space-occupying mass. Five different surgical techniques have been reported for treatment of pseudo-odontoma in prairie dogs [41–43]. Extraction of maxillary incisor teeth is the least complex but may not be possible when tooth root apexes are severely deformed or adhered to alveolar bone. In these cases, extraction can be performed by means of a dorsal rhinotomy approach or ventrally (intraorally) by a transpalatal approach. An additional technique recently described includes rhinotomy by means of a lateral approach with the goal of debulking the mass and creating an accessory nostril. Permanent rhinostomy by means of a monolateral or bilateral dorsal approach has also been described.

Cardiac disease

Cardiac disease, including cardiomyopathy, has been described in African Hedgehogs and prairie dogs [17,26]. Diagnosis was by means of radiographs and ultrasonography. Most reports are anecdotal, but there are a few brief descriptions of the use of drugs like furosemide, enalapril, and digoxin. The author was able to find limited published information regarding the doses of these drugs used in these patients (Table 6). The overall prognosis is reported to be poor.

Selection of therapeutic agents in sugar gliders, African hedgehogs, and prairie dogs

Drug dosages for these species are largely anecdotal, but many are based on years of clinical experience. Several formularies suggest dosages for common therapeutics in these species, and selected dosages are reported in Table 6. Dosages for drugs not listed here or reported elsewhere are typically extrapolated from similar species and used with caution while carefully monitoring the patient.

Table 6
Common therapeutic drug dosages for sugar gliders, African Hedgehogs, and prairie dogs

Drug	Sugar glider	African Hedgehog	Prairie dog
Amoxicillin	30 mg/kg PO divided q 12–24 hours	15 mg/kg PO, SQ, IM q 12 hours	Do not use
Enrofloxacin	5 mg/kg PO, SQ, IM q 12 hours	2.5–5.0 mg/kg PO, IM q 12 hours	5–10 mg/kg PO, IM q 12 hours
Trimethoprim/ sulfamethoxazole	15 mg/kg PO q 12 hours	30 mg/kg PO, SQ, IM q 12 hours	15–30 mg/kg PO, SQ q 12 hours
Metronidazole	25 mg/kg PO q 12 hours	20 mg/kg PO q 12 hours	20 mg/kg PO q 12 hours
Butorphanol	0.5 mg/kg IM q 8 hours	0.2–0.4 mg/kg SQ q 8 hours	0.2–2.0 mg/kg SQ, IM q 4 hours
Buprenorphine	0.01–0.03 mg/kg IM	0.01–0.03 mg/kg IM	0.01–0.03 mg/kg IM
Diazepam	0.5–1.0 mg/kg IM	0.5–2.0 mg/kg IM	3–5 mg/kg IM
Midazolam	0.25–0.05 mg/kg IM[a]	0.25–0.05 mg/kg IM[a]	0.25–0.05 mg/kg IM[a]
Calcium gluconate 23%[a]	100–150 mg/kg IV	100–150 mg/kg IV	100–150 mg/kg IV
Furosemide	2–4 mg/kg[a]	2.5–5.0 mg/kg PO, SQ, IM q 8 hours	1–4 mg/kg SQ, IM q 4–6 hours
Enalapril	0.5 mg/kg[a]	0.5 mg/kg PO q 24 hours	0.5 mg/kg[a]
Doxapram	2 mg/kg IV[a]	2 mg/kg IV[a]	2–5 mg/kg IV
Epinephrine	0.003 mg/kg IV[a]	0.003 mg/kg IV[a]	0.003 mg/kg IV

Note that dosages for prairie dogs are extrapolated from those used in rodent species in general.

Abbreviations: IM, intramuscular; IV, intravenous; PO, by mouth; q, every; SQ, subcutaneous.

[a] Marla Lichtenberger, personal communication, 2006.

Data from Carpenter J. Exotic animal formulary. 3rd edition. St. Louis (MO): Elsevier; 2005; except where indicated.

References

[1] Ness RD, Booth R. Sugar gliders. In: Quesenberry KE, Carpenter JW, editors. Ferrets, rabbits and rodents, clinical medicine and surgery. St. Louis (MO): Saunders; 2004. p. 330–8.
[2] Delaney C. Practical marsupial medicine. Proc Assoc Ex Mammal Vet Conf. San Antonio; 2006. p. 51–60.
[3] Tocidlowski M. Histoplasmosis outbreak at the Houston zoo. Proc Am Assoc Zoo Vet 2003;141–8.
[4] Raymond JT, White MR. Necropsy and histopathologic findings in 14 African hedgehogs (Atelerix albiventris): a retrospective study. J Zoo Wildl Med 1999;30(2):273–7.
[5] Miller DL, Styer EL, Stobaeus JK, et al. Thyroid C-cell carcinoma in an African pygmy hedgehog (Atelerix albivenris). J Zoo Wildl Med 2002;33(4):392–6.
[6] Wellehan JF, Southorn E, Smith DA, et al. Surgical removal of a mammary adenocarcinoma and a granulosa cell tumor in an African pygmy hedgehog. Can Vet J 2003;44(3): 235–7.

[7] Ramos-Vara JA, Miller MA, Craft D. Intestinal plasmacytoma in an African hedgehog. J Wildl Dis 1998;34(2):377–80.
[8] Ramos-Vara JA. Soft tissue sarcomas in the African hedgehog (Atelerix albiventris): microscopic and immunohistologic study of three cases. J Vet Diagn Invest 2001;13(5):442–5.
[9] Fukuzawa R, Fukuzawa K, Abe H, et al. Acinic cell carcinoma in an African pygmy hedgehog (Atelerix albiventris). Vet Clin Pathol 2004;33(1):39–42.
[10] Peauroi JR, Lowenstine LJ, Munn RJ, et al. Multicentric skeletal sarcomas associated with probably retrovirus particles in African hedgehogs (Atelerix albiventris). Vet Pathol 1994; 31(4):481–4.
[11] Rivera RY, Janovitz ED. Oronasal squamous cell carcinoma in an African hedgehog (Erinaceidae albiventris). J Wildl Dis 1993;28(1):148–50.
[12] Raymond JT, Clarke KA, Schafer KA. Intestinal lymphosarcoma in captive African hedgehogs. J Wildl Dis 1998;24(4):801–6.
[13] Raymond JT, Garner M. Mammary gland tumors in captive African hedgehogs. J Wildl Dis 2000;36(2):405–8.
[14] Raymond JT, White MR, Janovitz EB. Malignant mast cell tumor in an African hedgehog (Atelerix albiventris). J Wildl Dis 1997;33(1):140–2.
[15] Helmer PJ. Abnormal hematologic findings in an African hedgehog (Atelerix albiventris) with gastrointestinal lymphosarcoma. Can Vet J 2000;41(6):489–90.
[16] Mikaelian I, Reavill DR, Practice A. Spontaneous proliferative lesions and tumors of the uterus of captive African hedgehogs (Atelerix albiventris). J Zoo Wildl Med 2004;35(2): 216–20.
[17] Ivey E, Carpenter JW. African hedgehogs. In: Quesenberry KE, Carpenter JW, editors. Ferrets, rabbits and rodents, clinical medicine and surgery. St. Louis (MO): Saunders; 2004. p. 339–53.
[18] Raymond JT, Garner MM. Cardiomyopathy in captive African hedgehogs (Atelerix albiventris). J Vet Diagn Invest 2000;12(5):468–72.
[19] Graczyk TK, Cranfield MR, Dunning C, et al. Fatal cryptosporidiosis in a juvenile captive African hedgehog (Atelerix albiventris). J Parasitol 1998;84(1):178–80.
[20] Raymond JT, Williams C, Wu CC. Corynebacterial pneumonia in an African hedgehog. J Wildl Dis 1998;34(2):397–9.
[21] Graesser D, Spraker T, Dressen P, et al. Wobbly hedgehog syndrome in African pygmy hedgehogs (Atelerix spp.). J Exotic Pet Med 2006;15(1):59–65.
[22] Wheler CL, Grahn BH, Pocknell AM. Unilateral proptosis and orbital cellulitis in eight African hedgehogs (Atelerix albiventris). J Zoo Wildl Med 2001;32(2):236–41.
[23] Riley P, Chomel B. Hedgehog zoonosis. Emerg Infect Dis 205;11(1).
[24] Allison N, Chang TC, Steele KE, et al. Fatal herpes simplex infection in a pygmy African hedgehog (Atelerix albiventris). J Comp Pathol 2002;126(1):76–8.
[25] Lennox A. Firsthand encounter with Monkeypox. Exotic DVM 2003;5(4):15.
[26] Funk R. Medical management of Prairie dogs. In: Quesenberry KE, Carpenter JW, editors. Ferrets, rabbits and rodents clinical medicine and surgery. St. Louis (MO): Saunders; 2004. p. 266–73.
[27] Capello V, Gracis M. Dental diseases. In: Lennox AM, editor. Rabbit and rodent dentistry handbook. Lake Worth (FL): Zoological Education Network; 2005. p. 113–63.
[28] Miwa Y, Matsunaga S, Nakayama H, et al. Spontaneous lymphoma in a Prairie dog (Cynomys ludovicianus). J Am Anim Hosp Assoc 2006;42(2):151–3.
[29] Mouser P, Cole A, Lin TL. Maxillary osteosarcoma in a Prairie dog (Cynomys ludovicianus). J Vet Diagn Invest 2006;18(3):310–2.
[30] Garner M, Raymond J, Toshkov I, et al. Hepatocellular carcinoma in black tailed prairie dogs (Cynomys ludivicianus): tumor morphology and immunohistochemistry for hepadnavirus core and surface antigens. Vet Pathol 2004;41(4):353–61.
[31] Une Y, Tatra S, Nomura Y, et al. Hepatitis and hepatocellular carcinoma in two prairie dogs (Cynomys ludovicianus). J Vet Med Sci 1996;58(9):933–5.

[32] Phalen D. Prairie dogs: vectors and victims. Seminars in Avian Exotic Pet Medicine 2004; 13(2):105–7.
[33] LaMoret WW, O'Leary DP, Booker ML, et al. Increase dietary fat content accelerates cholesterol gallstone formation in the cholesterol-fed prairie dog. Hepatology 1993;18(6): 1498–503.
[34] Dierenfield E, Thomas D, Ives R. Comparison of commonly used diets on intake, digestion, growth and health in captive sugar gliders (Petaurus breviceps). Journal of Exotic Pet Medicine 2006;15(3):218–24.
[35] Antinoff N. Small mammal critical care. Vet Clin North Am Exot Anim Pract 1998;1(1): 153–75.
[36] Lichtenberger M. Shock, fluid therapy, anesthesia and analgesia in the ferret. Exotic DVM 2005;7(2):24–31.
[37] Available at: Murdock NE, www.Oxbowhay.com. Accessed June 2006.
[38] Fossum TW. In: Small animal surgery. 2nd edition. St. Louis (MO): Mosby; 2002. p. 76–7.
[39] Available at: www.rocksolidherpetoculture.com. Accessed January 2007.
[40] Capello V. Application of the cranial vena cava venipuncture technique to small exotic mammals. Exotic DVM 2006;8(3):51–5.
[41] Brown SA. Surgical removal of incisors in the rabbit. J Small Exotic Anim Med 1992;1(4): 150–3.
[42] Crossley DA. Small mammal dentistry (part I). In: Quesenberry KE, Carpenter JW, editors. Ferrets, rabbits and rodents: clinical medicine and surgery. 2nd edition. St. Louis (MO): Saunders; 2004. p. 370–9.
[43] Wagner R, Johnson D. Rhinotomy for treatment of odontoma in prairie dogs. Exotic DVM 2001;3(5):29–34.

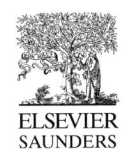

Emergency Care of Reptiles

David Martinez-Jimenez, LV MSc*,
Stephen J. Hernandez-Divers, BVetMed, DZooMed
(Reptilian), MRCVS, DACZM

Department of Small Animal Medicine and Surgery, College of Veterinary Medicine, University of Georgia, Athens, GA 30602-7390, USA

Because most reptile emergencies are secondary to inappropriate husbandry or diet, it is imperative that the clinician be familiar with the common reptile species kept in captivity, their husbandry and nutritional requirements, handling, and potential dangers. For more detailed descriptions the reader is referred to major reptile texts or earlier issues in this *Veterinary Clinics* series [1–3].

The veterinarian can use critical care knowledge gained from small animal medicine and apply it to reptiles. Principles of fluid therapy, cardiopulmonary monitoring, and resuscitation are similar. Well-practiced clinical techniques are important for the critical patient, which is often less forgiving than the healthy reptile. The last part of this article focuses on common emergency presentations.

Biologic concepts

Orders of reptiles (Chelonia, Crocodilia, Rhynchocephalia, and Squamata) are morphologically distinct, and several features have critical care importance. Most reptiles have a three-chambered heart (except for the crocodilians), and all possess metanephric kidneys [4]. The major nitrogenous waste product of terrestrial reptiles is uric acid, although ammonia and urea may be produced in greater quantities than uric acid in some aquatic species, particularly turtles.

---

* Corresponding author. Lawndale Veterinary Hospital, 4314 Lawndale Drive, Greensboro, NC 27455.
  E-mail address: davidmjvet@hotmail.com (D. Martinez-Jimenez).

Veterinarians treating reptiles, even if only on an emergency basis, should take a special interest and become familiar with the common species kept in captivity. Client education is important, and written handouts save time, ensure completeness, and prevent misunderstanding. Comprehensive and accurate booklets that cover the most common species are available from various herpetologic societies (eg, Herpetological Society, 2001 N. Clark St., Chicago, IL, 60614 or Zoological Society Network, PO Box 541749, Lake Worth, FL, 33454-1749).

History and physical examination

Owners should be instructed on the phone to secure their reptile in an escape-proof, ventilated, and insulated container (eg, pillowcase within a pet carrier). The precise species should also be determined to permit husbandry and diet research before arrival. The veterinarian should be aware that some reptile species are venomous and that special training and requirements are necessary to accept such animals.

Clinical evaluation starts with a detailed history and physical examination, the details of which have been previously published in this series [1,5].

If the reptile is not stable, the clinician should proceed to cardiopulmonary-cerebral resuscitation (CPCR) as given below. If the reptile seems stable, the clinician should place the reptile in a warm incubator (set to within the preferred optimum temperature zone of the species in question) while taking the history (Fig. 1).

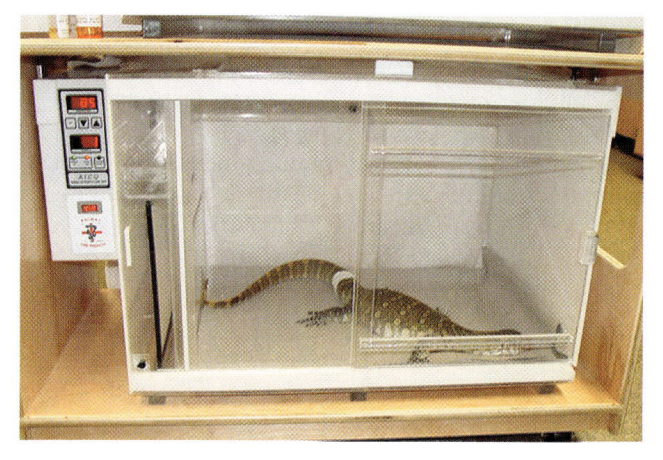

Fig. 1. Nile monitor in an animal intensive care unit that allows increasing temperature gradually by maintaining a set temperature and humidity.

Temperature

Correction of metabolic derangements in reptiles is an important first step in their critical care. Reptiles being ectotherms rely on external heat and behavior for thermoregulation. Compromised, inactive reptiles should be closely monitored for hyper- and hypothermia during hospitalization [6–9]. Each species has their preferred optimal temperature zone (POTZ) necessary for optimal metabolic processes, including digestion, healing, reproduction, and immune system function. POTZ can be found in specialized reptile medicine, exotic formularies, and on the internet (www.anapsid.org) [3,10].

Except in the case of CPCR, no reptile should be given any medications before reaching their POTZ. Medications have little effect on a cold reptile. Rapid warming may not be advisable, however, because it may cause further compromise. Warming is therefore done by slowly increasing the temperature of the incubator to the reptile's POTZ over 4 to 6 hours. For emergency care, the animal intensive units from Lyon Technologies Inc. (www.lyonelectric.com) maintain a set temperature and humidity, whereas plastic or fiberglass vivaria (eg, Vision cages) can be used with suitable lighting and heating devices (www.lllreptile.com or www.kingsnake.com/visionherp/).

A thermal gradient should be created according to the species' POTZ [3,10]. Sick reptiles have often been reported to seek higher temperatures (behavioral fever), and therefore should be provided with a temperature range at the higher end of the POTZ [11,12]. Digital thermometers at both ends of the enclosure and a hydrometer should be used for monitoring purposes. An indoor/outdoor digital thermometer is a convenient alternative to the common reptile thermometers and hydrometers. A good range for most reptiles is 24°C–29°C (75°F–85°F), until the species-specific temperature range can be obtained [13]. Lethal environmental temperatures for reptiles (except diurnal desert species) are those greater than 38°C (100°F), but lower temperatures can still be fatal. Hyperthermia is manifested by abnormal behavior, open mouth breathing, gasping, and tachypnea [14]. Most species do well at humidity levels of 50% to 70%, but without proper ventilation this can lead to bacteria and fungus overgrowth in the cage [3]. Depending on the species' requirements, full spectrum UV light should also be considered in the hospital enclosure for psychologic benefits, even though any effects of bone metabolism are unlikely to be significant during a short hospital stay.

Cardiopulmonary-cerebral resuscitation

In an emergency situation, a rapid systematic (but often brief) physical examination can be performed. Initial assessment should be performed to determine cardiovascular and respiratory stability, mentation, and evidence of trauma or blood loss. The reptile should be examined for breathing, and when no respiratory excursions are noted, CPCR should be initiated. The clinician should follow basic life support with the ABC (airway, breathing, circulation) approach of CPCR. Secure a patent airway by opening the mouth of the reptile. The glottis is located at the base of the tongue in the rostral oral cavity. Most reptiles can be easily intubated, and 100% oxygen should be initiated using an Ambubag (Ridge Medical, Lombard, IL) or ventilator (Small Animal Ventilator, Vetronics, Lafayette, IN) connected to an oxygen outlet or anesthesia machine. Positive pressure ventilation is commenced at a rate of 4 to 6 breaths per minute, whereas peak positive pressure ventilation should not exceed 8 cm H_2O [15]. The heart is not easily auscultated using a standard stethoscope; however, electronic stethoscopes and Dopplers are often more rewarding. Electrocardiography (ECG) can be used to identify electrical activity and should not be performed in cold reptiles, because identification of the waves' boundaries can be challenging [16]. It should be noted that dead reptiles may continue to exhibit cardiac electrical activity for many hours after CNS collapse, whereas mere handling and restraint may also induce ECG artifacts. The alligator clips from the ECG leads can be attached to hypodermic needles and then placed appropriately through the skin (Table 1) [17]. The snake's heart is located in the upper third of the body length and the leads can be attached cranial and caudal to the heart. In lizards and turtles, the leads can be attached to the front limbs and right rear limb as in dogs and cats. The heart is located within the shell of turtles and under the boney sternum in lizards and therefore heart compressions cannot be performed. Except for the crocodile, reptiles lack a functional diaphragm. Although there have been no studies that have investigated reptile CPCR, many biologists have studied the reptilian heart, its functions, and neuroendocrine control mechanisms, which should be appreciated [18–22].

If no heart beat is detected, epinephrine (Table 2) is administered endotracheally with a catheter inserted down the endotracheal tube if intravenous (IV) or intraosseous (IO) access is not possible. For endotracheal administration the dose of emergency drugs should be doubled and diluted with sterile saline to 1 mL/100 g body weight to facilitate delivery of drug to vascular respiratory tract. Administration of doxapram (see Table 2) [23–26] can be given in cases of severe respiratory depression or arrest, and although its effect in reptiles has not been critically assessed, profound and immediate effects have been noted following IV administration. Reptiles typically have slow heart rates (30–100 bpm); however, in cases of true bradycardia, atropine is likely to be effective [20,27]. If hypovolemia is suspected because of blood loss or severe dehydration, an IV or IO catheter should be placed (see later discussion on catheter placement) and fluids administered (see later discussion on fluid therapy). The effectiveness of resuscitation can be assessed with the use of a Doppler probe placed at the base of the heart or peripherally to detect blood flow. The Doppler probe can also be placed over a distal artery to assess pulse quality or determine systolic blood pressure (see section onshock, blood pressure, and fluid resuscitation). Trends in

Table 1
Lead placement in the reptilian patient

Group	Lead placement	Comment
Ofidia	Self-adhering cutaneous skin electrodes designed for humans are placed approximately two heart-lengths cranial and caudal to the heart.	
Sauria	In lizards with the heart located caudal to pectoral girdle (eg, monitors and tegus), electrodes are placed either in limbs or torso. Lizards with heart located at the level of the pectoral girdle (eg, skinks, iguanas, chameleons, and water dragons), electrodes should be placed in the cervical region.	Stainless steel hypodermic needles or loops of stainless steel suture material can be used to attach the alligator clips.
Chelonian	Leads can be placed on limbs; however, placement of the cranial leads on the skin lateral to the neck and medial to the forelimbs is more rewarding. Leads can be attached to dermal bone after drilling holes in the carapace; however, this is a very invasive technique.	Limb lead placement is often adequate but problematic to interpretation because of frequently small surface voltages.
Crocodilian	Use of limb electrodes or torso electrodes is appropriate.	Use same limb lead placement as in lizards.

blood lactate and pH may be useful to assess improvement in circulatory status.

The clinician should be reminded that reptiles have an ability to convert to anaerobic metabolism, and this can result in brain and tissue survival even after many hours of hypoxia. Even without a beating heart, the reptile can be warmed and continued on IV or IO fluids. There are reports of reptiles recovering after many hours of arrest with supportive care (ie, heat, oxygen, and fluids). Research studies have proven that turtle hearts are tolerant of global ischemia, and that they can recover completely on reperfusion without any indication of ischemia- or reperfusion-related injury [28].

Turtles also have an extraordinary ability for the brain to tolerate anoxia based on many factors [29]. Anoxia tolerance is caused by enhanced glycogen stores, increased antioxidant capacities, and elevated heat shock protein [30]. There is a long-term survival at basal levels of ATP expenditure [30]. The heat shock proteins have an important protective function against ischemia and anoxia in the mammalian brain; however, unlike mammalian brains, turtles have very high levels of heat shock proteins [29,31]. There is a rapid upregulation of neuronal processes in the turtle when oxygen becomes available [29,31]. The authors have seen reptiles, believed on initial presentation to be deceased, respond to supportive care over several hours.

Table 2
Common emergency drugs used during cardiopulmonary resuscitation in reptiles

Agent	Dosage	Species/Comments
Epinephrine	0.5 mL/kg IV, IO, IT	Concentration 1:1000; on IT, use 2 times the IV dose and dilute with sterile saline at 1 mL/100 g body weight to facilitate delivery of drug to the bronchus
Atropine	0.01–0.04 mg/kg IM, IV, IO [23] 0.2 mg/kg SC, IM [24]	Generally used in bradycardia; extrapolation from mammals; may not increase heart rate in green iguanas [25]
Doxapram	5 mg/kg IV, IO, IM	Respiratory stimulant [93]
Calcium gluconate	100 mg/kg IV, IO, IM every 8 h [26]	Hypocalcemic muscle tremors, seizures or flaccid paresis; switch to oral calcium once patient is stable

Abbreviations: IM, intramuscularly; IO, intraosseously; IT, intratracheally; IV, intravenously; SC, subcutaneously.

Shock, blood pressure, and fluid resuscitation

Blood volume in healthy reptiles varies from 4% to 8%, which is lower than in mammals [32,33]. Approximately 75% of the body weight is water, except in turtles, in which the presence of the carapace reduces the value to that found in mammals by approximately 66% [34]. Reptiles have an equal distribution of intracellular and extracellular fluid compartments, which is different than that seen in mammals and birds (in which the intracellular space contains 60% of fluid and the extracellular contains 40% of the total fluid volume). Approximately 30% of the extracellular fluid exists in the intravascular space and 70% within the interstitial space [34]. The principles of water movement and fluid therapy are similar to that in other species. Fluid choice (ie, crystalloids and colloids) is presented in the article by Lichtenberger elsewhere in this issue; however, it should be noted that the osmolarity of reptile plasma is typically lower than that of mammals, and consequently solutions osmotically balanced for mammals (eg, 0.9% normal saline) are likely to be hypertonic for reptiles and may further deplete the intracellular compartment (Table 3) [35]. In addition, many arid species of reptiles physiologically cope with dehydration by coping with major elevations of plasma osmolarity that would be fatal to mammals [36].

Blood pressure in reptiles is controlled by mechanisms similar to those described in mammals [37–41]. Hypovolemia secondary to intravascular volume loss produces a profound baroreceptor response. The increase in sympathetic nervous system stimulation leads to an increase in heart rate, increase in heart contractility and increase in systemic vascular resistance [37–41], but there are several differences in this response seen in reptiles compared with mammals and birds.

Table 3
Plasma osmolarity and electrolytes of selected reptile species

Order	Species	Plasma concentrations in mOsm/L				
		Na$^+$	K$^+$	Cl$^-$	HCO$_3^-$	Osmolarity
Crocodilia	American alligator	141	3.8	112	20	284
Chelonia	Red-eared slider	113	4.2	80	NA	260
	Greek tortoise (summer)	115	4.5	95	NA	290
	Greek tortoise (hibernation)	156	3.9	125	NA	404
	Desert tortoise (summer hydrated)	122	5.3	86	NA	291
	Desert tortoise (summer dehydrated)	150	3.8	120	NA	334

Because of the lack of complete data, the authors decided to list only those species in which most of the information was completed. For more information, refer to Bentley [35].

Abbreviation: NA, not available.

Being ectotherms, normal blood pressure in reptiles may be more profoundly affected by environmental stresses such as habitat and temperature outside the POTZ. This greater variability may originate from a reptile's poor ability to regulate normal homeostasis in a cold environment, thereby decreasing the energetic cost of thermoregulation. Heart rate and blood pressure are significantly higher during heating than during cooling [22]. The reptile's ability to mount an appropriate sympathetic response to hypovolemia requires a warm environment. The reptile should be maintained at its POTZ during fluid therapy [42–44].

There is a great variation in heart rate and blood pressure between the different species of reptiles [34,45]. Chelonians tend to have the lowest mean arterial pressure (15–40 mm Hg), whereas some lizards (eg, chameleons) have resting mean arterial pressures similar to mammals (60–80 mm Hg) [45]. In the green iguana, the resting systemic arterial pressure is reported to be 40 to 50 mm Hg [45]. A study in green iguanas under anesthesia at 1% isoflurane describes a systolic mean pressure of 43 ± 7 mm Hg and diastolic mean pressure of 29 ± 4 mm Hg [46]. Snakes have been reported to have an allometric relationship between arterial blood pressure and body mass. As body mass increases, so does blood pressure [45].

Monitoring blood pressure in reptiles during fluid resuscitation and anesthesia is valuable. Indirect systolic Doppler blood pressure has been measured in several species of reptiles using techniques similar to those used in small mammals (M.K. Lichtenberger, personal communication, 2006). Unpublished data (Hernandez-Divers, 2007) involving blood pressure and arterial blood gas determinations in research iguanas at the University of Georgia, however, have indicated serious discrepancies between direct and indirect pressure measurements. Further studies are needed to compare direct to indirect blood pressure measurements in reptiles.

Direct pressure monitoring using the carotid and femoral arteries have been shown to be accurate and consistent and to correlate with baroreceptor reflex studies and previously published results, whereas indirect measurements have been highly variable in comparison [46]. As direct blood pressure monitoring is likely to be difficult in practice, indirect monitoring using a Doppler monitor (Parks Medical, Aloha, OR) may be the only practical option. Clinicians are advised to be skeptical of the pressure values obtained, and like pulse oximetry, it is probably advisable to pay attention to the trend rather than an individual result.

In chelonians, the cuff is attached at the highest point of the front leg and the probe detects blood flow on the brachial artery at the palmar aspect of the radius and ulna (Fig. 2). The cuff is inflated to suprasystolic blood pressure and slowly released until the first sound is heard. The first sound is the measure of indirect systolic blood pressure. The caudal artery at the tail can be used in large male chelonians. In chameleons, bearded dragons, iguanas, and other lizards, the blood pressure can be measured using the front leg as described for chelonians (Fig. 3). In snakes, the cuff is placed just distal to the cloaca and the probe detects blood flow from the caudal tail artery. Indirect systolic blood pressures have been reported between 40 and 90 mm Hg (M.K. Lichtenberger, personal communication, 2006). Direct pressure studies in conscious green iguanas at 28°C, however, have indicated normal resting heart rates of 48 ± 2 bpm and mean arterial blood pressures of 51 ± 2 mm Hg, with a range of 30 to 63 mm Hg (Hernandez-Divers, unpublished data, 2007).

Reptiles can maintain hemodynamic stability despite substantial hemorrhage because of the rapid shift of interstitial fluid into the vascular space [33,38]. Some snakes withstand 4% graded hemorrhage until the cumulative deficit is 32% of the blood volume, and they are able to maintain their initial blood volume throughout hemorrhage. Typically, 50% to 60% of the hemorrhaged deficit is transferred from the interstitium to the circulation

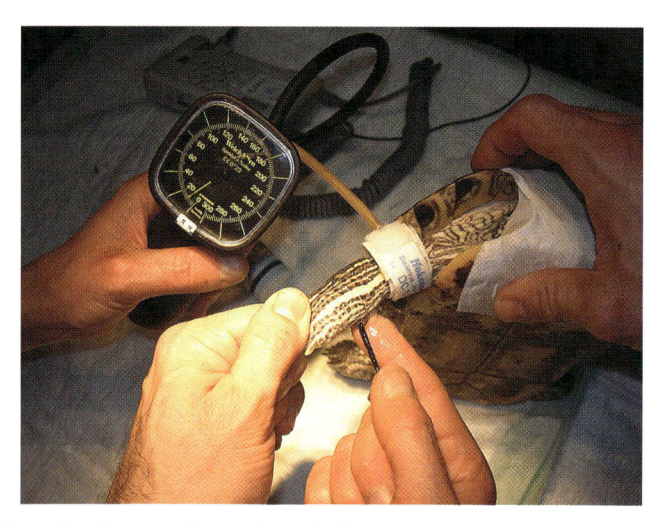

Fig. 2. Indirect blood pressure in a red-eared slider. (*Courtesy of* Marla Lichtenberger, DVM, Mequon, WI.)

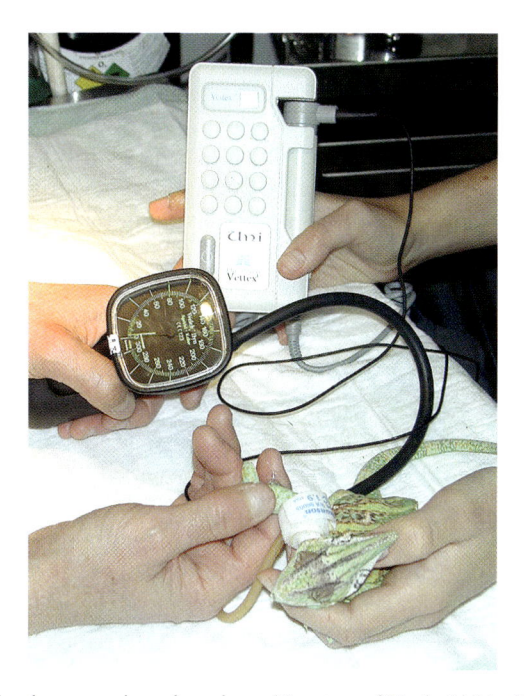

Fig. 3. Indirect blood pressure in a chameleon. (*Courtesy of* Marla Lichtenberger, DVM, Mequon, WI.)

throughout hemorrhage [33,38]. Major fluid shifts between the intravascular and interstitial compartments thus significantly compensate for hypovolemia, but in some species do not result in a well-regulated arterial blood pressure [38]. IV or IO fluid therapy using crystalloids and colloids is therefore important for the treatment of hypovolemia in reptiles (fluid therapy with crystalloids and colloids is discussed in the article by Lichtenberger elsewhere in this issue).

Perfusion deficits are assessed using blood pressure and heart rate. The mouth and cloaca can be examined for color and capillary refill time; however, heart rates vary and are temperature-dependent. Based on allometric scaling, heart rate in reptiles under its preferred temperature zone (PTZ) has been mathematically calculated: $HR = 33.4 \times W_{kg}^{-0.25}$. For that reason, IO or IV fluids should be administered after warming the patient. Bolus doses of crystalloids (5–10 mL/kg) with colloids (3–5 mL/kg) can be given IV or IO until blood pressure is detected in the normal range for the species. Fluids given IV or IO should also be warmed to mid-POTZ before administration. Some colloids such as oxyglobin (hemoglobin-based oxygen carrier) also have the added advantage of carrying oxygen to the tissue [44]. The use of blood transfusions in reptiles has been anecdotally reported [47].

Dehydration

Once the perfusion deficits and body temperature have been restored, hydration can be assessed. The blood pressure should be within the normal resting range. The parameters used for assessing hydration include mucous membrane moisture, skin elasticity, position of the ocular globe, and packed cell volume (PCV) and total protein (TP). The skin turgor is of limited value in judging dehydration in reptiles because of their highly keratinized and often thickened integument. There is a large range in PCV and TP within Reptilia, typically 20%–35% and 3 to 7 g/dL, respectively. So unless the species-specific or preferably the individual's normal PCV and TP are known, a single PCV/TP result has little value for assessing dehydration. Serial measurements, however, can be useful for assessing response to therapy. Dehydration should be suspected in any reptile that presents with a history of poor husbandry methods (eg, chameleons provided with a water bowl instead of a water dripper or misting system).

Many reptiles have a high tolerance for dehydration and increases in plasma sodium and osmolarity. They are able to restore plasma sodium through increased thirst and excretion of sodium from salt glands. Reptiles with a urinary bladder are able to reabsorb water from the bladder along a concentration gradient. Dehydration deficits should be restored using a crystalloid with an osmolality comparable with normal reptile plasma (varies between 250 and 290 mOsm/L). The normal plasma sodium concentration varies with different species, but is generally between 142 and 165 mmol/L [36]. Use of common mammalian isotonic crystalloids (normal saline, 308 mOsm/L; Plasmalyte-A [Baxter, Deerfield, IL], 294 mOsm/L; Normosol-R [Abbott, North Chicago, IL]) cannot be recommended, because undiluted these fluids are hypertonic for reptiles. Jarchow's modification (two parts 2.5% dextrose in 0.45% saline and one part LRS, 278 mOsm/L) has been specifically recommended for reptiles in the past [47]. The additional dextrose seems to be beneficial, and once metabolized provides a net water gain that is particularly useful, given that most reptiles present with water deficiencies. There may be little or no benefit from this self-made fluid, however, when commercially available 2.5% dextrose in half-strength LRS (264 mOsm/L) is used as a replacement fluid. For meeting maintenance requirements, 2.5% dextrose in 0.45% saline (280 mOsm/L) also seems acceptable. Additional dextrose is given intravenously if the blood glucose is especially low. Reptiles produce lactate and use anaerobic metabolism during anoxia. Blood lactate levels also increase during shock with inadequate tissue perfusion. Lactate is rapidly metabolized to bicarbonate in the liver when tissue oxygen delivery is restored. Concerns over the use of lactate-containing fluids aggravating acidosis are unfounded in any animal with appropriate liver function. Fluid deficits can be replaced over 12 to 36 hours when lost acutely or more commonly over 48 to 96 hours for the chronically dehydrated reptile. Maintenance fluid requirements in reptiles are 5 to 15 mL/kg/day because of their slow metabolic rate and variable resistance to insensible fluid losses. Maintenance fluids are given orally when the reptile is able to assimilate oral nutrition and by soaking the reptile in warm fluids (note that some desert species resist bathing). Water absorption may take place through the cloaca during freshwater soaks and is a useful way of providing maintenance needs [36].

Drug administration

The intramuscular route is most commonly used in reptiles for drug administration. Historically hind limb and tail muscles have been avoided because of the renal portal system and concerns of first-pass effect through the kidneys. Studies have shown, however, that this is probably more of a theoretical concern and of limited clinical importance [48,49]. The renal portal system is also under control of the autonomic nervous system in poultry [50]. With sympathetic stimulation, the blood is shunted from the tail and hind limbs to the vena cava by way of closure of a valve on the iliac vessels. Under cholinergic stimulation, the valve is opened and blood is shunted from the tail and hind limbs through the kidneys. Most reptiles during illness, shock, and stress have a strong sympathetic response, and blood is then shunted away from the kidneys directly to the vena cava. The epaxial muscles provide a suitable injection site in snakes. In lizards, the muscle mass of the forelimb (triceps and biceps), hind limb, and tail can be used. In chelonians, the injections are most often administered in the deltoid or triceps muscles. The cranial surface of the foreleg should be avoided because of the proximity to the radial nerve and risk for damage to this nerve.

Vascular access: catheterization and blood collection

Intravascular catheter placement is (sub)order-specific and may require a cut-down technique. Table 4 [51,52] summarizes the sites for catheterization [53]. Catheterization of the coccygeal vein and abdominal vein is mostly performed without direct visualization. The jugular vein can be visualized in some turtles and tortoises; however; jugular catheterization in squamates often requires a skin incision and blunt dissection (Fig. 4). When lizards, crocodilians, or chelonians are poorly perfused and veins cannot be visualized, the IO access is used. The IO catheter can be placed into the tibial medullary cavity of lizards and crocodilians (Fig. 5). In chelonians, it may be possible to catheterize the plastrocarapacial bridge, but care is required not to penetrate into the coelom, and the size of the target is species-specific and may be nonexistent in some patients [54]. An IO catheter should not remain in place for longer than 72 hours. The catheter site should be aseptically prepared and a sterile technique performed. Spinal needles (20-, 22-, and 25-gauge 1.5 in) should be used. If a spinal needle is not readily available,

Table 4
Vascular and intraosseous catheterization sites commonly used in the reptile patient

Species	Catheter site	Comment
Snakes	Jugular vein	Right jugular larger than the left; lateral incision is made 4–7 scutes cranial to the heart and at the junction between ventral and lateral scutes
	Heart	Appropriate-sized catheter is directed toward the heart; once flush is obtained, style is removed and catheter is advanced as further as it goes
Chelonians	Jugular vein	Right jugular vein preferentially
	Bony bridge	Controversial as to whether it communicates with the vasculature or the coelomic cavity [51]
Lizards	Cephalic vein	Requires a cutdown procedure at the dorsal surface of the antebrachium from lateral to medial
	Ventral coccygeal vein [52]	Similar principle as that of blood sampling, but the vascular catheter stays in place
	Femur, humerus, or tibia	Similar principle as that in small animals
Crocodilian	Ventral coccygeal vein [52]	Similar principle as that of blood sampling, but the vascular catheter stays in place
	Femur, humerus, or tibia	Similar principle as that in small animals

hypodermic needles of similar gauge can be used, but can block on insertion [55]. Once it is placed and the catheter seated, antimicrobial ointment can be applied around the entry site. The catheter can be secured with a thick, padded, noncompressing bandage that encompasses the hub of the catheter and the limb distally. Catheters can be sutured in place.

A range of sites are available for blood collection (Table 5). The ventral tail vein is most commonly used in lizards. The ventral abdominal vein on the ventral abdominal midline just deep to the abdominal muscles and jugular vein are recommended as alternative sites. In turtles and tortoises, venipuncture from the jugular vein is easily performed if the head can be restrained in an extended position. If this is not possible, the (post)occipital sinus, subcarapacial sinus, supravertebral sinus, coccygeal vein, or brachial plexus can be used. Cardiocentesis is an option in snakes, but again the ventral tail vein is preferred. The amount of blood that can be safely removed is 0.4% to 0.8% of the reptile's total blood volume [32,33] and is placed in microtainer blood collection tubes (Becton Dickinson and Company,

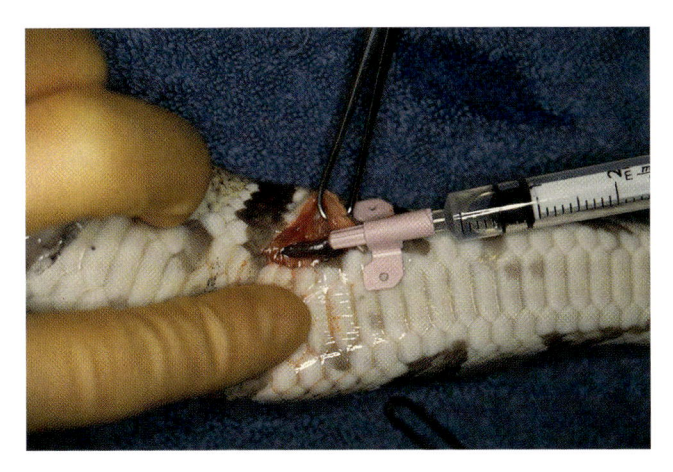

Fig. 4. Skin incision and blunt dissection is often required for jugular catheterization in the squamate. Jugular catheterization in a ball python.

Rutherford, NJ). Blood smears are made with fresh blood, because anticoagulants may alter cell morphology and staining. There is no single preferred anticoagulant for reptilian hematology, and it is likely that anticoagulant predilection may be taxa-specific. If volume permits, blood for hematology should be collected in ethylenediaminetetraacetic acid and lithium heparin unless a definite anticoagulant of choice has been identified [56–64]. If in doubt, collect into heparin. Because of rapid plasma chemistry changes, samples for biochemistry should be centrifuged immediately.

Variations in hematology and plasma biochemistry may be caused by a myriad of factors. It is therefore recommended to document blood values from all healthy reptiles at routine health examinations, which can then be

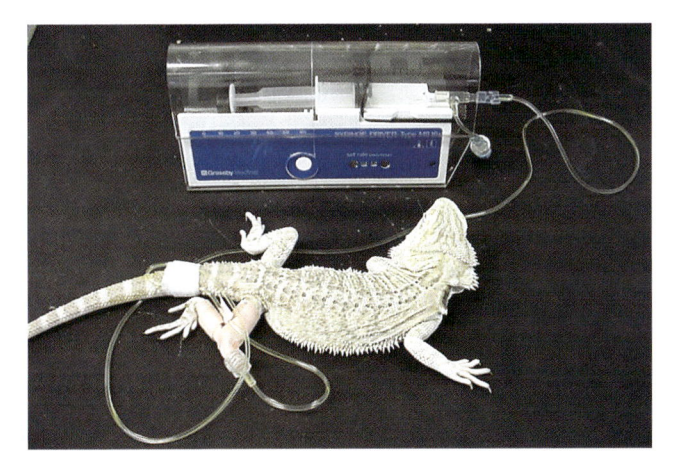

Fig. 5. Intraosseous catheter placed and secured in the tibial medullary cavity of a bearded dragon. Fluid is delivered by way of a syringe pump.

Table 5
Summary of blood collection sites

Group	IV site	Comment
Snakes	Cardiocentesis	Heart should be located (in the second quadrant) and stabilized between the thumb and the index finger; this approach should be performed under anesthesia and in animals weighing no less than 300 g
	Caudal (tail) vein	Needle is advanced until touching vertebrae and then retracted slowly with gentle aspiration
	Jugular vein	Requires cut-down techniques.
	Palatine–pterygoid veins	Reserved for larger patients; often severe bruising; not recommended
Chelonian	Jugular vein	Runs along the neck (usually right is larger) from the dorsal side of the tympanic membrane to the lateral side of the neck
	Dorsal coccygeal (tail) vein	Usually very small volumes, high risk for lymphatic contamination
	Cardiocentesis	Not very practical or safe; access through the plastron or axillary region
	Occipital sinus	Caudal to the occipital process and midline; very useful sinus that originates from the jugular vein
	Subcarapacial sinus	Below the first vertebral scutes of the carapace; it is safe and easy but gets easily lymph-contaminated
Lizards	Caudal (tail) vein	Along the midline and ventral to the vertebral column
	Ventral abdominal vein	Along ventral midline; it should be performed under anesthesia, it is fragile
	Jugular vein	From the tympanic membrane to the point of the shoulder
	Cephalic	Requires cut-down
Crocodilian	Supravertebral vessel	Located just caudal to the occipital and just dorsal to the spinal cord
	Ventral coccygeal vein	Similar to that in *Squamata* (lizards and snakes)

used to assess the animal during illness. A secondary option is careful extrapolation from published data [2,3,10].

Clinical tests of value in the critical patient

At the time of presentation, PCV, plasma protein, and glucose should be determined at a minimum. A blood smear for cell morphology, estimated

WBC count, and differential should be undertaken. Estimated total WBC can be performed by counting 100 WBC in 10 fields at 40× magnification and then multiplying the average by 2000. If a sufficient blood sample is obtained, a complete blood cell count and biochemical panel is recommended to help direct treatment. The Abaxis VetScan machine (Abaxis, Union City, CA) can run a biochemistry profile on just 0.2 mL of whole heparinized blood.

Pulmonary gas exchange is difficult to accurately calculate in reptiles because of heterogeneous gas distribution in their lungs, arrhythmic breathing pattern, extrapulmonary gas exchange, and cardiac and pulmonary vascular shunts, all of which can cause variation in blood gas composition [65]. End tidal CO_2 read by a capnograph during intermittent pressure ventilation may not be a reliable indicator of adequate ventilation in aquatic reptiles, because it may underestimate Pv_{CO2} [66]. The authors, however, have found pediatric mainstream capnography to be extremely valuable in monitoring ventilation. The i-STAT (Sensor Devices, Inc.; Waukesha, WI), which is commonly used in small animals, has not been validated with reptiles but may be useful [67].

Pulse oximetry measures the hemoglobin absorbance and uses the ratio of oxyhemoglobin to deoxyhemoglobin to determine the percent saturation of hemoglobin [68]. Unfortunately, it is often difficult to obtain a reliable pulse wave, and the information provided for the hemoglobin saturation (SO_2) is based on the mammalian oxyhemoglobin dissociation curve. Diethelm suggests the use of the pulse oximeter as a valid tool for SO_2 determination in the green iguana [69], and it has been found useful in other reptile species [70–72]. In several studies in which SO_2 was directly compared with blood gas values, however, the pulse oximeter was deemed inaccurate [70,72]. It remains unclear at this time whether pulse oximetry or hand-held blood-gas analyzers are accurate monitoring devices for use in reptiles.

Reptile urine is always isosthenuric (1.005–1.010), but it can still provide valuable information. Renal urine passes through the urodeum of the cloaca and into the colon or, if present, the bladder. Bladder urine is therefore seldom sterile. In addition, postrenal modification of urine occurs in the cloaca, colon, or bladder. Urinalysis and microscopic evaluation (eg, erythrocytes, leukocytes, cellular or protein casts, and parasites) can assist assessing health status and direct the diagnostic plan [5].

Microbiologic samples from wounds should be collected and submitted for cytology and culture/sensitivity before starting antimicrobial therapy. Immediate inhouse cytology (Diff quick) and Gram stains can be helpful in guiding antimicrobial therapy until culture and sensitivity results are forthcoming [73].

Diagnostic imaging (eg, radiography, ultrasonography) can assist diagnosis but may have to be postponed until the patient is stable. Rarely the reptile patient requires immediate surgical intervention (eg, penetrating injury). Radiographs of the chelonian should include a horizontal beam cranial to caudal view to evaluate the lungs (ie, pneumonia). Radiographs should be evaluated for bone density, foreign bodies, obstructive lesions, hepatomegaly, renomegaly, uroliths, pneumonia, and other signs of disease, including osteomyelitis, articular gout, soft tissue mineralization, pre- and postovulatory stasis, coelomic mass, and coelomic effusion. If plain radiography is unrevealing or if there is a suspected gastric obstruction/mass, contrast-enhanced radiography can be performed. Contrast radiographs may take hours to days to complete in some species [74]. Maintaining the animal at the high end of its POTZ is important for normal gut motility. Because of the risk for barium sulfate desiccating in the digestive tract and resulting in intestinal obstruction, Omnipaque (iohexol) 240 mg/mL (Nycomed Inc., Princeton, NJ) is preferred [75]. Ultrasonography can also provide useful information (eg, hepatic aspiration, coelomic fluid collection, gastrointestinal function, reproductive tract assessment, and so on.) [75]. A proposal for standardization of echocardiography in snakes has been recently put forth [76].

If pneumonia is suspected, a transtracheal wash or percutaneous lung wash is indicated for sample collection before starting antibiotic treatment. The sample should be evaluated by direct wet mount, stained cytology, and bacterial/fungal culture and sensitivity testing [5]. A volume equal to 0.5% to 1% body weight of sterile saline (0.5–1 mL/100 g) is delivered into the trachea/lungs with a red rubber catheter (Sherwood Medical, Norfolk, NE) of appropriate size, and the patient should be gently rotated before retrieving the sample into a sterile container [77].

Treatment and nutritional support

The goals of emergency treatment are to return the patient to its preferred body temperature, to maintain fluid status and cardiorespiratory function, and pain management. Antimicrobial therapy should be based on the identification of an infectious agent by cytology, Gram stain, culture, and sensitivity. Most common infections in reptiles are caused by gram-negative and anaerobic microorganisms. Common antimicrobial therapies used with critical reptiles are described in Table 6. Carpenter [10] and Mader [3] are good resources for further information regarding dosages and treatment.

Once the patient has been stabilized, further diagnostics can be initiated, including additional blood tests, fecal evaluations, radiography, endoscopy, and so on.

Nutritional support should follow rehydration once the animal is stable. It is therefore seldom part of critical care but rather of prolonged medical treatment. Enteral supplementation to a functional gastrointestinal tract can be performed by means of assisted syringe feeding, orogastric feeding, pharyngostomy, or gastrotomy. The specific treatment depends on the patient's calculated energy needs, which should be carefully determined (Table 7). Cachexic patients should receive only 10% to 20% of their daily energy requirements for the first few days, and then be gradually increased to the

Table 6
Antimicrobials commonly used with critical reptile patients

Antibiotic	Dosage	Comments
Enrofloxacin	Snakes and lizards: 5 mg/kg SC; IM every 24–48 h Chelonians: 5–10 mg/kg	Causes muscle necrosis if given repeatedly IM or SC; good gram-negative spectrum, but no anaerobic spectrum
Ceftazidime	20 mg/kg IM, IV every 72 h	Excellent gram-negative spectrum and some gram-positive and anaerobic spectrum
Ticarcillin	50–100 mg/kg IM every 24 h	Good gram-positive spectrum and some gram-negative and anaerobic spectrum; restricted to well-hydrated patients
Metronidazole	20 mg/kg PO every 24–48 h	Good anaerobic spectrum

Abbreviations: IM, intramuscularly; IV, intravenously; PO, orally; SC, subcutaneously.

energy goal to avoid refeeding syndrome or overloading an atrophied gastrointestinal tract [5,78].

Gavage feeding can be used for short-term feeding of most reptiles. Esophagostomy tubes can be placed in animals that are difficult to gavage feed (such as tortoises) or if long-term supplementation is required. The

Table 7
Food calculation

Food	Calories (Kcal/mL Kcal/g)	Protein (%)	Carbohydrates (%)	Fat (%)	Ca:P ratio	Osmolality (mOsm/kg)
Emeraid I	2	—	—	—	—	—
Emeraid II	1.53	—	—	—	—	—
Ensure	1	18	13	9	1.2:1	—
Hills a/d	1.3	—	—	—	—	—
Isocal	1.06	13	50	37	1.2:1	270
Oxbow CCF	0.65	16	55	3.2	2:1	—
Earthworm	4.65	49.9	—	5.8	1.9	—
Cricket	5.4	55.3	—	30.2	0.31	—
Mealworm	6.53	52.8	—	35	0.11	—

To calculate the basal energy requirement (BER): basal metabolic rate (BMR) = K (Wkg$^{0.75}$) = kcal/day, where K is 10, the energy constant for reptiles, and Wkg is the body weight in kg.

To calculate the maintenance energy requirement (MER): MER = BMR × f = kcal/day, where f is the energy factor: physical inactivity = 0.25 – 0.5, starvation = 0.12 – 0.725, hypometabolism = 0.25 – 0.98, elective surgery = 1.0 – 1.2, mild trauma = 1.0 – 1.2, severe trauma = 1.2 – 1.5, growth = 1.2 – 1.8, sepsis = 1.0 – 1.5.

To calculate the volume of formula required and schedule: MER ÷ kcal/mL (nutritional formula chosen) = mL of formula per day. Total number of daily meals (as per DVM discretion) = meals/day. Volume to be fed at each meal = mL/day ÷ number of daily meals.

technique has been described previously [79]. The indwelling esophagostomy tube placement is performed under local or light general anesthesia, and the tube should be measured and marked so that the tip of the tube is within the stomach. A red-rubber catheter or nasogastric tube is used. The head is extended and a hemostat is placed through the mouth into the pharynx. The tips of the hemostat are tented lateral against the esophagus ventral to the jugular vein. A small incision over the points of the hemostats permits the instrument to be forced through the skin. The tube is grasped and pulled back through the incision and redirected caudally down the esophagus and into the stomach. A Chinese finger suture is used to close the skin incision and attach the tube to the patient. The open end of the tube is taped or sutured to the dorsum of the body or shell.

Analgesia and anesthesia

Patients should be physiologically stable before induction of anesthesia, because all anesthetics produce some degree of cardiopulmonary depression. For a detailed description of reptile anesthesia, the reader is directed to major reviews on the subject [45,80,81]. In general, if anesthesia is essential for a critical patient, isoflurane or sevoflurane by mask is recommended for snakes and lizards, but injectables may be required for chelonians and crocodilians. Local anesthesia may be a viable option over general anesthesia for minor procedures (eg, catheter cut-down, esophagostomy tube placement). Analgesia must never be ignored, even in reptiles that seem unresponsive to painful stimuli.

Analgesics

- Morphine: 0.05 to 4 mg/kg intramuscularly (IM), intracutaneously (IC) [82], subcutaneously (SC) [81] every 12 hours. A dosage of 1.5 and 6.5 mg/kg SC in red-eared slider [83] and 1 and 1.5 mg/kg IM has been used by the authors in sliders with excellent results (unpublished data). Greater than 0.1 mg/kg IM in green iguana [84].
- Butorphanol: 0.2 to 2 mg/kg SC, IM, IV every 12 to 24 hours [81]. At 1.5 mg/kg and 8 mg/kg IM in green iguana [84]. Doses of 2.8 and 28 mg/kg SC did not provide adequate analgesia in red-eared slider [83].
- Buprenorphine: 0.02 to 0.2 SC, IM every 12 to 24 hours [81]. Buprenorphine was found to be not effective at 0.02 and 0.1 mg/kg in green iguana [84].
- Meperidine: 1 to 4 mg/kg IC [82], IM [85] every 12 to 24 hours (not in snakes [86]).
- Carprofen: 1 to 4 mg/kg orally, SC, IM, IV every 24 hours [81].
- Meloxicam: 0.1 to 0.2 mg/kg IM or IV every 24 to 48 hours [81] or 0.2 mg/kg IM or IV every 48 hours (Hernandez-Divers, unpublished data).

Some opioids seem to be ineffective in reptiles [83,84,87]. Although endogenous opioids and opioid receptors have been evaluated in reptiles, there is little information about pain perception and its alleviation [83,88–90]. The administration of opioids has not been associated with significant changes in behavior (eg, sedation) or physiologic parameters (eg, heart rate, respiration rate) [46]. Sladky, however, reports respiratory depression when using morphine at 1.5 mg/kg SC in red-eared sliders [83]. Morphine and meperidine have been used in crocodiles, demonstrating onset of action at 30 minutes and duration of effect lasting 2.0 to 2.5 hours [82]. Greenacre's study has contradictory results in which butorphanol was effective at 1.5 mg/kg and 8.0 mg/kg IM but not at 4.0 mg/kg IM [84].

Local anesthetics (eg, lidocaine, bupivacaine) provide complete anesthesia by interrupting nervous conduction and may be beneficial when the critical nature of a patient precludes general anesthesia (eg, IO catheterization, external coaptation of a fracture). In the absence of reptile-specific data, generally accepted toxic doses should not be exceeded (eg, bupivacaine 0.25% <2 m/kg, lidocaine 2% without epinephrine <2 mg/kg). Lidocaine (2 mg/kg) mixed with bupivacaine 0.25% (1 mg/kg) is commonly used. The combination of lidocaine and bupivacaine locally infiltrated at the surgery site can help to reduce or negate the need for anesthetic drug in critical patients. A dose-dependent "epidural" anesthesia has been described in the red-footed tortoise (*Geochelone carbonaria*) with lidocaine at approximately 4 to 8 mg/kg that provided an anesthetic period of 45 to 85 and 60 to 206 minutes [91].

Nonsteroidal anti-inflammatory drugs (NSAIDs) act by modulating nociception in the periphery and the spinal cord. The unknown actions of NSAIDs in the central and peripheral nervous system of reptiles may result in unpredictable variations in duration, potency, and side effects of the drugs used. All precautions with NSAID use in small mammals should be followed in reptiles (ie, avoid in poorly perfused, dehydrated reptiles with renal or gastrointestinal disease). Use NSAIDs primarily in the well-hydrated patient or for the stable reptile patient requiring analgesia following discharge. There have been no published studies evaluating NSAIDs in reptiles; however, unpublished pharmacokinetic data in iguanas has indicated that 0.2 mg/kg meloxicam IM or IV maintains appropriate blood levels for 36 to 48 hours (Hernandez-Divers, unpublished data, 2007).

The use of dissociative anesthetics and potent alpha-2 agonists should be carefully considered and is best avoided in critical reptiles. Some anesthetic protocols for critical patients are summarized:

- Chelonians
    - Premedication: butorphanol (1–2 mg/kg) IM [81] or buprenorphine (0.1–1.0 mg/kg) IM [92] or butorphanol (0.4 mg/kg) or morphine (1.5 mg/kg) + midazolam (2 mg/kg) IM [93]
    - Induction: IV or IO propofol to effect (often 2–12 mg/kg) [81]
    - Maintenance: isoflurane or sevoflurane

- Lizards
    - Premedication: butorphanol (1–4 mg/kg) IM [81] or morphine (1.5 mg/kg)
    - Induction: IV or IO propofol to effect (often 5–10 mg/kg) or isoflurane 5% (may result in prolonged induction time if breath holding)
    - Maintenance: isoflurane [94,95] or sevoflurane [95]
- Snakes
    - Premedication: butorphanol (1–4 mg/kg) IM or morphine (1.5 mg/kg)
    - Induction: isoflurane 5% or sevoflurane 8% in induction chamber (eg, tube or sealed bag), or IV propofol to effect (often 3–8 mg/kg)
    - Maintenance: isoflurane or sevoflurane

Common emergency presentations

Respiratory emergencies

True respiratory emergencies are limited and usually are a manifestation of a chronic condition or acute trauma. Common respiratory emergencies in reptiles are obstructive processes within the oropharynx and trachea from infectious granulomas (eg, abscess), foreign bodies or neoplasia (eg, tracheal chondroma), pneumonia, and drowning [14,96]. Road traffic accidents involving chelonians frequently cause severe shell trauma that may involve the carapace and underlying lungs. Clinical signs in reptiles may be subtle and difficult to recognize [96]. Clinical signs may include nasal discharge, oral discharge, glottal discharge, dyspnea, open-mouth breathing, crusted external nares (the presence of normal salt glands in some lizards can have the same effect), puffy throat, abnormal posturing, blowing bubbles, sneezing, and increased respiratory sounds.

Oxygen supplementation by way of face mask may be beneficial as short-term management [96]. Endotracheal intubation or tracheostomy tube placement should be attempted in severe cases. Endotracheal tube selection should be performed according to species and size. Current recommendations for ventilatory support include 2 to 6 breaths per minute using tidal volumes ranging from 15 to 30 mL/kg, with a peak airway pressure less than 8 cm H_2O.

Drowning is more common in chelonians but may occur in any reptile with access to water. Marine turtles can drown when incidentally entangled in shrimp nets or fishing gear. Live turtles that have been submerged under water for extended periods may present comatose without a deep pain or corneal reflex. CPCR protocols described earlier should be used in cases of cardiac or respiratory arrest. Once intubated, the turtle should be placed with its head down to drain fluid from the lungs. Suctioning from the endotracheal tube may be of benefit. Intermittent positive-pressure ventilation with oxygen and warming may assist in reviving the turtle. Blood gas and lactate levels should be monitored during treatment to assess success of treatment (eg, decreasing levels of lactate and improvement in the acidosis).

If pneumonia is suspected, a tracheal wash or percutaneous lung wash should be performed for sample collection and agent isolation. The reptile should be well perfused and hydrated (see section on fluid therapy). Antimicrobial choice should be based on Gram stain and cytology while awaiting culture and sensitivity results (Table 7).

Cardiovascular emergencies

The most common cardiovascular emergency is severe hemorrhage, which should be controlled with pressure, radiosurgery, or ligation of vessels [14]. The clinical signs for other cardiovascular diseases are nonspecific, such as malaise, anorexia, weight loss, change in skin color, and ultimately death. Other signs include swelling in the area of the heart (cardiomegaly, pericardial effusion), peripheral edema, ascites, cyanosis, and ecchymosis. Congenital cardiovascular anomalies have also been reported, most commonly in the neonate, and are associated with the myocardium or great vessels [97].

Electrocardiography can assist in the diagnosis but should not be performed in hypothermic reptiles, because identification of complexes and wave boundaries can be challenging [16]. Lead placement is (sub)order specific (see Table 5) [17].

Neurologic emergencies (ataxia, paresis, convulsions)

Neurologic signs such as lethargy and depression can be difficult to objectively evaluate. Moribund is usually obvious but can be difficult to differentiate from death. A complete neurologic examination should be performed. Clinical signs may be related to improper husbandry (including diet deficiencies, such as thiamine deficiency in snakes fed frozen-thawed fish or any one of several metabolic bone diseases), head trauma, intoxication (eg, organophosphates, heavy metals), infection or infestation, metabolic disease, and neoplasia. Spastic tremors and fasciculations are commonly present with severe calcium:phosphorus ratio imbalances.

Nutritional or renal secondary hyperparathyroidism (calcium:phosphorus ratio imbalances)

Clinical signs of secondary hyperparathyroidism include anorexia, dysphagia, ileus, listlessness, partial to complete lack of truncal lifting, and fibrous swellings of the mandible, limbs, and tail. Loss of bone density, skeletal deformities (eg, scoliosis, bowing) and pathologic fractures are common. In severe cases, muscular twitching, spasm, and paralysis are usually evident.

Nutritional secondary hyperparathyroidism is most commonly seen in young, growing reptiles owing to improper care. Herbivorous, insectivorous, and omnivorous reptiles are usually affected because of lack of proper husbandry (eg, lack of UV light) and diet (eg, lack of nutritional supplement, balanced diet, lack of owner knowledge). Carnivorous reptiles (eg, snakes) are less commonly seen with these signs, because they typically feed on balanced whole prey.

Reproductive activity (in previously normal females) may unmask signs of hypocalcemia (fasciculations and tremors) because of the current high calcium demands and borderline diet and husbandry. In these cases a complete physical examination, blood analysis including ionized calcium (1.47 ± 0.105 mmol/L in green iguanas [98]), and radiography are recommended. In cases of hypocalcemia (nutritional or renal related, Ca:P <1), temperature, fluid, and electrolyte support are the most immediate concerns. In iguanas, a Ca:P ratio of 1:1 or less than 1 indicates calcium deficiency, phosphorus excess, or inadequate vitamin D_3 (from deficiencies in diet, lighting, temperature, or severe kidney disease), and therefore it should be carefully investigated. If tetany is present, calcium gluconate 10% can be administered at 100 mg/kg (IM, intraceolomicly) every 6 hours, or given IV or IO to effect, and then orally [99]. Injectable calcium therapy is painful and can be detrimental to the kidneys at high doses [99]. Slow IV calcium administration to effect is preferred. In cases of hyperphosphatemia, parenteral calcium may predispose to soft tissue mineralization because of increases in the solubility index.

In adult reptiles, renal secondary hyperparathyroidism is more common. The cause for renal disease is likely to be multifactorial, such as low humidity, excessive protein intake, over-supplementation with vitamin D_3, and so on.

Hyperphosphatemia is often the first plasma chemistry abnormality seen with renal failure. Advanced cases may show an increase in plasma uric acid (or urea in aquatic species). Treatment is based on supportive care (nutrition and fluid therapy for chronic renal failure), and correcting the electrolyte imbalance (hyperphosphatemia and hypocalcemia). Oral phosphate binders (aluminium hydroxide, Amphojel) between meals and allopurinol (20–50 mg/kg orally every 24 hours) can be added to the treatment regimen [100]. A study in green iguanas demonstrated that a dose of 25 mg/kg every 24 hours of allopurinol decreased uric acid by 41% to 45% in hyperuricemic lizards [101]. Fluids are initially given as described in the section on fluid therapy and then using twice maintenance for diuresis until normal.

Gastrointestinal tract emergencies

Gastrointestinal foreign bodies

Ingestion of foreign bodies can be common in reptiles, especially in those permitted to free roam [102,103]. Lithophagy or geophagy may be associated with improper diet or husbandry. In mild to moderate cases, medical treatment may include correcting dehydration and electrolyte imbalances, assisted feedings, mineral oil (5 mL/kg), and petroleum laxatives mixed with water. Nonresponsive cases or those with an obvious complete obstruction, however, require surgery [14,103].

Regurgitation or vomiting

Regurgitation and vomiting can be easily confused in reptiles. Often the problem tends to be vomiting and can be related to husbandry: inappropriate diet size or amount, temperature, and postprandial handling. Rule-outs should include stomatitis, gastroenteritis (parasitic, viral, bacterial, or fungal), gastrointestinal stasis, and luminal or extraluminal gastrointestinal obstruction (eg, granuloma, neoplasia, abscess, foreign body). After a complete physical examination, hematology and biochemistry, fecal examination, and plain and contrast-enhanced radiography are recommended. Gastroscopy may assist diagnostic and, if needed, biopsies can be obtained.

Integumental emergencies

The most common skin emergencies are chemical and thermal burns, bites, and traumatic wounds (eg, abrasions, hit by car, and so on) [102]. Thermal burns are more commonly encountered when reptiles are kept in cages with a poorly protected heat source, including hot rocks or heating bulbs. Bite wounds are often serious and deep. These may occur when snakes are fed live animals (eg, rodents) but are also seen during ecdysis or in lethargic, sick, and aestivating reptiles.

Hemorrhage should be controlled and perfusion corrected with fluid therapy. Analgesia should be provided accordingly. Primary or delayed closure or secondary intention healing of wounds should be determined. Primary wound closure is appropriate for noncontaminated wounds of less than 6 to 12 hours of duration [104]. The methods for initial wound care and treatment in small animals are also applicable to reptiles [104]. If culture and sensitivity tests are to be performed, samples should be obtained before wound treatment. Wounds should be protected until the patient is fully examined and stable. Once the patient is stabilized, the wounds should be thoroughly assessed (skeletal, vascular, and neural integrity), débrided, and profusely cleaned. Sterile saline is a good option for wound flushes. Wounds should be reassessed periodically for tissue viability and further tissue debridement (surgical, mechanical by wet-to-dry bandages).

Prophylactic antimicrobial is controversial. Although there is no evidence of its benefit in properly debrided and drained wounds, systemic antimicrobials might be recommended for severe injuries [105–107]. Initial drug choice should be based on wound Gram stain and knowledge of likely organisms and sensitivities. Attention should be given to gram-negative pathogens (amikacin, ceftazidime, enrofloxacin) and the anaerobes (metronidazole, chloramphenicol). Combination therapy (eg, clindamycin and enrofloxacin;

ciprofloxacin and clindamycin; or ceftazidime and metronidazole) may be warranted in most cases of prey bites.

Burns, thermal or chemical, should be profusely irrigated with sterile saline solution. Treatment varies depending on the degree of the burn. First-degree burns benefit from cold-water rinses or cold compresses. Ice should not be used, because it could cause freeze damage to the tissue. Blisters should not be broken, because they can get infected. Second-degree burns should be debrided and treated daily. Topical creams such as silver sulfadiazine (Silvadene cream, Monarch Pharmaceuticals Inc., Bristol, TN) should be applied and systemic antimicrobial therapy started to prevent infection. Ticarcillin (50–100 mg/kg IM every 24 hours) and ceftazidime (20–30 mg/kg IM every 48–72 hours) are often considered the initial drugs of choice, but Gram stains should help direct therapy [108]. Analgesia and fluid therapy should also be provided accordingly. Third-degree and fourth-degree burns require similar treatment as for second-degree, but they require intensive care and carry a grave prognosis [108].

Cloacal prolapse and reproductive emergencies

Three different systems terminate at the cloaca (reproductive, urinary, and gastrointestinal). Prolapsed tissue should therefore be examined closely and identified. In cases of severe damage from chronic exposure or trauma it can be difficult to distinguish tissue origin. The rectum/colon and the salpinx are tubular organs with a lumen; however, the salpinx is striated longitudinally, whereas the others are smooth. The bladder (most lizards and all turtles), if still intact, is a fluid-filled, sac-like structure. If exposed for a long time, the bladder may become devitalized and rupture, thus appearing as thin, shredded tissue. The phallus and hemipenis are mushroom-like copulatory structures ranging from pink to black in color. Prolapse treatment varies depending on the cause and the presenting nature of the condition, but in some cases irrigation, lubrication, and occlusive bandaging using clear wrap can be used overnight while the patient is stabilized for anesthesia and surgery the next day.

Cloacal prolapse is often secondary to poor management or a disease process, and further diagnostics are recommended. Prolapse of the salpinx or oviduct can occur as a result of egg binding/dystocia/retained eggs or fetuses, hypocalcemia, salpingitis, neoplasia, or intra-coelomic disease or mass effects. In most cases, the urinary bladder prolapses as a result of cystitis (eg, urolithiasis, infection). Prolapse of the colon is usually the result of tenesmus (eg, colitis, endoparasites, foreign body/fecaliths, renomegaly, improper management, hypocalcemia, or physical deformities). Prolapse of the phallus or hemipenis is usually the result of infection and inflammation secondary to trauma (eg, sex probing), chronic sexual activity, constipation, or neurologic dysfunction. Prolapsed organ reduction can be accomplished using high concentration dextrose solutions to shrink edematous tissues or through surgery.

Dystocia is usually related to unfit animals and improper husbandry conditions (eg, deficient temperature, humidity, nesting place, and the like). Radiography and ultrasonography are indicated to determine if the dystocia is preovulatory (unshelled ova) or postovulatory (shelled eggs or fetuses). Although dystocia in mammals and birds typically requires urgent surgical intervention, reptiles can be stabilized over several days before embarking on surgery unless severe bacterial coelomitis is evident.

Septicemia

Septicemia is a serious condition that should be treated aggressively with systemic antibiotics. Blood cultures should be performed whenever it is suspected and before being on antibiotics. Clinical signs vary from generalized petechiae to depression and seizures. Osteoarthropathy lesions may develop 22 to 36 months after an episode of septicemia [109].

Egg yolk coelomitis is another important condition. It has been reported in several species of lizards, and these patients often respond well to supportive treatment and surgical intervention.

Summary

True acute emergencies are not common, because most presentations relate to a near terminal presentation of a chronic condition. Unfortunately there are still numerous limitations confronting the emergency clinician when dealing with reptiles, including limited knowledge base, species-specific peculiarities, and unfamiliar reptile anatomy and physiology. Similar principles and techniques used in small animal medicine can be applied to reptiles. An understanding of reptilian physiology and anatomy, however, is fundamental if the best emergency care is to be provided.

References

[1] Divers S. Clinical evaluation of reptiles. Vet Clin North Am Exot Anim Pract 1999;2: 291–331.
[2] Girling S, Raiti P. BSAVA manual of reptiles. 2nd edition. Quesgeley (UK): BSAVA; 2004.
[3] Mader DR. Reptile medicine and surgery. 2nd edition. Philadelphia: Elsevier Saunders Inc.; 2006.
[4] Jacobson E. Reptiles. Vet Clin North Am Exot Anim Pract 1987;17:1203–26.
[5] de la Navarre B. Common procedures in reptiles and amphibians. Vet Clin North Am Exot Anim Pract 2006;9:237–67.
[6] Seebacher F, Franklin CE. Physiological mechanisms of thermoregulation in reptiles: a review. J Comp Physiol B 2005;175:533–41.
[7] Batholomew G, Tucker V. Control of changes in body temperature, metabolism, and circulation by the agamid lizard, *Amphibolurus barbatus*. Physiol Zool 1963;36:199–218.
[8] Grigg G, Seebacher F. Field test of a paradigm: hysteresis of heart rate in thermoregulation by a free-ranging lizard (*Pogona barbata*). Proc Roy Soc Lond B 1999;266:1291–7.
[9] Seebacher F, Grigg G. Changes in heart rate are important for thermoregulation in the varanid lizard, *Varanus varius*. J Comp Physiol B 2001;171:395–400.

[10] Carpenter JW. Exotic animal formulary. 3rd edition. Philadelphia: Elsevier Saunders Inc.; 2005.
[11] Bernheim H, Kluger M. Fever and antipyresis in the lizard *Diposaurus dorsalis*. Am J Physiol 1976;231:199–218.
[12] Warwick C. Observations on disease-associated preferred body temperatures in reptiles. Appl Anim Behav Sci 1991;28:375–80.
[13] Rossi J. Biology and husbandry. In: Mader DR, editor. Reptile medicine and surgery. 2nd edition. Philadelphia: Elsevier Saunders Inc.; 2006. p. 25–41.
[14] Boyer L. Emergency care of reptiles. Vet Clin North Am Exotic Anim Pract 1998;1:191–206.
[15] Wang T, Smits A, Burggren W. Pulmonary function in reptiles. In: Gans C, Gaunt A, editors. Biology of the reptilia. Ithaca (NY): Society for the Study of Amphibians and Reptiles; 1998. p. 297–374.
[16] McDonald H. Methods for physiological study of reptiles. In: Gans C, editor. Physiology A. London: Academic Press Inc.; 1976. p. 19–126.
[17] Murray M. Cardiopulmonary anatomy and physiology. In: Mader DR, editor. Reptile medicine and surgery. 2nd edition. Philadelphia: Saunders Elsevier Inc.; 2006. p. 124–34.
[18] Yungin K, Parckchang S. Effects of acetylcholine, vagal stimulation and tyramine on the isolated atria of the tortoise. J Pharm Pharmacol 1965;17:356–61.
[19] Burggren W. Influence of intermittent breathing on ventricular depolarization patterns in the chelonian reptiles. J Physiol 1978;278:349–64.
[20] Ball D, Hicks J. Adrenergic and cholinergic response of ventricular muscle from the turtle, *Trachemys (Pseudemys) scripta*. Comp Biochem Physiol A Physiol 1996;113:135–41.
[21] de Vera L, Gonzalez J, Pereda E. Relationship between cortical electrical and cardiac autonomic activities in the awake lizard, *Gallotia galloti*. J Exp Zool 2000;287:21–8.
[22] Seebacher F, Franklin CE. Integration of autonomic and local mechanisms in regulating cardiovascular responses to heating and cooling in a reptile (*Crocodylus porosus*). J Comp Physiol [Br] 2004;174:577–8.
[23] Messonier S. Formulary for exotic pets. Vet Forum 1996;13:46–9.
[24] Rossi J. Emergency medicine of reptiles. Proc North Am Vet Conf 1998;799–801.
[25] Pace L, Mader D. Atropine and glycopyrrolate, route of administration and response in green iguana (*Iguana iguana*). Proc Assoc Rept Amph Vet 2002;79–84.
[26] Bennett R. Management of common reptile emergencies. Proc ARAV 1998;67–72.
[27] Wang T, Taylor E, Andrade D, et al. Autonomic control of heart rate during forced activity and digestion in the snake *Boa constrictor*. J Exp Biol 2001;204:3553–60.
[28] Wasser J, Meinertz E, Chang S. Metabolic and cardiodynamic responses of isolated turtle hearts to ischemia and reperfusion. Am J Physiol 1992;262:437–43.
[29] Lutz P, Milton S. Negotiating brain anoxia survival in the turtle. J Exp Biol 2004;207:314–7.
[30] Bickler P. Effects of temperature and anoxia on regional cerebral blood flow in turtles. Am J Physiol 1992;262:538–41.
[31] Prentice H, Milton S, Scheurle D, et al. The upregulation of cognate and inducible heat shock proteins in the anoxic turtle brain. J Cereb Blood Flow Metab 2004;24:826–8.
[32] Smits A, Kozubowski M. Partitioning of body fluids and cardiovascular responses to circulatory hypovolaemia in the turtle, *Pseudemys scripta elegans*. J Exp Biol 1985;116:237–50.
[33] Smits A, Lillywhite H. Maintenance of blood volume in snake: transcapillary shifts of extravascular fluids during acute hemorrhage. J Comp Physiol [Br] 1985;155:305–10.
[34] White F. Circulation. In: Gans C, Dawson W, editors. Physiology A. New York: Academic Press; 1976. p. 275–334.
[35] Bentley P. Osmoregulation. In: Gans C, editor. Physiology A. London: Academic Press Inc.; 1976. p. 365–412.
[36] Minnich H. The use of water. In: Gans C, editor. Biology of the reptilia, Physiology C. London: Academic Press Inc.; 1982.

[37] Burggren W, Farrell A, Lillywhite H. Vertebrae cardiovascular systems. In: Dantzler W, editor. Handbook of physiology section 13; comparative physiology. New York: Oxford University Press; 1997. p. 254–67.
[38] Lillywhite H, Pough F. Control of arterial pressure in aquatic sea snake. Am J Physiol 1983; 244:R66–73.
[39] Stephens G, Shirer H, Trank J, et al. Arterial baroreceptor reflex control of heart rate in two species of turtle. Am J Physiol 1983;244:544–52.
[40] Chiu K, Wong V, Chan M, et al. Blood pressure homeostasis in the snake, *Ptyas korros*. Gen Comp Endocrinol 1986;64:300–4.
[41] Crossley D, Hicks J, Altimiras J. Ontogeny of baroreflex control in the American alligator. J Exp Biol 2003;206:2895–902.
[42] Stinner J, Ely D. Blood pressure during routine activity, stress, and feeding in the black racer snakes. Am J Physiol 1993;264:79–84.
[43] Farrell A. Introduction to cardiac scope in lower vertebrates. Can J Zool 1991;69: 1981–4.
[44] Lichtenberger M. Principles of shock and fluid therapy in special species. Semin Avian Exotic Pet Med 2004;13:142–53.
[45] Mosley C. Anesthesia and analgesia in reptiles. Semin Avian Exotic Pet Med 2005;14: 243–62.
[46] Mosley C, Dyson D, Smith D. The cardiovascular dose-response effects of isoflurane alone and combined with butorphanol in the green iguana (*Iguana iguana*). Vet Anaesth Analg 2004;31:64–72.
[47] Mader DR, Rudloff E. Emergency and critical care. In: Mader DR, editor. Reptile medicine and surgery. 2nd edition. Philadelphia: Saunders Elsevier Inc.; 2006. p. 533–48.
[48] Holz P, Barker I, Burger J, et al. The effect of the renal portal system on pharmacokinetic parameters in the red-eared slider. J Zoo Wildl Med 1997;28:386–93.
[49] Holz P, Burger J, Pasloske K, et al. Effect of injection site on carbenicillin pharmacokinetics in the carpet python, *Morelia spilota*. J Herpetol Med Surg 2002;12:12–6.
[50] Akester A. Radiographic studies of the renal portal system in the domestic fowl (*Gallus domesticus*). J Anat 1964;98:365–76.
[51] Heard D. Perioperative supportive care and monitoring. Vet Clin North Am Exot Anim Pract 2000;3:587–615.
[52] Wellehan FX, Lafortune M, Gunkel C. Coccygeal vascular catheterization in lizards and crocodilians. J Herpetol Med Surg 2004;14:26–8.
[53] Hernandez-Divers S. Diagnostic techniques. In: Mader D, editor. Reptile medicine and surgery. 2nd edition. Philadelphia: Elsevier Saunders Inc.; 2006. p. 490–532.
[54] Jenkins JR. Diagnostic and clinical techniques. In: Mader DR, editor. Reptile medicine and surgery. Philadelphia: Saunders; 1996. p. 264–76.
[55] Briscoe JA, Syring R. Techniques for emergency airway and vascular access in special species. Semin Avian Exotic Pet Med 2004;13:118–31.
[56] Harr KE, Raskin RE, Heard DJ. Temporal effects of 3 commonly used anticoagulants on hematologic and biochemical variables in blood samples from macaws and Burmese pythons. Vet Clin Pathol 2005;34:383–8.
[57] Dotson TK, Ramsay EC, Bounous DI. A color atlas of blood cells of the yellow rat snake. Compend Contin Educ Pract Vet 1995;17:1013–26.
[58] Lamirande EW, Bratthauer AD, Fisher DC, et al. Reference hematologic and plasma chemistry values of brown tree snakes (*Boiga irregularis*). J Zoo Wildl Med 1999;30:516–20.
[59] Salakij C, Salakij J, Apibal S, et al. Hematology, morphology, cytochemical staining, and ultrastructural characteristics of blood cells in king cobras (*Ophiophagus hannah*). Vet Clin Pathol 2002;31:116–26.
[60] Muro J, Cuenca R, Pastor J, et al. Effects of lithium heparin and tripotassium EDTA on hematologic values of Hermann's tortoises (*Testudo hermanni*). J Zoo Wildl Med 1998; 29:40–4.

[61] Marks SK, Citino SB. Hematology and serum chemistry of the radiated tortoise (*Testudo radiata*). J Zoo Wildl Med 1990;21:342–4.
[62] Hanley CS, Hernandez-Divers SJ, Bush S, et al. Comparison of the effect of dipotassium ethylenediaminetetraacetic acid and lithium heparin on hematologic values in the green iguana (*Iguana iguana*). J Zoo Wildl Med 2004;35:328–32.
[63] Stacy BA, Whitaker N. Hematology and blood biochemistry of captive mugger crocodiles (*Crocodylus palustrus*). J Zoo Wildl Med 2000;31:339–47.
[64] Martinez-Jimenez D, Hernandez-Divers SJ, Floyd TM, et al. Comparison of the effects of dipotassium ethylenediaminetetraacetic acid and lithium heparin on hematologic values in yellow-blotched map turtles (Graptemys flavimaculata). J Herpetol Med Surg; in press.
[65] Wood S, Lenfant C. Respiration: mechanics, control and gas exchange. In: Gans C, editor. Physiology A. London: Academic Press Inc.; 1976. p. 225–74.
[66] Chittick E, Stamper M, Beasley J, et al. Medetomidine, ketamine, and sevoflurane for anesthesia of injured loggerhead sea turtles: 13 cases (1996–2000). J Am Vet Med Assoc 2002;221:1019–25.
[67] Heard D. Critical care monitoring. Vet Clin North Am Exotic Anim Pract 1998;1:1–10.
[68] Alexander C, Teller L, Gross J. Principles of pulse oximetry. Theoretical and practical considerations. Anaesth Analg 1989;68:368–76.
[69] Diethelm G, Mader D, Grosenbaugh D. Evaluating pulse oximetry in the green iguana (*Iguana iguana*). Proc ARAV 1998;11–2.
[70] Bennett R, Schumacher J, Hedjazi-Haring K. Cardiopulmonary and anesthetic effects of propofol administered intraosseously to green iguanas. J Am Vet Med Assoc 1998;212:93–8.
[71] Moon P, Stabenau E. Anesthetic and postanesthetic management of sea turtles. J Am Vet Med Assoc 1996;208:720–6.
[72] Anderson N, Wack R, Calloway L. Cardiopulmonary effects and efficacy of propofol as an anesthetic agent in brown tree snakes, *Boiga irregularis*. Bull Assoc Reptilian Amphibian Vet 1999;9:9–15.
[73] Hernandez-Divers S. Reptile critical care in emergency practice. Presented at the 11th International Veterinary Emergency and Critical Care Symposium 2005;87–93.
[74] Raiti P. Colonic obstruction in a red-eared slider (*Trachemys scripta elegans*). Proc ARAV 2006;75.
[75] Silverman S. Diagnostic imaging. In: Mader DR, editor. Reptile medicine and surgery. 2nd edition. Philadelphia: Saunders Elsevier Inc.; 2006. p. 471–89.
[76] Schilliger L, Dominique T, Pouchelon J-L, et al. Proposed standardization of the two-dimensional echocardiographic examination in snakes. J Herpetol Med Surg 2006;16:76–87.
[77] Murray MJ. Pneumonia and lower respiratory tract disease. In: Mader DR, editor. Reptile medicine and surgery. 2nd edition. Philadelphia: Saunders Elsevier Inc.; 2006. p. 865–77.
[78] Donoghue S. Nutrition. In: Mader DR, editor. Reptile medicine and surgery. 2nd edition. Philadelphia: Saunders Elsevier Inc.; 2006. p. 251–98.
[79] Bonner B. Chelonian therapeutics. Vet Clin North Am Exot Anim Pract 2000;3:257–332.
[80] Machin K. Fish, amphibian, and reptile analgesia. Vet Clin North Am Exot Anim Pract 2001;4:19–33.
[81] Schumacher J, Yelen T. Anesthesia and analgesia. In: Mader DR, editor. Reptile medicine and surgery. Philadelphia: Saunders Elsevier Inc.; 2006. p. 442–52.
[82] Kanui TI, Hole K. Morphine and pethidine antinociception in the crocodile. J Vet Pharmacol Ther 1992;15:101–3.
[83] Sladky KK, Paul-Murphy J, Miletic V, et al. Morphine, but not butorphanol, causes analgesia and respiratory depression in red-eared slider turtle (*Trachemys scripta*). Proc AAZV 2006;274–5.
[84] Greenacre C, Takle G, Schumacher J, et al. Comparative antinociception of morphine, butorphanol, and buprenorphine versus saline in the green iguana (*Iguana iguana*), using electrostimulation. J Herpetol Med Surg 2006;16:88–92.

[85] Heard DJ. Principles and techniques of anesthesia and analgesia for exotic practice. Vet Clin North Am Small Anim Pract 1993;23:1301–27.
[86] Bennett R. A review of anesthesia and chemical restraint in reptiles. J Zoo Wildl Med 1991; 22:282–303.
[87] Heard DJ. Reptile anesthesia. In: Heard DJ, editor. Analgesia and anesthesia. Philadelphia: W.B. Saunders Company; 2001. p. 83–117.
[88] Kanui T, Hole K, Miaron J. Nociception in crocodiles: capsaicin instillation, formalin and hot plate tests. Zoolog Sci 1990;7:537–40.
[89] Liang Y, Terashima S. Physiological properties and morphological characteristics of cutaneous and mucosal mechanical nociceptive neurons with A-delta peripheral axons in the trigeminal ganglia of crotaline snake. J Comp Neurol 1993;328:88–102.
[90] Dela Iglesia J, Martinez-Guijarro F, Loper-Garcia C. Neurons of the medial cortex outer plexiform layer of the lizard: Golgi and immunocytochemical studies. J Comp Neurol 1994; 341:184–203.
[91] Fontenelle J, Carvalho do Nascimento C, Lozano Cruz M, et al. Anesthesia epidural em jabuti piranga (Geochelone carbonaria). Presented at the Anais do IV congresso e IX encontro da ABRAVAS 2000. Sao Pedro, Brazil.
[92] Bennett R, Divers S, Schumacher J. Anesthesia. Bull Assoc Reptilian Amphibian Vet 1999; 9:20–7.
[93] Bennett R. Reptile anesthesia. Semin Avian Exotic Pet Med 1998;7:30–40.
[94] Mosley C, Dyson D, Smith D. Minimum alveolar concentration of isoflurane in green iguanas and the effect of butorphanol on minimum alveolar concentration. J Am Vet Med Assoc 2003;222:1559–64.
[95] Barter L, Hawkins M, Brosnan R, et al. Median effective dose of isoflurane, sevoflurane, and desflurane in green iguanas. Am J Vet Res 2006;67:392–7.
[96] Schumacher J. Reptile respiratory medicine. Vet Clin North Am Exotic Anim Pract 2003;6: 213–31.
[97] Murray MJ. Cardiology and circulation. In: Mader DR, editor. Reptile medicine and surgery. 1st edition. Philadelphia: Saunders; 1996. p. 95–104.
[98] Dennis P, Bennett R, Harr K, et al. Plasma concentration of ionized calcium in healthy iguanas. J Am Vet Med Assoc 2001;219:326–8.
[99] Mader D. Metabolic bone disease. In: Mader D, editor. Reptile medicine and surgery. 2nd edition. Philadelphia: Saunders Elsevier Inc.; 2006. p. 841–51.
[100] Mader D. Gout. In: Mader DR, editor. Reptile medicine and surgery. Philadelphia: Saunders Elsevier Inc.; 2006. p. 793–800.
[101] Hernandez-Divers S, Martinez-Jimenez D, Latimer K, et al. Effects of allopurinol on plasma uric acid level in normo- and hyperuricaemic green iguanas (*Iguana iguana*). J Herpetol Med Surg; in press.
[102] Wellehan FX, Gunkel C. Emergent diseases in reptiles. Semin Avian Exotic Pet Med 2004; 13:160–74.
[103] Rivera S, Crane MM, McManamon R. Medical and surgical treatment of gastric foreign bodies in newly imported impressed tortoises (*Manouria impressa*). Proc ARAV 2006;78–82.
[104] Mitchell M, Diaz-Figueroa O. Wound management in reptiles. Vet Clin North Am Exot Anim 2004;7:123–40.
[105] Underman R. Bite wounds inflicted by cats and dogs. Vet Clin North Am Small Anim Pract 1987;17:195–207.
[106] August J. Dog and cat bites. J Am Vet Med Assoc 1988;193:1394–8.
[107] Cowell A, Penwick R. Dog bite wounds: a study of 93 cases. Compend Contin Educ Pract Vet 1989;11:313–20.
[108] Mader D. Thermal burns. In: Mader DR, editor. Reptile medicine and surgery. Philadelphia: Saunders Elsevier Inc.; 2006. p. 916–23.
[109] Kiel J. Spinal osteoarthropathy in two southern copperheads. J Zoo Am Med 1977;8:21–4.

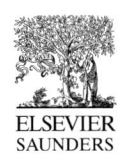

Amphibian Emergency Medicine

Leigh Ann Clayton, DVM, DABVP-Avian*, Stacey R. Gore, DVM

Department of Animal Health, National Aquarium in Baltimore, 501 East Pratt Street, Baltimore, MD 21202-3194, USA

There are more than 4,000 species of animals in the class Amphibia, which is divided into three orders: Anura (frogs and toads), Caudata (salamanders, newts, and sirens), and Gymnophiona (caecelians) [1]. Anurans and caudatans are most commonly kept in captivity and are the focus of this discussion, though concepts presented here apply to caecilians also. Interested readers are referred to a more detailed review of caecilian medicine [2]. A brief review of amphibian biology is presented. General concepts of amphibian emergency medicine are discussed; including a review of patient selection, appropriate history, and helpful equipment. Physical examination procedures, general treatment and critical care support, and diagnostic techniques are presented. Finally, common conditions and specific treatment options are discussed.

Amphibian biology review

Amphibians occupy a wide range of environmental niches and are found on every continent except Antarctica. They are found most frequently in tropical, semitropical, and temperate areas, though some range into desert and arctic environments [1]. Environmental needs can vary widely between species; some amphibians may be fully aquatic, some semiaquatic, and others are fully terrestrial. Terrestrial and semiaquatic species when on land need high ambient humidity levels to maintain adequate hydration. All amphibians are ectotherms and use behavioral means to adjust body temperature. During periods of environmental extremes, some species either hibernate (enter a dormant state during cold weather in winter) or estivate

---

* Corresponding author.

E-mail address: lclayton@aqua.org (L.A. Clayton).

(enter a dormant state during hot weather in summer). Compared with reptiles, amphibians generally require cooler temperatures for optimal health.

Amphibian adults are carnivorous or insectivorous and consume invertebrate prey, such as insects or worms, and vertebrate prey, such as rodents, fish, and other amphibians [3]. There is wide species variability in natural diet consumption [3]. Amphibians typically hunt rather than scavenge and eat live, moving prey. They generally do not hunt immobile food items, though they may inadvertently ingest foreign material along with a meal.

Amphibian eggs are typically laid in and hatch in water, and the larval (neonatal) stage is aquatic. Neonatal amphibians generally undergo significant anatomic and physiologic changes across body systems as they mature in a process known as metamorphosis [4]. The resulting juvenile and adult stages may be aquatic, semiaquatic, or terrestrial. Metamorphosis is most pronounced in anurans, in which the larval (tadpole) form has no physical similarity to the adult form and is less pronounced in most caudatans [4].

Caudatans are somewhat lizard-like in body form and typically have a cylindric, elongated body with a well-developed, laterally flattened tail and four similarly sized legs, though some species have reduced limb development. Some species, such as the axolotl (*Ambystoma mexicanum*), maintain larval features such as gills into adulthood (neotony). Anurans typically have a rounded, short body with no tail and four legs. The hind legs are typically longer than the front legs, and in most terrestrial species this is pronounced [4].

The skin is typically smooth with no scales or hair and is thin [4]. Toad species may have thickened skin with prominent ridges or mounds. Some arboreal species produce a waxy secretion to coat the skin and the skin feels thickened in these animals also [5]. Many amphibian species either produce or assimilate toxins in the skin, such as the poison arrow dart frogs (Dendrobatids) [5]. Other species, such as the cane toad (*Bufo marinus*), have specialized glands that are easily visible on the dorsum caudal to the head. When stressed, the toad actively secretes the toxin and can project it several feet [5]. Most toxins are not fatal to humans or other animals unless ingested in large quantities or delivered into the circulatory system, but they readily cause mucous membrane irritation with topical contact [4]. The skin of most amphibians is thin and it plays an active role in respiration and fluid and electrolyte balance in most species [4–6]. The skin must remain moist for effective cutaneous respiration [6]. Although adult anurans have well-developed sac-like lungs, adults of some caudatans may still rely primarily on gills for respiration [4,5]. Amphibians have a three-chambered heart (two atria, one ventricle), and in caudatans the interatrial septum is also typically incomplete [4,5]. Amphibians seem to have a renal–portal system similar to reptiles, and blood from the caudal part of the body may be directed through the kidneys [5,6]. Amphibians have an extensive lymphatic system, and anurans have large subcutaneous lymph sacs. Specialized areas of this system ("lymph hearts") circulate lymphatic fluid back to the vascular system and beat up to 60 bpm [6]. The vascular system seems to be "leaky," with more than 50 times the plasma volume being recirculated through the lymphatic system in a 24-hour period [6].

Proper captive husbandry for any amphibian species should reflect the species' biologic needs in the wild and is important because amphibians depend on environmental conditions, such as temperature and humidity, to maintain basic homeostasis [7,8]. Because these needs can vary considerably between species, generalizations regarding what constitutes optimal husbandry for all amphibians are difficult. For most species, ambient humidity levels should be higher than 70% [7]. Substrate needs vary between species, but commonly used materials include live moss, various soils, and peat moss. Organic substrates retain moisture and help maintain humidity. Sterile products, however, should ideally be used to reduce the possibility of disease introduction. Amphibians tend to be reclusive, because many species are prey for other vertebrates and therefore adequate hiding areas must be provided. Various substances can be used for this, including plants, organic substrate, opaque containers, and cork-bark. Terrestrial amphibians should be provided with access to water in a shallow dish, a "bog" area of the tank, or a shallow pool [7]. This helps maintain enclosure humidity and provides opportunities for hydration, although some arboreal species can be maintained without free-standing water. Semiaquatic amphibians should be provided with larger pools that cover 40% to 60% of the tank bottom. Any pool areas should have gently sloped edges to allow easy egress. The enclosure should have a temperature gradient within the species preferred range. Fully aquatic amphibians should typically be held in aquarium systems similar to those used for freshwater fishes [7]. The tank should have a water pump for water circulation and mechanical and biologic filtration. Water should generally be at neutral pH, have minimal salts (less than 2 ppt), and have no ammonia or other nitrogen compounds or chlorine. Basic testing kits are available at aquarium hobby stores. Some species may benefit from exposure to UV A and B light. Information on captive husbandry recommendations is available on-line at such sites as www.caudata.org and www.anapsid.com. In addition, a good review for interested clinicians is available [7].

Patient selection and overall considerations

Amphibian medicine is an emerging field; this is particularly true of emergency medicine and critical care. There is little published information in peer-reviewed journals regarding pet amphibian medicine; case studies, case series, mortality reviews in captive animals, clinical research, and pharmacologic studies are sporadic. The skills, medications, and protocols used in mammalian emergency and critical care, however, are applicable to ill amphibians. Clinicians experienced with companion animal critical care can apply the basic concepts of fluid support and treatment of shock to amphibian patients.

Routine (wellness) veterinary care is rarely provided to most amphibians; therefore animals presented to the veterinarian are typically ill and are frequently presented in an emergency situation. Even in collections or pets that are closely monitored by experienced owners, it can be difficult for caregivers to appreciate subtle signs of illness in these species. Animals are often in the end stages of a severe, chronic disease or condition; in these instances reversing the process is nearly impossible. The clinician has more success in managing animals that are presented for acute processes, such as trauma, or in the early stages of a disease when they are still exhibiting normal to dull reactions to the environment. In the experience of the authors, animals that present obtunded, stuporous, or comatose have a grave prognosis and rarely recover. If supportive care is started and no improvement is seen within 24 to 48 hours, further care is generally not beneficial. As application of standard critical care techniques expands, however, success rates may increase.

Owner goals for veterinary care can vary extensively. Although amphibians are held as pets, and owners may seek care for an individual animal, many owners maintain large collections as a personal hobby or for commercial interest, and even pure "pet" owners often have multianimal collections. In these instances, management of the entire collection may take precedence over individual animal care. This herd-health aspect of veterinary care is much more important in amphibian medicine than in traditional pet medicine and must not be overlooked when interacting with owners. In cases in which the prognosis is grave for an individual animal, the clinician can have a significant, positive impact on remaining animals through identification and correction of husbandry deficiencies and treatment of infectious diseases. In these cases or in cases in which supportive care of an individual failed, a complete necropsy with histology and ancillary testing combined with a thorough history and review of husbandry often allows the clinician to make recommendations that benefit remaining collection animals.

Hospital equipment

Although basic equipment appropriate for amphibian emergency care is typically available in most veterinary hospitals, particularly if other pet exotic animals are routinely seen [9,10], more specialized equipment should be obtained if the clinician wishes to focus on amphibian medicine. Many amphibians kept in private collections are small (<30 g) and thus require small-gauge needles (25–30 gauge) and syringes (insulin or tuberculin types). Alcohol should not be used on amphibian skin (ie, when preparing sites for injection). Sterile saline is an appropriate alternative to clean the skin. Iodine-containing compounds should be avoided. Micropipettes are ideal for appropriate topical and oral medication dosing in extremely small animals (<10 g) (Fig. 1). Endotracheal tubes for small patients can be

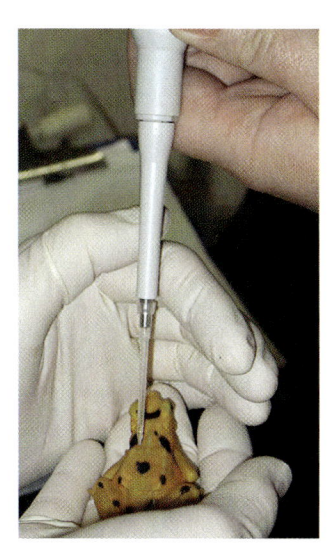

Fig. 1. Topical medication administration using a micropipette in a Panamanian golden frog, *Atelopus zeteki*.

made from mammalian intravenous (IV) catheters or red rubber catheters. IV needles used for injections can be used as intraosseous (IO) catheters. A scale accurate to at least one tenth of a gram is needed for appropriately medicating and monitoring weight changes in these patients. Dilutions of standard medications are often needed, and appropriate diluents for commonly used drugs should be available. For example, ivermectin is ideally diluted with propylene glycol to obtain a uniform suspension.

Gloves (powder-free) should be worn when handling amphibians to protect the clinician from any toxins secreted by the amphibian, to protect from possible zoonotic pathogens and to help protect the amphibian skin from trauma. Gloves should be moistened before handling [10]. Magnification allows a detailed examination of the eyes, nares, and skin in small animals and can be obtained with head loops, ophthalmoscopes, and magnifying glasses. Appropriate oral gags help in opening the mouth for examination or medication administration. Guitar picks work well to atraumatically open the mouth (VA Poole, personal communication, 2006) and are widely available at music stores, on-line, or as donations. Waterproof paper available at office stores works well in animals weighing less than 30 g and can be precut into small squares and disposed of after use (Fig. 2). In all cases, the clinician should use firm, steady pressure and be careful not to break the jaw or damage surrounding skin. The flat, narrow edge of the object being used to open the mouth should be inserted between the lip edges at the tip of the mouth or along the lateral edge and gently used to slightly pry open the mouth; it can then be moved fully into the oral cavity if needed.

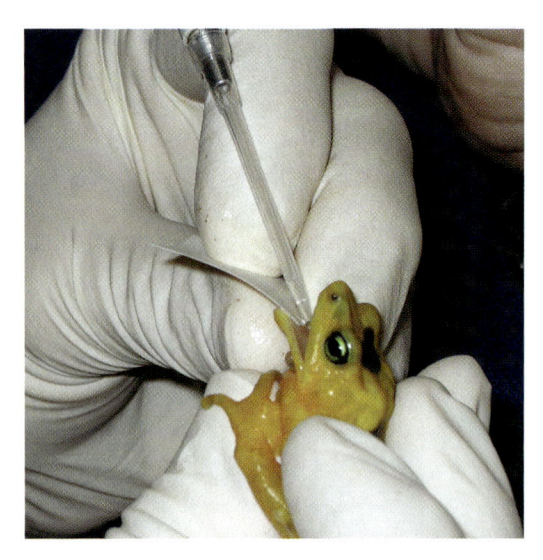

Fig. 2. Oral medication administration using a waterproof paper oral gag and a micropipette in a Panamanian golden frog, *Atelopus zeteki*.

Appropriate water is needed for managing amphibians. Water directly from the tap should not be used, because the chlorine, chloramines, or other dissolved substances (such as lead) can cause health problems. Aging water (holding it in a container at room temperature) for 24 hours allows chlorine to dissipate [9], though other contaminants may remain. Tap water may also be passed through an activated carbon filter to clean it for use [9]. Stocking appropriate fluids for soaking amphibians is important for managing hospital cases and for home use on discharge. "Amphibian ringers" solution can be made by mixing the recommended salts (weighed on a gram scale) in distilled or carbon-filtered water [11]. The base chemicals can be ordered from chemical supply companies such as VWR (www.vwr.com/index.htm), Fisher-Scientific (www1.fishersci.com/index.jsp), or Sigma-Aldrich (www.sigmaaldrich.com/Local/SA_Splash.html) and kept in the clinic. The dry salts should be American Chemical Society (ACS) grade to ensure purity. Topical fluids are discussed in the General Treatment Techniques section.

Appropriate hospital tanks should be available for maintaining animals in the clinic or at home with the owners. The enclosure should have a tight-fitting, ventilated lid and smooth, see-through sides to allow monitoring. Plastic carriers with vented tops (available in pet stores) are appropriate (Fig. 3), as are plastic food storage containers (available at grocery stores) with ventilation holes made in the lid or side; holes should be made from the inside out to prevent rough edges within the enclosure. All containers should be disinfected and thoroughly rinsed after use.

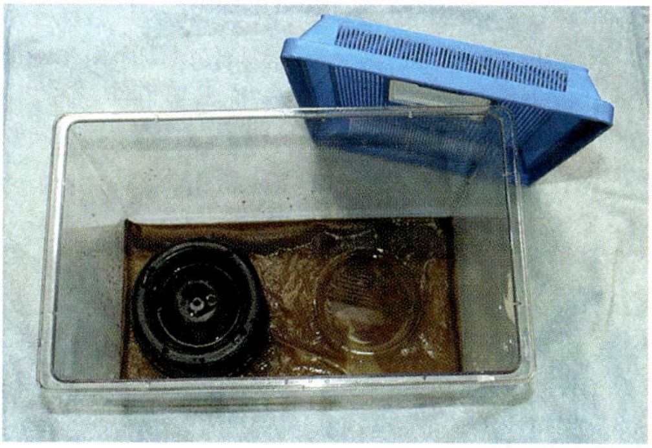

Fig. 3. Hospital enclosure with moistened paper towel, shallow pool of water, and hide box made from plastic plant pot turned upside down with a hole cut in side. Ventilated top is removed to show the inside of the enclosure.

Hospital enclosures for terrestrial amphibians should contain wet paper towels (ideally nonbleached) lining the bottom and a hide structure made of an easily cleaned or disposable substance; commercial plastic hide structures available at pet stores, small plastic plant pots placed upside down with a hole cut along the rim for entry, and small cardboard containers also work well. Hide structures allow the amphibian to retreat to a more confined space with reduced visual cues and may reduce stress. A shallow dish of water is sometimes included to increase rehydration opportunities [12,13]. This primary hospital tank can be placed within standard hospital animal cages. Many amphibians are normally kept in elaborate tanks with high organic loads in the home setting. These are inappropriate for housing ill amphibians. The high organic load increases the chance of bacterial, fungal, or parasitic disease, hinders the movement of weak animals, and makes tracking appetite and fecal production difficult. Appropriate temperature should be achieved by adjusting the ambient temperature around the hospital tank. Appropriate ambient temperatures vary by species, but a range of 23.8°C to 26.7°C (75°F to 80°F) is appropriate for many animals commonly encountered in the pet trade [9]. Species needs should be confirmed. As a rough guide, lowland tropical species should be housed at the high end of this range, and temperate, subtropical, and tropical montane species maintained at the low end [9]. Focal heat lights or ceramic heat lamps should not be placed directly over the cage, because they can cause drying. Heat pads may be placed along the back of the tank or under part of the tank. In all cases, actual temperatures should be closely monitored in all areas of the tank (tank bottom and higher in tank if amphibian can climb) to ensure adequate temperature is maintained. High ambient humidity is needed to maintain hydration and should be at least 50% but more ideally 70% to 90% [12]. Plastic wrap can be placed loosely over the top of the hospital enclosure to increase humidity within the cage. The cage substrate should be kept moist at all times; frequent misting of the tank helps maintain humidity. If oxygen support is needed, the hospital tank can be placed within a standard oxygen cage.

Hospital enclosures for aquatic amphibians require dechlorinated, fresh water (ideally of similar pH and temperature to the home tank water) or water from the home tank (if water quality is appropriate) with a submersible structure to provide a hide. Plastic aquarium plants also work well for hiding purposes. Stable ambient air and water temperatures are important; the range given above is also generally appropriate for aquatic species [9]. If supplemental oxygen is needed for support it can be gently bubbled into the water. An aquarium air stone is ideal for creating the small bubbles that enhance oxygen diffusion, but bubbling by way of a small line such as a red rubber catheter can also be helpful. It is important to monitor water quality parameters for aquatic species. Water quality guidelines for freshwater fish are generally appropriate for amphibians; these include a near-neutral pH and nonmeasurable (using home test kits) levels of ammonia and nitrate. A basic water quality test kit can be used to evaluate the home tank's water quality and to evaluate water used in hospital enclosures. Home test kits should be able to measure pH, hardness, alkalinity, chlorine, ammonia, nitrite, and nitrate. Products made by Hach Company (www.hach.com) and La Motte Chemicals (www.lamotte.com) have been recommended [9].

History

Detailed husbandry information is mandatory, because amphibians depend on environmental conditions to maintain basic homeostasis [8]. Whenever possible, it is beneficial to have the client bring in the entire enclosure for evaluation. Enclosure pictures are helpful if the primary enclosure cannot be moved. Husbandry records, such as cage temperature, humidity, water quality, water change frequency, and eating habits, should also be reviewed when they are available. The clinician should also review information on apparently healthy animals and the sick individual.

The history should include questions about the individual animal being presented and general information about the owner's collection, such as numbers of animals and species housed. The history should also include the age of the animal, how long the animal has been with the client, and if animals have been brought into the collection in the recent past (30–90 days). Quarantine protocols should be evaluated if such additions have been made. Many owners do not quarantine new animals and infectious disease can be a problem. Disease information should include clinical signs, duration, progression, and number of animals affected. Activity level, eating patterns, and defecation frequency should be discussed. If multiple animals are affected, a schematic representation of the physical locations and dates of cases is helpful when reviewing the disease process.

The husbandry information should include a review of cage type, cage substrate, cage cleaning frequency and methods, water quality and source, temperature, humidity, light source, and light cycle. Detailed dietary information is also important. This should include types of prey fed, where prey is purchased, diet fed to prey items, frequency of feeding, timing of feeding, and type and frequency of supplementation. Most amphibians are fed live invertebrate prey. If prey are not fed and cared for properly, their poor nutritional value predisposes amphibians to disease. In addition, nutritional supplements (primarily calcium) are needed when feeding invertebrates to amphibians. Clients should be asked about medication administration (such as antibiotics available in pet stores) or possible exposure to toxins in the enclosure (such as plant food), the room (such as aerosol cleaners), or on food items (such as pesticides in wild-caught invertebrate foods).

Physical examination

The examination should begin with visual observation to evaluate respiratory effort and obtain a respiratory rate and to evaluate the animal's coloration, body condition, body posture, ambulatory ability, and responsiveness to novel environmental factors. This examination can often be completed with the animal in the transport carrier. A physical examination should be conducted quickly and efficiently. A firm, consistent grip is needed to prevent escape of the animal and possible damage to the integument and skeletal system. Small, fully transparent containers may be used to hold the animal to allow a detailed evaluation of movement, general attitude, and dermal condition without the need for handling. Many anuran species expand with air when stressed, and this can make palpation difficult. Magnification may be needed for full evaluation of the skin, nares, and eyes in small species. Transillumination may be helpful in small species to evaluate for organ size, coelomic fat pads, and egg masses. Limbs should be palpated for fractures or boney abnormalities. A complete dermal examination should include evaluation of the foot pads and rostrum and the skin on the body. Dehydration is common in ill amphibians; animals may feel tacky and have obvious skin tenting or sunken eyes. Anurans normally urinate when handled but may not do so if dehydrated [12]. Many amphibians normally have pale oral cavities and mucous membranes, but circulatory abnormalities may be appreciated by reduced prominence of the lingual or central abdominal vein if these can be visualized [12]. Shock should be assumed in animals with signs of significant dehydration or reduced mentation (obtunded, stuporous, or comatose). A heart rate may be obtained visually in some animals (the apical beat is seen caudal to the xiphoid in anurans) or by using a Doppler flow monitor to hear the beat. Ultrasound may also be used to evaluate cardiac contractions in larger animals. In general, anesthesia is not needed to complete a physical examination on amphibians presented for emergency care. More detailed reviews of physical examinations and restraint techniques are available [10,14].

General treatment techniques

General emergency support

Animals that are obtunded, stuporous, or comatose have a grave prognosis, as do animals in cardiorespiratory arrest. Emergency supportive care as used in mammals can be initiated while a history is being obtained and the prognosis discussed with the owners. Basic emergency management of all cases may include appropriate thermal support, fluid support, oxygen administration, and a clean hospital tank. Antibiotic administration should be started in most cases pending diagnostic results, as sepsis is a common finding in ill amphibians. Animals that are seizuring (tetany), have muscle fasciculations, or are paretic or paralyzed should be started on calcium administration pending diagnostics because of the prevalence of hypocalcemia resulting from dietary deficiency. If toxin exposure is suspected, appropriate antidotes should be given when possible (eg, atropine for organophosphate toxicity). Amphibians can be easily intubated and ventilation supported with room air or oxygen and an ambu-bag. The trachea is very short [3,4], and care is needed to maintain the tracheal location and inflate both lungs. Vascular fluid support in anurans can be provided readily with IO fluids. In-dwelling IV catheters are difficult to place in most species, but bolus fluids are easily administered into the ventral tail vein of caudatans. Although clinicians may apply standard mammalian emergency supportive protocols in amphibian cases, it is important to keep the animal's skin moist at all times and to make sure ambient local temperature around the animal is appropriate.

Standard mammalian emergency resuscitation medications can also be used in amphibians; in the authors' experience, doxapram seems to act as a general stimulant in many species and may be more useful than in mammalian medicine. Doses for emergency drugs and some commonly used medications are provided in Table 1, but clinicians should review current formularies for broader options [11,15] and check the literature for updated information.

Routine fluid support in terrestrial species

Fluid support is important, because the rate of evaporative water loss through the skin is far greater in amphibians than in terrestrial vertebrates. Dehydration is common in ill amphibians (Fig. 4) [12]. In some species the skin is also involved in osmoregulation and in respiration [6]. Unlike in other terrestrial vertebrates, transdermal fluid support is a viable rehydration option in all cases. Even in species such as toads that have reduced

Table 1
Commonly used medications and emergency drugs

Drug	Dose	Indication
Amikacin	5 mg/kg IM, SC, ICe every 24-48 h [15]	Broad spectrum antibiotic
Atropine	0.03 mg/kg IM [13]	Slow heart rhythm
	0.1 mg SC, IM as needed [15]	Organophosphate toxicity
Calcium gluconate	100 mg/kg IM, IV, SC, ICe every 12–24 h [11]	Hypocalcemic tetany, metabolic bone disease
Dopram	5 mg/kg IM, IV [13]	Respiratory/general stimulant
Enrofloxacin	5–10 mg/kg PO, SC, IM every 24 h [15]	Broad spectrum antibiotic
Epinephrine 1:1000	0.2–0.5 mL IM, ICe, IV, IC [15]	Cardiac arrest
Fenbendazole	50 mg/kg PO every 24 h × 3–5 d, repeat in 14–21 d [15]	Nematodiasis
Itraconazole	0.01% 5 min bath every 24 h × 11 d [15]	Chytridiomycosis antifungal
Ivermectin	0.2–0.4 mg/kg[a] PO, SC, repeat in 14 d [15]	Nematodiasis
Vitamin B$_1$ (thiamine)	25–100 mg/kg IM, ICe [11]	Neurologic signs (paresis)
Vitamin B complex	1 mL/gallon bath [11]	Spindly leg syndrome (tadpole, froglet)

Abbreviations: IC, intracardiac; ICe, intracoelomicly; IM, intramuscularly; IV, intravenously; PO, orally; SC, subcutaneously.

[a] The lower dose of 0.2 mg/kg is used in the authors' practice.

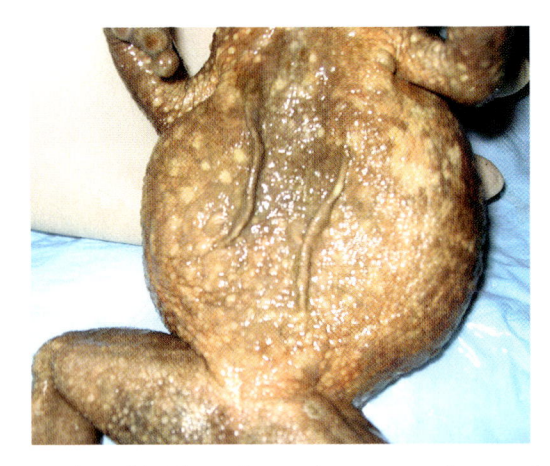

Fig. 4. Severe dehydration with skin tenting on the ventrum of a smooth-sided toad, *Bufo guttatus*.

generalized transdermal fluid exchange, specialized areas ("patches") on the ventral thigh allow fluid uptake [3]. Ideally, fluids (transdermal and injectable) would be selected after evaluating the dehydration status and electrolyte balance of each animal; however, this level of evaluation is often impossible because of the small size and lack of normal values for most species.

Topical fluid administration for rehydration and fluid maintenance should always be the first step in supportive care and should be done concurrently with more direct methods used in cases of severe dehydration and shock. Transdermal absorption methods are less stressful to the animal, allow normal physiologic processes to work, and may decrease the risk for fluid overload. In many cases, topical fluids are sufficient for adequate rehydration. Dehydrated terrestrial amphibians generally benefit from being placed in isotonic to hypotonic (as compared with normally hydrated animals) solutions. Various rehydration soaking solutions have been proposed [11], many of which were developed in a research setting rather than for clinical care. A partial list of amphibian fluid solutions is provided in Table 2. Any fluid that is hypo-osmotic or isotonic to normal amphibian plasma should help with rehydration. Normal plasma osmolality varies with species, but 200 to 250 mOsm is considered typical for healthy amphibians [11]. Animals may also present with excessive fluid retention in the body cavity or lymph sacs; soaking in hypertonic fluid baths has been proposed to reduce fluid accumulation in these cases and can be used in conjunction with manual removal. In reality, it seems difficult to effect this change in the clinical setting in the authors' experience. In either scenario, weights should be obtained before and after soaking to document responsiveness to fluid administration. Variable soaking schedules are used by the authors, typically for 60 minutes 1 to 2 times daily. In some cases, 24-hour exposure to the fluid

Table 2
Amphibian soaking solutions

Category	Solution name	Ingredients (if applicable)	Notes/reference
Hypotonic	Saline 0.6%		[11]
	Steinberg's solution	3.4 g NaCl, 0.05 g KCl, 0.05 g CaCl$_2$, 0.205 g MgSO$_4$, 0.56 g Tris in 1 L distilled water	Use HCl as needed to balance pH to 7.4 [11]
	Fresh water		Carbon-filtered
Isotonic	LRS and dextrose 5%	4 parts lactated Ringer's solution and 1 part dextrose 5%	Use fluids for IV use [11]
	Reptile Ringer's	1 part lactated Ringer's solution and 1 part dextrose 2.5% in NaCl 0.45%	Use fluids for IV use [12]
	Amphibian Ringer's	6.6 g NaCl, 0.15 g KCl, 0.15 g CaCl$_2$, 0.2 g NaHCO$_3$ in 1 L distilled water	[11]
Hypertonic	5% Whitaker-Wright	5 mL stock solution[a] to 95 mL distilled water	[11]
	10% Whitaker-Wright solution and higher	10 mL stock solution to 90 mL distilled water or greater concentrations up to full strength	[11]

[a] Whitaker-Wright stock solution (ie, 100% Whitaker-Wright solution): 113 g NaCl, 8.6 g MgSO4, 4.2 g CaCl2, 1.7 g KCl in 1 L distilled water. Use Trizma (7.4) base (fish grade) buffer to adjust pH to 7.0 to 7.3 [11].

(at very shallow depth) is used rather than bolus soaking at slightly deeper depth. If animals are severely debilitated or paralytic, clinicians must make sure the nares and mouth are not under water during soaking or aspiration may occur. In these cases, injectable methods of fluid administration may be more appropriate.

Various injectable fluids are available in most small animal clinics for attempted treatment of severe dehydration or shock. The ideal fluid for use in amphibians is unknown and, as with conventional pet emergency care, likely varies with each patient and disease process. The authors typically use a reptile Ringer's solution (equal parts 2.5% dextrose in 0.45% sodium chloride + lactated Ringer's solution) for rehydration in severely dehydrated animals and attempted treatment of shock [11]. A "shock dose" bolus of 5 to 10 mL/kg IO or IV is used and repeated as needed. In less debilitated animals (such as paralytic animals that cannot safely be soaked), a fluid dose of 10 to 20 mL/kg/d intraceolomicly (ICe) or into the lymph sacs is used for support. Other crystalloid fluids such as lactated Ringer's solution (LRS), Normosol-r, or Plasma-lyte A may be considered, though they are typically slightly hypertonic to normal amphibian plasma [11]. It has been theorized that lactated Ringer's solution could contribute to undesirable acidosis in amphibians because of the extremely slow clearance time for lactic acid in these species [11]. The authors have not used administration of colloids (such as hetastarch) routinely but would consider doing so in appropriate cases. The authors are unaware of in-depth clinical research on ideal fluid types and resuscitation volumes in debilitated amphibians. Given the extremely poor prognosis and relative lack of information on clinical management of amphibians in severe shock or circulatory collapse, experienced emergency clinicians would seem to be justified in applying knowledge gained in companion animal critical care to critical care of amphibians in cases in which owners are interested in this type of management.

Subcutaneous (SC) injections in amphibians are actually injections into the extensive lymphatic system [12,16]. This space is most accessible dorsally and along the lateral body wall and thigh area in anurans, and these locations are appropriate for fluid administration (Fig. 5). ICe fluid administration can also be effective. The animal should be held to allow body organs to fall away; a caudal and ventral injection site on the lateral body wall is preferred by the authors to avoid the pulmonary system and mid-line abdominal vein.

Direct administration of fluid into the vascular system by way of IO or IV injection can be attempted in animals with severe dehydration or circulatory collapse from other causes (such as thermal shock or blood loss). In anurans, IO catheters may be used to provide an in-dwelling catheter for direct access to the vasculature. The authors most frequently use the hind limb, with normograde placement into the tibiafibula (Fig. 6), but retrograde placement into the femur is also possible. Standard IV needles are appropriate for most animals. The catheter may be left in place for continued fluid

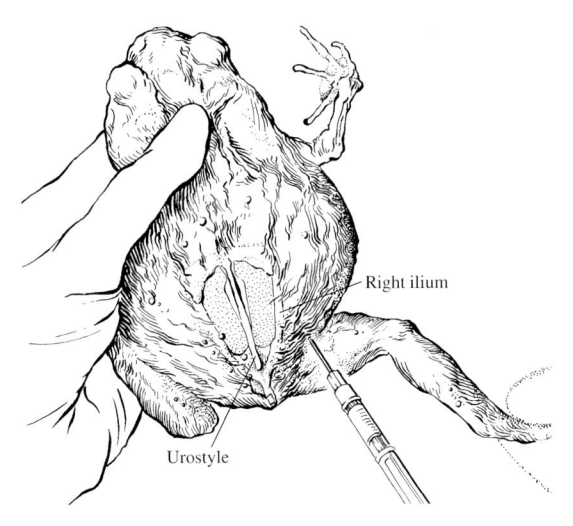

Fig. 5. Location for dorsal lymph sac injections in an anuran. (*Courtesy of* Devon Nykaza, Baltimore, MD.)

and medication administration. IV fluid administration is possible, though in-dwelling catheter placement is not common in the clinical setting. In caudatans, a vein runs ventral to the spine of the tail and in debilitated animals is easily used for bolus fluid administration. Amphibians also have a midline abdominal vein that may be used for bolus injections.

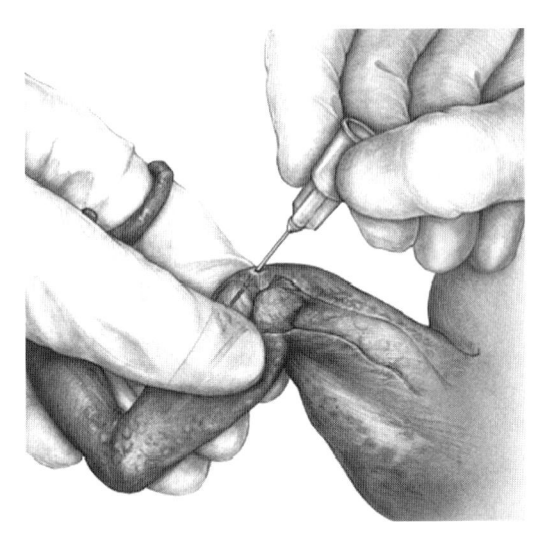

Fig. 6. Placement of an interosseous catheter in the left tibiafibula in an anuran. (*Courtesy of* Kate Burnett, Baltimore, MD.)

Oral (PO) fluids may also be given, but this is not a primary method of rehydration used by the authors given the effectiveness of the transdermal route. Most anurans swallow when fluids are placed into the caudal mouth/cranial esophagus. Typically the glottis closes spontaneously and aspiration is not a problem unless the animal is severely debilitated. Orogastric gavage is easily accomplished, owing to the short, straight esophagus and wide mouth in most species.

Routine fluid support in aquatic species

Fully aquatic species still require fluid support. Amphibians live in fresh water, which is hypo-osomotic to the animal; fluid thus diffuses across the permeable skin (and gills in some species) into the animal and the excess fluid must be excreted (primarily by the kidneys) while conserving electrolytes [6]. In critically ill amphibians and in animals with severe skin disease, the mechanisms of electrolyte conservation and fluid excretion may become disrupted and fluid overload can occur. These animals typically suffer from excessive fluid retention and loss of electrolytes in the disease state [6,12]. Increasing the osmolarity of the water to more closely match that of the animal theoretically reduces the fluid burden. The simplest method of providing this support is to place the animal in isotonic fluid solutions, such as those used for soaking ill terrestrial amphibians [11]. This seems to be most helpful as a prophylactic measure, because once fluid overload develops correction is difficult [6,11].

Medication administration

Medications are most commonly administered topically, orally, and by intramuscular (IM) or SC/lymph sac injection. Topical administration seems to be a viable method to deliver certain medications systemically, particularly in small amphibians with permeable skin. This method is unlikely to deliver adequate amounts to toads or waxy tree frogs in which the skin is less permeable. Topical medications may be delivered in water as baths or dips for aquatic species. In all cases of topical administration, clinicians should monitor for any signs of discomfort (such as wiping at the area with a hind leg) or changes in skin color (darkening, lightening, or erythema) and re-evaluate use if these develop. Appropriate oral or topical dosing in small species requires a micropipette. IM injections are typically delivered into the large muscles of the front or hind limb. In limbless caudatan species, the epaxial musculature can be used. ICe and lymph sac injections should be administered as for fluids. The clinician must balance many factors when determining the appropriate administration route, including patient size and condition, the number of animals to be treated, staff skills, and medication pharmacokinetics and volume.

A short list of commonly used medications is provided (see Table 1). There is, however, variety among amphibians and no drug has been tested on all species. When treating a large group of animals with a medication that the clinician has not used before, a few animals should be tested initially and observed for potential signs of toxicity. Clinicians should consult more complete formularies whenever possible [11,15].

Nutritional support

Nutritional support is critical in debilitated amphibians. Force-feeding liquid or gel diets during the initial stages of recovery is recommended. Adult amphibians are carnivorous/insectivorous and should be fed moderate- to high-protein diets. Amphibian/reptile commercial diets are becoming available and are appropriate for supportive feeding. For example, Mazuri produces Amphibian & Carnivorous Reptile Gel (Mazuri Diets, PMI Nutrition, LLC., St. Louis, MO) that is sold as a powder. When the product is mixed with boiling water and cooled it forms a gel, and when mixed with lukewarm water it forms a liquid gruel. Gel diets may be cut into small blocks and placed into the animal's mouth; this often initiates a swallow reflex. Gruels or liquid diets can be gavage fed. If specialized diets are unavailable, products routinely used in mammal care may be substituted. For example, CliniCare Canine/Feline (Abbott Laboratories, Abbott Park, IL) has been used in the authors' practice with success. Semisolid diets such as Hill's Prescription Diet Canine/Feline a/d (Hill's Pet Nutrition, Inc., Topeka, KS) have also been recommended [12]. The authors are unaware of studies on optimal supportive care diets. In the authors' practice, liquid diets (CliniCare or Mazuri Amphibian & Carnivorous Reptile Gel gruel) are generally used for supportive feeding. Initial feedings are dilute and fed at a dose of 1% of body weight (10 mL/kg). An excellent review of supportive feeding techniques and energy requirement formulas is available [17]. As animals stabilize, the diet is not diluted excessively and the amount fed is increased. Successful weight gain has been achieved in these patients by feeding 2% to 3% of body weight (20–30 mL/kg) daily or every other day, depending on species and the condition of the individual. Commonly used diets with some basic nutritional information are listed in Table 3. As animals recover strength, fresh prey items should be placed in the enclosure. These items can be force-fed to the patient also, but most amphibians readily start hunting when they have recovered enough to properly process

Table 3
Supportive care diets

Product	Protein	Fat	Fiber	Calories
Mazuri Amphibian & Carnivorous Reptile Gel	55%	15%	1%	3.2 kcal/g (powder)
Mazuri Insectivore Diet	28%	12%	13%	3.2 kcal/g
CliniCare Feline/Canine	8.2% (min)	5.1% (min)	0.05% (max)	1 kcal/mL
Hill's Canine/Feline a/d	8.5% (min)	5.2% (min)	0.5% (max)	1.1 kcal/g

prey items. The prey items should be fed a well-balanced diet and either gut-loaded with a high calcium food or coated with calcium supplement before feeding.

Analgesia, anesthesia, and euthanasia

Pain management is appropriate in trauma or postoperative cases. It is not, however, a first-line therapy in most animals presented for emergency veterinary care. There are few published papers on pain management in clinical settings. Opioid receptors are present in amphibians, and experiments have demonstrated efficacy of opioid analgesics in the research setting, though the clinical applicability of this research is unknown [18]. In the authors' practice, buprenorphine at 0.02 mg/kg IM, SC, or PO has been used without negative side effects. Nonsteroidal anti-inflammatory drugs are also used in amphibian medicine. In the authors' practice, meloxicam (Metacam; Boehringer Ingelheim, Vetmedia, Inc., St. Joseph, MO) 0.2 mg/kg IM or PO has been used without obvious negative short-term side effects.

Although not typically needed in the emergency setting, general anesthesia is possible in amphibians. Techniques used to monitor mammals are applicable to amphibians. Heart rate is easily monitored using a Doppler probe over the heart or visualization of the apical beat. A transesophageal stethoscope could be tried in larger animals, but the authors have no direct experience with this. Pulse oximetry is not validated in amphibians but may have usefulness in measuring peripheral pulses or monitoring trends in oxygen saturation. Electrocardiography (ECG) can be used in amphibians, but alligator clips should not be placed directly on the animal. The authors are also unaware of studies on the usefulness of end tidal CO_2 monitoring in amphibians but would encourage interested clinicians to attempt monitoring amphibians of sufficient size. Amphibians have significantly lower heart rates than similarly sized mammals, and rates of 20 to 60 are commonly recorded in the authors' practice in sedated animals. The authors work to keep the heart rate at a level close to that at induction or that at initial loss of pain reflex.

Tricaine methanesulfonate (MS-222, Finquel; Argent Chemical Laboratories, Redmond, WA) or inhalant isoflurane are commonly used for anesthesia procedures. MS-222 comes as a powder. Anesthetic solution is made by mixing the powder (measured by weight) with nonchlorinated water. Sodium bicarbonate powder at equal weight to the MS-222 powder should be added to help buffer the solution. Effective anesthetic doses vary significantly with species and even for individuals within the same species and are expected to vary with temperature at which the animal is kept. General guidelines are given here, but it is advisable to start with lower doses and increase as needed until the animal reaches the appropriate plane of anesthesia. Nonanesthetic water should be available to dilute the induction solution to reduce the plane of anesthesia and to transfer the animal into during recovery (aquatic, semiaquatic) or wash the animal (terrestrial). Terrestrial or semiaquatic species can typically be dosed at 1 to 3 g (by weight)/L [15]. Aquatic species may need lower doses, such as 0.2 g (by weight)/L.

Induction with gas isoflurane is typically at 5% in oxygen delivered by way of face mask or chamber induction and is used primarily for terrestrial amphibians, such as toads, in the authors' practice (Fig. 7). Many animals attempt to breath-hold; gentle stimulation encourages continued respiration. A solution made from K-Y jelly (3.5 mL), water (1.5 mL), and liquid isoflurane (3.0 mL) has been described, but the authors have no primary experience with the solution [15]. The authors have no direct experience with sevoflurane but would consider using this inhalant anesthetic also. Amphibians often take 10 to 30 minutes for induction and recovery, but rates can vary significantly with species, type of illness, temperature, and protocol. It is common to witness an excitement phase during induction.

Recent work at the authors' practice with ketamine (50 mg/kg) and medetomidine hydrochloride (Domitor; Pfizer Animal Health, Exton, PA) (0.15–0.2 mg/kg) IM in several smooth-sided toads (*Bufo guttatus*) has been promising. Inductions were smooth with loss of reflex at 20 minutes and stable heart rates. The animals were reversed with atipamezole hydrochloride (Antisedan, Pfizer Animal Health) at equal volume to medetomidine IM with return to mobility at approximately 20 minutes. This protocol, however, has been used in only a handful of animals of one species in relatively healthy animals. No extensive trials have been conducted in the authors' practice.

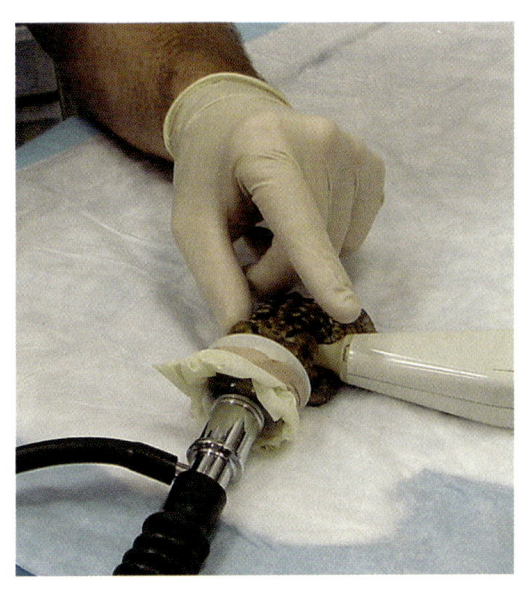

Fig. 7. Inhalent mask isoflurane anesthesia and Doppler heart rate monitoring in a juvenile marine (cane) toad, *Bufo marinus*.

Euthanasia is sometimes required. Standard barbiturate overdose as used in small animal practice is the method of choice in amphibians, and the drug is typically injected into the vascular system or into the peritoneal cavity. Euthanasia solutions can be painful and can cause tissue changes and complicated histology. It is recommended to dilute the drug with water or saline to reduce these complications. An overdose of MS-222 can be used for smaller amphibian patients. If the animal is relatively alert, inducing general anesthesia before medication administration can further reduce potential discomfort. Pithing the animal after loss of all reflexes and heart rate ensures that all neuronal activity has stopped.

General diagnostic techniques

Fecal analyses

Direct and fecal floats should be done on nearly all ill amphibians, because parasitic disease is common [19]. In anorexic animals, force-feeding may be necessary before obtaining a fecal. In the authors' experience, nematode infection is the most common cause of parasitic disease. Lungworm (*Rhabdias* spp) infection is considered pathogenic and typically causes morbidity and mortality in individual animals and collections (Fig. 8). The parasite is readily transmissible between animals. Eggs are passed in the feces after being expelled from the trachea and swallowed. On fecal examination these nematode ova are indistinguishable from those of common intestinal nematodes. Intestinal nematodes (*Aplectana* spp, *Cosmocerca* spp, and *Cosmocercoides* spp) are considered less pathogenic in amphibians, though high loads may be associated with disease. Intestinal protozoa are common and generally not a source of disease. Fecal cytology may be helpful to evaluate

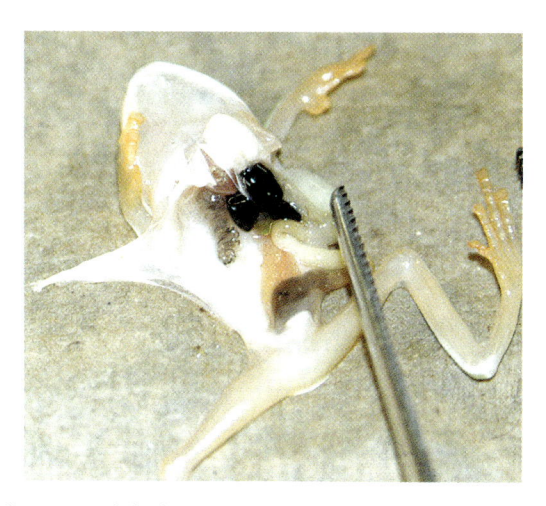

Fig. 8. Lungworm infection in a black-eyed treefrog, *Agalychnis moreletti*.

for cells, improperly digested foods, and yeast or other fungi. Budding yeast in a fresh fecal sample is abnormal. Clinicians must keep in mind that feces pass through the common cloaca, and any material collected may represent or include discharge from the reproductive or urinary tracts.

Bloodwork

Blood can be obtained from most species using various sites, though sedation may be needed if animals are struggling. In anurans, the lingual venous plexus and midline abdominal vein are recommended [20]. In caudatans, the ventral tail vein is most commonly used [20]. Cardiocentesis may also be used in all amphibians [20] and is commonly used in research facilities. An appropriately sized needle (generally 25–27 gauge) is inserted into the apex and blood is taken from the ventricle. Lithium heparin is the preferred anticoagulant, because it does not lyse red cells [20]. Even if only a small sample is obtained, evaluation of a blood smear can help the clinician appreciate changes associated with sepsis (such as bacteria) or neoplasia [20,21]. Chemistries may be run in-house or sent out as for other exotic patients following the clinics standard practice. Cage side machines and avian/reptile rotors using less than 0.2 mL of whole blood (VetScan; Abaxis Inc., Union City, CA) are ideal for obtaining the most information from small samples. Normal blood values for amphibians are largely undefined, but preliminary references exist for a small number of species [15,20,22,23]. Hemogram and biochemistry values can vary significantly based on age, sex, and season of the year, among other environmental factors [20], and this makes easily defining normal values challenging. A few broad generalizations can be attempted, such as anuran hematocrits tend to be less than 30% [15,20] and amphibian blood glucose values tend to be less than 50 mg/dL [20].

Cytology/histology/culture

Samples of material from lesions or masses should be collected for cytology. Skin scrapes or impression smears of external lesions should be performed, and fine-needle aspirates should be obtained from masses. Samples of internal masses found at endoscopy or surgery should also be collected [24]. Cytology is recommended even if histology is being submitted, because many amphibian lesions are secondary to parasitic, bacterial, or fungal infection, and cytology is useful in guiding treatment. Fluid aspirated from animals with lymph sac fluid accumulation or body cavity effusion should also be evaluated using standard fluid analysis techniques. Direct examination (wet mount) or Diff Quick-type and Gram staining should be routinely completed on all samples. In addition, acid-fast stains should be used because of the frequency of environmental mycobacterial infection. In some cases, acid-fast stains may not stain mycobacterial organisms. Nonstaining rod structures should be further evaluated and a different acid-fast stain should be tried. Infection with the fungus *Batrachochytrium dendrobatidis*, the etiologic agent of chytridiomycosis, may cause generalized skin sloughing (most easily seen with the animal put in fresh water); wet mount or Gram stain evaluation of the sloughed skin may demonstrate the organism (BR Whitaker, MS, DVM, personal communication, 2005).

A complete gross necropsy with ancillary cytology often allows a clinician to identify likely causes of mortalities. Histology should be submitted whenever possible to confirm the diagnosis and assist the clinician in understanding amphibian diseases. An excellent review of the amphibian necropsy is available [16].

Cultures may be helpful in eliciting disease etiologies. Although gram-negative bacterial infections are common, gram-positive infections may also occur. Cytology may guide preliminary treatment and dictate which cultures are appropriate (aerobic, anaerobic, mycobacterial, or fungal). Fungal and mycobacterial cultures can be attempted but require a laboratory familiar with growing these organisms. Blood cultures can be run in cases in which systemic bacterial infection is suspected. Sensitivities also help guide the clinician to choose appropriate medications.

Diagnostic imaging

Diagnostic imaging is helpful in amphibian cases [25]. Radiographs are most useful to look for bone fractures or malformations (ie, consistent with trauma or metabolic bone disease), evidence of osteomyelitis, and gastrointestinal changes consistent with foreign object ingestion or gastric impaction. Radiographs may also demonstrate evidence of pulmonary tissue thickening. There is limited radiographic contrast in the normal amphibian abdomen and generally no sharp distinction between the liver, intestines, fat pads, and reproductive organs. Small species can be better imaged using mammography machines or mammography film in combination with standard radiograph machines. Dental machines and film can be used for evaluating small patients if mammography equipment is unavailable.

Intestinal contrast agents can be used as in mammalian medicine. Contrast agents may be delivered directly to the stomach by means of an orogastric tube. Contrast agents may allow for diagnosis of intestinal obstruction or motility disorders. In addition, contrast agents visually define the gastrointestinal tract, which may allow the clinician to appreciate abnormalities in the size of other organs. For instance, an enlarged liver may displace the gastrointestinal tract dorsally on a lateral view.

Ultrasound can be easily used in amphibians. Because of the small size of many species, probes of 10 MHz or higher are most useful for evaluating organ size and structure. Ultrasound guidance can be used to allow fine-needle aspiration of coelomic masses or fluid. Aquatic species can be easily imaged with the probe held underwater, away from the body, as ultrasound waves are conducted well through water.

CT and MRI can also be used in amphibians to help delineate masses and better define other diagnostic findings, though these techniques are not routinely used in most facilities.

Endoscopy/exploratory surgery

Coelomic or gastric endoscopy can be performed on amphibians as in other animals [24,26]. Rigid endoscopes or thin fiberscopes can be used in many species to visualize the stomach and cloaca and the coelomic cavity. The short, wide esophagus makes gastric endoscopy easy to accomplish. Endoscopy can also be used to visualize the glottis, trachea, bronchi, and lungs in animals of sufficient size. Exploratory surgery may be used for diagnostics and treatment.

Common conditions

General presenting signs

Amphibians may present with a wide range of clinical signs. Common presenting complaints include anorexia, lethargy/collapse, trauma (eg, fractures and internal bleeding), dehydration (particularly if animals escaped from their primary enclosure), paralysis/paresis, dermatologic conditions (eg, sloughing skin, ulceration, lacerations, masses/growths, or erythema), lymph sac fluid accumulation (subcutaneous edema), tissue prolapse through the cloaca, and abdominal distention. As with all animals, healthy animals suffering a traumatic event or other acute process (eg, gastric or intestinal obstruction from foreign body) generally have the best chance of responding to care. In addition, animals presented early in the course of illness with mild signs are typically more responsive to care. A list of presenting complaints and possible differentials with diagnostic and empiric supportive care recommendations is provided in Table 4.

There is a wide variety of disease processes in amphibians. Some of the more common diseases or conditions are reviewed here.

Parasitic disease

The presence of organisms or ova in a fecal sample is not a sufficient indicator of disease. Many healthy amphibians have low parasite burdens, and some organisms are nonpathogenic (ie, opalinid ciliates). Familiarity with parasite burdens in healthy animals can help the clinician evaluate the significance of fecal findings. Heavy parasite loads may occur in debilitated animals or may represent a primary disease condition. In thin, unthrifty animals or in animals with clinical conditions potentially related to parasites, such as rectal prolpase (Fig. 9) and positive fecal results, deworming

Table 4
Common presenting signs with recommended diagnostics and supportive care

Presenting signs	Partial differential list	Initial diagnostics	Initial supportive care
Anorexia with weight loss/emaciation	Inappropriate husbandry (temperature, food items, cage structure, water quality, overcrowding) Infectious (bacterial, fungal, parasitic, viral—tends to be more acute) Visual deficit (corneal lipid deposits, central nervous system) Hypovitaminosis A (short tongue syndrome) Metabolic disease (liver/kidney failure) Nutritional secondary hyperparathyroidism (NSHP) caused by jaw deformities, leg fractures, or hypocalcemia causing loss of ability to capture prey Neoplasia Gastrointestinal foreign body (may be more acute)	History/species review Fecal (direct, float, cytologies) Radiographs (possible contrast) Skin scrape/ cytology/ chytrid evaluation (especially if skin sloughing present or other animals affected) Ultrasound Blood work	Fluid support Hospital caging Nutritional support Antibiotics Calcium and vitamin B complex administration Deworming for nematodes after initial supportive care started if animal severely debilitated (consider premedication with anti-inflammatories)
Edema (subcutaneous or lymph accumulation)	Infectious (bacterial, fungal, parasitic, viral) Metabolic (kidney/liver failure)	History/species review Fecal (direct, float, cytologies) Fluid aspiration and analysis (cytologies and cultures)	Hypertonic fluid soaks (weigh animal pre- and post-soak to ensure fluid is moving in proper direction)

	Cardiac failure or lymph heart failure	Blood work	Hospital caging
	Hypocalcemia (NSHP)	Radiographs	Nutritional support if anorexic
	Ova retention (generally apparent as abdominal distension)		Antibiotics
			Calcium administration
	Physiologic (eg, female *Atelopus zeteki* during breeding season)		
Paresis/paralysis	*Mentation normal*	History/species review	Hospital caging
	NSHP (long bone or spinal fractures).	Radiographs	Calcium and thiamine supplementation
	Trauma Infectious (bacterial, viral)	Blood work	Pain medication (if fractures).
	Thiamine deficiency	Fecal	Nutritional support if anorexic or cannot capture prey
	Mentation abnormal		
	Infectious (bacteria, viral, fungal)		
	Severe NSHP/hypocalcemia		
	Severe dehydration		
	Neoplasia		
	Metabolic (renal/liver failure)		
	Toxin (organophosphate, other)		
Collapse/sudden death	Infectious (bacterial, fungal, viral, parasitic)	History/species review	Evaluate other animals in collection and husbandry standards
	Toxin (organophosphate, ammonia, nitrate, chlorine, cleaning agents)	Necropsy with appropriate ancillary testing	
	Traumatic		
	Improper husbandry (temperature or hydration extremes)		
	Gastric overload/impaction		

(*continued on next page*)

Table 4 (*continued*)

Presenting signs	Partial differential list	Initial diagnostics	Initial supportive care
Skin ulceration	Traumatic (especially rostrum/limbs) Infectious (bacterial, parasitic, fungal, viral) Neoplasia	History/species review Skin scrape (direct/cytologies) Culture (bacterial and fungal) Biopsy	Topical treatment (cleaning with chlorhexadine solution and medication such as silver sulfadine or orabase) Antibiotics (if suspect secondary sepsis) Antifungals (if suspect secondary infection) Cage modification to prevent further trauma/possible hospital cage
Skin color change	Infectious (bacterial—red leg syndrome, parasitic, fungal, viral) Toxin Topical irritant Dehydration	History/species review Skin scrape (direct/cytologies/cultures) Chytrid PCR evaluation Fecal	Antibiotics (if suspect sepsis) Antifungal Fluid support Hospital cage Nutritional support
Body distention	Infectious (bacterial, parasitic, viral, fungal) Metabolic (renal/liver failure) Cardiac failure Neoplasia Ova retention Atonic bladder NSHP	Coelomocentesis and fluid analysis Fluid cytology and cultures Radiographs Fecal Ultrasound	Coelomocentesis as needed Hospital tank Hypertonic soaks (weigh pre- and post-soaks to ensure correct fluid movement) Antibiotics Antifungals Deworming Nutritional support

Tissue prolapse from cloaca	Identify organ (cloaca, intestine, bladder, reproductive) Infectious (parasitic, fungal, bacterial) Ova retention Neoplasia	Cytology of tissue (direct, other) Fecal Radiographs Colonoscopy Cultures	Clean tissue with sterile saline Hypertonic solution (dextrose 50%) to reduce edema Replace and apply a purse string suture if animal is large enough Deworm Antibiotics Analgesia
Masses	Bacterial disease (mycobacteria, other bacteria) Fungal disease (typically saprophytic organisms) Neoplasia Viral disease (Lucke herpesvirus) Parasitic cyst	Fine-needle aspirate and cytology Culture Biopsy Radiographs	Surgical removal if possible Antibiotics Antifungal

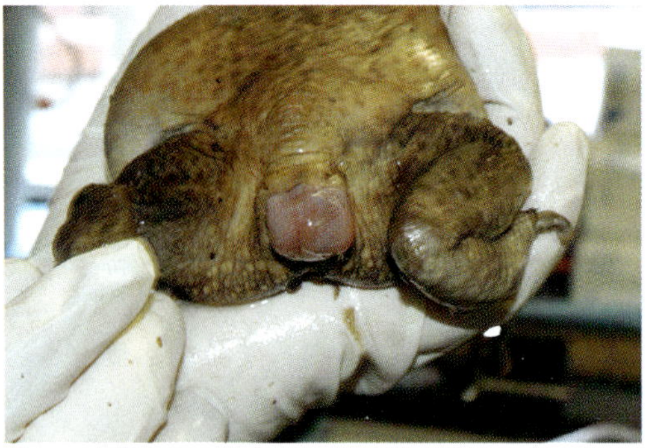

Fig. 9. Rectal prolapse in a smooth-sided toad, *Bufo guttatus*.

is recommended. In debilitated animals, supportive measures with fluids and prophylactic antibiotics before and in conjunction with deworming may improve response to therapy. Nutritional support should be provided if animals are not eating or seem underweight. In some cases, the authors have used anti-inflammatories (primarily meloxicam) in an attempt to reduce the inflammatory reaction to dead parasites.

Nematodes are the most common cause of clinical parasitic disease. Other organisms such as cestodes, flukes, and acanthocephalans are reported less commonly in captive amphibians [19]. Fenbendazole and ivermectin are commonly used in the United States for nematodiasis treatment. Possible ivermectin toxicity has been reported anecdotally and therefore proper dosing is critical. The authors have not seen ivermectin toxicity in any of a wide variety of South or North American amphibians when the drug was dosed at 0.2 mg/kg.

In conjunction with antiparasitic medication, the enclosure should be broken down and cleaned to decrease parasitic loads in the environment. The substrate should be replaced and any cage furniture disinfected and thoroughly rinsed or discarded. Plants should be replaced, because the potting soil may contain large amounts of parasite ova or larvae. If the plants need to be kept, the root ball should be thoroughly rinsed and the plant repotted in new soil.

Bacterial disease

Bacterial infections in amphibians are common [27]. Bacterial infections may be localized (eg, in a wound, ulceration, abscess, or osteomyelitis site) or systemic. Localized infections should be debrided, cultured, and have cytologies done. Underlying etiologies may include inappropriate caging (ie, causing skin trauma during normal movement or feeding or focal irritation secondary to escape attempts), cutaneous parasitic disease, bite wounds (from cage mates or prey items), or traumatic lacerations. A biopsy may be appropriate for certain lesions or if lesions are not responding to treatment. Systemic antibiotics are frequently indicated and are ideally based on cytology and culture results. First-line antibiotics are typically those appropriate for gram-negative infections, such as fluoroquinolones. Healthy amphibians are capable of mounting an effective response to localized infection, and treatment is often successful, even in cases of severe osteomyelitis. In addition to antibiotic administration, topical wound care is often beneficial in treating skin wounds. Infected wounds should be left to heal by second intention. Wound cleaning with 0.9% saline or 0.05% chlorhexidine solution followed by application of 1% silver sulfadiazine every 24 to 48 hours is commonly used in the authors' practice. Other products to enhance wound healing, such as becaplermin (Regranex gel 0.01%; Ortho-McNeil Pharmaceutical, Inc., Raritan, NJ), may also be tried.

Systemic infection (sepsis) may be secondary to a local injury, gastrointestinal irritation, or general immunosuppression. It may indicate husbandry problems or the presence of a virulent strain in a collection. Any findings of bacterial infection should prompt a review of husbandry. If multiple animals are in the enclosure, they should all be evaluated for signs of lethargy and erythema, and group treatment may be appropriate. Aquatic systems should have water quality evaluated. Gram-negative bacteria, such as *Aeromonas* spp, *Pseudomonas* spp, *Citrobacter* spp, and *Salmonella* spp, among others, have historically been associated with amphibian septic events. Chlamydia and gram-positive bacterial infections have also been reported [27]. Any systemic bacterial or viral infection may cause erythema (red leg syndrome); ancillary testing is mandatory. Cultures of blood, lymph fluid, coelomic fluid, and wounds are recommended in suspected septic animals.

Initial treatment of sepsis should include broad-spectrum antibiotic administration and the supportive care measures discussed earlier (appropriate thermal support, fluid support, and oxygen administration). In many cases, multiple antibiotics are needed in the early stages of disease to provide appropriate treatment for gram-negative, gram-positive, and anaerobic infections [12]. Antibiotics should be administered by way of injectable or oral routes in animals suspected to be septic during the initial phase of treatment.

Mycobacterial infections are common in amphibians. These are typically acquired from environmental (or atypical) *Mycobacterium* present in the enclosure soil or water. Mycobacterial infections typically cause granulomatous lesions in internal organs but skin lesions are also possible. Infection is often limited to an individual animal, and in such cases is secondary to immunosuppression or excessive environmental levels of the organism. In some collections, however, certain strains may produce aggressive infections that spread between animals. Acid-fast staining is recommended in all cases in which cytology or histology is run. In general, animals diagnosed with mycobacterial infection should be euthanized to prevent further spread in the environment and to other animals. In addition, there may be some risk for zoonotic transmission.

Fungal disease and chytridiomycosis

Fungal disease is also common in amphibians. Granulomatous infection is typically with saprophytic soil fungi, such as pigmented fungi that cause chromomycosis, or fungi of the orders Mucorales and Entomophthorales associated with zygomycosis [28]. Fungal infections are often localized to granulomas within the skin or internal organs; there can be multiple fungi and granulomas in one animal. In these cases, immunosuppression secondary to environmental stress (such as suboptimal temperatures) should be suspected and husbandry reviewed in detail. Other forms of stress (such as another disease process or overcrowded caging) or exposure to extremely high fungal loads should also be considered. Generalized fungal dermatitis with *Candida* spp or other fungal organisms may also develop and can be fatal.

Fungal disease is often ultimately fatal, even if it seems localized on initial presentation. Excision and systemic antifungal treatment can be attempted, but treatment frequently fails in the long term. Focal fungal dermatitis secondary to skin trauma may be more successfully managed with the use of topical or systemic antifungal agents such as itraconazole in conjunction with appropriate wound care.

Aquatic amphibians may develop "water mold" (saprolegniosis) infections as is described in fish. These appear as white, fluffy growths on the animal and are typically secondary to skin trauma. Increasing the salinity of the water to 1 to 2 ppt can reduce the fungal lesions and help with osmoregulation (N Mylniczenko, DVM, personal communication, 2006), though treatment in isotonic soaking solutions may also work. In deep lesions, more aggressive therapy such as with malachite green (67 mg/L) for 15 seconds (maximum) may be attempted [28].

Batrachochytrium dendrobatidis is a pathogenic fungal organism that causes mortalities in captive and wild amphibians [28]. The fungus disrupts the skin, leading to severe dehydration and death. Acute mortality is often the presenting sign and multiple animals in an enclosure can be dead within a few days. Chytridiomycosis may be diagnosed using cytology and histology, especially in clinical cases. Subjectively, in clinical cases the fungus causes the skin to slough in broad sheets, which is most easily seen by placing the animal in fresh water (BR Whitaker, MS, DVM, personal communication, 2006). A commercial PCR test (Pisces Molecular, Boulder, CO) is also available and is particularly useful for screening subclinical and carrier animals. In cases of suspected outbreak, all animals in the enclosure and other possibly exposed animals in adjacent enclosures should be treated with itraconazole soaks. When possible, adjusting ambient temperature may help slow the progression of the disease. In one study, elevating the ambient temperature to 37°C (98.6°F) allowed 100% survival after experiment infection with the chytrid organism, while other infected frogs held at constant 8°C (46.4°F) or 20°C (68°F) temperature and fluctuating 13.5°C to

23.2°C (56.3°F–73.8°F) temperature did not survive [29]. The species' normal temperature range should be kept in mind, however, when adjusting housing temperature, because temperature ranges far outside normal ranges stress amphibians.

Viral disease

A few viral diseases, including iridovirus, ranavirus, and herpes viral infections have been well described in amphibians [30]. These infections seem to be less commonly identified or reported in captive, pet amphibian medicine. Animals often present acutely moribund or with red leg syndrome, and collection mortality rates may be high. Treatment should be aimed at general supportive care, antibiotics to control secondary infections, and reviewing husbandry and quarantine procedures.

Gastrointestinal obstruction/foreign bodies

Gastrointestinal obstruction and foreign body ingestion is common in amphibians, particularly in toads. Amphibians may ingest substrate material with a meal and this material may lead to gastric or intestinal impaction or perforation. Foreign objects of a larger size, such as coins or stones, may also be ingested. Inappropriate husbandry conditions can also hinder digestion of normal food items. For instance, if the temperature is too cool and the intestinal transit time is reduced, food may become necrotic within the gastrointestinal tract. This causes excessive gas production and can lead to bloat [17]. Impaction can also develop if indigestible parts of prey, such as fur or chitin, accumulate in the intestinal tract. Contributing factors may include inappropriate husbandry conditions, dehydration, or disease. Some amphibians are prone to over-eating, which can result in severe, life-threatening gastric distention. Obstruction is diagnosed as in small animal medicine, using history, physical examination findings, and diagnostic imaging.

Gastrointestinal distention, whether from overeating or gas production, can lead to secondary shock and collapse, as is seen in dogs with gastric dilatation. Treatment involves removing the obstruction and general supportive care. Surgical correction may be needed, particularly if items are in the intestines. Because of the wide mouth and straight, short esophagus in anurans and many caudatans, orogastric lavage or retrieval with forceps or endoscopy may be productive. The exact treatment depends on the actual disease process and condition of the animal. In cases of intestinal impaction with nondigestible food items, correcting husbandry conditions, providing fluid support, and treating underlying disease (such as parasitic infection) may allow the animal to re-establish normal motility and pass the material. In cases of acute gastric or intestinal obstruction, supportive care and surgical or endoscopic removal are typically needed.

Metabolic bone disease (nutritional secondary hyperparathyroidism)

Metabolic bone disease seems to be common in amphibians, particularly in growing anurans. In the authors' experience, this condition is typically secondary to inappropriate prey item calcium:phosphorous ratio, though other nutritional and environmental factors (such as lack of exposure to UV light) may play a role [17]. Animals may present in various states. Lameness or ambulation changes may be recognized secondary to fractures of long bones or spinal deformity. Soft (rubber jaw) or deformed jaws may be evident; jaws may hang open in some animals. In other cases, generalized tetany or paresis is the presenting sign and poor intestinal motility may occur. In most animals, radiographs are helpful in diagnosis, because boney changes (eg, fractures, healing fractures, poor bone density, or bone deformity) are typically present.

Animals with mild forms of the disease may respond well to supportive care and calcium supplementation. Animals that present in tetany or with paralysis have a much poorer prognosis, though treatment can be successful. In animals with ambulation problems, the skin should be monitored closely for evidence of secondary trauma. If skin lesions are present, antibiotics should be used to prevent secondary infection. The caging may need to be adjusted to prevent further injury (eg, using bubble wrap to pad the cage bottom). Other supportive measures include nutritional support of anorexic animals, fluids in debilitated individuals, vitamin D3 supplementation, and confining to a small hospital tank until bone lesions have healed [17]. Treatment with supplemental calcium should be continued until bone density is normal (up to 6 weeks or more) [17]. The veterinarian should review the diet to ensure all insect prey items are of good nutritional value and are supplemented adequately with calcium. Husbandry, such as adequate exposure to ultraviolet light, should also be reviewed.

Trauma

Traumatic lesions include bone fractures, internal bleeding, wounds, and desiccation. Animals that were healthy before the event have a greater chance of recovery. Supportive care should be instituted on a case-by-case basis based on the actual physical examination findings. Closed fractures can be managed conservatively in many cases by confining the animal to a small hospital tank that limits mobility. Open fractures with small wounds benefit from topical wound care and prophylactic antibiotic administration. Larger wounds may need primary closure if possible. Fixation methods are poorly described in amphibians, but internal and external fixation can be attempted if needed. Internal bleeding may be secondary to blunt trauma (such as being stepped on). Supportive care with fluids as described and confinement to a hospital cage can be successful in helping animals recover from blood loss.

Renal disease

Renal disease in amphibians is poorly described in the clinical literature but seems to be common in the experience of these authors and others (N Mylniczenko, DVM, MS, personal communication, 2006). Animals with end-stage disease often demonstrate bloating or edema and may be lethargic or have a poor appetite. Antemortem diagnosis is exceedingly challenging in most cases and diagnosis is generally made at necropsy. An excellent review of amphibian renal disease is available [31].

Summary

Amphibian emergency medicine can be rewarding, though individual animals often present at the end stage of a chronic disease process and treatment may not be successful. The clinician may still have a significant impact on any remaining animals in the owner's collection by reviewing husbandry to identify areas for improvement. Timely diagnostic testing and appropriate supportive care should be used to identify disease conditions and assist in animal recovery.

References

[1] Wright KM. Taxonomy of amphibians kept in captivity. In: Wright KM, Whitaker BR, editors. Amphibian medicine and captive husbandry. Malabar (Kerala): Krieger; 2001. p. 3–14.
[2] Mylniczenko ND. Caecilians (Gymniophona, Caecilia). In: Fowler ME, Miller RE, editors. Zoo and wild animal medicine. 5th edition. St. Louis (MO): Elsevier Science; 2003. p. 40–5.
[3] Wright KM. Diets for captive amphibians. In: Wright KM, Whitaker BR, editors. Amphibian medicine and captive husbandry. Malabar (Kerala): Krieger; 2001. p. 63–72.
[4] Wright KM. Anatomy for the clinician. In: Wright KM, Whitaker BR, editors. Amphibian medicine and captive husbandry. Malabar (Kerala): Krieger; 2001. p. 15–30.
[5] Helmer PJ, Whiteside DP. Amphibian anatomy and physiology. In: O'Malley B, editor. Clinical anatomy and physiology of exotic species. Edinburgh (UK): Elsevier Saunders; 2005. p. 3–14.
[6] Wright KM. Applied physiology. In: Wright KM, Whitaker BR, editors. Amphibian medicine and captive husbandry. Malabar (Kerala): Krieger; 2001. p. 31–4.
[7] Barnett SL, Cover JF, Wright KM. Amphibian husbandry and housing. In: Wright KM, Whitaker BR, editors. Amphibian medicine and captive husbandry. Malabar (Kerala): Krieger; 2001. p. 35–61.
[8] Reichenbach-Klinke H, Elkan E. Techniques of investigation. In: The principal diseases of lower vertebrates (diseases of amphibians, book II). The British Crown Colony of Hong Kong: T.F.H; 1965. p. 209–19.
[9] Whitaker BR, Wright KM, Barnett SL. Basic husbandry and clinical assessment of the amphibian patient. Vet Clin North Am Exot Anim Pract 1999;2(2):265–90.
[10] Whitaker BR, Wright KM. Clinical techniques. In: Wright KM, Whitaker BR, editors. Amphibian medicine and captive husbandry. Malabar (Kerala): Krieger; 2001. p. 89–110.
[11] Wright KM, Whitaker BR. Pharmacotherapeutics. In: Wright KM, Whitaker BR, editors. Amphibian medicine and captive husbandry. Malabar (Kerala): Krieger; 2001. p. 309–30.

[12] Crawshaw GJ. Amphibian emergency and critical care. Vet Clin North Am Exot Anim Pract 1998;1(1):207–31.
[13] Hadfield KH, Whitaker BR. Amphibian emergency medicine and care. Sem Avian Exot Pet Med 2005;14(2):79–89.
[14] Wright KM. Restraint techniques and euthanasia. In: Wright KM, Whitaker BR, editors. Amphibian medicine and captive husbandry. Malabar (Kerala): Krieger; 2001. p. 111–22.
[15] Wright KM. Amphibians. In: Carpenter JW, editor. Exotic animal formulary. 3rd edition. St. Louis (MO): Elsevier Saunders; 2005. p. 33–52.
[16] Pessier AP, Pinkerton M. Practical gross necropsy of amphibians. Sem Avian Exot Pet Med 2003;12(2):81–8.
[17] Wright KM, Whitaker BR. Nutritional disorders. In: Wright KM, Whitaker BR, editors. Amphibian medicine and captive husbandry. Malabar (Kerala): Krieger; 2001. p. 73–87.
[18] Stevens CW. Opiod analgesia research in amphibians: from behavioral assay to cloning opiod receptor genes. In: Proceedings of the 13th Annual Conference of the Association of Reptilian and Amphibian Veterinarians. Baltimore (MD): 2006. p. 9–15.
[19] Poynton SL, Whitaker BR. Protozoa and metazoa infecting amphibians. In: Wright KM, Whitaker BR, editors. Amphibian medicine and captive husbandry. Malabar (Kerala): Krieger; 2001. p. 193–221.
[20] Wright KM. Amphibian hematology. In: Wright KM, Whitaker BR, editors. Amphibian medicine and captive husbandry. Malabar, Kerala: Krieger; 2001. p. 129–46.
[21] Stacy BA, Parker JM. Amphibian oncology. Vet Clin North Am Exot Anim Pract 2004;7(3): 673–95.
[22] Cooper JE. Urodela (Caudata, Urodela): salamanders, sirens. In: Fowler ME, Miller RE, editors. Zoo and wild animal medicine. 5th edition. St. Louis (MO): Elsevier Science; 2003. p. 33–40.
[23] Crawshaw G. Anurans (Anura, Salienta): frogs, toads. In: Fowler ME, Miller RE, editors. Zoo and wild animal medicine. 5th edition. St. Louis (MO): Elsevier Science; 2003. p. 22–33.
[24] Wright KM. Surgical techniques. In: Wright KM, Whitaker BR, editors. Amphibian medicine and captive husbandry. Malabar, Kerala: Krieger; 2001. p. 273–83.
[25] Stetter MD. Diagnostic imaging of amphibians. In: Wright KM, Whitaker BR, editors. Amphibian medicine and captive husbandry. Malabar (Kerala): Krieger; 2001. p. 253–72.
[26] Bertelsen M, Crawshaw G. 5-minute guide to amphibian disease. Exotic DVM 2003;5(2): 23–6.
[27] Taylor SK, Green K, Wright KM, et al. Bacterial diseases. In: Wright KM, Whitaker BR, editors. Amphibian medicine and captive husbandry. Malabar (Kerala): Krieger; 2001. p. 159–79.
[28] Taylor SK. Mycoses. In: Wright KM, Whitaker BR, editors. Amphibian medicine and captive husbandry. Malabar (Kerala): Krieger; 2001. p. 181–91.
[29] Woodhams DC, Alford RA, Marantelli G. Emerging disease of amphibians cured by elevated body temperature. Dis Aquat Organ 2003;55:65–7.
[30] Green DE. Pathology of amphibia. In: Wright KM, Whitaker BR, editors. Amphibian medicine and captive husbandry. Malabar (Kerala): Krieger; 2001. p. 401–85.
[31] Cecil TR. Amphibian renal disease. Vet Clin North Am Exot Anim Pract 2006;9(1):175–88.

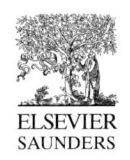

Emergency Care of Invertebrates

Daniel Dombrowski, MS, DVM[a],*, Ryan De Voe, DVM, MSpVM, DACZM, DABVP-Avian[b]

[a]*North Carolina Museum of Natural Sciences, 11 West Jones Street, Raleigh, NC 27601, USA*
[b]*North Carolina Zoological Park, Asheboro, NC 27205, USA*

Most recognized animal species lack a backbone. As a group, invertebrates are extremely diverse in their morphology and natural history, with varying degrees of phylogenetic relations. Invertebrates are becoming increasingly popular in the pet trade and as display animals in zoos and museums. Some keepers develop emotional attachments to their invertebrate pets, especially those that are long-lived, such as tarantulas. Several species are rare or carry significant monetary worth. These more rare species may be legitimate conservation concerns, making captive maintenance and propagation especially important.

Although not a traditional area of focus for veterinary medicine, there is a growing need for veterinarians to be able to treat invertebrates. Most veterinarians faced with invertebrate patients are intimidated by the fact that these animals differ so greatly from mammals in their anatomy and physiology. Little to no time is spent in veterinary curricula in the United States on teaching invertebrate medicine. To the contrary, most US veterinarians learn extensively about the role invertebrates play in causing vertebrate disease. The veterinarian is taught methods to eradicate the invertebrate rather than to preserve it.

A wide variety of invertebrates are used as research subjects in the laboratory and the field. Good data often depend on the use of healthy animals. Veterinarians may be asked to be involved in maintenance of research colonies, especially when disease outbreaks occur. Invertebrates are not currently covered by the US Animal Welfare Act or animal welfare regulations; therefore, approval by an institutional animal care and use committee (IACUC) is typically not required by most institutions [1]. Invertebrates are not likely to be continued to be excluded by the Animal Welfare

* Corresponding author.
E-mail address: dan.dombrowski@ncmail.net (D. Dombrowski).

Act. Therefore, laboratory animal veterinarians are likely to be required to become more familiar with their medicine.

The intent of this article is to provide an introduction to the general concepts of practicing veterinary medicine on nonvertebrates, with a particular focus on issues of critical care. Unfortunately, it is well beyond the scope of this work to cover all invertebrate species.

In the authors' opinions, the best approach to the practice of clinical medicine on these nontraditional species is first to have a general understanding of their clinical similarities to the more familiar vertebrates and also some level of comfort with their unique anatomies and physiologies. Remember that a good history and physical examination should always initiate any clinical evaluation. Although the practice of invertebrate medicine as a whole is in its infancy in many aspects, there are an increasing number of interesting and valuable references available to the practitioner, such as *Lewbart's Invertebrate Medicine*, *Williams' Biology and Pathology of the Invertebrate Eye*, *Cooper's Invertebrate Anesthesia*, *Cooper's Emergency Care of Invertebrates*, and *Frye's Captive Invertebrates* [2–6].

Invertebrate taxonomy

The group of organisms collectively referred to as "invertebrates" comprises essentially all the nonvertebrate organisms in the animal kingdom that do not belong to the subphylum Vertebrata (phylum: Chordata). This artificial grouping of organisms includes animals that have vastly differing anatomies and physiologies. Everything from a sponge to a grasshopper to a tunicate is included under this heading. For the purposes of this article, only those select species that are encountered in the pet trade or are commonly used for educational exhibits and programming are discussed. Extensive resources on disease and other medical issues of agriculturally important species are available and well beyond the scope of this work. A general overview of invertebrate taxonomy is presented in Table 1.

Laws and regulations

As a reminder to the practitioner, there are many laws and regulations to be considered before obtaining and keeping invertebrates [2]. Unfortunately, many people are unaware of these rules, and violations commonly occur. It is recommended that practitioners encourage their clients to contact the appropriate local, state, and federal agencies. The major federal agencies that have jurisdiction over invertebrate species in the United States include the US Department of Agriculture, Animal and Plant Health Inspection Service (USDA: APHIS); US Fish and Wildlife Service (USFWS); and National Oceanic and Atmospheric Administration, National Marine Fisheries Service (NOAA-NMFS). These agencies can all be accessed by means of the Web and can direct additional questions to the appropriate sources.

Table 1
Taxonomic grouping of invertebrate species commonly encountered in zoos, aquariums, and the pet trade (kingdom: Animalia)

Phylum	Class	Common name
Arthropoda	Arachnida	Scorpions, spiders, tailless whip scorpions, vinegaroons, wind scorpions
	Chilopoda	Centipedes
	Diplopoda	Millipedes
	Insecta	Butterflies, grasshoppers, honeybees, stick insects
	Merostomata	Horseshoe crabs
	Malacostraca	(Subphylum: Crustacea) Crabs, crayfish, lobsters
Cnidaria	Anthozoa	Corals, sea anemones
Echinodermata	Asteroidea	Sea stars
	Echinoidea	Sea urchins
	Holothuroidea	Sea cucumbers
	Ophiuroidea	Brittle stars
Mollusca	Gastropoda	Sea slugs, snails
	Bivalvia	Clams, mussels, oysters, scallops
	Cephalopoda	Cuttlefish, octopus, squid

For a complete listing of known species and their taxonomy, see the book by Ruppert et al [24].

Concepts of critical care

The key to providing appropriate care to invertebrate species lies in following the basic tenets of emergency medicine and understanding the natural history of the species. Examination, diagnosis, and treatment of invertebrate patients is infinitely possible if veterinarians use common sense and apply their knowledge of cardiovascular and nutritional support and treatment of traumatic and infectious disease to these unique animals. Husbandry-related problems, as with many reptile and amphibian patients, are the most common reason for presentation of invertebrates to veterinarians, emphasizing the need for knowledge of natural history. If the specimen is not too debilitated, most disorders can be corrected by providing an appropriate habitat (including temperature, humidity, and light cycle) and diet.

Anamnesis and physical examination

A good history with invertebrates should include all the usual information that you would gather for a vertebrate species plus the origin of the animal (wild caught or captive propagation), how long it has been in captivity if it is wild caught, how it is housed (in a group or singly), and the captive husbandry procedures of the keeper. The clinician should also determine if this is a herd medicine case or an individual animal to be treated. Information collected should include a description of the enclosure (size, configuration, and material), substrate and cage furniture, environmental conditions (temperature, light cycle, and humidity), and diet (content and feeding frequency). It is also important to determine if the enclosure is in an area in which exposures to chemicals, environmental extremes, or vibrations are possible. Obviously, it is useful for the veterinary clinician to have some concept of appropriate husbandry for the various invertebrate species encountered. Husbandry recommendations are beyond the scope of this article; however, the interested clinician can find information on spiders and other arthropods on the World Wide Web [7] and on the American Tarantula Society's Web site [8]. Information on the care of aquatic invertebrates can also be found [9].

The physical examination obviously varies considerably between different species; however, the same concepts should be applied as with traditional veterinary patients. If the animal is aquatic, make sure to examine and evaluate its behavior in the water before disturbing it. Anesthesia may be necessary for a thorough physical examination of some invertebrates, such as spiders, myriapods, and crabs.

Invertebrate anatomy

There is no basic anatomic design for invertebrates, because many widely variable taxa are lumped into this artificial grouping. It should be readily apparent to the casual observer that an anemone, arthropod, and snail share few anatomic similarities. For specific questions regarding the anatomy of invertebrate species, the clinician is advised to review other texts.

One generalization that can be made is that most invertebrates possess a somewhat open circulatory system that bathes the tissues in hemolymph. Hemolymph is the invertebrate equivalent of vertebrate blood and contains many of the same basic elements. Invertebrates do not have red or white blood cells but instead have amebocytes that are involved in hemostasis and immune function. The type of respiratory pigments used by invertebrate species varies. Some species possess hemoglobin or other iron-containing molecules, such as chlorocruorins, and hemerythrins for oxygen transport. Many species use hemocyanin (a copper-containing molecule) for gas transport.

Most invertebrate species possess a hemocoel (a body cavity containing the visceral organs that is continuous with the circulatory system). The heart is a contractile organ that directs flow of hemolymph through the hemocoel and the rest of the body. This relatively open circulatory system makes serious hemorrhage possible with injuries anywhere on the body wall.

The pulmonary anatomy of invertebrates is drastically different from that of vertebrates. Many aquatic species possess gills of varying structure. Other aquatic species as well as some small terrestrial species use cutaneous respiration. Terrestrial snails have a structure analogous to a lung, which is formed by the mantle wherein gas exchange takes place. Most terrestrial arthropods respire by means of book lungs or tracheae. Book lungs are composed of many lamellae that increase the surface area for gas exchange. Gases enter and leave the book lung by way of spiracles by means of passive diffusion. The spiracles are typically found on the ventral surface of the abdomen. Most of the commonly kept chelicerae (scorpions and tarantulas) possess book lungs. Tracheal systems are used by most insects and consist of a system of branching tubes of decreasing size called tracheoles that come in contact with tissues in their terminal stages. Gas enters the tracheal system from the environment by way of spiracles found on the thoracic and abdominal segments, which variably possess filters or muscular flaps capable of closing the openings and decreasing water loss. Gas exchange takes place in the tracheoles.

Fig. 1 illustrates the basic anatomy of a tarantula. This is a reasonable representation of the anatomy of most arthropods.

Anesthesia

Completing a physical examination, collecting samples, and administering treatments on an invertebrate can be difficult or dangerous with a conscious patient. Judicious use of anesthesia is important when dealing with these species for their safety as well as that of the handlers. Most terrestrial arthropods can be effectively anesthetized using isoflurane or sevoflurane, which is available in most veterinary clinics. Induction can usually be accomplished with 5% isoflurane, after which the gas percentage can be titrated to effect. The authors have not used sevoflurane with invertebrate species but assume that it can also be used effectively. It is important to understand that the respiratory openings of most arthropods are not found on the head but on the body at various locations. Masks over the head of arthropods are obviously not effective to maintain anesthesia. Measures can be taken to deliver gas directly to the respiratory openings (Fig. 2) or to

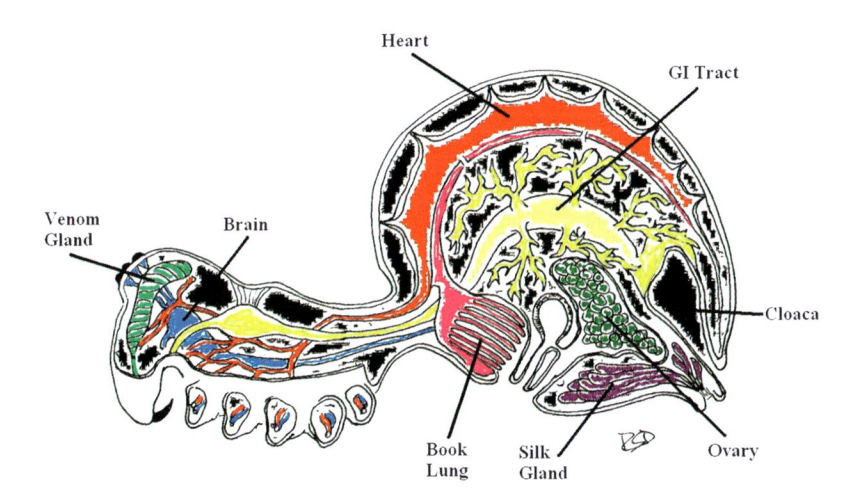

Fig. 1. Internal features of a female tarantula seen in sagittal section. GI, gastrointestinal.

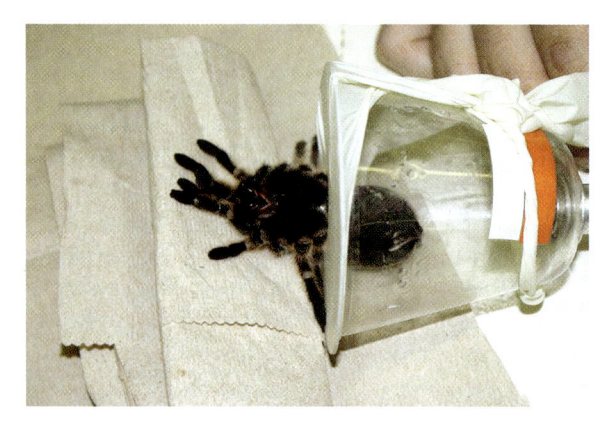

Fig. 2. A face mask with an examination glove diaphragm is used to deliver anesthetic gas to the book lungs of this Chilean Rose tarantula (*Grammostola rosea*). The tarantula's abdomen is contained within the mask. The book lungs are located on the ventral abdomen or opisthoma. (*Courtesy of* Michelle Mehalick, DVMc.)

configure an anesthesia chamber that allows manipulation of the specimen while inside [10].

Monitoring can be a challenge. Many invertebrates experience asystole when anesthetized but recover without incident. Methods for detection of cardiac movement have been described but are not clinically feasible in most cases [11]. Also, respiration occurs by means of passive diffusion in many species; thus, respiratory excursions are not normally present. In the authors' experience, it is rare to lose healthy arthropods under anesthesia despite lack of monitoring capabilities. It is best to keep the anesthetic levels as low as possible to achieve immobilization and not to assume that an invertebrate is dead until it displays rigor or shows signs of deterioration (eg, odor, liquefaction).

Therapeutics

There are few published drug doses for invertebrates and even fewer with pharmacokinetic data to support their use. For this reason, the invertebrate clinician is often required to make an educated guess as to the most appropriate dosage regimen for a particular species. Realizing the limitations of this approach, the authors typically base invertebrate drug doses on those published for other terrestrial and aquatic invertebrates.

Harmless or sturdy invertebrates can be manually restrained for administration of medications. If the process of medicating is deemed potentially stressful or dangerous, anesthesia should be considered.

Oral medications can typically be administered by using a syringe to apply liquid to the mouth parts or mouth area. It is difficult or impossible to ensure complete ingestion of the medication; thus, the clinician should be satisfied if a significant portion of the dose seems to have been ingested.

Oral ingestion of fluids can be encouraged in most terrestrial arthropods by placing them on a slant with their mouth area in a shallow dish of water. There is no danger of aspiration or inhibition of respiration if only the mouth area is in contact with the fluid, because the respiratory openings of most arthropods are found ventrally or laterally in the caudal portion of the body.

Medications can also be injected into the hemocoel of many invertebrates. In tarantulas, medications are often delivered directly into the heart because it is easily accessible in the dorsal abdomen. Care should be taken to use as small a needle as possible to avoid creation of a significant defect in the exoskeleton. If a defect is created, it can usually be sealed with a small amount of cyanoacrylate.

Hospitalization

If an invertebrate requires hospitalization, it is important that it be held in a safe escape-proof enclosure. Small plastic aquaria with locking lids lined newsprint or paper toweling usually suffice for most terrestrial arthropods. The substrate can be moistened depending on the species and its medical needs. Aquatic invertebrates obviously pose additional challenges and should be managed like fish in regard to water quality and aeration. Adequate hide areas should be provided to all animals.

It is advisable to keep hospitalized invertebrates in the temperatures ranges they are accustomed to. If this information is not known or the clinician is unfamiliar with husbandry for the species, the authors advise keeping hospitalized invertebrates at a moderate temperature (70°F–75°F). Most invertebrates can handle cooler temperatures much more readily than those that are too warm.

Light intensity and activity around the hospital cage should also be a concern. Most invertebrates prefer subdued lighting and become easily stressed with too much commotion going on around their enclosures.

Common disorders across taxa

Chemical intoxication

It is important to realize that invertebrates kept in captivity are not immune to the chemicals used by human beings to kill those in the environment that are viewed as pests. On more than one occasion, significant losses have occurred in large arthropod collections when pesticides were applied in close proximity to the collection. Flea control products that are inadvertently introduced to pet invertebrates can be quite lethal. Often, death from chemical intoxication in invertebrate species is quite rapid, leaving no time for reaction. If the specimen lives long enough to allow it, treatment should consist of supportive care (eg, fluids, nutrition, environmental). The prognosis is typically guarded to poor [12].

Traumatic injuries in arthropods

Trauma leading to a cracked or damaged exoskeleton can be a major issue in a large heavy-bodied arthropod or a freshly molted animal that is dropped onto a hard surface. Rough handling and inappropriate caging are usually to blame for traumatic injury of arthropods. Some arthropods, most notably terrestrial tarantulas [12,13], are exceptionally fragile and can incur severe damage to the abdomen with even minor trauma. Because of the open circulatory system of most arthropods, even a seemingly insignificant defect in the exoskeleton can lead to loss of hemolymph and a quick death if not addressed. With injured animals that have recently molted and do not have actively hemorrhaging wounds, the authors find it helpful to place them in a dark quiet chamber and leave them undisturbed for 12 to 24 hours. Temperature should be maintained in the range that the animal is normally exposed to. These actions allow the exoskeleton to harden completely, and, often, no further interventions are necessary. Dampened coconut husk or a layer of damp paper towels can help to increase the humidity of the chamber and reduce evaporative fluid loss of the animal. Note that it is important to avoid using chlorinated tap water with invertebrates. One should always choose dechlorinated water, reverse-osmosis water, or distilled water.

If hemolymph is actively flowing from a lesion, efforts should be made to stop it with gentle pressure by means of a gauze sponge or cotton-tipped applicator. After the bleeding is stopped, the affected area can be carefully dried and repaired with cyanoacrylate glue or paraffin wax. Anesthesia may be required for safe and accurate repair [14]. Suturing of injuries to the exoskeleton may be possible in some cases, but in most cases, this is likely to prove difficult or ineffective. One of the authors (DD) has used an acrylic fingernail and cyanoacrylate glue to stabilize a fractured exoskeleton in a millipede (Fig. 3). Fluid replacement may be necessary depending on the extent of hemolymph loss. After treatment, the animal should be placed in a dark humid enclosure for recovery.

Trauma to limbs can result in hemorrhage that is difficult to control. In these cases, most arthropods can be induced to autotomize the affected limb. Autotomy of limbs is an active process and can only be induced in conscious animals. Generally, the leg can be grasped near where it attaches to the body, and traction can be applied. When the leg breaks free, muscular spasms help to stop significant loss of hemolymph. If needed, the resultant defect can be sealed with cyanoacrylate glue or wax [12]. Loss of limbs, in general, may not be detrimental to the organism. If the animal is in an early life stage and continues to ecdyse, it usually regrows limbs. Adult arthropods that are in their last molt, stage, or instar do not regrow limbs.

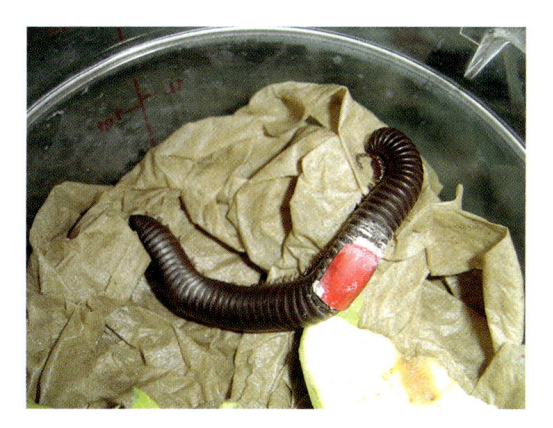

Fig. 3. Acrylic nail and cyanoacrylate glue were used to repair a fracture of the exoskeleton in this giant millipede.

Some adult arthropods have specific morphologic characteristics that identify them as being in their last molt, but many show no outward evidence.

Dysecdysis

Dysecdysis is an important problem of captive arthropods. Causes of dysecdysis include trauma of critical tissues in earlier life stages, infectious disease, dehydration, and existing deformities of the exoskeleton or any disorder that causes weakness in the specimen making it incapable of escaping the shed exoskeleton or exuvia. Attempts to free an arthropod from a retained exuvia are usually unsuccessful, because the new exoskeleton is pliable and easily damaged. Interventions during ecdysis should be performed as salvage procedures, understanding that the prognosis is guarded to poor. Parenteral fluids can be administered to an arthropod experiencing dysecdysis in case dehydration plays a part in the etiology. Placement in a humid environment may also help. Mild detergent solutions or glycerin can be used to soften the retained exuvia and loosen it from the animal, using care to avoid the book lungs or spiracles. The exuvia can be carefully trimmed with fine scissors and teased away with cotton-tipped applicators. If a single limb is entrapped, the exuvia can be trimmed, leaving only the portion directly attached to the limb. If deemed necessary, the affected limb can later be autotomized after the new exoskeleton hardens and allowed to regenerate during the next ecdysis.

Retained bands of exoskeleton may cut into the body of arthropods, resulting in loss of hemolymph or creating an infection on the body. Efforts can be made to soften the retained exoskeleton to make it more amenable to removal or to allow the animal to survive until it undergoes its next molt. Topical antibiotics or antifungals may be necessary to control infection. Triple-antibiotic ointment and clotrimazole have been used with some success with terrestrial arthropods. These medications should be applied sparingly using cotton-tipped applicators or syringes.

Arthropods that do not ecdyse properly may be left with deformities to their exoskeleton. For example, if a butterfly pupa is left on a flat surface or confined to a small enclosure and has no structure to climb and hang from as a newly emerged butterfly, it is not able to extend and dry its wings properly. The result is an otherwise normal healthy adult butterfly with small wrinkled wings. This animal may be suitable for breeding stock by hand pairing but is unlikely to be able to fly or oviposit properly (if it is a female butterfly).

Arachnids

The two most commonly encountered arachnids in veterinary practice are scorpions and spiders. Other arachnids that are less commonly seen but are sometimes kept by zoologic institutions, museums, and specialized collectors include the Wind and Whip scorpions from the orders Solifugae and Uropygi, respectively. Most spiders seen in veterinary practice are in the group commonly referred to as tarantulas (Fig. 4), and most scorpions are the African emperor scorpion *Pandinus imperator* (Fig. 5). Arachnids are diverse in the habitats they inhabit; therefore, generalizations regarding husbandry requirements are difficult. One commonality is that all arachnids are carnivorous, although prey preference may differ between species [15]. Care manuals for the commonly kept species are available [13,16].

Handling tarantulas to facilitate examination and therapy can be problematic. Many species, such as the commonly kept Mexican Red-Knee (*Brachypelma smithii*) and Chilean Rose-Hair (*Grammostola rosea*) tarantulas, are usually quite docile and amenable to handling but can cause problems

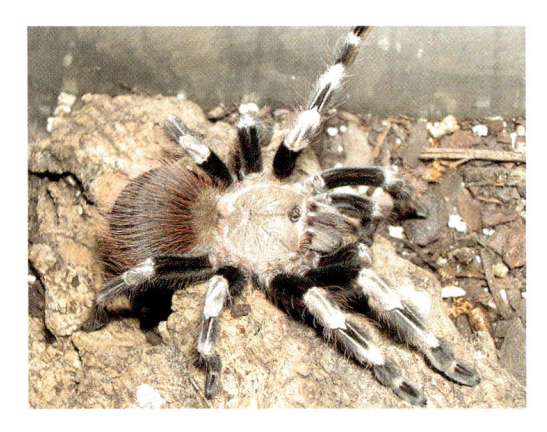

Fig. 4. Brazilian Red and White tarantula (*Nhandu chromatus*). These spiders are hardy and readily available in the pet trade.

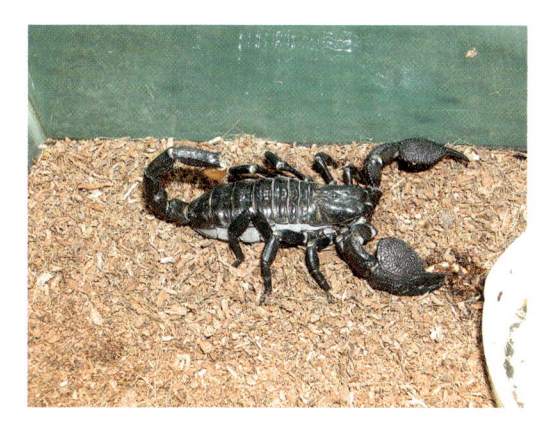

Fig. 5. Emperor scorpions (*Pandinus imperator*) are by far the most common scorpion seen in the pet trade.

because of possession of urticating hairs that are shed from the opisthosoma or abdomen [12,13]. Urticating hairs are not actually hair but setae that are part of the exoskeleton. Tarantulas that have urticating hairs kick them off when they feel threatened. These hairs can cause serious allergic reactions when they come in contact with skin or are inhaled. Urticating hairs can also cause severe ocular lesions [17]. Gloves should be worn when handling tarantulas and care used to avoid introduction of hairs to the eyes. Some tarantula species are quite aggressive and capable of delivering painful bites, necessitating that precautions be taken for handler safety. The aggressive nature of an individual can be assessed by gently prodding the spider's forelimbs with a soft probe [12,13]. Other species, although not necessarily aggressive, are nervous, flighty, and fast. These species can easily escape or injure themselves during handling episodes. Many of the arboreal species fall into this category. In general, examinations are best performed under anesthesia or with the spider in a clear plastic container.

Scorpions are capable of inflicting injury to handlers by pinching with the pedipalps or delivering stings. Most of the commonly kept scorpion species, including the Emperor scorpion, have stings that are comparable in effect to a bee sting. Other species such as the Death Stalker (*Leiurus quinquestriatus*) and members of the genus *Centruroides* have dangerous stings that can potentially cause fatalities [16,18]. In general, examination and treatment of a scorpion are best performed by using a clear plastic container or judicious use of anesthesia. Brief restraint for movement between containers and other innocuous manipulations can be accomplished by gently grasping the scorpion by the tail proximal to the telson with atraumatic forceps [18].

In general, arachnids are extremely hardy and rarely experience disease if proper husbandry and diet are provided. It is not uncommon to encounter extremely debilitated tarantulas and scorpions that have recently been obtained through the pet trade. Many arthropods are kept by unscrupulous dealers in small containers without food or water for extended periods before sale. If they are not too severely debilitated, these animals often respond readily to improved husbandry and provision of food and water. Extremely weak arachnids can be encouraged to drink by placing their mouths in a shallow dish of water, using care not to submerge the book lungs. Many also accept prekilled insects as food if placed near their mouths. Parenteral fluids can be administered as well by means of direct injection into the hemocoel or heart (Fig. 6). The authors recommend 0.9% saline or lactated Ringer's solution administered at a dose of 15 to 25 mL/kg.

Oral nematodiasis caused by parasites in the family Panagrolaimidae has recently been observed to cause morbidity and mortality in captive tarantulas. Clinical signs consist of lethargy, anorexia, or a white discharge from the mouth (the mouth in tarantulas is found at the base of the chelicerae). Microscopic examination of swabs from the oral cavity shows masses of small motile nematodes. Treatments with benzimidazoles have proven ineffective or toxic to this point. There is also a zoonotic potential with these nematodes, making euthanasia of affected specimens warranted [12,19].

Understanding the normal molting process is important for the veterinarian treating a tarantula. When a tarantula prepares to molt, it flips into dorsal recumbency for 12 to 24 hours. This is normal and should not be interpreted as a sign of disease. The old carapace is sloughed, the exoskeleton splits on the dorsal surface of the abdomen, and the spider escapes the exuvia while in the upside-down position. The new exoskeleton is quite soft immediately after ecdysis and requires several hours to days to harden properly. The spider is quite vulnerable while going through ecdysis and should be disturbed as little as possible.

Mites are occasionally seen to infest arachnids, although their clinical significance is sometimes difficult to determine. In large numbers, it is

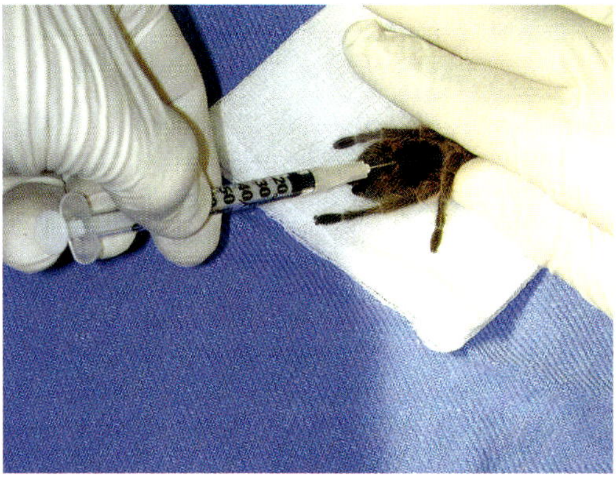

Fig. 6. An injection delivered into the heart of a Chilean Rose tarantula. The heart is a tubular structure found on midline in the dorsal abdomen.

theoretically possible that they may cause irritation or potentially interfere with gas exchange in the book lungs. Mites can be removed mechanically with a soft brush while the arachnid is anesthetized. Predatory mites (*Hypoaspis miles*) are commercially available and have been used by some keepers effectively to control mites. The predatory mites die out when their food source has been depleted [12].

Bacterial and fungal infections have been reported in arachnids. In some cases, an obvious cutaneous lesion is easily identified. In other cases, external lesions are not obvious. Hemolymph should be collected for cytology and culture in all ill arachnids in an effort to identify septicemia. Whereas the significance of some bacterial and fungal isolates from the gastrointestinal tract or exoskeleton is debatable, it is likely that any microorganism found in an appropriately obtained sample of hemolymph is significant [12]. The authors have noted that the hemocytes in ill and suspected septic tarantulas seem "toxic," showing poikilocytosis and vacuolization (as compared with presumed normal tarantula hemocytes). Treatment of suspected and confirmed bacterial or fungal infection can be with topical or systemic administration of drugs. Dosing is empiric, with little pharmacokinetic data available. The authors have administered enrofloxacin (Baytril) at a dose of 10 mg/kg by mouth or injected into the hemocoel daily with no apparent signs of toxicity.

Veterinarians are sometimes asked to evaluate alopecia on the abdomen or opisthosoma of tarantulas. As previously mentioned, loss of these urticating hairs is the result of the animal reacting to perceived threats. Remember that urticating hairs are not true hairs but setae that arise from the exoskeleton. Animals that have acutely developed patchy loss of abdominal hairs should be placed in a less stressful situation, but no other actions are necessary. The hairs do not grow back until the next molt [12].

Centipedes and millipedes (myriapods)

The subphylum Myriapoda is made up of arthropods with many legs. Centipedes and millipedes are the most commonly encountered animals in this group. Myriapods are found in moist terrestrial habitats throughout the temperate and tropical regions of the world and are relatively common captives. Centipedes and millipedes are easily distinguished, because centipedes have a single pair of legs per body segment, whereas the body segments are fused in millipedes, forming diplosegments that each possess two pairs of legs [20]. It is important to distinguish between the two, because millipedes are typically herbivorous and centipedes are carnivorous. In addition, centipedes are capable of delivering extremely painful venomous bites (especially those in the genus *Scolopendra*), and millipedes do not typically bite. Serious complications are unlikely with a centipede bite, although anecdotal accounts of human deaths are reported, and it is at least an extremely painful experience that sometimes necessitates a trip to the emergency room. Extreme caution is recommended when working with these species. Some millipedes possess repugnatorial glands that are located laterally on the body wall. Chemicals capable of causing staining, irritation, and burns are emitted from these glands as a defense mechanism [20,21]. It is advisable to wear gloves and avoid transferring these secretions to mucous membranes when handling millipedes [21].

Myriapods have internal anatomy similar to insects. The hemocoel is large and extends throughout most of the body. This anatomic feature should theoretically allow for easy collection of hemolymph or administration of fluids into the vascular space. In some millipedes, a large air cell is present in the dorsal coelom; therefore, any injections or aspirates should be attempted in the ventral regions [21]. Small-gauge needles (27–30 gauge) should be used to collect samples or inject drugs. Needles should be introduced between body segments, and extreme care should be taken with centipedes to avoid damage to their relatively delicate exoskeleton.

Many myriapods are sensitive to desiccation, especially the centipedes. Several anatomic and physiologic features may explain this sensitivity. The first is that many myriapods lack the waxy waterproofing layer found on the exoskeleton of most terrestrial arthropods. Second, in some species, the spiracles of the respiratory system are not capable of closing and serve as a constant source of water loss. Finally, centipedes secrete mainly ammonia and only a small amount of uric acid as nitrogenous waste products, resulting in relatively inefficient water conservation (millipedes are mostly uricotelic and lose less water with excretion) [20,21]. For these reasons, maintaining appropriate fluid balance is paramount in maintaining captive myriapods and in treatment of an ill centipede or millipede. Careful questioning regarding husbandry is recommended to assess the potential for dehydration.

Bacterial and fungal infections are seen with some frequency in myriapods. Infections are typically the result of inappropriate husbandry conditions or injuries to the exoskeleton that allow the microorganisms to gain access. Typical signs include lethargy and anorexia as well as cutaneous manifestations, such as softening of the exoskeleton and discoloration [21]. If a bacterial or fungal infection is suspected, hemolymph can be collected for cytology and culture [22]. Treatment can be attempted with empiric dosing of antimicrobials or ideally based on the results of culture.

Mites are commonly encountered on millipedes and tend not to be pathogenic. To the contrary, some have suggested that these mites may even be beneficial to the millipede by eating debris that accumulates in the crevices of the exoskeleton. Treatment is usually not recommended [21]. If the mite infestation is deemed excessive or the millipede is showing obvious signs of discomfort, measures can be taken to reduce the mite population. The millipede can be gently washed with water to remove mites. Materials in the environment that may harbor mites should be discarded and replaced.

Another option for mite removal is to anesthetize the millipede with isoflurane and brush the mites off with a small brush (the mites are anesthetized as well). Essential oils have shown some efficacy in controlling mites that infest honeybee hives and may have utility in treating acariasis in other arthropod species [23].

Insects

Insects are one of the largest groups of animals on earth, including more than twice the known number of species of all other taxa combined [24]. Several orders in the class Insecta, including Lepidoptera (butterflies and moths), Orthoptera (grasshoppers and roaches), Hymenoptera (honeybees), and Coleoptera (beetles), are of increasing importance in the pet trade and in zoos and aquariums. Many of these animals are used for educational programs and as exhibit animals because of their great diversity and shock value for the public. Although insect medicine may sound like a new concept to many veterinarians in the United States, as pointed out by Cooper [14], information on insect disease is not as rare as it may seem. He goes on to point out that veterinary medicine curricula in many European countries include the study of economically important species and there is much published information to be found in non-English journals [14].

Important aspects of adult insect anatomy include a general body design of three distinct segments (head, thorax, and abdomen). They also have three pairs of walking legs and many have two pairs of wings attached to the middle body segment (thorax). They can have a multitude of different types of mouth parts, including sucking, chewing, or sponging mouth parts. Some adult insects (eg, species of silk moths) do not feed as adults.

There are several aspects of insect anatomy and physiology that may be unfamiliar to the practitioner but are extremely important to consider in cases of emergency care. Insects have a hard chitinous exoskeleton instead of an internal bony skeleton. They do not have true hair as in mammals but actually have hair-like structures called setae. They have an open circulatory system with the main pumping organ (heart) situated in the dorsal abdomen of the organism rather than in the ventral thorax. Their central nervous system is located ventrally rather than dorsally. Insects, along with other arthropods, have hemolymph rather than blood that carries free oxygen–binding molecules and blood cells called hemocytes.

In general, husbandry varies considerably for different species of insects. Many are extremely sensitive to too little or too much moisture. Temperatures outside of their normal ranges can lead to stress and decreased ability to feed. Improper environmental conditions quickly lead to problems, including ill health and death [14]. A good history and physical examination should be the first step in identifying husbandry problems.

Bacterial, fungal, and viral diseases of insects can be recognized and diagnosed with the same basic tools as used for more conventional species.

Clinical signs of infectious disease in insects include lethargy, anorexia, diarrhea, weakness, irregular pigmentation of their exoskeleton, liquefaction, and dysecdysis. Wet mounts of fluids, direct smears, touch impressions, and fine-needle aspirates for staining and cytology can all be performed antemortem on individual specimens. A thorough gross necropsy with histopathologic examination is recommended postmortem for colonies or cultures. As with all live animal collections, a good quarantine and preventative medicine protocol can go a long way toward herd health management.

Parasitic diseases are also common in insects. A protozoal disease that has been recognized as a major problem in Milkweed butterflies, particularly Monarchs, is a neogregarine called *Ophryocystis elektroscirrha* (Oe); this intracellular apicomplexan organism has an affinity for the hypodermal tissues of the butterfly larvae and pupae, eventually forming spores in the tissue that become the scales of the adult butterfly [25]. These spores are cast onto host plants of the larvae as adult female butterflies lay their eggs or feed on nectar of flowering host plants. The butterfly eggs hatch, and the first instar caterpillars begin to feed and ingest the spores. After the spores are ingested, they release sporozoites that penetrate the intestinal wall of the caterpillar gut. They go through two vegetative states wherein they undergo asexual replication inside the gut tissue [26]. After the caterpillars mature through five instars and pupate, the parasites undergo sexual reproduction and form spores inside the pupae. These spores are concentrated in the areas that form the scales of the developing butterfly. After the adult butterfly emerges from its pupal case, the spores are easily spread from the beating wings and abdomen of the butterfly (Fig. 7). Spores can be shed by male and female butterflies. Contaminated male butterflies can infect female

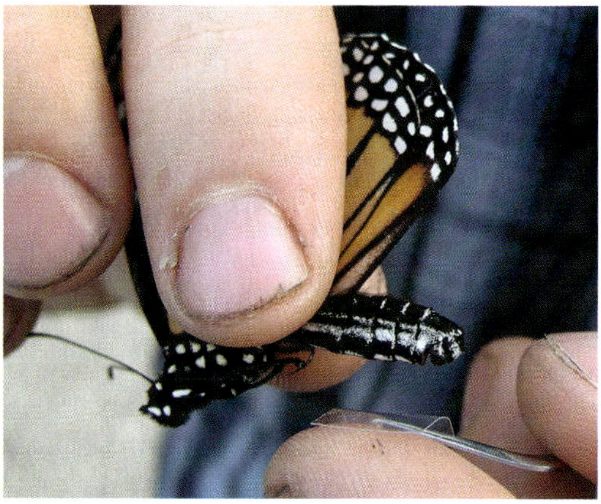

Fig. 7. One of the authors samples a Monarch butterfly for the presence of *Ophryocystis elektroscirrha*. This can easily be done by applying a small piece of transparent tape to the ventral abdomen and then examining the tape under a light microscope at ×100 magnification. (*Courtesy of* Debbie Corpuz, DVM.)

butterflies casually or during copulation. Over time, multiple generations of butterflies promote the accumulation of spores within the environment and on the host plants. Current known treatments for this disease include depopulating the culture and disinfecting the environment with a 10% bleach solution. Some butterfly farmers also report washing their plants and Monarch eggs in 10% bleach with some success.

Crustaceans

When considering subjects for invertebrate medicine, one might overlook the hermit crab; however, this crustacean is by far one of the most common pet invertebrates kept in the United States. There are two species of terrestrial hermit crabs commonly imported as pets: the Purple Pincher (*Coenobita clypeatus*) native to the Caribbean and the Ecuadorian crab (*Coenobita compressus*). These animals are sold from coastal beach shops and pet stores by the thousands up and down the eastern coast of the United States. Like other crustaceans, they are arthropods and share all the arthropod features, including an exoskeleton, segmented body, jointed appendages, and open circulatory system with hemolymph and hemocytes. Hermit crabs respire by means of gills and have two prominent appendages modified into claws. The most notable characteristic of hermit crabs is probably their unique adaptation of carrying the shells of dead gastropods for protection and shelter.

As with most other invertebrates, proper husbandry is the key to keeping terrestrial hermit crabs healthy in captivity. They should be housed in a relatively large enclosure with a substrate that is at least twice as deep as the hermit crab's shell is tall. The animal should be able to dig in and be completely covered by substrate. This is extremely important during ecdysis, because the crab encloses itself in a small cavity under the substrate and needs to leave the safety of its gastropod shell to molt. The substrate should be moist. A mixture of ground coconut husk and beach sand works well. It is also important to offer a shallow dish of fresh water. An additional dish with seawater is generally recommended. Crabs need a variety of empty gastropod shells of the appropriate size to choose from. They also use climbing structures and cover in their enclosures. There are many commercial diets available. The authors also recommend offering some dried fruit and freeze-dried shrimp.

The most common medical emergencies with hermit crabs tend to involve dysecdysis or damage to freshly molted animals. If their substrate is not deep enough or inadequate for burrowing, they molt on the surface. These animals tend to have difficulty in ecdysing properly. They may not be able to shed their exoskeleton completely. They frequently lose legs and claws in the process. Animals that attempt to ecdyse on the surface are also left vulnerable to other crabs in the cage while they are still soft. Their fresh exoskeletons take approximately 24 hours to harden fully.

A common presentation for an injured hermit crab is when an owner does not see his or her pet for a while and decides to dig it up. This inevitably happens on the same day that the crab is molting and is still too soft to handle. If a soft crab is handled, damage may be done to the exoskeleton that can only be corrected by the next molt.

Hermit crabs presented for fractured exoskeletons should be handled carefully, particularly if they are freshly molted. Hermit crabs should never be forcibly removed from their protective shells. They should be isolated from other animals and placed in a dark chamber with adequately moistened substrate. Soft crabs should be left undisturbed as much as possible for their first 12 to 24 hours and allowed to harden fully. An attempt should be made to repair fractures or damage that is severe or actively leaking hemolymph. The affected area can be dried and repaired with a small amount of cyanoacrylate glue. These animals should be isolated from other tank mates until they are fully recovered or have gone through an additional normal molt.

Corals

Corals and anemones (Fig. 8) represent the most commonly kept captive species of the phylum Cnidaria. They are cylindric organisms with a basic gross polyp structure consisting of a pedal disk, body, oral disk, and tentacles. They have a mouth that is connected by a pharynx to a blind-ended digestive sac called the gastrovascular cavity. True anemones (*Actinaria*) live as single polyps, and many true stony corals (scleractinians) exist in colonies

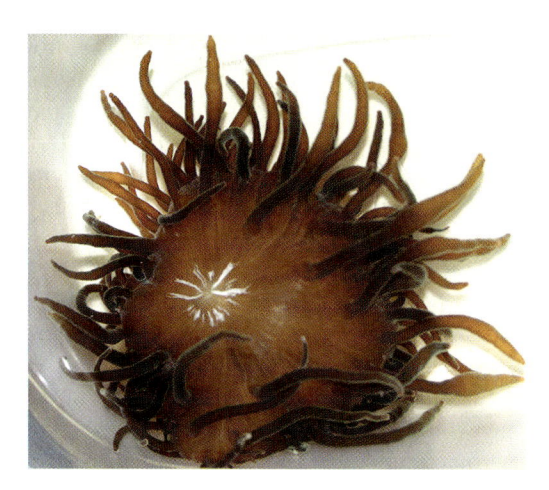

Fig. 8. A common pet trade species, the Green Bubble Tip sea anemone (*Entacmaea quadricolor*), is prepared for a physical examination. This photograph illustrates some basic cnidarian anatomy, including the mouth, oral disc, and tentacles.

made up of multiple polyps sharing a continuous calcium carbonate skeleton. Most possess intracellular algal symbionts called zooxanthellae that give them their radiant colors and supply them with some portion of their nutritional needs. Although not fully understood, zooxanthellae photosynthesis is thought to enhance coral calcification rates [27].

It is important for the clinician to remember that anemones and corals posses poisoned stinging cells called nematocysts. They also secrete a multitude of other toxic biocompounds. Examination gloves should always be worn when handling them. Corals or anemones should always be transported in single specimen bags or containers to avoid unnecessary damage caused by their chemical warfare. In most cases, if two different species or specimens of corals or anemones are in contact with each other for even a short period, tissue damage occurs.

Although, coral reef tanks have been popular with public aquariums and zoos for many years, we have only recently begun to understand the needs of coral species well enough to maintain them successfully in small home aquaria (Fig. 9). Today, many species are commonly kept and even captive raised and propagated by home hobbyists. The captive propagation of corals is called "fragging" and can be as simple as breaking or cutting off pieces or "frags" of a healthy animal and securing them to some sort of substrate. This process is similar to plant propagation by means of cuttings. Aquarium-safe epoxies or cyanoacrylate adhesives can be used in the tank to secure coral frags. Some nonstony or soft corals can be cut and secured to the substrate by means of monofilament fishing line successfully. After 5 to 10 days, the line can be removed and the coral is secure.

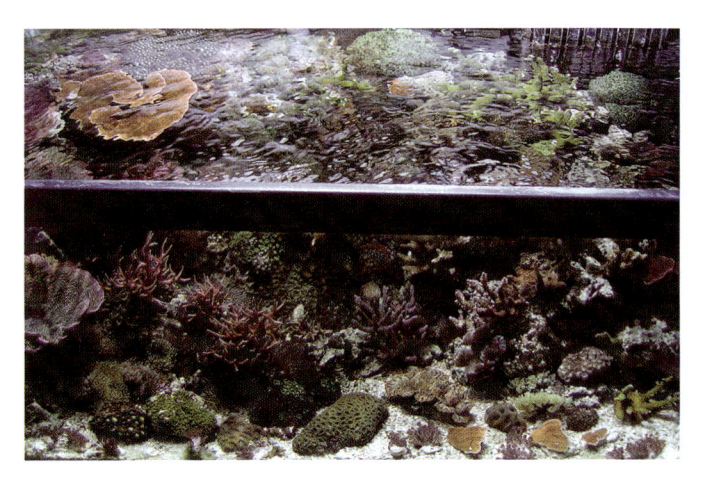

Fig. 9. A typical 40-gal coral reef aquarium with a 20-gal sump, protein skimmer, and a 400-W metal halide canopy maintained in the home of a hobbyist. Many of these corals have been grown from captively propagated frags traded among hobbyists.

As with many other invertebrate species, the key to keeping healthy coral is proper husbandry. The clinician should have a basic understanding of water quality and chemistry as with aquatic vertebrates. Additional parameters that are important with coral and anemone health include lighting; temperature; flow; nutrient load in the aquarium; and stability of pH, salinity, and alkalinity. Generally, conditions that favor the growth of green, brown, or macro algae are not ideal for most corals or anemones. A good history for these animals should include information on all these parameters and on the age and history of the system.

It is always wise to recommend quarantining new corals in a separate system before adding them to an established tank. Abrupt changes in temperature, pH, or even light intensity can shock the animals and cause tissue sloughing and death. A slow drip of the new aquarium water by means of small-diameter tubing into a separate container with the specimen and its original water can help to acclimate the animal to new water chemistries slowly. Remember to always discard transport water to avoid adding unwanted pathogens or toxins to established tanks.

The clinician should approach coral medicine as with any other animal. Careful observations and an open mind are the keys to a successful diagnosis. Infectious diseases may be caused by bacterial, fungal, protozoal, or metazoan agents. One of the authors has even seen a distressed anemone with a sea spider infestation. The following are just a few of the emergency problems commonly encountered by coral reef hobbyists.

Loss of normal color or "bleaching" is an event observed in natural coral reefs and in reef aquariums. Bleaching is caused by the expulsion of zooxanthellae, tiny symbiotic algal organisms, from the cells of the coral. It is generally thought to be more of a disease syndrome than a specific disease. Causes of this syndrome in captive corals may not be the same as in natural coral reefs. It is also not necessarily synonymous with death; however, it is usually a sign that immediate action should be taken. Bleaching or loss of color in captive corals and anemones can be caused by improper illumination: too high an intensity of light or an improper spectrum. Bleaching can be observed in new animals shocked with an abrupt change in lighting or in well-established animals as aquarium bulbs age and light spectra drift over time. Bleaching events in natural reefs have been tied to increased temperatures and infections with *Vibrio* sp [28]. Finally, it is important to remember that in some cases, shaded portions of healthy coral specimens (eg, *Montipora capricornis*) may be pale or appear bleached but are, in fact, healthy and can return to normal color if "fragged" and exposed to regular light levels. As a rule, changes to lighting sources or intensities should be done gradually over increasing time intervals, and aging bulbs should be replaced regularly to ensure a proper spectrum.

Rapid tissue necrosis is a syndrome of natural coral reefs characterized by the apparent melting away of the soft tissues from the calcareous skeleton. This syndrome or one similar to it is commonly seen with recently shipped or transported captive specimens, especially when they are exposed to high temperatures. If corals are moved from one tank to another without acclimation, they may experience rapid changes in temperature, pH, or other system parameters and be more prone to illness. This disease has been associated with *Vibrio vulnificus* in natural coral reefs; however, as Stoskopf [28] points out, Koch's postulates have not been fulfilled. If a clinician suspects a syndrome like rapid tissue necrosis or observes soft tissue sloughing, one would expect further diagnostics to be useful. Although the clinician's experience with these species may be limited, wet mounts, impression smears, Gram stains, and culture and sensitivity would all be reasonable. After acquiring diagnostic samples, it is recommended that the specimen be debrided of all affected tissue. The remaining healthy coral can be fragged, secured to substrate with marine epoxy or cyanoacrylate adhesives, and moved to an isolation system with appropriate lighting and water flow for further treatment.

A disease of captive corals know as "red bug" is thought to be caused by a copepod, *Tegastes acroporanus*, which seems to be an obligate parasite on certain species of stony corals in the genus *Acropora*. Infected corals can present with decreased growth rates, loss of normal vibrant color, bleaching, or death of tissue. Hobbyists may report a change in coral behavior over time with decreased polyp extension or decreased feeding response. The parasites appear as tiny red spots (Fig. 10) that are mobile on the surface of the coral and just visible to the naked eye. The use of a dissecting microscope is extremely helpful in identifying these organisms. Under the microscope, they appear as yellow laterally compressed crustaceans with an anterior red spot. Some corals seem to be unaffected by the presence of the parasites, but others seem to be more agitated and decline in health over time.

Although there are no published peer-reviewed studies to date, milbemycin oxime (Interceptor) has been successfully used off-label by hobbyists as a bath at varying doses and time intervals to treat red bug. One of the authors has used a one-time 24-hour bath treatment of milbemycin oxime at

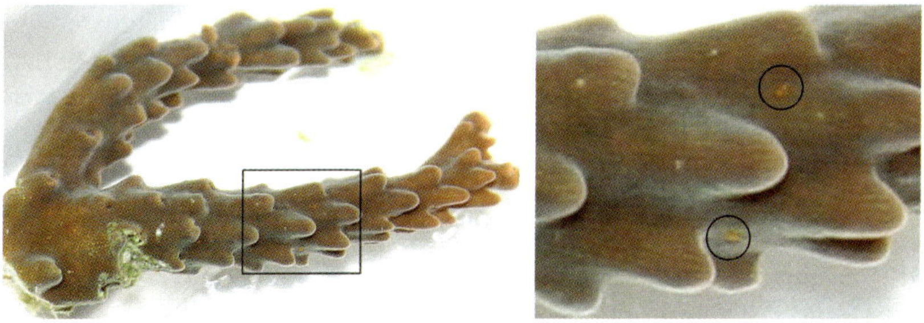

Fig. 10. *Acropora* sp frag presented for physical examination that was found to be infested with tiny copepods. This coral was diagnosed with red bug. (*Courtesy of* Michelle Mehalick, DVMc.)

a dose of 0.0152 mg/L in an isolation tank according to a protocol posted to an Internet Web site by Eric Hugo Boreman [29] modified from an original protocol posted by Dustin Dorton [30]. As suggested by Boreman on his Web site, the author removed all *Acropora* species from the main display tank and placed them in an isolation tank for 1 week. This allowed time, without any host species present, to rid the main tank of free red bug parasites. After one bath treatment and 7 days of isolation, all the corals were returned to the display tank with minimal loss and no detectable reoccurrence of red bug within at least 3 months. It is important, however, to note that many crustaceans and polychaetes died in the isolation tank during the treatment. Other hobbyists have reported varying success with variations of this method, including reoccurrence of the parasite. The clinician should note that it is always important with any bath treatment of aquatic species to monitor the specimens closely for stress and be ready to discontinue treatment if necessary.

Mollusks

Mollusks are represented by gastropods (snails and slugs), bivalves (clams and oysters), and cephalopods (octopi and squid). All are aquatic, inhabiting fresh water and saltwater, with the exception of some species of terrestrial snails and slugs. Because of the aquatic nature of most species, the health of mollusks is directly related to water quality [31]. As with fish, the first action when disease is suspected in an aquatic mollusk should be a comprehensive water analysis. Typically, water quality that is appropriate for fish should be appropriate for aquatic mollusks, although exact requirements vary according to species.

Methods for collecting hemolymph have been described for various species of mollusks in other publications [22,32]. Collection of hemolymph for cytologic evaluation and culture should be considered in all ill gastropods. Cytology of hemolymph can be challenging, because few veterinary clinicians and pathologists are familiar with invertebrate cell types and no easily accessible literature is available on the subject. Observation of bacteria, fungi, or other potentially infectious organisms on cytology or isolation by means of culture may help to direct treatment attempts.

The described diseases that affect gastropods are mostly restricted to those that affect the commercially important species of abalone (*Haliotis* sp). Withering foot disease, caused by *Candidatus Xenohaliotis californiensis* a rickettsial-like organism is seen in wild and farmed abalone. The organism infects the digestive gland and causes a wasting syndrome [33]. Oxytetracycline injections have proven effective in treatment of withering foot disease [34].

Septicemia and death associated with gram-negative bacteria have been reported in gastropods and cephalopods. *Vibrio* species are the most commonly isolated bacteria and can cause morbidity and mortality in wild and captive populations [31,33].

As with other invertebrates, trauma is an important cause of morbidity and mortality in mollusks. Life-threatening shell fractures can occur in gastropods and bivalves. Repair of a shell fracture in an apple snail (*Pomacea* sp) with epoxy has been described [35]. If properly stabilized, these shell fractures can heal as new shell matrix is laid down by the animal's mantle. Trauma in captive cephalopods occurs frequently as a result of animals swimming into the walls of their tanks or damaging their delicate bodies on inappropriate materials within the tank. Lesions can range from bruising, abrasions, and ulcers that are at risk for infection to severe cuttlebone fractures in cuttlefish [31]. Injuries should be treated with antimicrobials to avoid infection, and measures should be taken to modify the environment to avoid further mishaps. Enrofloxacin can be administered at a dose of 5 mg/kg by mouth every 8 to 12 hours or by means of a 2.5-mg/L bath for 5 hours [31].

A self-mutilation disorder is described in captive octopuses. These animals actually mutilate and consume their arms. The etiology of the disease is unknown, but it seems to be transmissible. Affected octopuses also seem to experience neurologic dysfunction. No treatment has been identified, and the animals usually die in 1 to 2 days after onset of clinical signs [31].

Euthanasia

Euthanasia of terrestrial invertebrate species can be accomplished by inducing anesthesia with gas anesthetics followed by immersion in 70% ethanol, injection of pentobarbital into the hemocoel, or freezing. Aquatic invertebrates can be euthanized in the same fashion after immobilization with tricaine methanesulfonate (1–4 g/L), magnesium chloride (10%), or dilute ethanol (10%) [31]. Immersion in ethanol allows for the best postmortem examination. Live animals should not be placed directly into high concentrations of alcohol or frozen for humane reasons [12].

Summary

As a group, invertebrates are extremely diverse and make up a huge proportion of the animal kingdom. With their increasing popularity in the pet trade and use in educational facilities, there is a growing need for veterinarians to be able to work with them. A significant amount of medical literature pertaining to invertebrates exists but is found mainly in publications not frequently perused by clinical veterinarians. Clinicians are encouraged to familiarize themselves with the existing literature and to be innovative when challenged with invertebrate patients. Persistent application of sound medical principles to invertebrate cases should continue to push forward the frontiers of clinical invertebrate medicine.

Acknowledgments

The authors thank Greg Lewbart and Shane Christian for inspiring and facilitating their interest in invertebrate medicine. The authors also thank Claudia Dombrowski and Megan De Voe for tolerating the hordes of "invited" invertebrates that occupy their homes.

References

[1] Dombrowski DS. Laws, rules, and regulating agencies for invertebrates. In: Lewbart GA, editor. Invertebrate medicine. Ames (IA): Blackwell Publishing; 2006. p. 275–95.
[2] Lewbart GA, editor. Invertebrate medicine. Ames (IA): Blackwell Publishing; 2006.
[3] Williams DL. Biology and pathology of the invertebrate eye. Vet Clin North Am 2002;5(2): 407–15.
[4] Cooper JE. Invertebrate anesthesia. Vet Clin North Am 2001;4(1):57–67.
[5] Cooper JE. Emergency care of invertebrates. Vet Clin North Am 1998;1(1):251–63.
[6] Fry FL. Captive invertebrates; a guide to their biology and husbandry. Malabar (FL): Krieger Publishing; 1992.
[7] Available at: www.insecthobbyist.com.
[8] Available at: www.atsh.org.
[9] Available at: www.saltaquarium.about.com.
[10] Melidone R, Mayer J. How to build an invertebrate surgery chamber. Exotic DVM 2005; 7(5):8–10.
[11] Coelho FC, Amaya CC. Measuring the heart rate of the spider, Aphonopelma hentzi: a non-invasive technique. Physiol entomol 2000;25:167–71.
[12] Pizzi R. Spiders. In: Lewbart GA, editor. Invertebrate medicine. Ames (IA): Blackwell Publishing; 2006. p. 143–68.
[13] Breene RG. Concise care guide for the 80 plus most common tarantulas. Carlsbad (NM): American Tarantula Society; 2000.
[14] Cooper JE. Insects. In: Lewbart GA, editor. Invertebrate medicine. Ames (IA): Blackwell Publishing; 2006. p. 205–19.
[15] Anderson DT. The chelicerata. In: Anderson DT, editor. Invertebrate zoology. New York: Oxford University Press; 2001. p. 325–49.
[16] Rubio M. Scorpions: a complete pet owner's guide. Barron's Educational Series. New York: Hauppauge; 2000.
[17] Shrum KR, Robertson DM, Baratz KH, et al. Keratitis and retinitis secondary to tarantula hair. Arch Ophthalmol 1999;117(8):1096–7.
[18] Frye FL. Scorpions. In: Lewbart GA, editor. Invertebrate medicine. Ames (IA): Blackwell Publishing; 2006. p. 169–78.
[19] Pizzi R, Carta L, George S. Oral nematode infection of tarantulas. Vet Rec 2003;152(22): 695.
[20] Tait NN. The myriapoda. In: Anderson DT, editor. Invertebrate zoology. New York: Oxford University Press; 2001. p. 275–91.
[21] Chitty JR. Myriapods (centipedes and millipedes). In: Lewbart GA, editor. Invertebrate medicine. Ames (IA): Blackwell Publishing; 2006. p. 195–204.
[22] Williams DL. Sample taking in invertebrate veterinary medicine. Vet Clin North Am 1999; 2(3):777–801.
[23] Allam SFM, Hassan MF, Risk MA, et al. Utilization of essential oils and chemical substances alone or in combination against Varroa mite (Varroa destructor), a parasite of honeybees. Bulletin OILB/SROP 2003;26(1):273–8.
[24] Ruppert EE, Fox RS, Barnes RD. Invertebrate zoology, a functional evolutionary approach. 7th edition. Belmont (CA): Brooks/Cole- Thomas Learning; 2004.

[25] McLaughlin RE, Myers J. Ophryocystis elektroscirrha sp. n., a neogreganine pathogen of the Monarch Butterfly Danaus plexippus (L.) and the Florida Queen Butterfly D. gilippus berenice Cramer. J Protozool 1970;17(2):300–5.
[26] Altizer SM, Oberhauser KS. Effects of the protozoan parasite Ophryocystis elektroscirrha on the fitness of the monarch butterflies (Danaus plexippus). J Invertebr Pathol 1999; 74(1):76–88.
[27] Muller-Parker G, Elia CF. Interactions between corals and their symbiotic algae. In: Birkeland C, editor. Life and death of coral reefs. New York: Chapman and Hall; 1997. p. 96–112.
[28] Stoskopf MK. Coelenterates. In: Lewbart GA, editor. Invertebrate medicine. Ames (IA): Blackwell Publishing; 2006. p. 19–51.
[29] Available at: http://www.ericborneman.com/Tegastes-content/Research.html. Accessed September 13, 2006.
[30] Discussion forums for Reefs.org and Advanced Aquarist Online Magazine. Reefs.org Bulletin Board. Available at: http://www.reefs.org/phpBB2/viewtopic.php?t=45859. Accessed September 13, 2006.
[31] Scimeca JM. Cephalopods. In: Lewbart GA, editor. Invertebrate medicine. Ames (IA): Blackwell Publishing; 2006. p. 79–90.
[32] Sminia T. Gastropods. In: Ratcliffe NA, Rowley AF, editors. Invertebrate blood cells, vol. 1. New York: Academic Press; 1981. p. 191–232.
[33] Smolowitz R. Gastropods. In: Lewbart GA, editor. Invertebrate medicine. Ames (IA): Blackwell Publishing; 2006. p. 65–78.
[34] Friedman CS, Trevelyan G, Robbins TT, et al. Development of an oral administration of oxytetracycline to control losses due to withering syndrome in cultured red abalone Haliotis rufescens. Aquaculture 2003;224:1–23.
[35] Lewbart GA, Christian LS. Repair of a fractured shell in an apple snail. Exotic DVM 2003; 5(2):8–9.

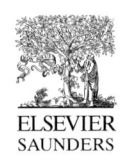

Emergency and Critical Care of Fish

Catherine A. Hadfield, MA, VetMB, MRCVS[a],*,
Brent R. Whitaker, MS, DVM[a,b],
Leigh Ann Clayton, DVM, DABVP-Avian[a]

[a]*National Aquarium in Baltimore, Pier 3, 501 East Pratt Street, Baltimore, MD 21202, USA*
[b]*Center of Marine Biotechnology, University of Maryland, 701 East Pratt Street, Baltimore, MD 21202, USA*

A great variety of fish species are kept in private and public aquaria and ponds. These fish can be divided into two main groups: the bony teleosts (eg, freshwater koi carp and marine clownfish) and the cartilaginous elasmobranchs (eg, dogfish and stingrays). Most true fish emergencies seen by clinicians involve teleosts showing acute morbidity or mortality in freshwater or marine aquaria or outdoor freshwater ponds.

Fish emergencies are often first communicated over the telephone. A history should be taken, and immediate recommendations can be given, particularly increasing aeration, assessing water quality, and providing suitable water. Whenever possible, an on-site visit is recommended to examine the fish and their environment and to provide emergency care, although the fish may be brought into the practice. Further diagnostics under manual or chemical restraint may be necessary to reach a diagnosis, and necropsies can be useful. Although the immediate needs of the animals depend on the case, a thorough evaluation of the environment is usually required to identify the primary cause.

Fish health and the environment: an overview

Fish are completely dependent on their aquatic environment. The water is their source of oxygen and is where waste products (eg, ammonia, carbon dioxide) are released. Their respiratory surfaces (gills) are bathed in water; thus, the composition of the water, including essential ions (eg, sodium,

---

* Corresponding author.
E-mail address: khadfield@aqua.org (C.A. Hadfield).

chloride, magnesium, calcium, bicarbonate, hydrogen) and toxins (eg, ammonia, chlorine, copper), is critical. The water also dictates the temperature of these ectotherms. Life support equipment is used to maintain these parameters within an appropriate range; in a simple tropical freshwater system (eg, guppies, tetras), this usually includes a water pump or air pump, filter, and heater. A basic understanding of these factors is essential in fish emergency medicine.

Water parameters

Most parameters (dissolved oxygen [DO], ammonia, nitrites, salinity, pH, alkalinity, hardness, and temperature) can be measured using equipment available from large pet stores or aquarium stores. Some of the larger manufacturers of equipment and commercial assays are Tetratest (Blacksburg, Virginia), Salifert (Holland), and Aquarium Pharmaceuticals (Chalfont, Pennsylvania). All these parameters need to be suitable for the species in the system, but some general ranges exist (Table 1). More information can be obtained from various sources [1–5]. For all these variables, acute fluctuations are more disruptive than gradual changes. Acute fluctuations are more likely to occur in smaller systems.

- DO: oxygen is taken up across the gills and used for respiration. DO in the water is in equilibrium with atmospheric oxygen at air-water interfaces. Adequate DO throughout a body of water depends on movement of the water; in closed (self-contained) systems, this usually requires air pumps or water pumps. Some oxygen is also produced in planted aquaria and ponds during daylight by photosynthesis. DO is lowest in water showing little or no turbulence, high temperatures, high salinities, and high organic load. This is a particularly common problem in

Table 1
Essential water parameters

Parameter	Ideal values	Abnormal values
Unionized ammonia	<0.02 ppm	>0.2 ppm
Nitrites	<0.1 ppm	>0.5 ppm
DO	>6 ppm (>85% saturated)	<4 ppm
pH	Marine 7.5–8.5 Freshwater 6.5–7.5	Acute changes or outside the species' range
Salinity	Marine 30–35 ppt Brackish 5–20 ppt Freshwater <3 ppt	Acute changes or outside the species' range
Temperature	Tropical 22–30°C (70–85°F) Temperate 15–22°C (60–70°F) Cold 7–15°C (45–60°F)	Acute changes or outside the species' range

Note that ppm = mg/L and ppt = g/L.
Abbreviations: DO, dissolved oxygen; ppt, parts per thousand.

outdoor ponds during the summer; DO is decreased by the high temperatures, high organic loads (heavy plant or algae growth, water evaporation, or falling leaves) and is lowest in the morning before photosynthesis starts again. One further factor that decreases DO is formalin, a treatment commonly available to hobbyists. DO meters and assays are not owned by many hobbyists but are recommended for clinicians with moderate fish case loads. They must be used on-site. When DO cannot be measured, it should be assumed to be low with these predisposing factors.
- Ammonia and nitrites: ammonia is the primary nitrogenous waste product of fish and is toxic to fish. No ammonia should be present in the water. It should be removed with partial water changes or used by the nitrogen cycle. The nitrogen cycle involves bacteria that oxidize ammonia to nitrites and then to less toxic nitrates. Nitrates are then used by plants and algae and are eventually ingested by fish. These essential bacteria can be found localized in biologic filters and on every surface in the aquarium (eg, in the gravel, on the décor). Ammonia is found when these bacteria are overloaded (eg, overstocking, overfeeding, infrequent water changes to remove the toxin) or damaged (eg, antibiotic baths, salinity changes, copper treatment). Total ammonia and nitrites can be measured using commercial assays, and water samples can be taken off-site for analysis (Fig. 1). The measurable total ammonia nitrogen (TAN) is actually composed of unionized and ionized ammonia (NH_3 and NH_4^+) in equilibrium. The unionized form is the soluble and toxic form and increases with high temperature and pH; therefore, although any ammonia is detrimental, this is particularly damaging when combined with high temperature and pH.

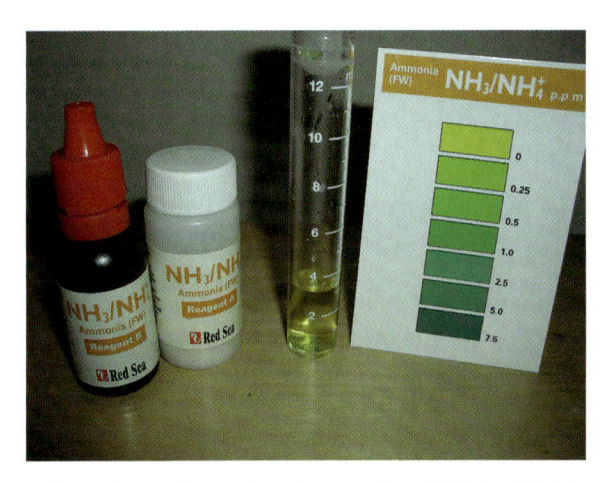

Fig. 1. Ammonia colorimetric assay ("test kit"); low TAN.

- Salinity: this is a measurement of all the salts in the water, and along with pH, alkalinity, and hardness, affects the ionic balance of the fish. Fish are adapted to live within specific salinity ranges. Salinity can be measured using a handheld refractometer but is more accurately measured using a conductivity meter.
- pH: this is the inverse log of the hydrogen ion concentration. Fish are adapted to live within specific ranges, which are often slightly alkaline for marine fish and slightly acidic for some freshwater fish (eg, Amazonian species). High pH increases the proportion of toxic unionized ammonia. pH can be measured using commercial assays.
- Alkalinity and hardness: alkalinity (also known as KH) is a measure of the anion concentration (eg, bicarbonate) and provides an assessment of the buffering capacity of the water. Low alkalinity means the pH is more likely to fluctuate rapidly away from neutral. Hardness (also known as GH) is a measure of the cation concentration (eg, magnesium, calcium); these are essential minerals in fish. Alkalinity and hardness can be measured using test kits, but they fluctuate less than the other variables and, if established, do not need to be measured in every case.
- Temperature: high temperatures increase the proportion of toxic ammonia and decrease DO. Temperature also affects disease susceptibility, food intake, and drug pharmacokinetics. It must be measured on-site.

Equipment to maintain water quality

The equipment used to maintain an appropriate and stable environment is clinically important [2,3,6].

- Pumps (water and air): water pumps produce water flow through the system and filters. Air pumps aerate the water and generate water flow.
- Filters (biologic, mechanical, and chemical): all systems should have biologic filters containing media with a high surface area for colonization by bacteria involved in the nitrogen cycle (eg, canister filters, undergravel filters, fluidized beds). It takes several weeks for these bacteria to become established in a new or damaged filter. Any environmental change that affects this bacterial fauna (eg, antibiotic baths, acute temperature or salinity changes) inhibits its ability to oxidize toxic ammonia. Systems may also have mechanical filters (eg, protein skimmers [also called foam fractionators], sand filters) that entrap particulate matter (eg, fecal material). Systems may have chemical filters (eg, activated carbon, zeolite) that bind potential toxins (eg, ammonia, copper). Ultraviolet sterilizers or ozone may be present on more elaborate systems to destroy potential toxins or pathogens.
- Lights: these should provide a suitable light spectrum, intensity, and photoperiod.
- Heaters and chillers: these may be required to provide a stable and appropriate water temperature.

All these life support systems must be suited to the size and design of the system and require regular monitoring and maintenance [2,3,6]. Malfunctions in any of these can directly alter environmental parameters and cause mortality. A common problem with hobbyists is obstructed or damaged biologic filters disrupting the nitrogen cycle and permitting ammonia to increase. Power outages can cause heaters and chillers to fail, allowing acute temperature fluctuations, and can cause pumps to fail, which reduces DO and stops filtration. Electrical shorts leading to stray current in the water and ozone malfunctions may also cause fish emergencies.

Regardless of the equipment on the system, all closed systems should be on a partial water change schedule to remove wastes and replace salts used by the animals. A total of 10% to 20% of the water volume should be replaced weekly with chlorine-free water of suitable temperature, salinity, and pH. Chlorine-free water is obtained by treating water with sodium thiosulphate (the main constituent of "water conditioners" available at pet stores), by using spring water, or by off-gassing tap water in a container for 24 hours before use. Larger aquarium systems may use activated carbon or reverse osmosis to remove chlorine and chloramines. No system should receive 100% water changes because this would acutely alter environmental conditions for the fish and biologic filter.

Other environmental factors

Overstocking or attempting to maintain incompatible species or life stages is common and can lead to trauma or competition; this should be the first differential in any trauma case [1]. Overstocking or overfeeding fish, particularly with a biologic filter that is not yet established, worsens water quality, thus increasing ammonia and nitrites in the water. This "new tank syndrome" is the most common problem seen with hobbyists.

Recent animal introductions (eg, within the past month) increase the risk of poor water quality and an outbreak of bacterial or protozoal disease, particularly when no quarantine program exists. A minimum recommended quarantine is 30 days of observation in an isolated system.

Nutritional requirements are not well established for most fish species. Common problems include obesity in some fish and emaciation and specific nutritional deficiencies in others, which is often attributable to competition or providing an inappropriate diet [7].

History

Because many problems result from an inappropriate environment, a history should be obtained during the first client contact, which is often over the telephone. A "fish emergency form" allows staff at the practice to collect pertinent information and provide the client with immediate instruction. Important information includes the following:

- Animals affected: species, size, and maturity; clinical signs, onset, and progression; and morbidity and mortality rates
- Other species in the system: fish, invertebrates, live plants, or others
- Recent animal introductions: species, their sources, and quarantine protocols
- System information: enclosure type (eg, outdoor/indoor, closed/open, marine/brackish/freshwater, cold/temperate/tropical), size, time in operation, life support (eg, pumps, filtration, lighting, heaters/chillers), and décor
- Water source and turnover: source (eg, tap water, well water, natural sea water), additions (eg, water conditioners, salt mixes), frequency and volume of water changes, date of most recent water change
- Water quality: target and current values of DO, ammonia, nitrites, nitrates, salinity, and pH if known (see Table 1)
- Temperature: target and current values if known (see Table 1)
- Feeding records: recent food intake and routine dietary information (food items, method and frequency of feeding, supplements, food storage)
- Additives: recent treatments or chemicals added to the aquarium or pond (eg, products containing copper, formalin, organophosphates, or tetracyclines that are commonly available from pet stores and aquarium stores)
- Possible contaminants: (eg, drips of condensation from air handling units or other structures above aquaria, recent aerosol treatments around aquaria, recent pesticide or fertilizer treatments around ponds)

Responses also help to evaluate the experience level of the aquarist.

Immediate responses

The following advice is generally applicable and can be provided over the telephone:

1. Provide additional aeration by adding air pumps and air stones and increasing water flow (Fig. 2). Use air that is not contaminated by aerosols, such as cigarette smoke or exhaust fumes.
2. Measure water temperature (see Table 1).
3. Measure water quality parameters: DO, ammonia, nitrites, salinity, and pH (see Table 1). If the owner is unable to do this, recommend that he or she brings 1 L of tank water to the veterinary clinic or local aquarium store within 1 to 2 hours for analysis of ammonia, nitrites, salinity, and pH. For later analysis of other toxins, freeze 1 L of water in a plastic bottle.
4. If possible, change 50% of the system volume with water that is similar in temperature, salinity, and pH and is chlorine-free. Conduct additional water changes as needed. If the water cannot be changed or a known toxin cannot be removed (eg, fertilizer contamination of a pond), the fish should

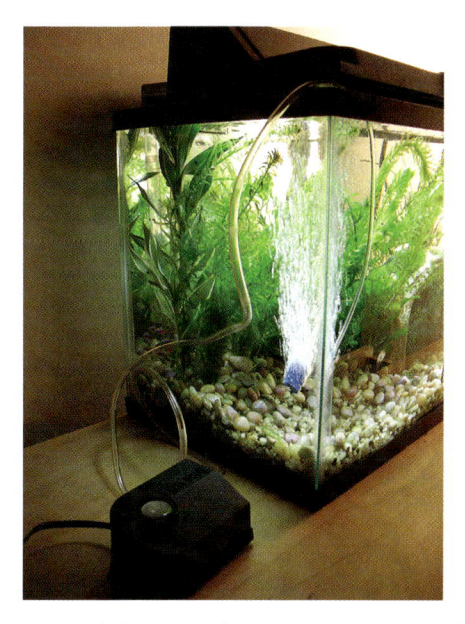

Fig. 2. Air pump and air stone to increase oxygen content of the water.

be moved to a different aquarium with water of a suitable temperature, salinity, and pH. When moving fish, it is important to acclimate them gradually; place each fish in a bag or bucket with enough water from the original tank to cover the fish, gradually mix in the water from the new system over approximate 20 minutes, and then transfer the fish to the new tank.
5. Confirm that life support systems (eg, pumps, filters, lights, heaters, chillers) are operating normally. Correct any obvious malfunctions.
6. Stop feeding for a few days to improve water quality.
7. Isolate affected fish and any fish being traumatized by tank mates, using partitions or floating baskets.
8. Remove dead fish, place them in a bag with a little tank water, and chill at 2°C to 4°C (35°F–39°F). Unless an on-site visit is possible, transport the fish as soon as possible to the clinic for necropsy.

Consultation and clinical examination

The best approach is for a properly equipped veterinarian [8] to visit the system. When an on-site visit is not possible, affected fish may be brought into the practice.

Transport

For transport, a sturdy plastic bag or bucket with a lid should be filled one third with tank water (enough to cover the fish), with only one fish per container. Bags should then be filled with air or oxygen, tied off, placed in a second bag to reduce the risk of a leak, and transported in a cooler to reduce temperature fluctuations. A portable air pump should be available in case animals show signs of respiratory distress and if transport is likely to be more than 1 hour. Because many hobbyists do not have such pumps, support staff should be prepared to provide aeration of the transport container immediately on the patient's arrival, using a portable air pump and disposable air stone. It can be useful to maintain some 10- to 20-gallon aquaria with filter capacity, heaters, pumps, and air stones for short-term care of some species. Extensive hospitalization facilities [9] are rarely required, however, because most cases are best managed with the animals in their original system.

Examination

The fish should be examined to assess the degree of support required. Soft-woven hoop nets or nylon stretchers may be used for initial restraint [10]. When handling is required, wear nonpowdered latex gloves to prevent damage to the mucus and epithelium and to protect against zoonoses. Be aware of hazards (eg, spines of stingrays, stonefish, and catfish; scalpels of surgeonfish); many of these animals are best handled under chemical restraint. The following should be evaluated in all fish:

- Responsiveness: most species should be aware of disturbances in the water and try to swim away.
- Respiration: fish in respiratory distress may be seen "piping" or gasping at the air-water interface or congregating at water inlets or areas of turbulence. Increased movement (rate or effort) of the sites of water inflow (eg, mouth in teleosts, mouth and spiracles in elasmobranchs) or water outflow (eg, operculum in teleosts, gill slits of elasmobranchs) is indicative of respiratory distress. Depressed respirations are shown by decreased movement of these structures.
- Swimming behavior: abnormalities include fish that rub against structures because of skin irritation ("flashing"), schooling fish that are isolated from the group, and animals that are resting on the substrate when the species normally swims.
- Body condition: healthy fish should have sufficient epaxial muscle to produce a slightly convex profile without prominent vertebrae; most species should not have a "neck" behind the head.
- Visible abnormalities: examine the mouth, eyes, gills, skin, fins, coelom, and vent for discoloration (eg, pallor, hyperemia, petechiae), increased mucus, ulcers, masses, or evidence of trauma. Gills should be bright red, with sharp primary lamellae that divide easily (Fig. 3). Abnormal gills may be pale or have areas of gray (eg, necrosis) or brown discoloration (eg, with nitrite toxicity). The primary lamellae may stick together if edematous.

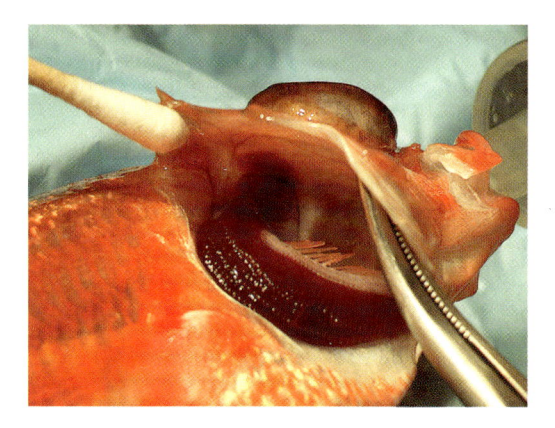

Fig. 3. Normal gills show sharp primary lamellae in an anesthetized squirrelfish with exophthalmos.

Emergency care

Resuscitation

Respiration can be assessed as discussed previously, and heart rate can be determined using Doppler or Brightness-mode ultrasound and electrocardiograms. Although the heart may continue to beat after cessation of opercular movement, resuscitation is rarely successful unless the arrest is attributable to an acute stressor or an overdose of anesthetic. The "ABC's" of mammalian resuscitation can be used to direct the resuscitative efforts.

- 'Airway' (A): oxygenated water needs to flow over the gills in a cranial-caudal direction to allow respiration (mouth to operculum in teleosts). To clear this pathway, any obstruction in the oral cavity or gill cavity should be removed, including sediment.
- 'Breathing' (B): oxygenation can be improved by increasing water flow over the gills by forcing water into the oral cavity (by hand, by syringe, or using a pump to recirculate the water) or by manually swimming the animal forward through the water column [11]. Concurrently, the oxygen partial pressure in the water should be increased using air stones connected to air pumps (see Fig. 2) or cylinders with compressed room air (1–2 L/h for each liter of water) [3]. Compressed oxygen can be used but the increase in partial pressure of oxygen may lead to toxicity, which can present with depressed respiration and neurologic signs. Alternatively, the fish can be placed in a closed container with an oxygen-enriched atmosphere (eg, bagged with one-third water and two-thirds oxygen) [8].
- 'Circulation' (C): if opercular movement has ceased and the heart is not beating, the authors believe that cardiac compressions are unlikely to be successful because of anatomic features of the area and severe hypoxia.

Emergency drugs and restoring fluid balance

A variety of medications are available for initial support. Most drugs and doses have been extrapolated from other vertebrate classes (Table 2); however, their use should be based on fish physiology. Acute stress in fish triggers the release of catecholamines and corticosteroids, which cause a transient hyperglycemia followed by prolonged hypoglycemia [12], and changes in gill permeability that alter ion regulation across the epithelium, with loss of electrolytes in freshwater fish and loss of water in marine fish [13,14]. Strenuous activity (particularly capture and transport of large elasmobranchs) increases lactate production, resulting in hypoxemia and acidosis [15–17].

Consequently, in freshwater fish, it is often useful to increase salinity to 2 to 3 parts per thousand (ppt; g/L) to decrease osmotic stress. One level tablespoon of sodium chloride per US gallon increases salinity by approximately 3 ppt. Table salt may be used, but the clinician should confirm the constituents, because many "low-sodium table salts" are actually potassium chloride [18]. Some plant and fish species are anecdotally considered sensitive to salinity treatments, but recent evidence suggests that some (eg, *Corydoras* catfish) may be able to tolerate 0.5 to 2 ppt [19].

In marine fish, it is probably most useful to administer fluids to restore volume and correct acid-base balance [13]. Fluids may be given orally into the upper gastrointestinal tract, intracoelomically, or intravenously

Table 2
Emergency drug doses that may be used in fish

Drug	Dose	Comments
Atropine sulfate	0.03 mg/kg IV, IC, IM	Tx of bradycardia
Atropine sulfate	0.1 mg/kg IV, IC, IM prn	Tx of organophosphate or organochlorine toxicity [7]
Butorphanol	0.4 mg/kg IM	Analgesia [43]
Calcium gluconate	0.1 mg/kg slow IV	Tx of hypocalcemia [15]
Doxapram	5 mg/kg IV, IC, IM, topically to gills prn	Tx of respiratory depression [7] Hyperactivity has been seen in elasmobranchs [21]
Epinephrine (1:1000)	0.2 mL/kg IV, IC, IM	Tx of cardiovascular collapse
Fluid therapy	10–30 mL/kg PO 20–60 mL/kg IV, ICe	See text for more details [13]
Flunixin meglumine	0.3 mg/kg IM once per week	NSAID [7]
Sodium acetate	40 mEq/L of IV fluids at 20–30 mL/kg/h IV	Tx of acidosis in elasmobranchs secondary to severe exertion [21]
Sodium bicarbonate	1 mEq/L of IV fluids	Tx of acidosis in elasmobranchs, risk of iatrogenic alkalosis (authors)
Sodium thiosulphate	7–10 mg/L as long-term bath	Tx of chlorine toxicity [8]
Whole blood from conspecific	4 mL/kg IV through in-line filter	Tx of severe hemorrhage [23–25]

Abbreviations: IC, intracardiac; ICe, intracoelomic; IM, intramuscular; IV, intravenous; NSAID, nonsteroidal anti-inflammatory drug; PO, oral; prn, repeat as needed; Tx, treatment.

(see Table 2). For oral administration, dechlorinated fresh water can be used. This is the least invasive route and is usually well tolerated in conscious fish; parenteral routes may require chemical restraint. For parenteral administration in marine fish, crystalloids, such as lactated Ringer's solution (LRS) or 2.5% dextrose and 0.45% saline, potentially together with colloids, can be used [13]. For marine elasmobranchs, fluids that more closely match their high plasma osmolality (900–1100 mOsm/kg) and high plasma urea, sodium, and chloride are recommended. "Elasmobranch-Ringer's" solution can be made using sodium chloride (10 g/L), $NaHCO_3$ (0.1 g/L), and urea (26 g/L) in LRS to reach an osmolality of 960 mOsm/kg (authors' preference), although other protocols exist [20]. The solution should be sterilized by passing through a 22-μm filter before intravascular or intracoelomic use.

In acidotic elasmobranchs, with point-of-care evaluation of the acid-base status (eg, i-STAT chemical analyzers, Abbott Laboratories, East Windsor, New Jersey) and no improvement after aggressive fluid therapy, sodium bicarbonate or sodium acetate may be used (see Table 2) but carry a risk of iatrogenic alkalosis [21,22]. Fluid therapy is the recommended treatment for acidosis. With acute hemorrhage, blood transfusion from a conspecific may be used (see Table 2) [23–25].

Further diagnostics

Unless the cause of the problem is already apparent from the history and initial examination, further diagnostics are indicated. Many diagnostics can be done under manual restraint, including skin scrapes, aspirations, and diagnostic imaging; many fish species can be manually restrained out of water for up to 60 seconds, and some species (eg, seahorses, frogfish) remain very still when handled. Chemical restraint is recommended for some diagnostics (eg, gill biopsy and blood sampling in teleosts) and for more active species and potentially dangerous species (eg, stonefish, surgeonfish).

Chemical restraint

Although many anesthetics are available [11,26–28], tricaine methanesulfonate (MS-222, Finquel; Argent Chemical Laboratories, Redmond, Washington) is the most commonly used because it is straightforward and approved by the US Food and Drug Administration (FDA) for food fish. MS-222 comes as a soluble white powder. It should be buffered with sodium bicarbonate (1:1 ratio by dry weight), especially in compromised fish and in water of low alkalinity to prevent a drop in pH and to reduce the loss of bacteria and ectoparasites [29,30]. MS-222 and bicarbonate should be dissolved in a container of tank water to provide the anesthetic solution; using tank water avoids acute environmental changes for the fish. For marine species, MS-222 at a rate of 80 to 120 mg/L is usually adequate, whereas many freshwater species need higher doses starting at 100 mg/L. In all cases, MS-222 should be used to effect. Additional aeration with an air pump and air stone should always be provided. Wear gloves when handling this drug or the medicated water.

During induction, fish usually go through a period of hyperactivity before they lose the righting reflex and stop moving their fins, resulting in lateral or ventrodorsal recumbency. Once response to tactile stimuli is lost but ventilation is strong, the fish can usually be handled safely. If continuous flow of water over the gills is provided by a syringe or pump, the animal can be handled out of the water (Fig. 4). With excessive anesthetic depth, there is depression of ventilation and cardiovascular collapse; if this occurs, the fish should be moved immediately to the recovery water and ventilated. Recovery should be in unmedicated tank water, and the affected fish should be isolated from tank mates to prevent aggression.

Alternative anesthetics that are useful for larger animals include intramuscular ketamine, with or without medetomidine or xylazine, and intravenous propofol [11,26–28]. Clove oil is another bath anesthetic used in the trade but is not currently approved by the FDA.

Diagnostic samples

Once the fish is manually or chemically restrained, samples can be collected as follows:

- Skin scrapes: obtain skin scrapes using a coverslip or the back of a scalpel blade running cranial to caudal in sheltered areas, such as under the pectoral fins. Scrapes should also be taken from any lesions. These

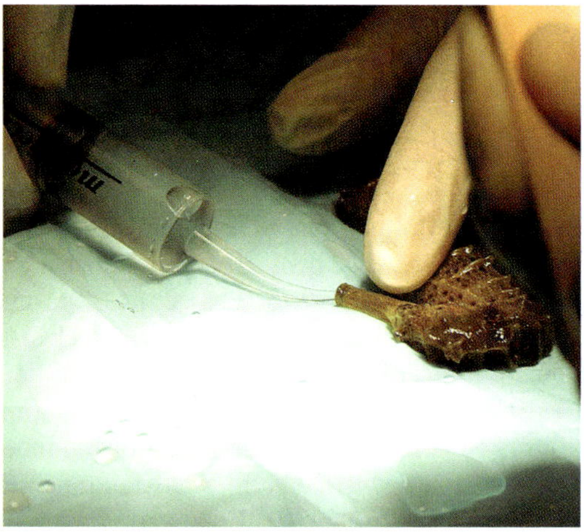

Fig. 4. A syringe is used to pass water through the oral cavity and over the gills of an anesthetized Lined Seahorse.

should be placed under a coverslip with a drop of tank water and examined as soon as possible using ×40 to ×400 magnifications. Abnormalities include increased mucus, ectoparasites (especially ciliates), and abnormal bacteria (eg, *Flexibacter columnaris*). Fin biopsies (clips taken from the distal end of fins) may also prove useful.
- Gill biopsies: cut off a few millimeters at the tips of the primary lamellae, and examine as soon as possible under a coverslip using ×40 to ×400 magnifications (Figs. 5–7). Abnormalities include increased mucus, epithelial hyperplasia (a nonspecific response to toxins or to infectious or particulate irritants), gas emboli in blood vessels, and ectoparasites (especially ciliates and trematodes). Some fish (eg, many sharks, rays, eels) require endoscopic or laryngoscopic guidance to visualize the gills for biopsy [31], whereas others have inaccessible gills (eg, seahorses, pipefish).
- Aspiration: aspiration of masses and aspiration of fluid in the coelom or gas in the swim bladder can be diagnostic and therapeutic. Cytologic examination (Gram, Diff-Quik, and modified Ziehl-Neelsen), and culture and sensitivity testing should be considered. In teleosts, fine-needle aspirates of the cranial kidney can be obtained by way of the opercular cavity. In elasmobranchs, cerebrospinal fluid samples [32] may be useful [33,34].
- Blood samples: blood can be drawn from the caudal vein or heart. The caudal vein runs just ventral to the vertebrae in the peduncle or tail. It is approached laterally (just below the lateral line, if present) or through the ventral midline caudal to the anal fin (Fig. 8). Intracardiac samples can be taken from teleosts and elasmobranchs in the ventral midline just cranial to the pectoral girdle; 1.5-inch needles may be required in fish weighing more than a few kilograms (Fig. 9). Recommended anticoagulants include commercially available blood tubes with liquid heparin in teleosts [35], dry ethylenediaminetetraacetic acid (EDTA) in sharks

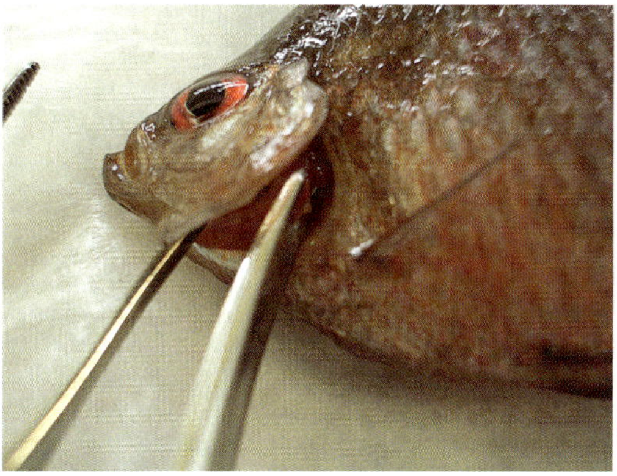

Fig. 5. Gill biopsy in an anesthetized Bleeding Heart Tetra.

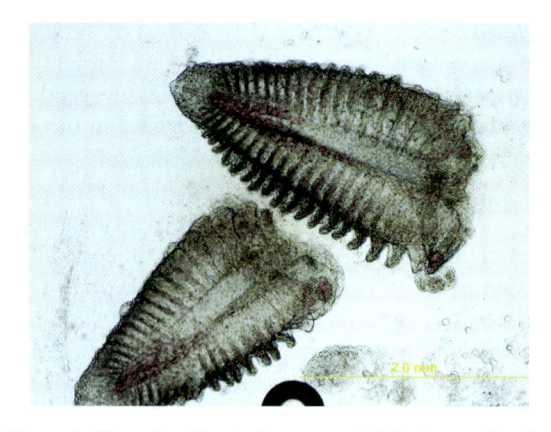

Fig. 6. Normal gills under direct microscopy (original magnification, ×40).

[36], and dry heparin in rays (authors' preference). The most useful samples include the following:
- Blood cultures [37]
- Blood smears for white blood cell estimates and differentials and for bacterial Gram stains [7,36].
- Packed cell volume using hematocrit tubes
- i-STAT analysis (EC8+ and EC7+ cartridges) to allow point-of-care evaluation of acid-base balance, calcium, glucose, and muscle enzymes (creatine kinase [CK] and lactate dehydrogenase [LDH]) [15,38]

Reference values are extremely limited; thus, blood from a healthy conspecific or serial samples are helpful.

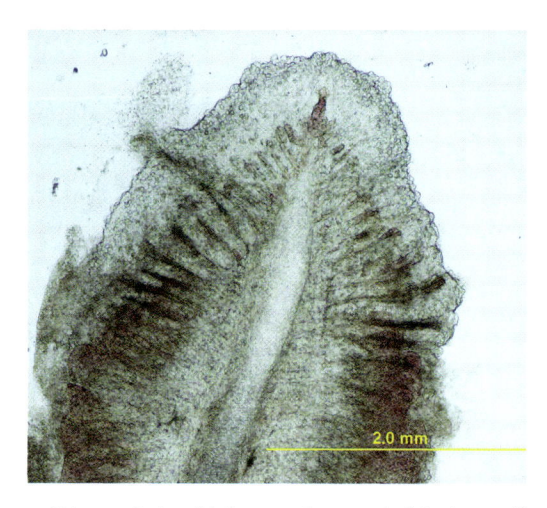

Fig. 7. Severe gill hyperplasia with increased mucus (original magnification, ×40).

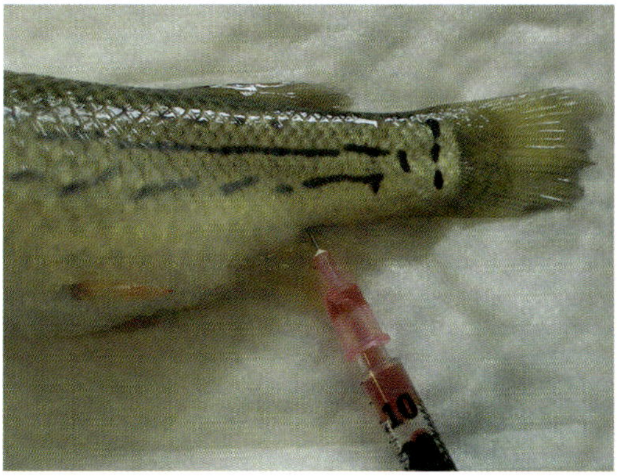

Fig. 8. Intravenous access in an anesthetized Striped Killifish.

- Diagnostic imaging: radiography should be considered if there is coelomic distention ("dropsy"), buoyancy or swimming disorders, or possible foreign body ingestion. Wrap plates in plastic to prevent water damage to the film. Positive contrast agents can be used for gastrointestinal assessment. Ultrasound is useful to evaluate animals with coelomic distention and gives better soft tissue definition in fish compared with plain radiography. The ultrasound probe can be used through water, alleviating the need for ultrasound gel.

Surgery and analgesics

Exploratory coeliotomy and rigid laparoscopy are useful to diagnose or remove internal masses and in the management of egg retention or swim bladder disorders [39–42]. Fish with external masses are also presented frequently in clinical practice, and incisional or excisional biopsies can be performed for diagnosis and treatment.

Analgesia should be used with any invasive procedure or trauma. Many fish species do have opioid receptors, and butorphanol can have behavior-sparing effects in koi carp after surgery [43]; this is one of the more commonly used analgesics in fish. Local infiltration of lidocaine and nonsteroidal anti-inflammatory drugs, such as flunixin, has also been used. Doses are usually extrapolated from other vertebrate classes, because pharmacokinetic data are lacking (see Table 2).

Necropsy

Necropsies should be performed on any mortality. Fish autolyze rapidly, however, resulting in the loss of primary pathogens and proliferation of secondary organisms (including various bacteria and the protozoa *Tetrahymena* spp and *Uronema* spp) that confuse the necropsy results [44]. Frozen

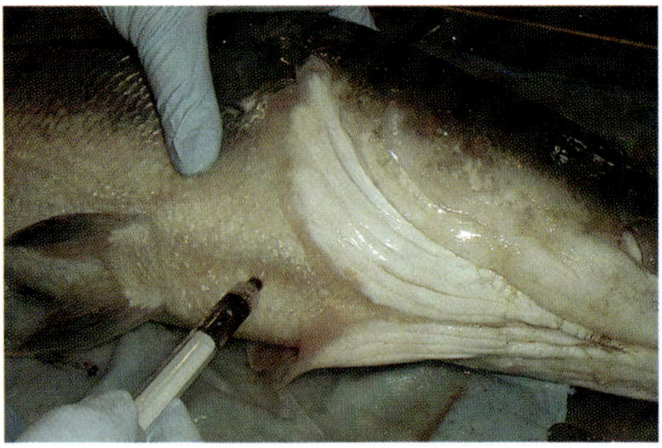

Fig. 9. Intracardiac access in an anesthetized Striped Bass.

and formalin-fixed autolyzed fish also provide much less information [44]. Therefore, although animals with an unknown time of death may still provide useful information (eg, *Cryptocaryon* spp under the epithelium after autolysis has begun), animals should ideally be examined within 1 hour if stored at room temperature or within 6 hours at 2°C to 4°C. Useful samples include the following [44,45]:

- Skin scrapes and gill biopsies as described previously
- Squash preparation of internal viscera and the gastrointestinal tract examined by direct microscopy under a coverslip with a drop of normal saline; these wet mounts can be invaluable in fish. Abnormalities include bacteria, protozoan or metazoan parasites, and granulomas.
- Impression smears from the liver, kidney, spleen, and any lesion stained with Diff-Quik, Gram, and modified Ziehl-Neelsen stains. Abnormalities include bacteria and protozoan or metazoan parasites.
- Additional samples: cultures (often, kidney and brain) should be taken as indicated. "Blood agar plates" (trypticase soy agar [TSA] with 5% sheep's blood) can be used, although aerobic swabs can be sent to outside laboratories that accept fish samples. Tissues are usually collected in 10% buffered formalin for histopathologic examination (although acid fixatives, such as Bouin's, may be preferable in fish [46]). Paired tissue samples can be frozen for viral ($-70°C$, $-94°F$) or contaminant ($-20°C$, $-4°F$) analysis. Samples may be saved for electron microscopy, and Trump's fixative can be used [44]. Because these results may take several weeks, initial treatment must be based on the history, examination findings, and direct and stained cytologic examinations.

Euthanasia

Euthanasia of moribund fish should be considered for diagnostic and humane reasons. Euthanasia of one or two affected fish should also be considered when tank mates may be at risk and no diagnosis exists. Euthanasia options approved by the American Veterinary Medical Association are buffered MS-222 at more than 500 mg/L for at least 15 minutes after loss of opercular movement; cranial concussion followed by decapitation and double pithing (spinal cord and brain); and pentobarbital at 100 mg/kg by intravascular, intracardiac, or intracoelomic injection, ideally after sedation [47]. Freezing is inappropriate in all situations.

General treatment principles

Before discussing specific emergency conditions, there are some important treatment principles that apply in every situation.

1. Provide ideal water parameters, and monitor these closely. Additional aeration should be continued throughout the clinical course of the disease.
2. When considering the route of administration, take into account the whole system. It is important to consider which animals need treatment, what parts of the system may affect the treatment, and what parts of the system may be damaged by the treatment. Potential routes of administration are as follows:
   - Parenteral: intravascular, intracoelomic, and intramuscular routes ensure delivery but can be impractical in large systems or with small fish and have no effect outside the animal. Intravascular injections have been described previously. Intracoelomic injections are usually given in the caudal coelom, and in one study, indwelling catheters were successfully maintained in koi for up to 6 days [48]. Intramuscular injections should be given into the epaxial musculature lateral to the dorsal fin in teleosts and sharks (Fig. 10) and into the pectoral fins of rays; they can usually be done under manual restraint. The authors rarely use any skin disinfection; alcohol, in particular, damages the skin and mucus of fish.
   - Oral: oral medications can be provided to a group of fish in food items (eg, inside prey or in medicated gel foods) if the fish are eating; however, plasma levels are unpredictable. Oral medications can also be provided to individual fish by tube feeding.
   - Immersion: medications can be added to the water ("long-term bath"), such as copper, formalin, or some antibiotics. In these cases, the whole system is being treated, including the biologic filter, plants, and invertebrates, and these may be damaged by the treatment (Table 3) [49–59]. Many of these medications are also removed by chemical filters, ultraviolet sterilizers, and ozone, and these need to be taken off the system during treatment. Alternatively, the fish can be moved into a smaller container with medicated tank water for a shorter

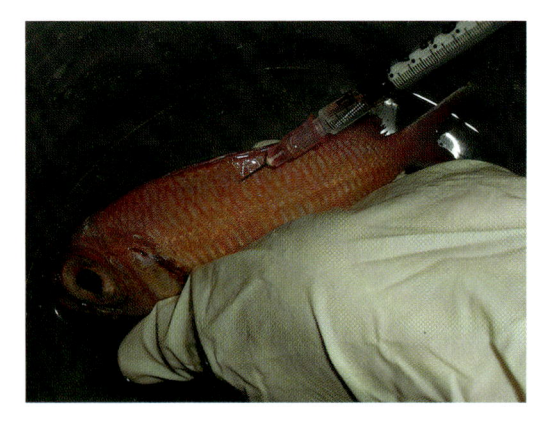

Fig. 10. Intramuscular injection in a Blackbar Soldierfish.

treatment period (bath or dip), such as antibiotic potentiators or hypo- and hypersalinity dips.

Note that FDA approval exists for few medications and only under specific uses (eg, florfenicol [Aquaflor] in medicated feed for *Edwardsiella ictaluri* in catfish); further information on this topic can be obtained from the FDA web site [60].

3. Provide optimal nutrition. There is evidence that supplementation with vitamin C beyond the minimum dietary requirement can improve immune function and decrease the effects of stressors (often, 200–1000 mg/kg of feed) [61,62]. Feeding can be encouraged using a diversity of food items (including live foods), decreasing competition from tank mates, and providing ideal environmental conditions. If fish are inappetent, the need for ongoing nutritional or fluid support must be assessed, because a positive caloric balance may improve immune function and anorexia in marine fish may lead to dehydration [13]. A tube passed orally into the upper gastrointestinal tract can be used to provide fluids, medications, and food (eg, ground food items; feline critical care diets; Mazuri omnivore gel (Purina Mills Inc., St. Louis, Missouri), which remains liquid if mixed with cold water; Fig. 11). During tube feeding, the opercular cavities should be checked regularly to ensure that particulate matter does not occlude the gill filaments. Knowledge of the gastrointestinal anatomy is useful to determine food volume, because some fish (including cyprinids, such as goldfish) lack a true stomach. Approximately 10 to 30 mL/kg can be used as a baseline, however [13]. Placement of a gastrostomy tube has been reported in a Green Moray Eel to allow nutritional support with reduced handling stress [63].

4. Closely monitor the animals and the system during treatment and after resolution. Because of the enormous range of fish species and environmental conditions, it is important to monitor closely for any clinical

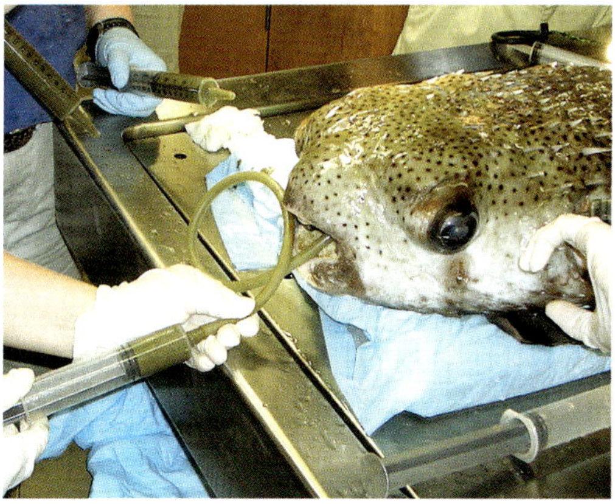

Fig. 11. Syringe feeding an anesthetized Spotfin Porcupine fish using Mazuri omnivore gel food.

changes during treatment. Reassess immediately if adverse effects are seen under treatment. Even after resolution of clinical signs, the animals should continue to be monitored, because secondary problems may occur after stressors.

Common environmental emergencies

The most common environmental diseases that present with sudden morbidity or mortality include ammonia and nitrite toxicity, low DO, temperature and pH changes, chlorine and copper toxicity, and gas supersaturation.

Ammonia and nitrite toxicity

High ammonia and high nitrites are most often attributable to failure of the biologic filter to process the load present (eg, because of overstocking, overfeeding, infrequent water changes, or damage to the filter) and are common with new hobbyists. Clinical signs consistent with ammonia toxicity and nitrite toxicity include respiratory distress, discoloration, neurologic signs, secondary infections, and mortality. In particular, nitrite toxicity causes brown discoloration of the blood (and therefore gills) attributable to methemoglobinemia.

Treatment should include daily 30% to 50% water changes until parameters are within normal limits, increased aeration, decreased stocking and feeding, removal of excess organic matter (eg, nets over ponds in the fall), and a review of the life support equipment. A slight reduction in water temperature decreases the proportion of toxic ammonia. Adding low levels of salt to freshwater systems decreases osmotic stress and decreases nitrite uptake, because chloride and nitrite ions directly compete for uptake at the gills (see Table 3).

Low dissolved oxygen

Low DO is usually attributable to inadequate aeration, increased temperature, increased salinity, excessive organic load, or recent formalin treatment. Clinical signs are the same as for ammonia and nitrite toxicity, with respiratory distress, discoloration, neurologic signs, secondary infections, and mortality.

Treatment should include increased aeration and water flow, decreased stocking and feeding, removal of excess organic matter, and a review of the life support equipment. A slight reduction in water temperature increases DO. If the cause cannot be resolved (eg, a large pond in midsummer), the fish may need to be moved to a different system.

Other toxicities

Chlorine and chloramine toxicity are common and are usually due to using untreated tap water but can be secondary to disinfection with a product containing chlorine (eg, bleach). In freshwater species, morbidity has been seen at 0.02 ppm and mortality at 0.04 ppm [10,64,65]; tap water may contain up to 2 ppm [66].

Copper toxicity is common and is most often attributable to inappropriate dosing; copper products are common algicides and parasiticides available for use in aquaria and ponds and have a narrow therapeutic index (see Table 3). Toxicity is most likely in a poorly buffered system (ie, in which alkalinity is low), especially with a sudden drop in pH or when a copper product has been added as a bolus, because both cause levels of free copper ions to transiently exceed toxic levels. In addition, copper toxicity may occur when source water is supplied through copper piping. Elasmobranchs seem particularly susceptible to copper toxicity, possibly because of differences in gill uptake [67].

Pesticides (eg, organophosphates, carbamates), herbicides, and fertilizers are possible toxins in outdoor ponds that can leach into the water from surrounding land. Formalin is a potential toxin used to treat aquaria or ponds, and paraformaldehyde is a crystalline precipitate that forms in formalin over time and is extremely toxic. Aerosolized toxins, such as cigarette smoke, can be concentrated by air pumps in indoor aquaria and can potentially reach toxic levels.

Clinical signs with most toxins are nonspecific, including neurologic signs, respiratory distress, and acute mortality. Diagnosis is often obtained from the history, although water levels of some of these toxins may be measured. Commercial assays are available for chlorine (eg, by Spectrapure, Tempe, Arizona) and copper (eg, by Aquarium Pharmaceutical or Salifert), but for analysis of other toxins, a toxicology laboratory should be used.

Table 3
Possible treatments for infectious disease

Drug	Dose	Comments
Enrofloxacin	5–10 mg/kg IM or PO SID to EOD	Antibiotic: pharmacokinetics for IM and PO dose in Atlantic Salmon [49] and Red Pacu [50], IM dose in Leopard Sharks [51], PO dose in Rainbow Trout [52]
Ceftazidime	22 mg/kg IM q 3–4 days	Antibiotic [53]
Florfenicol	10–50 mg/kg PO SID to BID	Antibiotic: pharmacokinetics in Korean Catfish [54], koi and gourami [55], Red Pacu [56], Rainbow Trout [57], and Atlantic Salmon [58,59]
	40 mg/kg IM q 5 days	Pharmacokinetics in bamboo sharks [32]
Trimethoprim sulfamethoxazole	960 mg/10 US gallons as 6–8-hour bath SID for 5–7 days with 50% water change between Tx, or 30 mg/kg PO SID	Antibiotic: tablet dissolves in water [7,53]
Sodium chloride	Increase by 1–3 ppt for >3 week bath	To reduce osmotic burden, and decrease bacterial, fungal, and ectoparasite loads in freshwater and brackish fish; hypo- and hypersalinity dips also possible [7,8,68]
Copper sulfate	Gradually increase over 3–5 days by infusion to 0.18–0.20 ppm Cu^{2+} for 21-day bath	Toxic to invertebrates (including ectoparasites, except invasive *Uronema* spp), many plants, and elasmobranchs; use with care in juveniles and novel species and not if alkalinity <50 ppm; measure daily; gradually remove with carbon filter or zeolite and water changes
Formalin (37% formaldehyde)	25 ppm bath for 24 hours (1 mL per 10 US gallons) or 100 ppm for 1-hour bath; may need to repeat	Toxic to invertebrates (including ectoparasites) and elasmobranchs; use with care in scaleless fish, juveniles, fish with skin lesions, and novel species; increase aeration; carcinogenic; found in "malachite green"
Trichlorfon (Dylox)	0.25 mg/L of active ingredient as 1-hour bath followed by 50% water change; repeat q 3–7 days	Organophosphate for metazoan ectoparasites; use with care in novel species; human health and safety issues for use and disposal; use protective wear and prepare in fume hood; raise pH to 11 for disposal [7]

(*continued on next page*)

Table 3 (*continued*)

Drug	Dose	Comments
Praziquantel	10 mg/L 3-hour bath, 2 mg/L indefinite bath, or 400 mg per 100 g of food or 400 mg/kg PO SID for 5–7 days; may need to repeat	Tx for trematodes and cestodes (authors, [7]); problems reported in some marine elasmobranchs [21] and catfish [7]

Abbreviations: BID, twice daily; EOD, every other day; IM, intramuscular; PO, oral; ppt, parts per thousand; q, every; SID, once daily; Tx, treatment.

Treatment consists of stopping the chemical addition or contamination and removing the toxin using partial water changes. The chemical can also be removed using activated carbon or zeolite. In cases of chlorine toxicity, sodium thiosulphate can be added (see Table 2). In cases of organophosphate toxicity, atropine may be used (see Table 2). In cases in which the toxin cannot be removed, the fish should be moved to a different system.

Gas supersaturation

Gas supersaturation (gas bubble disease) occurs when gases, usually nitrogen, become abnormally concentrated in the water. In an aquarium, this is usually attributable to a leak in, or upstream of, a water pump that pulls in air and forces it into solution under pressure. Clinical signs include gas emboli in the periorbital tissues, anterior chamber of the eye, or vessels of the fins and gills as well as acute mortality. Total gas pressure in the water can be recorded using specialized equipment; however, the cost of this equipment can be prohibitive. Even without these meters, the characteristic lesions should prompt a careful investigation of the water pumps.

For treatment, the source of gas supersaturation must be identified and stopped as soon as possible. Agitating the water and substrate increases the release of compressed gases. Animals may be treated with a carbonic anhydrase inhibitor, such as acetazolamide, and fine-needle aspiration of gas accumulations, but treatment of animals showing acute clinical signs is rarely successful and prevention with good system maintenance is essential.

Common infectious disease emergencies

Infectious diseases that acutely affect fish are usually caused by bacteria or protozoa, although metazoa and viruses should be considered. Morbidity from fungal pathogens is less common and often secondary to damage to the skin. In all cases, further information should be sought after emergency therapy has been given [7,46,68].

Bacterial diseases

Acute bacterial septicemia is common and usually secondary to other stressors. Causative agents are often gram-negative bacilli (eg, *Vibrio* spp and *Photobacterium damselae* in marine fish, *Aeromonas* spp and *Edwardsiella ictaluri* in freshwater fish), although gram-positive bacilli and cocci can cause acute disease [7,68,69]. Signs include petechiae, hyperemia, ulceration, ocular pathology (eg, keratitis, uveitis, exophthalmia), coelomic distention, respiratory distress, neurologic signs, mortality, organomegaly, and necrosis. Diagnosis is by means of clinical signs; direct and stained cytologic examination to identify the distribution, shape, motility, and staining of the bacteria; histopathologic examination; and culture and sensitivity testing. Note that some bacteria (*Clostridium* spp and *Vibrio* spp) appear to be commensal in elasmobranchs [70].

Treatment usually includes antibiotics (see Table 3), which should be given parenterally whenever possible to ensure delivery and reduce the risk of antibiotic resistance. Some antibiotics can be given orally in food items if a fish is eating or by tube feeding. Bath and dip treatments are also available but do have the potential to damage the biologic filter. In the emergency setting, the first-choice antibiotic should have a gram-negative spectrum, a practical method of application, and be based on pharmacokinetic data whenever possible (see Table 3). Once culture and sensitivity results are available, the antibiotic should be changed if indicated.

Protozoal diseases

Protozoal parasites are common causes of acute morbidity and mortality, particularly when animals have been recently added without a quarantine period and with high stocking densities and poor water quality. Mortalities can be sudden and dramatic in number. Some protozoal parasites of marine species that present acutely are the ciliates *Cryptocaryon irritans* (marine ich or white spot), *Brooklynella hostilis* and the more invasive *Uronema marinum*, and the nonmotile flagellate *Amyloodinium ocellatum* (coral fish disease). Common protozoal parasites of freshwater species are the ciliates *Ichthyophthirius multifiliis* (freshwater ich; Fig. 12), *Chilodonella* spp and the more invasive *Tetrahymena corlissi* in tetras and guppies, and the nonmotile flagellate *Oodinium* spp. Diagnosis is usually made using skin scrapes and gill biopsies. Some protozoal parasites, such as *Uronema* spp and *Tetrahymena* spp, may be nonpathogenic on the skin, however, and are more significant if found in muscle or viscera.

Treatment may include copper sulfate, formalin, salinity changes, or temperature changes (see Table 3) and depends on knowledge of the life cycle of the parasite and the system components. For example, bath treatments for marine or freshwater ich target the free-living stage (theront) of the parasite, because the encysted trophozoites, which are found under the epithelium,

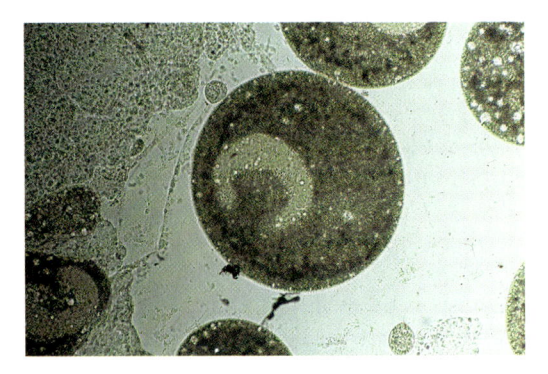

Fig. 12. Protozoan *Ichthyophthirius multifiliis* (freshwater ich) on direct microscopy (original magnification, ×400).

are resistant. Some species, such as invertebrates, are sensitive to these treatments and may be moved to a different tank and monitored closely while the original tank is treated.

Metazoan and microsporidian parasites

Metazoan parasites rarely cause acute mortality, but some exceptions exist. The monogenean trematodes *Dactylogyrus* spp and *Gyrodactylus* spp have direct life cycles and can build up rapidly, causing local damage to gills and skin, respectively. Diagnosis is usually made by skin scrapes and gill biopsies (Fig. 13). Treatment may include praziquantel, formalin, organophosphates, copper sulfate, or salinity changes (see Table 3) and depends on the parasite life cycle and the system components.

Microsporidian parasites are usually responsible for chronic disease, but one agent in goldfish is commonly presented in clinical practice: *Hoferellus* (*Mitaspora*) spp causing polycystic kidney disease and coelomic distention. Diagnosis may involve ultrasound or fine-needle aspiration of the cranial kidney, but the parasite is most often diagnosed at necropsy by the presence of white or yellow cysts (xenomas), which result from cellular hypertrophy around the gram-positive intracellular spores. Treatment is usually depopulation and disinfection.

Viral diseases

Most known viral pathogens are from the fish-farming and koi industries. Some viruses that can cause acute morbidity or mortality include lake trout and koi herpesviruses and two rhabdoviruses: viral hemorrhagic septicemia and spring viremia of carp (notifiable in the United States and United Kingdom). Diagnosis is by history and clinical signs (similar to those of bacterial septicemia), histopathologic examination, virus isolation, virus neutralization, polymerase chain reaction (PCR), and electron microscopy [71,72].

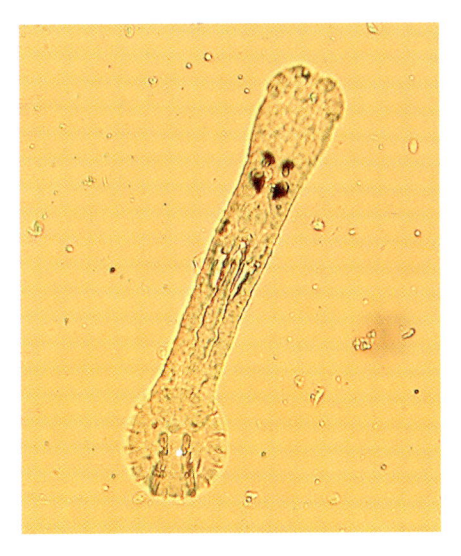

Fig. 13. Monogenean gill trematode *Dactylogyrus* on direct microscopy (original magnification, ×40).

Diagnosis for some viral pathogens requires specific US Department of Agriculture–accredited laboratories [72]. Submission protocols can be obtained from state veterinarians. Treatment usually consists of depopulation and disinfection.

Trauma

Trauma commonly occurs when incompatible animals are housed together. Trauma may also be caused by predators around ponds, jumping out of tanks, or contact with tank décor (especially in flighty fish, such as needlefish or barracuda), or it may follow transport or handling. Fish show remarkable healing when provided with ideal environmental conditions and generally require less wound management than mammals. The skin forms an essential barrier to the environment, however; thus, the risk of electrolyte changes and secondary infections should be assessed [46,73]. Secondary infectious diseases are most commonly bacterial and fungal; in particular, water mold (eg, *Saprolegnia* spp) can present dramatically as white to green cotton-like material on a wound.

Skin wounds and ulcers should be flushed and debrided with sterile saline or dilute chlorhexidine. Wounds can be closed primarily using nonabsorbable monofilament suture material and surgical adhesives. When primary closure is not possible, a water-resistant ointment, such as Orabase without benzocaine (Soothe-N-Seal, Colgate, Canton, Masssachusetts) can be used. Formation of granulation tissue may be promoted using the wound dressing Vet BioSISt (Cook Veterinary Products, Bloomington, Iowa) [74,75] or the topical angiogenic growth factor becaplermin (Regranex; OrthoMcNeil, Raritan, New Jersey) [76].

Corneal ulcers should be treated to reduce the risk of subsequent perforation. Gentle debridement with saline, followed by a topical antibiotic, drying, and then application of a thin layer of Orabase may be used [77].

Prophylactic antibiotics are advisable, and immersion baths in an antibiotic with a potentiator (Tricide; Molecular Therapeutics, Riverbend Laboratories, Athens, Georgia) may significantly reduce the risk of antibiotic resistance [78,79]. Freshwater fish can be kept in a long-term low-salinity bath to reduce electrolyte losses (see Table 3). The cause of the trauma must be identified and addressed.

Summary

Fish emergencies are most commonly attributable to inappropriate environmental conditions and primary or secondary infectious disease or trauma. A logical sequence of history and immediate responses, evaluation of the animals and their environment, and further diagnostics should establish the cause, allowing appropriate treatment. Management changes may be required to prevent recurrence.

References

[1] Tucker CS. Water analysis. In: Stoskopf MK, editor. Fish medicine. Philadelphia: WB Saunders; 1993. p. 166–97.
[2] Mohan PJ, Aiken A. Water quality and life support systems for large elasmobranch exhibits. In: Smith M, Warmolts D, Thoney D, et al, editors. The elasmobranch husbandry manual: captive care of sharks, rays and their relatives. Columbus Zoo, Columbus (OH): Biological Survey; 2004. p. 69–88.
[3] Beleau MH. Tropical fish medicine: evaluating water problems. Vet Clin North Am Exot Anim Pract 1988;18:293–304.
[4] Available at: www.fishbase.org.
[5] Available at: www.aquariumfish.net.
[6] Plunkett SJ. Pet fish. In: Plunkett SJ, editor. Emergency procedures. 2nd edition. Philadelphia: WB Saunders; 2000. p. 430–4.
[7] Stoskopf MK. Fish medicine. Philadelphia: WB Saunders; 1993.
[8] Lewbart GA. Emergency and critical care of fish. Vet Clin North Am Exot Anim Pract 1998; 1:233–49.
[9] Stoskopf MK. Hospitalization. In: Stoskopf MK, editor. Fish medicine. Philadelphia: WB Saunders; 1993. p. 98–112.
[10] Francis-Floyd R. Clinical examination of fish in private collections. Vet Clin North Am Exot Anim Pract 1999;2:247–64.
[11] Brown LA. Anesthesia and restraint. In: Stoskopf MK, editor. Fish medicine. Philadelphia: WB Saunders; 1993. p. 79–90.
[12] Wedemeyer GA, Barton BA, McLeay DJ. Stress and acclimation. In: Schreck CB, Moyle PB, editors. Methods in fish biology. Bethesda (MD): American Fisheries Society; 1990. p. 451–89.
[13] Greenwell MG, Sherrill J, Clayton LA. Osmoregulation in fish. Mechanisms and clinical implications. Vet Clin North Am Exot Anim Pract 2003;6:169–89.

[14] Groff JM, Zinkl JG. Hematology and clinical chemistry of cyprinid fish. Vet Clin North Am Exot Anim Pract 1999;2:741–76.
[15] Mylniczenko ND, Kinsel M, Young F, et al. Lessons from a case of capture myopathy in a pelagic silky shark (*Carcharinus falciformis*). In: Proceedings of the Annual Conference of the American Association of Zoo Veterinarians. Minneapolis (MN); 2003. p. 211–6.
[16] Claiborne JB, Edwards SL, Morrison-Shetlar AI. Acid-base regulation in fishes: cellular and molecular mechanisms. J Exp Zool 2002;293:302–19.
[17] Varela RA, Krum H, Lewbart GA, et al. A fish out of water: a glimpse into the 5-minute office exam. In: Proceedings of the 32nd Annual Conference of the International Association of Aquatic Animal Medicine. Tampa (FL); 2001. p. 26–7.
[18] Maclean B. Ornamental fish. In: Meredith A, Redrobe S, editors. BSAVA manual of exotic pets. Gloucester (MA): BSAVA; 2002. p. 267–79.
[19] Murphy R, Lewbart GA. Salt tolerance in the callichthyid catfish, *Corydoras aeneus*. In: Proceedings of the 26th Annual Conference of the International Association of Aquatic Animal Medicine. Mystic (CT); 1995. p. 15–6.
[20] Andrews AJC, Jones RT. A method for the transport of sharks for captivity. Journal of Aquariculture and Aquatic Sciences 1990;5(4):70–2.
[21] Stamper MA, Miller SM, Berzins IK. Pharmacology in elasmobranchs. In: Smith M, Warmolts D, Thoney D, et al, editors. The elasmobranch husbandry manual: captive care of sharks, rays and their relatives. Columbus Zoo, Columbus (OH): Biological Survey; 2004. p. 447–66.
[22] Ross LG, Ross B. Anesthetic and sedative techniques for aquatic animals. 2nd edition. Oxford (UK): Blackwell Science Ltd; 1999.
[23] Hadfield CA, Haines AN. Cross-matching of blood in elasmobranchs, followed by a transfusion trial in Atlantic stingrays (*Dasyatis sabina*). In: Proceedings of the 36th Annual Conference of the International Association of Aquatic Animal Medicine. Seward (AK); 2005. p. 77–8.
[24] Pica A, Cristino L, Sasso FS, et al. Haematopoietic regeneration after autohaemotransplant in sublethal X-irradiated marbled electric rays. Comp Haem Int 2000;10(1):43–9.
[25] Sakai DK, Okada H, Koide N, et al. Blood type compatibility of lower vertebrates: phylogenetic diversity in blood transfusion between fish species. Dev Comp Immunol 1987;11(1): 105–15.
[26] Stoskopf MK. Shark diagnostics and therapeutics: a short review. Journal of Aquariculture and Aquatic Sciences 1990;5(3):33–43.
[27] Stamper MA. Immobilization of elasmobranchs. In: Smith M, Warmolts D, Thoney D, et al, editors. The elasmobranch husbandry manual: captive care of sharks, rays and their relatives. Columbus Zoo, Columbus (OH): Biological Survey; 2004. p. 284–95.
[28] Harms CA. Anesthesia in fish. In: Fowler ME, Miller RE, editors. Zoo and wild animal medicine. Current therapy 4. Philadelphia: WB Saunders; 1999. p. 158–63.
[29] Callahan HA, Noga EJ. Tricaine dramatically reduces the ability to diagnose protozoan ectoparasite (*Ichthyobodo necator*) infections. J Fish Dis 2002;25(7):433–7.
[30] Fedewa LA, Lindell L. Inhibition of growth for select gram-negative bacteria by tricaine methane sulfonate (MS-222). J Herpetol Med Surg 2005;15(1):13–7.
[31] Murray MJ. Endoscopy in fish. In: Murray MJ, Schildger B, Taylor M, editors. Endoscopy in birds, reptiles, amphibians and fish. Tuttlinge, Germany: Endo-Press; 1998. p. 57–75.
[32] Zimmerman DM, Armstrong DL, Curro TG, et al. Pharmacokinetics of florfenicol after a single intramuscular dose in white-spotted bamboo sharks (*Chiloscyllium plagiosum*). J Zoo Wildl Med 2006;37(2):165–73.
[33] Stoskopf MK. Bacterial diseases of sharks. In: Stoskopf MK, editor. Fish medicine. Philadelphia: WB Saunders; 1993. p. 774–6.
[34] George A. Meningitis in captive lemon sharks, *Negaprion brevirostris*. In: Proceedings of the Annual Conference of the International Association of Aquatic Animal Medicine; 1981. p. 48.

[35] Houston AH. Blood and circulation. In: Schreck CB, Moyle PB, editors. Methods in fish biology. Bethesda (MD): American Fisheries Society; 1990. p. 273–333.
[36] Arnold JE. Hematology of the sandbar shark, *Carcharhinus plumbeus*: standardization of complete blood count techniques for elasmobranchs. Vet Clin Pathol 2005;34(2):115–23.
[37] Klinger R, Francis-Floyd R, Riggs A, et al. Use of blood culture as a non-lethal method for isolating bacteria from fish. J Zoo Wildl Med 2003;34(2):206–7.
[38] Harrenstein LA, Tornquist SJ, Miller-Morgan TJ, et al. Evaluation of a point-of-care blood analyzer and determination of reference ranges for blood parameters in rockfish. J Am Vet Med Assoc 2005;226(2):255–65.
[39] Lewbart GA, Stone EA, Love NE. Pneumocystectomy in a Midas cichlid. J Am Vet Med Assoc 1995;207:319–21.
[40] Harms CA, Lewbart GA. Surgery in fish. Vet Clin North Am Exot Anim Pract 2000;3:759–74.
[41] Stetter MD. Use of rigid laparoscopy in fish. In: Proceedings of the Annual Conference of the American Association of Zoo Veterinarians. Milwaukee (WI); 2002. p. 339–42.
[42] Murray MJ. Fish surgery. Seminars in Avian and Exotic Pet Medicine 2002;11(4):246–57.
[43] Harms CA, Lewbart GA, Swanson CR, et al. Behavioral and clinical pathology changes in koi carp (*Cyprinus carpio*) subjected to anesthesia and surgery with and without intra-operative analgesics. Comp Med 2005;55(3):221–6.
[44] Yanong RPE. Necropsy techniques for fish. Seminars in Avian and Exotic Pet Medicine 2003;12(2):89–105.
[45] Reimschuessel R. Postmortem examination. In: Stoskopf MK, editor. Fish medicine. Philadelphia: WB Saunders; 1993. p. 160–5.
[46] Groff JM. Cutaneous biology and diseases of fish. Vet Clin North Am Exot Anim Pract 2001;4:321–411.
[47] Beaver BV, Reed W, Leary S, et al. 2000 Report of the AVMA panel on euthanasia. J Am Vet Med Assoc 2001;218(5):669–96.
[48] Lewbart GA, Butkus DA, Papich MG, et al. Evaluation of a method of intracoelomic catheterization in koi. J Am Vet Med Assoc 2005;226(5):734–8.
[49] Stoffregen DA, Wooster GA, Bustos PS, et al. Multiple route and dose pharmacokinetics of enrofloxacin in juvenile Atlantic salmon. J Vet Pharmacol Ther 1997;20(2):111–23.
[50] Lewbart GA, Vaden S, Deen J, et al. Pharmacokinetics of enrofloxacin in the red pacu (*Colossoma bachypomum*) after intramuscular, oral and bath administration. J Vet Pharmacol Ther 1997;20:124–8.
[51] Rosonke B, Dover S. A study of enrofloxacin serum concentrations versus time in five leopard sharks. In: Proceedings of the 25th Annual Conference of the International Association of Aquatic Animal Medicine. Vallejo (CA); 1994. p. 60–1.
[52] Bowser PR, Wooster GA, St Leger J, et al. Pharmacokinetics of enrofloxacin in fingerling rainbow trout (*Oncorhynchus mykiss*). J Vet Pharmacol Ther 1992;15(1):62–71.
[53] Carpenter JW. Exotic animal formulary. Philadelphia: Elsevier; 2001.
[54] Park BK, Lim JH, Kim MS, et al. Pharmacokinetics of florfenicol and its metabolite, florfenicol amine, in the Korean catfish (*Silurus asotus*). J Vet Pharmacol Ther 2006;29(1):37–40.
[55] Yanong RPE, Curtis EW. Pharmacokinetics studies of florfenicol in koi carp and threespot gourami *Trichogaster trichopterus* after oral and intramuscular treatment. J Aquat Anim Health 2005;17:129–37.
[56] Lewbart GA, Papich MG, Whitt-Smith DW. Pharmacokinetics of florfenicol in the red pacu (*Piaractus brachypomus*) after single dose intramuscular administration. Journal of Veterinary Pharmacology and Therapeutics 2005;28(3):317–9.
[57] Pinault LP, Millot LK, Sanders PJ. Absolute oral bioavailability and residues of florfenicol in the rainbow trout (*Oncorhynchus mykiss*). Journal of Veterinary Pharmacology and Therapeutics 1997;20(1):297–8.

[58] Horsberg TE, Hoff KA, Nordmo R. Pharmacokinetics of florfenicol and its metabolite florfenicol amine in Atlantic salmon. J Aquat Anim Health 1996;8:292–301.
[59] Martinsen B, Horsberg TE, Varma KJ, et al. Single dose pharmacokinetic study of florfenicol in Atlantic salmon (*Salmo salar*) in seawater at 11°C. Aquaculture 1993;112:1–11.
[60] Available at: www.fda.gov/cvm.
[61] Falahatkar B, Dabrowski K, Arslan M, et al. Effects of ascorbic acid enrichment by immersion of rainbow trout (*Oncorhynchus mykiss*) eggs and embryos. Aquaculture Research 2006; 37(8):834–41.
[62] Chen R, Lochmann R, Goodwin A, et al. Alternative complement activity and resistance to heat stress in golden shiners (*Notemigonus crysoleucas*) are increased by dietary vitamin C levels in excess of requirements for prevention of deficiency signs. J Nutr 2003;133:2281–6.
[63] Kizer A. Percutaneous gastrostomy tube placement in a green moray eel. Exotic DVM 2005; 7(1):31–5.
[64] Bakal RS, Smith TS, Lewbart GA. Emergency care of a tancho koi (*Cyprinus carpio*) suffering from acute chlorine toxicity. In: Proceedings of the 26th Annual Conference of the International Association of Aquatic Animal Medicine. Mystic (CT); 1995. p. 13–4.
[65] Tompkins JA, Tasi C. Survival time and lethal exposure time for blacknose dace exposed to free chlorine and chloramines. Trans Amer Fish Soc 1976;105:313–21.
[66] Petty BD, Francis-Floyd R. Pet fish care and husbandry. Vet Clin North Am Exot Anim Pract 2004;7:397–419.
[67] Grosell M, Wood CM, Walsh PJ. Copper homeostasis and toxicity in the elasmobranch *Raja erinacea* and the teleost *Myxocephalus octodecemspinosus* during exposure to water-borne copper. Comp Biochem Physiol 2003;135(2):179–90.
[68] Noga EJ. Fish disease: diagnosis and treatment. St. Louis (MO): Mosby-Year Book Inc; 1996.
[69] Smith SA, Hughes KP, George R. Pathology associated with mixed bacterial infections in weedy sea dragons (*Phyllopteryx taeniolatus*) and leafy sea dragons (*Phycodurus eques*). In: Proceedings of the 33rd Annual Conference of the International Association of Aquatic Animal Medicine. (Portugal); 2002. p. 34–5.
[70] Grimes DJ, Brayton P, Colwell RR, et al. Vibrios as autochthonous flora of neritic sharks. Syst Appl Microbiol 1985;6:221–6.
[71] Szignarowitz BA. Update on koi herpesvirus. Exotic DVM 2005;7(3):92–5.
[72] Petty BD, Fraser WA. Viruses of pet fish. Vet Clin North Am Exot Anim Pract 2005;8:67–84.
[73] Fontenot DK, Neiffer DL. Wound management in teleost fish: biology of the healing process, evaluation and treatment. Vet Clin North Am Exot Anim Pract 2004;7:57–86.
[74] Travis EK, Mylniczenko ND, Greenwell MG. Treatment of traumatic mandibular symphyseal fracture and facial tissue loss in a laced moray eel. Exotic DVM 2004;6(5):31–5.
[75] Mylniczenko ND, Travis EK. Techniques using Vet BioSISt in aquatic animals. In: Proceedings of the Annual Conference of the American Association of Zoo Veterinarians. San Diego (CA); 2004. p. 107–10.
[76] Boerner L, Dube K, Peterson K, et al. Angiogenic growth factor therapy using recombinant platelet-derived growth factor (Regranex) for lateral line disease in marine fish. In: Proceedings of the Annual Conference of the American Association of Zoo Veterinarians. Minneapolis (MN); 2003. p. 200–1.
[77] Jurk I. Ophthalmic disease of fish. Vet Clin North Am Exot Anim Pract 2002;5:243–60.
[78] Ritchie BW, Wooley RE, Vaughan V. Use of potentiated antimicrobials in treating skin infections. In: Proceedings of the 36th Annual Conference of the International Association of Aquatic Animal Medicine. Seward (AK); 2005. p. 108–13.
[79] Wooley RE, Ritchie BW, Burnley VV. In vitro effect of a buffered chelating agent and neomycin or oxytetracycline on bacteria associated with diseases of fish. Dis Aquat Organ 2004; 59(3):263–7.

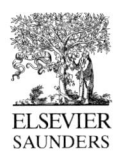

Index

Note: Page numbers of article titles are in **boldface** type.

A

Abalone, diseases affecting, 642

ABC's, of resuscitation, basic vs. advanced, 286, 290
    in fish, 655–656
    in rodents, 508

Abdominal examination, for emergency/critical care, of ferrets, 472–473, 484
    of rodents, 504

Abrasions, in pet birds, 368

Acetaminophen, caution with, in ferrets, 481, 484

N-Acetylcysteine, nebulized, for pet birds, 357
    for rodents, 512

Acid-base status, blood gas analysis of, 340–341
    in fish emergencies, 657, 661

Acidosis, in shock syndromes, 284–285, 287
    metabolic vs. respiratory, 341

Acropora sp. infestation, of corals, 641–642

Acute renal failure, in pet birds, 385–386, 388
    in rabbits, 451–452
    in rodents, 527–528

Acute stress response, in fish, 656

Adenocarcinoma, uterine, in rabbits, 449, 456

Adrenal disease, in ferrets, 468–470, 489–490, 496

Advanced life support, approach to, 286

African hedgehogs, blood chemistry data for, 550
    emergency and critical care procedures in, common reasons for, 534–536
    nutrition for, 539, 547–548
    stabilization principles for, 539–548
    therapeutic drug dosages for, 552–553
    hematologic data for, 549–550
    physiologic data for, normal, 541–542

Air exchange, in birds, 332–333, 367
    in fish, 659–660
    in invertebrates, 624–625
    in reptiles, 571
    in small mammals, 333

Air pump, for aquatic fish environment, 648–649
    in immediate emergency response, 652–653
    portable, 654

Air sac cannulation, in birds, 430–433
    in pet birds, 358
    in raptors, 408–409, 413

Air sacs, in bird respiratory system, 332, 366–369

Air stone, for aquatic fish environment, 653–654

Airway(s), of birds, 332–333
    large, 360–362
    small, 362–364
    upper, 359–360
    of fish, 655
    of small mammals, 333

Airway intubation, for cardiopulmonary-cerebral resuscitation, 287–290
    for emergency/critical stabilization, of exotic mammals, 540
    of raptors, 408–409
    of reptiles, 576–577
    of rodents, 508–510
    for inhalation anesthesia, in birds, 310–311, 341–342
    in small mammals, 309–311, 342
    surgical patients and, 313

Airway obstruction, during anesthesia, 342
    in birds, 430–431
    in ferrets, 472
    in pet birds, 360

Airway obstruction (*continued*)
  in raptors, 408–409
  in reptiles, 576
  mechanical ventilation and, 335

Airway support, for critically ill patients, exotic mammals as, 540
  fish as, 655
  reptiles as, 560
  rodents as, 508–512

Albendazole, for rabbits, 438, 458

Alkalinity (KH), in aquatic environment, for corals and anemones, 640
  for fish, 648, 650

Alkalosis, metabolic vs. respiratory, 341

Alopecia, in ferrets, 468, 473
  in tarantulas, 633

α_2-Agonists, for pain management, in small mammals, 297, 304

Alveoli, in small mammal respiratory system, 333

American Heart Association, CPCR guidelines of, 286, 288

Amikacin, for amphibians, 597

Aminoglycosides, nebulized, for pet birds, 356–357

Aminophylline, for raptors, 410

Ammonia, in aquatic fish environment, 647–650
  nitrogen cycle disruption and, 651
  toxicity of, 665–666

Amoxicillin, for exotic mammals, 553
  for ferrets, 482

Amphibians, emergency medicine of, **587–620**
  aquatic species fluid requirement, 602
  biology review for, 587–589
  common reasons for, 609–619
    bacterial disease, 614–615
    chytridiomycosis, 608, 616–617
    fungal disease, 616–617
    gastrointestinal, 617
    general presenting signs, 609–613
    metabolic bone disease, 617–618
    parasitic disease, 609, 614
    renal disease, 618–619
    trauma, 618
    viral disease, 617
  general diagnostic techniques for, 606–609
  general treatment techniques for, 596–606
  history taking for, 594–595
  hospital equipment for, 590–594
  husbandry and, 589, 594–595
  overall goals for, 589–590
  overview of, 587, 619
  patient selection in, 590
  physical examination for, 595–596
  taxonomy of, 587–589

Amphotericin B, nebulized, for pet birds, 356
  for rodents, 511

Anaerobic metabolism, in reptiles, 561
  in shock, 341

Analgesia/analgesia drugs, for emergency/critical care, in amphibians, 604
  in exotic mammals, 548–549
  in fish, 661
  in rabbits, 446–447
  in raptors, 398–399, 405, 407
  in reptiles, 574–575
  in rodents, 518, 520–521, 523
  for pain management, in birds, 311–312
    in exotic mammals, 549, 553
    in pet birds, 369–370, 374
    in small mammals, classes and agents of, 295–301
      constant rate infusions of, 305–306, 313–314
      dental blocks vs., 301–304
      for cesarean section, 312–313
      for critically ill surgical patient, 313–314
  multimodal plan for, 294

Anamnesis, in ferrets, 467, 470

Anemia, in ferrets, 491

Anemones, emergency care of, 638–642
  husbandry for, 639–640
  physical examination of, 638

Anesthesia/anesthetic drugs, cardiopulmonary arrest from, in birds, 287–289
  in small mammals, 288–290
  cardiovascular system monitoring for, in birds, 325, 331
  in invertebrates, 626
  for emergency/critical care, in amphibians, 604–605
    in exotic mammals, 548–549

INDEX 679

in fish, 657–658
in invertebrates, 625–626
in rabbits, 446–447
in raptors, 415
in reptiles, 575–576
of rodents, 502
for pain management, in birds,
 311–312
in small mammals, classes of,
 296–304
   dental block techniques
    and, 301–304
   epidural administration of,
    297, 300, 307–309
   for cesarean section,
    312–313
   for critically ill surgical
    patient, 313–314
   induction agents as,
    306–307
   inhalants as, 307
    intubation techniques
     for, 309–311
mechanical ventilation during, 332,
 334–336
respiratory system monitoring for, in
 birds, 336–342
in invertebrates, 626
in small mammals, 336–342

Anesthesia induction agents, for fish,
 657–658
for reptiles, 574–576
for small mammals, 306–307,
 312–313

Anesthesia induction techniques, for
 amphibians, 604–605
for birds, 333, 341–342
for invertebrates, 625–626
for small mammals, 333, 342

Anesthesia maintenance, in small mammals,
 agents for, 313–314
 techniques for, 333–336

Aneurysms, endometrial venous, in
 rabbits, 450

Angiotensin converting enzyme (ACE)
 inhibitors, for hypertension, in pet
 birds, 390–391

Animal introductions, into fish tanks,
 651–652

Animal Welfare Act, US, 621–622

Anorexia, in amphibians, 609–610
in ferrets, 468, 484
in pet birds, 385
in rabbits, 444, 447–449
in rodents, 523–524

Anoxia, reptile recovery ability from, 561

Antibiotic-associated enteritis, in rabbits,
 455

Antibiotics, in emergency/critical care, of
 amphibians, 596–597, 615
 of exotic mammals, 553
 of ferrets, 482–483
 of fish, 667–668, 672
 of pet birds, 365, 369, 374, 377,
  382–383
   nebulization of, 356–357
 of rabbits, 438, 458
   inappropriate, 455
 of raptors, 410–412
 of reptiles, 572–573
 of rodents, 511–512, 518, 520

Antihypertensive therapy, for pet birds,
 390–391

Apnea, during anesthesia, in birds, 333

Apnea monitors, 338

Aquatic environment. See *Water
 environment.*

Arachnids, emergency care of, 630–633. See
 also *Invertebrates.*
 husbandry for, 630–631

Arginine vasotocin (AVT), in pet birds, egg
 binding and, 375

Arrhythmias, cardiopulmonary
 resuscitation and, 286, 290
 during anesthesia, 331, 626
 ECG evaluation of, in birds, 328–331
  in raptors, 399
  in small mammals, 328–331
 hypovolemic shock causing, 277, 290

Arterial catheterization, for blood pressure
 monitoring, 320–321
 in reptiles, 563–564

Arthropods, exoskeleton of, dysecdysis of,
 629–630
  traumatic injuries of, 628–629
  in invertebrate taxonomy, 622–623,
   633

Ascites, coelomic, in pet birds, 364–366
 in ferrets, 468, 492

Aspergillosis, in pet birds, 368
 in raptors, 409

Aspiration emergencies, in birds, 427
 in rodents, 510

Aspiration samples, of ferrets, 478–479, 481
 of fish, 659
 of pet birds, 364–366

Aspiration samples (*continued*)
    of rabbits, 441–442
    of rodents, 527
Aspirin, for glomerular disease, in pet birds, 387
Ataxia, in reptiles, 577
Atherosclerosis, in pet birds, arterial, 388–390
    clinical diagnosis of, 389
    glomerular, 385
    treatment of, 389–390
Atropine sulfate, emergency indications for, in amphibians, 597
    in fish, 656
    in raptors, 410, 414
    in reptiles, 562
    in small mammals, 331
    for cardiopulmonary-cerebral resuscitation, 286, 288–289
Auscultation, for emergency assessments, of ferrets, 471–472
    of pet birds, 347, 358, 365
Avian species. See *Birds*.
    pet. See *Pet birds*.

B

Bacterial diseases, emergencies related to, in amphibians, 614–615
    in fish, 667–669
    in invertebrates, 633–636, 642
    in pet birds, 365, 377
    in rabbits, 448, 451–453, 456
    in raptors, 415
Bacterial pneumonia, in ferrets, 493
    in rabbits, 456
Bandaging techniques, in emergency/critical care, of birds, 419–425
    Ehmer type, 422–423, 425
    figure-of-eight, 423–425
    "football" type, 420, 422
    leg splint, 420–421, 423
    modified Robert Jones, 421–422
    overview of, 419–420
    plastic spica, 420–421, 423
    tape splint, 420–421
    Thomas-Schoeder splint, 422, 424
    of raptors, 399, 402, 404
Barium studies, in ferrets, 477
    in reptiles, 572
Basal cell tumors, in ferrets, 491

Basal metabolic rate (BMR), in rabbits, 445–446
Basic life support, approach to, 286
Batatrachochytrium dendrobatidis, in amphibians, 616–617
Beetles, emergency care of, 635–637
Benzodiazepines, for seizure control, in rodents, 522
β-Receptor agonists, for pet birds, 363
Bile acid assays, in pet birds, 351
Biopsy(ies), of fish, 661
    for necropsy, 662
    gill, 659
    of pet birds, renal, 385–386
    small airway, 363
Birds, bandaging techniques in, 419–425
    Ehmer type, 422–423, 425
    figure-of-eight, 423–425
    "football" type, 420, 422
    leg splint, 420–421, 423
    modified Robert Jones, 421–422
    overview of, 419–420
    plastic spica, 420–421, 423
    tape splint, 420–421
    Thomas-Schoeder splint, 422, 424
    critical care monitoring of, **317–344**
        blood pressure measurements, 323–325
        cardiac evaluation in, 326–332
        cardiovascular system components in, 318–326
        overview of, 317–318, 342–343
        perfusion parameters in, 317–326
        respiratory system during anesthesia, 333–342
    emergency stabilization of, **419–436**
        bandaging techniques for, 419–425
        endoscopy for, 426–427
        overview of, 419, 436
        surgical procedures for, 427–436
    endoscopy in, 426–427
    pain assessment in, 293–294
    pain management in, **293–315**
        analgesic drugs for, 311–312
        anesthetic drugs for, 311–312
        inhalants for, 307
        intubation techniques for, 310–311
        multimodal analgesia for, 294
        options for, 294–295
        overview of, 293–294
    pet, emergency and critical care of, **345–394**. See also *Pet birds*.

respiratory system components in, 332–333
shock in, **275–291**
    cardiopulmonary-cerebral resuscitation for, 287–289
    effectiveness of, 286–287, 289
    fluid resuscitation for, for dehydration deficits, 285
    plan for, 277–278, 281–282
    types of fluids in, 278–281
    glucocorticoids in, 284
    pathophysiology of, 275–276
    phases of, 276–277
    sodium bicarbonate in, 284–285
surgery in, 427–436
    air sac cannulation, 430–433
    coelom approaches, 428–429
    equipment for, 428–430
    esophagostomy tube placement, 433–434
    overview of, 427–428
    proventriculotomy, 435–436
    salpingohysterectomy, 433–435
    ventriculotomy, 435–436

Bite wounds, in pet birds, 368

Bivalve mollusks, emergency care of, 642–643

Bleaching, in corals, 640

Blood cultures, of fish, 660, 662

Blood gas analysis, cardiopulmonary-cerebral resuscitation and, arterial vs. venous, 287–288
    components of, 340
    essentials of, 341
    in reptiles, 560–561, 571
    lactate in, 341
    point-of-care, 340–341

Blood glucose level, in ferrets, 474

Blood group typing, in small mammals, 281

Blood loss, shock related to, 275–277
    uncontrolled. See *Hemorrhage.*

Blood pressure, central venous pressure, 317, 325–326
    direct monitoring of, 320–321
        in reptiles, 563–564
    Doppler monitoring of, 321–322
        hypovolemic shock and, 282
        in amphibians, 595, 604
        in birds, 323–325, 387
        in reptiles, 560, 563
        in rodents, 512–514
        in small mammals, 323
    in critically ill patients, birds as, 323–325
    measurement of, 320–326
    raptors as, 399
    reptiles as, 562–565
    small mammals as, 322–323, 325–326
    indirect monitoring of, 321–322
        in reptiles, 564–565

Blood pressure cuffs, for blood pressure monitoring, 322
    in birds, 323–324
    in reptiles, 564
    in rodents, 512–513
    in small mammals, 322–323

Blood sample collection, for critically ill patients, exotic mammals as, 549–550
    ferrets as, 475, 496
    fish as, 659–661
    pet birds as, 347–348
    rabbits as, 441
    raptors as, 400
    rodents as, 505–507

Blood transfusions, for exotic mammals, 544–545
    for fish resuscitation, 656
    for fluid resuscitation, of shock, 280–281
    for raptors, 400, 402–403, 414
    for rodents, 517

Blood work. See *Laboratory tests.*

Body distention, in amphibians, 609, 612

Body temperature, as critical care monitoring parameter, 319–320
    in critically ill patients, exotic mammals as, 546–547
    raptors as, 399–400
    reptiles as, 558–559, 563

Bone disease, metabolic. See also *Secondary hyperparathyroidism.*
    in raptors, 415
    in sugar gliders, 534–535

Bone marrow aspiration, in ferrets, 479

Bowel disease, proliferative, in ferrets, 485–486

Bradycardia, during anesthesia, 331

Breathing, in fish resuscitation, 655–656

Breathing circuits, for anesthesia maintenance, 333

Breathing patterns, emergency assessment of, in ferrets, 471–472
    in pet birds, 360–361, 363–364

Bronchi, in bird respiratory system, 332, 362, 366
    in small mammal respiratory system, 333
    of pet birds, anatomy and physiology of, 362
        emergency/critical care for, 362–364
        parenchymal disease and, 366
Bronchodilators, for pet birds, 358, 363
    for raptors, 412–413
    nebulized, for pet birds, 356–357
    for rodents, 511–512
Bupivacaine, local, for pain management, in birds, 312
    in reptiles, 575
    in small mammals, 297, 300–301
        critically ill surgical, 313–314
        dental block techniques for, 301–304
        epidural injections of, 300, 307–308
        with cesarean section, 313
Buprenorphine, for pain management, in exotic mammals, 549, 553
    in reptiles, 574
    in small mammals, 298
Burns, emergency/critical care for, in pet birds, 368–369, 371
    in reptiles, 579–580
    in rodents, 518, 520–521
Butorphanol, for pain management, in birds, 311
    in exotic mammals, 549, 553
    in fish, 656, 661
    in raptors, 410, 413
    in reptiles, 574
    in small mammals, 295–296, 298
Butterflies, emergency care of, 635–637

C

Caecelians, emergency medicine of, **587–620**. See also *Amphibians*.
Calcium, for cardiopulmonary-cerebral resuscitation, 286
    serum, in pet birds, 349–350
Calcium channel blockers (CCBs), for hypertension, in pet birds, 391
Calcium EDTA, for rabbits, 438, 457
    for raptors, 410

Calcium gluconate, emergency indications for, hyperkalemia as, 495
    in amphibians, 597
    in exotic mammals, 553
    in ferrets, 495
    in fish, 656
    in raptors, 410
    in reptiles, 562
Calcium:phosphorus ratio imbalance, in reptiles, 577–578
Calculi, renal, in ferrets, 470
    urinary, in rabbits, 453–454
    in rodents, 526–527
Canine distemper virus, in ferrets, 494
Capillary refill time (CRT), as critical care monitoring parameter, 319
    in raptors, 398–400
    in hypovolemic shock, 276–277
Capnography, in respiratory monitoring, 338–340
Capnometry, in respiratory monitoring, 338–340
Carbon dioxide, in respiratory monitoring, arterial, 340–341
    cardiopulmonary-cerebral resuscitation and, 287–288
    end-tidal, 287, 332, 338–340
Cardiac arrest. See *Cardiopulmonary arrest*.
Cardiac disease, emergencies related to, in ferrets, 468–470, 492–493
    in rabbits, 456–457
    in rodents, 522
Cardiac evaluation, ECG in, 330–331. See also *Electrocardiogram (ECG)*.
    in critically ill patients, 326–332
        ferrets as, 478
        pet birds as, 347, 365–366
Cardiac output, carbon dioxide excretion and, 287
    chest compressions for, 290
    critical care monitoring of, 317–318, 331–332
    hypovolemic shock impact on, 276, 280, 283
Cardiac rhythm, abnormalities of. See *Arrhythmias*.
    ECG evaluation of, 330–331
Cardiomyopathy, in African hedgehogs, 534–535, 552
    in ferrets, 329
    in rodents, 522

INDEX 683

Cardiopulmonary arrest, anesthesia
causing, in birds, 287–289
in small mammals, 288–290
hypovolemic shock causing, 277,
287–288
in ferrets, 471

Cardiopulmonary-cerebral resuscitation
(CPCR), for shock, 286–290
drugs for, 286–287
effectiveness of, 286–287
algorithm for evaluating,
288–289
goal of, 286
in birds, 287–289
in small mammals, 288–290
of reptiles, 558–562
of rodents, 508

Cardiopulmonary resuscitation (CPR), goal of, 286

Cardiovascular system, critical care
monitoring parameters for, 318–326
hypovolemic shock impact on,
275–277, 281–285
of amphibians, assessment of,
588–589, 595
of ferrets, diseases of, 492–493
examination of, 471–472
of reptiles, emergencies involving,
565–566, 577
of rodents, examination of, 512–513

Carprofen, for pain management, in
raptors, 410
in reptiles, 574
in small mammals, 297, 299

Catarrhal enteritis, epizootic, in ferrets, 485

Catheterization techniques, urinary. See
Urinary catheterization.
vascular. See *Intravenous access/
catheterization.*

Cefazolin, for raptors, 410

Ceftazidime, for fish, 667
for reptile, 573

Centipedes, emergency care of, 633–635

Central nervous system (CNS), critical care monitoring parameters and, 317–318

Central venous pressure (CVP), as critical
care monitoring parameter, 317,
325–326

Ceolomic space, of pet birds, physical
examination of, 347

Cephalexin, for ferrets, 482

Cephalopods, emergency care of, 642–643

Cerebral spinal fluid, in pet birds, collection technique for, 379

Cesarean section, analgesia/anesthesia for, in small mammals, 312–313

Charcoal, activated, for raptors, 410

Chelation therapy, for heavy metal
poisoning, in pet birds, 381

Chelonians, emergency care of, **557–585**.
See also *Reptiles.*

Chemical burns, in reptiles, 579–580

Chemical intoxication, emergency/critical
care for, in fish, 665–666, 668
in invertebrates, 627–628
in raptors, 409, 413–414

Chemical restraint, for emergency/critical
care, of exotic mammals, 550–551
of fish, 654, 657–658
of rodents, 502–503

Chemistries analysis, in emergency/critical
care, of amphibians, 607
of ferrets, 474–475
of pet birds, 348, 373–374
of reptiles, 566, 569–571

Chest compressions, in
cardiopulmonary-cerebral
resuscitation, 290

Chillers, for aquatic fish environment,
651, 653

Chinchillas, emergency and critical care of,
501–531. See also *Rodents.*
physiologic parameters for, 501–502

Chitosan, for atherosclerosis, in pet birds, 390

Chlamydophilosis, in pet birds, 382

Chloramphenicol, for ferrets, 482
for rodents, 518

Chlorhexidine, for bird surgery prep, 428

Chlorine-free water, for amphibians, 592, 594
for fish, 651, 653

Chlorine toxicity, in aquatic fish
environment, 666

Chlorpheniramine, for ferrets, 482

Chytridiomycosis, in amphibians, 608,
616–617

Circulation, emergency assessment of. See
Cardiovascular system; Perfusion entries.
in fish resuscitation, 656

Cisapride, for ferrets, 482
    for rabbits, 438, 449

Clams, emergency care of, 642–643

Clinical examination, assessment techniques for. See *Physical examination.*
    testing in. See *Diagnostic tests.*

Cloacal prolapse, in amphibians, 609, 613
    in pet birds, 376–378
    in reptiles, 580

Clostridium spp. overgrowth, in rabbits, 448, 455

Closure techniques, for wounds, in raptors, 402, 404

Cnidaria, emergency/critical care for, 638–642
    in invertebrate taxonomy, 622–623

Coagulopathies, in ferrets, 491–492

Coeliotomy, exploratory, in fish, 661

Coelomic cavity, of birds, surgical procedures for, 428–429, 435
        of pet birds, anatomy and physiology of, 364
            biopsy of, 363
            emergency/critical care for, 364–366, 373

Coelomic endoscopy, in amphibians, 609
    in birds, 427

Coelomocentesis, for ascites, in pet birds, 364–366

Colchicine, for glomerular disease, in pet birds, 387

Collapse, in amphibians, 609, 611

Colloid osmotic pressure (COP), in hypovolemic shock, 279–280

Colloid solutions, for fluid resuscitation, of shock, 279, 562, 565

Color change, in amphibians, 609, 612

Color loss, in corals, 640

Compensatory phase, of hypovolemic shock, 276

Computed tomography (CT), in amphibians, 609
    in pet birds, 353, 379–380
    in rabbits as, 442–443, 457–458

Constant rate infusions (CRIs), of analgesics, for small mammals, 305–306
            postoperative, 313–314

Contaminants, environmental. See *Toxins/toxicities.*

Contrast radiography, in ferrets, 477
    in reptiles, 572

Convulsions. See *Seizures.*

Copper sulfate, for fish, 667

Copper toxicity, in aquatic fish environment, 666

Coral reef aquarium, 639

Corals, emergency care of, 638–642
    husbandry for, 639–640

Corneal ulcers, in fish, 672

COX inhibitors, for pain management, in small mammals, 299

Crabs, hermit, emergency care of, 637–638

Cranial nerves (CN), evaluation with trauma, in pet birds, 378–379

Creatinine, serum, in ferrets, 474

Critical care monitoring, **317–344**
    amphibian challenges of, 604
    blood pressure measurement in, 320–326
    cardiac evaluation in, 326–332
    cardiovascular system components in, 318–326
    invertebrate challenges of, 626
    overview of, 317–318, 342–343
    perfusion parameters in, 317–326
    respiratory system components in, 332–342

Critical care/procedures, emergency perspectives of. See *Emergency care/procedures.*
    in exotic mammals, **533–555**
            anesthesia and analgesia for, 548–549
            common emergency presentations, 533–538
            diagnosis of, 549–552
            treatment of, 549–552
            emergency stabilization principles for, 539–548
            husbandry and, 539, 546–547
            nutrition and, 538–539, 547–548
            therapeutic drug dosages for, 552–553
    in fish, **647–675**
            clinical examination for, 653–655
            common emergency presentations, environment-related, 665–668

infection-related, 668–671
    treatment of, 667–669
    trauma-related, 671–672
  drugs for, 656–657
  environmental factors, 647–651, 665, 672
  fluids for, 656–657
  further diagnostics for, 657–663
  general principles of, 663–665
  history taking for, 651–652
  immediate responses as, 652–653
  resuscitation as, 655–656
in small mammal surgery, analgesia/anesthesia for, 313–314
of invertebrates, 623
of pet birds, **345–394**
  common reasons for, 358–391
    gastrointestinal disease, 382–384
    hypertension, 387–391
    mites, 371
    neurologic disease, 378–382
    renal disease, 384–387
    reproductive-related, 372–378
    respiratory-related, 358–369
    trauma, 369–372
  diagnostic testing in, 347–354
  history taking for, 346
  overview of, 345, 391
  physical examination for, 346–347
  procedures for, 354–358
  treatment protocols for, 369–372
  triage in, 345–346
of rabbits, **437–461**
  common reasons for, acute respiratory distress, 456
    anorexia, 444, 447–449
    cardiac disease, 456–457
    diarrhea, 454–455
    head tilt, 458–459
    heat stress, 459
    myiasis, 459
    neoplasia, 449, 456
    neurologic signs, 457
    paresis/paralysis, 457–458
    pregnancy toxemia, 459
    red urine, 455–456
    renal disease, 451–452
    urethral obstruction, 454
    urolithiasis, 453–454
    uterine disorders, 449–451
  diagnostic approaches to, 440–442
  dietary history in, 439
  drugs for, 437–439
  emergency stabilization importance in, 437–439
  physical examination for, 439–440
  therapeutic techniques for, 442–447
of rodents, **501–531**
  emergency presentations for, 518–528
  general supportive measures in, 513–518
  history taking for, 503
  overview of, 501–502, 528
  patient handling for, 502–503
  physical examination for, 503–505
  physiologic parameters in, normal, 501–502
  radiography for, 507–508
  restraint techniques for, 502–503
  sample collection for, 505–507
  triage of emergencies, 508–513

Crocodiles, emergency care of, **557–585**. See also *Reptiles*.

Crop fistulas, in pet birds, 371

Crop specimen examination, in pet birds, 346, 351–352

Crop stasis, in pet birds, 383–384

Crustaceans, emergency care of, 637–638

Crystalloid solutions, for fluid resuscitation, of dehydration, 566
    of shock, 278–279, 282, 562, 565

Cultures, in emergency/critical care, of amphibians, 608
    of fish, 660, 662
    of reptiles, 571–572, 577
    of rodents, 521

Cyst(s), prostatic, in ferrets, 494, 496

Cystocentesis, for rabbits, 441–442
    for rodents, 527

Cytology, in emergency/critical care, of amphibians, 607–608
    of reptiles, 571–572, 577

D

Decompensatory phase, of hypovolemic shock, 277
    early, 276–277

Defibrillation, external, in cardiopulmonary-cerebral resuscitation, 286

Degenerative disease, of spinal nerve roots, in rodents, 522–523

Degu, emergency and critical care of, **501–531**. See also *Rodents.*

Dehydration, in critically ill patients, amphibians as, 595–596, 598–602
exotic mammals as, 540–541
fluid resuscitation for, 281, 284–285
invertebrates as, 632, 634
pet birds as, 385
rabbits as, 440, 452, 459
reptiles as, 565, 632
rodents as, 14–15

Dental block techniques, for small mammals, 301–304

Dental disorders, emergency/critical care for, in rabbits, 437, 449–450
in rodents, 504–505, 508, 524

Dermatologic disorders. See *Integumentary system; Skin entries.*

Desication, of myriapods, emergency/critical care for, 634

Dexamethasone, for ferrets, 482
for raptors, 410

Dextran 70, for raptors, 410

Dextrose, for raptors, 410
for reptiles, 566
for rodents, 517

Diabetes, in ferrets, 490

Diagnostic tests, for critically ill patients, amphibians as, 606–609
exotic mammals as, 549–550
fish as, 659–661
pet birds as, 347–354
rabbits, 440–442
raptors as, 399–401, 415
reptiles as, 569–572
rodents as, 505–508, 521

Diarrhea, emergency/critical care of, in ferrets, 467–468
in pet birds, 384
in rabbits, 454–456
in rodents, 524

Diazepam, for exotic mammals, 553
for raptors, 410, 415
for small mammals, 296, 306–307

Diazoxide, for ferrets, 482

Diets, of critically ill patients, amphibians as, 588, 595, 603–604
arachnids as, 631–632
exotic mammals as, 538–539, 547–548
ferrets as, 465–466, 481
fish as, 651–652, 664–665
rabbits as, 439, 442–445, 448
diarrhea related to, 454–455
raptors as, 404–405
rodents as, 503, 517–518, 528
renal disease induced by, in pet birds, 385–386

Digoxin, for ferrets, 482

Dimercaptosuccinic acid (DMSA), for raptors, 410

Diphenhydramine, for ferrets, 482

Dissolved oxygen (DO), in aquatic fish environment, 647–648
low level of, 666

Diuresis therapy, for rabbits, 452, 454
for raptors, 411

Doppler monitoring, of blood pressure, hypovolemic shock and, 282
in amphibians, 595, 604
in birds, 323–325, 387
in reptiles, 560, 563
in rodents, 512–514
in small mammals, 323
materials for, 321–322

Doxapram (Dopram), for cardiopulmonary-cerebral resuscitation, 286–289
in emergency/critical care, of amphibians, 597
of exotic mammals, 553
of fish, 656
of raptors, 410
of reptiles, 560, 562

Drowning, emergency procedures for, in reptiles, 576–577

Drug formulary, for emergency and critical care, for CPCR, 286–287
of amphibians, 596–597
of birds, 286–287
of exotic mammals, 552–553
of ferrets, 481–484
of fish, 656–657, 667–668, 672
of rabbits, 437–439
of raptors, 407, 410–412
of reptiles, 560, 562
of small mammals, 286–287

Dysecdysis, in invertebrates, 629–630, 637

Dystocia, emergency/critical care for, in birds, 433–435
in pet birds, 372–376
in rabbits, 450–451
in reptiles, 580–581
in rodents, 525

E

Early decompensatory phase, of hypovolemic shock, 276–277

Early phase, of hypovolemic shock, 276

Echinodermata, in invertebrate taxonomy, 622–623

Echocardiogram, in birds, 326–328
    in small mammals, 327

Edema, in amphibians, 609–611

Egg binding, emergency/critical care for, in birds, 433–435
    in pet birds, 372–376
    in reptiles, 580–581

Egg laying emergencies, in pet birds, 372

Ehmer type bandage, for birds, 422–423, 425

Electrocardiogram (ECG), for cardiac evaluation, general inspection of, 330
    heart rate measurement, 330
    in amphibians, 604
    in birds, 328–331
    in ferrets, 478
    in raptors, 399
    in reptiles, 560–561, 577
    in rodents, 512–513
    in small mammals, 328–331
    leads for recording, 329–330
    rhythm evaluation, 330–331, 399

Electrocution, emergency procedures for, in raptors, 405–407
    in rodents, 518, 520–521

Electrosurgery, in birds, 430

Emaciation, emergency/critical care for, in amphibians, 609–610
    in raptors, 414

Emergency care/procedures, in birds, **419–436**
    bandaging techniques for, 419–425
    endoscopy for, 426–427
    overview of, 419, 436
    surgical procedures for, 427–436
  in exotic mammals, **533–555**
    anesthesia and analgesia for, 548–549
    common reasons for, 533–538
        diagnosis of, 549–552
        treatment of, 549–552
    husbandry and, 539, 546–547
    nutrition and, 538–539, 547–548
    stabilization principles of, 539–548

    therapeutic drug dosages for, 552–553
  in fish, **647–675**
    clinical examination for, 653–655
    common reasons for, environment-related, 665–668
        infectious disease, 668–671
            treatment of, 667–669
        trauma, 671–672
    consultation for, 653–655
    drugs for, 656–657
    environmental factors, 647–651, 665, 672
    fluids for, 656–657
    further diagnostics for, 657–663
    general principles of, 663–665
    history taking for, 651–652
    immediate responses as, 652–653
    resuscitation as, 655–656
  of amphibians, **587–620**
    aquatic species fluid requirement, 602
    biology review for, 587–589
    common reasons for, 609–619
        bacterial disease, 614–615
        chytridiomycosis, 608, 616–617
        fungal disease, 616–617
        gastrointestinal, 617
        general presenting signs, 609–613
        metabolic bone disease, 617–618
        parasitic disease, 609, 614
        renal disease, 618–619
        trauma, 618
        viral disease, 617
    general diagnostic techniques for, 606–609
    general treatment techniques for, 596–606
    history taking for, 594–595
    hospital equipment for, 590–594
    husbandry and, 589, 594–595
    overall goals for, 589–590
    overview of, 587, 619
    patient selection in, 590
    physical examination for, 595–596
  of ferrets, **463–500**
    anamnesis and, 467, 470
    anatomy in, 464–465
    biologic characteristics in, 464
    common reasons for, 484–498
        cardiovascular disease, 492–493
        endocrine disease as, 486–490

Emergency (*continued*)
    gastrointestinal disorders, 484–486
    heat stroke, 497–498
    hematopoietic disorders, 491–492
    immune-related disease, 497
    musculoskeletal disease, 497
    neoplasia, 490–491
    ophthalmologic disease, 498
    respiratory disease, 493–494
    trauma, 496–497
    urogenital disease, 494–496
  diagnostic approaches to, 474–479
  differential diagnosis for, 467–471
    clinical signs in, 467–470
    pathology in, 467, 471
  handling and restraint for, 466–467, 475
  husbandry for, 465–467
  nutrition and, 465–466
  overview of, 463, 498–499
  physical examination for, 471–473
  taxonomy terms and overview, 463–464
  therapeutics for, 479–484
    drug therapy as, 481–484
    physical interventions as, 479–481
  of invertebrates, **621–645**
    anamnesis and, 623–624
    anatomy representations in, 624–625
    anemone presentations for, 638–642
    anesthesia for, 625–626
    arachnid presentations for, 630–633
    centipede presentations for, 633–635
    common reasons for, 627–630
      chemical intoxication, 627–628
      dysecdysis, 629–630
      trauma, 628–629
    coral presentations for, 638–642
    critical care concepts in, 623
    crustacean presentations for, 637–638
    euthanasia for, 643
    hospitalization for, 627
    insect presentations for, 635–637
    millipede presentations for, 633–635
    mollusk presentations for, 642–643
    overview of, 621–622, 643
    ownership regulations and, 621–622
    physical examination for, 623–624
    taxonomy overview for, 622–623
    therapeutics for, 626–627
  of pet birds, **345–394**
    common reasons for, 358–391
      gastrointestinal disease, 382–384
      hypertension, 387–391
      mites, 371
      neurologic disease, 378–382
      renal disease, 384–387
      reproductive-related, 372–378
      respiratory-related, 358–369
      trauma, 369–372
    diagnostic testing in, 347–354
    history taking for, 346
    overview of, 345, 391
    physical examination for, 346–347
    procedures for, 354–358
    treatment protocols for, 369–372
    triage in, 345–346
  of rabbits, 437–439
  of raptors, **395–418**
    bandaging for, 402, 404
    common reasons for, 395, 405–409
      emaciation, 414
      infectious disease, 409, 415
      other presentations, 415
      respiratory disease, 407–409, 413
      toxin exposures, 409, 413–414
      trauma, 400–401, 405–407, 409
    drug formulary for, 407, 410–412
    euthanasia for, 415
    fluid administration sites for, 401–402
    fluid therapy for, 398–399, 402
    handling for, 395–396
    hospitalization for, 397
    monitoring techniques for, 399–400
    nutritional support for, 404–405
    overview of, 395, 415–416
    pain control for, 405
    patient assessment for, 397–399
    radiographs for, 400–401
    restraint for, 396–397
    sample collection for, 400
    stabilization therapies in, 398–399, 404

transfusion medicine for, 400, 402–403
triage for, 397–400
wound care for, 399, 402, 404
of reptiles, **557–585**
  analgesia for, 574–575
  anesthetics for, 575–576
  biologic concepts in, 557–558
  blood pressure in, 562–565
  cardiopulmonary-cerebral resuscitation in, 558–562
    drugs for, 560, 562
  clinical tests for, 570–572
  common reasons for, 576–581
    cardiovascular, 577
    cloacal prolapse, 580–581
    gastrointestinal, 578–579
    integumental, 579–580
    neurologic, 577
    nutritional, 577–578
    renal, 577–578
    reproductive, 580–581
    respiratory, 576–577
    septicemia, 581
  dehydration in, 565–567
  drug administration in, 567
  fluid resuscitation as, 562–565
  goals of, 572
  history taking for, 558
  nutritional support in, 572–574
  overview of, 557, 581
  physical examination for, 558–559
  shock in, 562–565
  vascular access for, 567–570
of rodents, **501–531**
  common presentations for, 518–528
    cardiac disease, 522
    gastrointestinal, 523–525
    miscellaneous conditions, 528
    neurologic, 522–523
    renal failure, 527–528
    reproductive, 525–526
    respiratory disease, 521–522
    trauma, 518–521
    urinary obstruction, 526–527
  diagnostic approaches to, 505–508, 521
  general supportive measures in, 513–518
  history taking for, 503
  overview of, 501–502, 528
  patient handling for, 502–503
  physical examination for, 503–505

physiologic parameters in, normal, 501–502
radiography for, 507–508
restraint techniques for, 502–503
sample collection for, 505–507
triage for, 508–513

Emergency drugs, in resuscitation/stabilization, cardiopulmonary-cerebral, 286–287
of amphibians, 596–597
of birds, 286–287
of exotic mammals, 552–553
of ferrets, 481–484
of fish, 656–657, 667–668, 672
of rabbits, 437–438
of raptors, 407, 410–412
of reptiles, 560, 562
of small mammals, 286–287

Emergency medicine. See *Emergency care/procedures.*

Enalapril, for exotic mammals, 553
for ferrets, 482

Encephalitozoon cuniculi, in rabbits, head tilt related to, 458–459
posterior paresis related to, 457–458
renal disease related to, 451–452

End-tidal carbon dioxide, cardiopulmonary-cerebral resuscitation and, 287–288
in respiratory monitoring, 332, 338–340, 604

Endocrine disease, in ferrets, differential diagnosis of, 468–470
emergencies involving, 486–490, 496

Endometrial venous aneurysms, in rabbits, 450

Endoscopy, emergency diagnostic, in amphibians, 609
in birds, 426–427
for airway management. See *Airway intubation.*

Endoscopy equipment, for birds, 426

Endotracheal tube (ET), emergency use of, in amphibians, 590–591
in birds, 310–311, 342
in ferrets, 309
in rabbits, 309–310, 437
in raptors, 408
in rodents, 509–510
in small mammals, 310, 342

Energy requirement, in rabbits, basal, 445–446
　illness factor of, 446

Enrofloxacin, in emergency/critical care, of amphibians, 597
　　of exotic mammals, 553
　　of ferrets, 482
　　of fish, 667
　　of invertebrates, 633, 643
　　of rabbits, 438
　　of raptors, 411
　　of reptiles, 573

Enteral feeding, for critically ill patients, exotic mammals as, 538–539, 547–548
　　pet birds as, 358
　　rabbits as, 442–445
　　raptors as, 404–405
　　reptiles as, 572–574

Enteritis, in ferrets, eosinophilic, 469, 486
　　epizootic catarrhal, 485
　　lymphocytic-plasmacytic, 469, 486
　in rabbits, antibiotic-associated, 455
　　mucoid, 455

Environment, acute management of. See *Hospitalization*.
　aquatic. See *Water environment*.
　housing. See *Husbandry*.

Environmental contaminants. See *Toxins/toxicities*.

Eosinophilic gastroenteritis, in ferrets, 469, 486

Epidural analgesia/anesthesia, for pain management, in reptiles, 575
　　in small mammals, drugs for, 297, 300, 307–308, 312–313
　　injection techniques for, 308–309

Epinephrine, emergency indications for, in amphibians, 597
　　in exotic mammals, 553
　　in fish, 656
　　in rabbits, 438
　　in raptors, 411
　　in reptiles, 560, 562
　for cardiopulmonary-cerebral resuscitation, 286, 288–290

Epizootic catarrhal enteritis (ECE), in ferrets, 485

Esophagostomy tube placement, in birds, 433–434

Etomidate, for ferrets, 482
　for small mammals, 296, 306, 312

Euthanasia, of amphibians, 605–606
　of invertebrates, 643
　of moribund fish, 663
　of raptors, 415

Exoskeleton, of arthropods, dysecdysis of, 629–630
　　infections of, 634–635
　　traumatic injuries of, 628–629
　of crustaceans, fractures of, 638
　of insects, 635

Exotic mammals, emergency and critical care procedures in, **533–555**
　　anesthesia and analgesia for, 548–549
　　common reasons for, 533–538
　　　diagnosis of, 549–552
　　　treatment of, 549–552
　　husbandry and, 539, 546–547
　　nutrition and, 538–539, 547–548
　　stabilization principles of, 539–548
　　therapeutic drug dosages for, 552–553

Exploratory surgery, in amphibians, 609

External defibrillation, in cardiopulmonary-cerebral resuscitation, 286

F

Famotidine, for ferrets, 482

Fecal examination, for amphibians, 606–607
　for ferrets, 473
　for pet birds, 346, 351–352, 384

Fecal impaction, in rodents, 525

Federal agencies, jurisdiction over invertebrates, 622

Feeding tubes. See also *Enteral feeding*.
　for birds, 433–434
　for rabbits, 442–445, 448

Fenbendazole, for amphibians, 597
　for rabbits, 438, 458

Fentanyl, for pain management, in small mammals, 296, 314
　　ketamine combined with, 313–314

Ferrets, anatomy of, 464–465
　biologic characteristics of, 464
　blood pressure monitoring in, 322–323, 325–326
　emergency medicine of, **463–500**
　　anamnesis and, 467, 470

background information for, 463–465
common reasons for, 484–498
cardiovascular disease, 492–493
endocrine disease, 486–490
gastrointestinal disorders, 484–486
heat stroke, 497–498
hematopoietic disorders, 491–492
immune-related disease, 497
musculoskeletal disease, 497
neoplasia, 490–491
ophthalmologic disease, 498
respiratory disease, 493–494
trauma, 496–497
urogenital disease, 494–496
diagnostic approaches to, 474–479
differential diagnosis for, 467–471
clinical signs in, 467–470
pathology in, 467, 471
husbandry for, 465–467
overview of, 463, 498–499
physical examination for, 471–473
physiologic values for, 464
taxonomy terms and overview, 463–464
therapeutics for, 479–484
drug therapy as, 481–484
physical interventions as, 479–481
handling and restraint of, 466–467, 475
nutrition for, 465–466
pain assessment in, 481
pain management in, analgesic drugs for, 295–305
anesthetic drugs for, 296–305
local administration of, 300–301
dental block techniques for, 301–304
epidural anesthesia for, 297, 300, 307–309
for emergency/critical care, 481
inhalants for, 307
intubation techniques for, 309
options for, 294
shock in, **275–291**. See also *Shock*.
cardiopulmonary-cerebral resuscitation for, 288–290
effectiveness of, 286–287, 289
fluid resuscitation for, for dehydration deficits, 285
plan for, 277–278, 282–284
types of fluids in, 278–281
glucocorticoids in, 284
pathophysiology of, 275–276
phases of, 276–277
sodium bicarbonate in, 284–285

Fetal abnormalities, in rabbits, 450–451

Figure-of-eight bandage, for birds, 423–425

Filters, for aquatic fish environment, 648–649, 653

Fipronil, for ferrets, 482

Fish, aquatic environment for, common emergencies of, 665–668
health dependent on, 647–648
health factors of, 651, 672
quality maintenance equipment for, 648, 650–651
water parameters for, 648–650
emergency and critical care of, **647–675**
clinical examination for, 653–655
common reasons for, environment-related, 665–668
infection-related, 668–671
treatment of, 667–669
trauma-related, 671–672
consultation for, 653–655
drugs for, 656–657
environmental factors, 647–651, 665, 672
fluids for, 656–657
further diagnostics for, 657–663
general principles of, 663–665
history taking for, 651–652
immediate responses as, 652–653
resuscitation as, 655–656

Fish and Wildlife Services (FWS), US, 622
reporting to, 413, 415

"Fish emergency" form, 652

Fish tanks, animal introductions into, 651–652
maintenance of. See *Water environment*.

Fistulas, crop, in pet birds, 371

Florfenicol, for fish, 667

Fluid and electrolyte balance, in rabbits, 445–446, 451

Fluid resuscitation, for critically ill patients, exotic mammals as, 540–541
fish as, 657
preoperative, in small mammals, 313

692 INDEX

Fluid resuscitation (*continued*)
    raptors as, 398–399, 414
    reptiles as, 566–567
  for shock, during surgery, 282
    in birds, 281–282
    in reptiles, 562–565
    in small mammals, 282–284
    plan for, 277–278
    types of fluids in, 278–281

Fluid support, for critically ill patients,
    amphibians as, 596–602
      exotic mammals as, 540–543
      rabbits as, 448, 452
      raptors as, 401–402
      rodents as, 514–517, 527–528

Flumazenil, for rabbits, 438

Flunixin meglumine, for fish, 656
  for small mammals, 299–300

"Football" type bandage, for birds, 420, 422

Foreign body ingestion/inhalation, in
    amphibians, 617
  in birds, 430–431, 435
  in ferrets, 484
  in raptors, 409, 413, 415
  in reptiles, 578–579
  in rodents, 521, 524

Formalin, for fish infections, 667

Fractures, emergency procedures for, in
    amphibians, 618
      in birds, 419–425
      in invertebrates, 628–629, 638, 643
      in pet birds, 368–369, 371–372
      in rabbits, 457
      in raptors, 405
      in rodents, 518–519

Frogs, emergency medicine of, **587–620**. See also *Amphibians*.

Frostbite, in raptors, 415

Fungal diseases, emergencies related to, in
    amphibians, 616–617
      in invertebrates, 633–636
      in pet birds, 356

Furosemide, in emergency/critical care, of
    exotic mammals, 553
    of ferrets, 482, 492–493
    of pet birds, 386
    of rabbits, 438, 457
    of raptors, 411

G

Gas bubble disease, 668

Gas exchange, physical. See *Air exchange; Airway(s)*.

physiological. See *Blood gas analysis*.

Gas flow, for anesthesia maintenance, 333

Gas supersaturation, in aquatic fish environment, 668

Gastric endoscopy, in amphibians, 609

Gastritis, *Helicobacter*, in ferrets, 469, 484–485

Gastroenteritis. See *Enteritis*.

Gastrointestinal disorders, emergency/
    critical care for, in amphibians, 617
    in ferrets, 484–486
      differential diagnosis of, 468, 470
      drugs in, 482–473
      examination for, 472–473
    in pet birds, 382–384
    in rabbits, 440, 446–449
    in reptiles, 578–579
    in rodents, 523–525, 617

Gastrointestinal distention, in amphibians, 617
  in rabbits, 440, 448

Gastrointestinal foreign body, in
    amphibians, 617
  in ferrets, 484
  in raptors, 409, 413
  in reptiles, 578–579

Gastrointestinal obstruction, in
    amphibians, 617
  in rabbits, 448
  in rodents, 523

Gastrointestinal stasis, in rabbits, 446–449
  in rodents, 523–524

Gastropods, emergency care of, 642–643

Gastrostomy tube, for rabbits, 445

Gerbils, emergency and critical care of, **501–531**. See also *Rodents*.
  physiologic parameters for, 501–502

Gill biopsies, of fish, 659

Gills, of fish, normal vs. hyperplastic, 659–660

Globe proptosis, in rodents, 519–520

Glomerulonephropathies, in pet birds, 385–387

Glottis, of pet birds, 360–361
    emergencies involving, 361–362

Gloves, for handling, of amphibians, 591
  of raptors, 396–397

Glucocorticoids, for shock syndromes, 284

Glucose, for cardiopulmonary-cerebral resuscitation, 286
 serum. See *Blood glucose level*.

Glycopyrrolate, for cardiopulmonary-cerebral resuscitation, 286

Gout, articular, in pet birds, 387

Grasshoppers, emergency care of, 635–637

Guinea pigs, emergency and critical care of, **501–531**. See also *Rodents*.
 physiologic parameters for, 501–502

H

Hair loss, in ferrets, 473
 in tarantulas, 633

Hamsters, emergency and critical care of, **501–531**. See also *Rodents*.
 physiologic parameters for, 501–502

Handling guidelines, for emergency/critical care, of amphibians, 591
  of ferrets, 466–467
  of rabbits, 439–440
  of raptors, 395–396
  of rodents, 502–503

Hardness, water, in fish environment, 648, 650

Head tilt, in rabbits, 458–459

Head trauma, emergency procedures for, in pet birds, 378–379
  in raptors, 400–401, 405–406
  in rodents, 518–519

Heart disorders. See *Cardiac disease*.

Heart function, in critically ill patients. See also *Cardiac entries*.
  evaluation of, 326–332
  perfusion parameters for, 317–326

Heart rate, as critical care monitoring parameter, 317–319
  ECG measurement of, 330
  in amphibians, 595
  reptiles variability of, 563, 565

Heart rhythm, abnormalities of. See *Arrhythmias*.
  ECG evaluation of, 330–331, 399

Heartworm disease, in ferrets, 493

Heat stress, in rabbits, 459

Heat stroke, in ferrets, 497–498
 in rodents, 528

Heaters, in aquatic environment, for amphibians, 593–594
 for fish, 648, 651

Heavy metal poisoning, in pet birds, 380–381
 in rabbits, 457
 in raptors, 413–414
 in rodents, 523

Hedgehogs. See *African hedgehogs*.

Helicobacter gastritis, in ferrets, 469, 484–485

Hematology analysis, in emergency/critical care, of ferrets, 474
 of pet birds, 348–349, 373–374
 of reptiles, 566, 570–571
 of rodents, 515, 517

Hematopoietic disorders, in ferrets, emergency/critical care for, 491–492
  examination for, 473

Hemocoel, in invertebrate anatomy, 624, 627, 634

Hemoglobin-based oxygen carrier (HBOC), for hypovolemic shock, 280

Hemoglobin glutamer-200, for raptors, 411

Hemoglobin saturation, arterial, in blood gas analysis, 340
 in pulse oximetry, 336–337

Hemolymph, in invertebrates, anatomy of, 624, 635
  collection techniques for, 633–634, 642

Hemolytic anemia, immune-related, in ferrets, 497

Hemorrhage, emergency/critical care for. See also *Shock*.
  in exotic mammals, 543–545
  in fish, 656
  in pet birds, 346, 369
  in rabbits, 450
  in reptiles, 564–565, 577, 579
  resuscitation indications in, 280–281

Hemostatic clips, for bird surgery, 429–430

Herd-health aspect, of veterinary care, 590

Hermit crab, emergency care of, 637–638

Hetastarch, for fluid resuscitation, in raptors, 411, 414
  of shock, 279–280, 282

History taking, for emergency/critical care, of amphibians, 594–595

History (*continued*)
	of ferrets, 467, 470
	of fish, 651–652
	of invertebrates, 623
	of pet birds, 346
	of rabbits, 439
	of reptiles, 558
	of rodents, 503

Honeybees, emergency care of, 635–637

Hormonal therapy, for egg binding, in pet birds, 374–376

Hospital enclosures, for amphibians, 592–594

Hospital equipment, for emergency/critical care, of amphibians, 590–594
	of rabbits, 437, 439

Hospital tanks, for amphibians, 592–593

Hospitalization, for emergency/critical care, of invertebrates, 627
	of raptors, 397
	of rodents, 513, 522

Housing. See *Husbandry*.

Human chorionic gonadotropin, for ferrets, 482

Human influenza virus, in ferrets, 467, 469, 493

Humidity regulation, for amphibians, 593–594
	for reptiles, 558–559

Husbandry, in emergency/critical care, of amphibians, 589, 594–595
	hospital equipment for, 590–594
	of anemones and corals, 639–640
	of arachnids, 630–631
	of exotic mammals, 538–539, 546–547
	of ferrets, 466–467
	of invertebrates, 623–624, 627, 635, 637
	of raptors, 397
	of rodents, 513–514

Hydrometers, for reptiles, 559

Hydromorphone, for pain management, in small mammals, 296, 298

Hypercalcinuria, in rabbits, 453–454

Hyperkalemia, in ferrets, 495

Hyperparathyroidism, nutritional (renal) secondary. See also *Metabolic bone disease*.
	in amphibians, 617–618
	in reptiles, 577–578

Hyperphosphatemia, in reptiles, 578

Hypertension, in pet birds, 387–391
	clinical consequences of, 388
	definition of, 387–388
	etiology of, 388–390
	pathophysiology of, 388
	primary (essential), 388–390

Hyperthermia, in critically ill patients, 320

Hypertonic replacement fluids, for hypovolemic shock, 278–279

Hypocalcemia, in pet birds, 381–382
	in reptiles, 578
	in rodents, 522

Hypoglycemia, in raptors, 415
	in rodents, 522

Hypoproteinemia, in pet birds, 351

Hypotension, in hypovolemic shock, 276, 282–283
	refractory, 284
	inhalation anesthesia causing, in birds, 311–312
	in small mammals, 314

Hypothermia, in critically ill patients, 319–320
	hypovolemic shock and, 281–283

Hypoventilation, during anesthesia, 335–336

Hypovolemia, in critically ill patients, exotic mammals as, 540–541, 549
	raptors as, 398–399
	reptiles as, 562–565
	inhalation anesthesia causing, in birds, 311–312
	in small mammals, 314

Hypovolemic shock, Doppler monitoring of, 282. See also *Doppler monitoring*.
	fluid resuscitation for, during surgery, 282
	in birds, 281–282
	in small mammals, 282–284
	plan for, 277–278
	types of fluids in, 278–281
	pathophysiology of, 275–276
	phases of, 276–277

Hypoxemia, mechanical ventilation causing, 335–336

Hypoxia, reptile recovery ability from, 561

Hysterectomy, in birds, 433–435
	in pet birds, 376–378

I

Idiopathic myofascitis, in ferrets, 497

Illness factor, of energy requirement, in rabbits, 446

Imaging, diagnostic. See *Radiography; Ultrasound.*
nuclear. See *Computed tomography (CT); Magnetic resonance imaging (MRI).*

Imidacloprid, for ferrets, 482

Immersion administration, of fish emergency treatments, 663–664, 672

Immune-related disease, in ferrets, emergencies involving, 472, 479, 497

Impression smears, for fish necropsy, 662

Incisor-premolar malocclusions, in rabbits, 449

Incubator, for critically ill patients, exotic mammals as, 546–547
    in hypovolemic shock, 281
    pet birds as, 347, 358
    rabbits as, 437
    raptors as, 408, 413

Infectious disease, emergencies related to, in amphibians, 594, 606–609, 614–617
    in ferrets, 467, 469, 484–485, 493–494, 498
        treatment of, 482–483
    in fish, 668–671
        treatment of, 667–669
    in invertebrates, arachnids as, 632–633
        corals as, 640–642
        insects as, 635–637
        mollusks as, 642–643
        myriapods as, 634–635
    in pet birds, 356, 360, 368, 374
        chlamydophilosis as, 382
    in rabbits, 448, 451–453, 456–459
    in raptors, 409, 415
    in reptiles, 572
    in rodents, 522

Influenza virus, human, in ferrets, 467, 469, 493

Infraorbital nerve block, for small mammals, 301–302

Infraorbital sinus, of pet birds, 359–360

Inhalation anesthesia, for birds, 333, 341–342
    agents for, 307, 311
    cardiopulmonary arrest from, 287–288
    intubation techniques for, 310–311
    for fish, 657–658
    for invertebrates, 625–626
    for small mammals, 313–314, 342
        agents for, 306–307
        cardiopulmonary arrest from, 288–290
        cesarean section and, 312–313
        intubation techniques for, 309–311

Inhalation therapy, for respiratory distress, in pet birds, 356–357
    in rodents, 511–512

Injury(ies). See *Trauma.*

Insects, anatomy of, 635
    emergency care of, 635–637

Insulin, for hyperkalemia, in ferrets, 495–496

Insulinoma, in ferrets, 486–488

Integumentary system, emergency/critical care for, in amphibians, 588, 598–600
    in ferrets, 491
    in fish, 671–672
    in reptiles, 579–580
    in rodents, 504

Intensive care unit, for reptiles, 558

Interstitial volume deficits, shock and, 275–278, 284–285
    in reptiles, 564

Intestinal torsion/intussusception, in rodents, 524

Intracardiac injections, for cardiopulmonary-cerebral resuscitation, 288

Intracoelomic injection, of fish emergency treatments, 663

Intracranial pressure, increased in birds, inhalation anesthesia causing, 311

Intramuscular injection, of emergency treatments, in amphibians, 602
    in fish, 663–664

Intraosseous (IO) catheterization, for critically ill patients, amphibians as, 591, 596, 600–601
    exotic mammals as, 541–545
    ferrets as, 476
    pet birds as, 354–355
    rabbits as, 440
    raptors as, 402–403
    reptiles as, 560, 567–569
    rodents as, 515–517

Intraperitoneal fluid administration, in exotic mammals, 543

Intratesticular block, for pain management, in small mammals, 303–304

Intravascular injection/infusions, for emergency/critical care, of fish, 663
　　of hypovolemic shock, 281–282
　　of invertebrates, 632
　　of raptors, 401–402
　　of reptiles, 560, 562, 567–569
　　of rodents, 515–517

Intravascular volume deficits, in hypovolemic shock, 275–277, 283

Intravenous (IV) access/catheterization, bandaging techniques for, in birds, 419–425
　　for critically ill patients, amphibians as, 591, 596, 600–601
　　exotic mammals as, 541–543
　　ferrets as, 475–476
　　fish as, 659–661
　　pet birds as, 355
　　rabbits as, 440
　　raptors as, 401–402
　　reptiles as, 560, 565

Intravenous (IV) infusions, for critically ill patients, exotic mammals as, 541, 546
　　fish as, 657
　　hypovolemic shock and, 277–281
　　invertebrates as, 632
　　raptors as, 410–411, 414

Intubation techniques, airway. See *Airway intubation*.
　　gastric. See *Feeding tubes*.

Invertebrates, anatomy of, 624–625
　　emergency care of, **621–645**
　　　　anamnesis and, 623–624
　　　　anemone presentations for, 638–642
　　　　anesthesia for, 625–626
　　　　arachnid presentations for, 630–633
　　　　background perspectives for, 622–624
　　　　centipede presentations for, 633–635
　　　　common reasons for, 627–630
　　　　　　chemical intoxication, 627–628
　　　　　　dysecdysis, 629–630
　　　　　　trauma, 628–629
　　　　coral presentations for, 638–642
　　　　critical care concepts in, 623
　　　　crustacean presentations for, 637–638
　　　　euthanasia for, 643
　　　　hospitalization for, 627
　　　　insect presentations for, 635–637
　　　　millipede presentations for, 633–635
　　　　mollusk presentations for, 642–643
　　　　overview of, 621–622, 643
　　　　physical examination for, 623–624
　　　　therapeutics for, 626–627
　　ownership laws and regulations, 621–622
　　taxonomy overview of, 622–623

Isoflurane, cardiopulmonary arrest from, 287
　　for anesthesia, in amphibians, 604–605
　　　　in birds, 311, 333
　　　　in exotic mammals, 548
　　　　in invertebrates, 625
　　　　in small mammals, 307, 313
　　for sedation, in exotic mammals, 551
　　for seizures, in raptors, 415

Isotonic replacement fluids, for dehydration, 566
　　for hypovolemic shock, 278–279, 282

Itraconazole, for amphibians, 597
　　for raptors, 411

Ivermectin, for amphibians, 591, 597
　　toxicity of, 614
　　for ferrets, 483, 493
　　for rabbits, 458

K

Ketamine, for anesthesia, in amphibians, 605
　　in fish, 658
　　in small mammals, 296, 304–305
　　　　diazepam combined with, 306–307
　　　　fentanyl combined with, 313–314

Ketoprofen, for raptors, 411
　　for small mammals, 297

Kidney disease. See *Renal disease*.

Kidney stones, in ferrets, 470

L

Laboratory tests, in emergency/critical care, of amphibians, 607–608
　　of exotic mammals, 549–550
　　of ferrets, 474–475
　　of fish, 659–661

of pet birds, 347–352, 373–374
of reptiles, 566, 569–571
of rodents, 515, 517

Lacerations, emergency/critical care for, in pet birds, 368, 370

Lactate, dehydration and, 566
in blood gas analysis, 341

Lactic acidosis, in shock syndromes, 284–285

Laparoscopy, in fish surgery, 661

Large airway, of pet birds, anatomy and physiology of, 360–361
emergency/critical care for, 361–362

Larynx, in bird respiratory system, 332, 360
emergency/critical care for, 361–362

Laws, on invertebrate ownership, 621–622

Lead poisoning, in rabbits, 457

Leg splint, for birds, 420–421, 423

Leuprolide acetate, for ferrets, 483

Level of consciousness, as critical care monitoring parameter, 319
in pet birds, 378
cardiopulmonary-cerebral resuscitation and, 287, 289

Lidocaine, local, for pain management, in birds, 312, 370
in fish, 661
in rabbits, 438
in reptiles, 575
in small mammals, 297, 300–301
critically ill surgical, 314
dental block techniques for, 301–304
epidural injections of, 300, 307–308
with cesarean section, 312–313

Life support systems, for aquatic fish environment, 648, 650–651
emergency management of, 663, 665
history in emergency assessment, 652
in immediate emergency response, 652–653

Lights, for aquatic fish environment, 649, 653

Liver function tests, in ferrets, 349, 474
in pet birds, 349

Lizards, emergency care of, **557–585**. See also *Reptiles*.

Local anesthetics, for pain management. See also *Bupivacaine; Lidocaine*.
in birds, 312
in reptiles, 574–575
in small mammals,
administration options for, 297, 300–301, 307
critically ill surgical, 314
dental block techniques for, 301–304
with cesarean section, 312–313

Low-flow oxygen, during anesthesia, in birds, 334

Lower airway, of ferrets, 472
of pet birds, 360–361
biopsy of, 363
emergency/critical care for, 361–362, 364

Lufenuron, for ferrets, 483

Lumbar spine fractures, in rabbits, 457

Lumbosacral (LS) space, epidural analgesia injection into, 308–309

Lung wash, in reptiles, 572, 577

Lungs, of ferrets, emergency/critical care for, 471–472, 481
of pet birds, anatomy and physiology of, 366–367
emergency/critical care for, 367–369
of rabbits, neoplasia of, 456

Lungworm infection, in treefrog, 606

Luxations, in rabbits, 457
in raptors, 399

Lymph nodes, in ferrets, aspiration of, 478–479
emergency examination of, 472

Lymphocytic-plasmacytic gastroenteritis, in ferrets, 469, 486

Lymphoma, in rabbits, 456

Lymphosarcoma, in ferrets, 468, 470, 490–491
mediastinal masses with, 493

M

Magnetic resonance imaging (MRI), in amphibians, 609
in pet birds, 354, 379–380

Magnification, for bird surgery, 430

Malnutrition, in pet birds, 351
  in raptors, 415
  in sugar gliders, 534–535

Malocclusions, dental, in rabbits, 449

Mandibular nerve block, for small mammals, 301–302

Mannitol, for raptors, 411

Manual manipulation, for egg binding, in pet birds, 375–376

Manual restraint, for emergency/critical care, of exotic mammals, 550–551
    of ferrets, 466–467, 475
    of fish, 654, 657–658
    of invertebrates, 626
    of raptors, 396–397
    of rodents, 502–503

Marbofloxacin, for rabbits, 438

Masks, for anesthesia induction, 333
  in invertebrates, 625–626
  for cardiopulmonary-cerebral resuscitation, 287–288

Mass(es), in amphibians, 609, 613
  mediastinal, in ferrets, 493
  in rabbits, 456

Mast cell tumors, in ferrets, 491

Maxillary nerve block, for small mammals, 302–303

Mean arterial pressure (MAP), direct monitoring of, 321
  in reptiles, 563
  indirect monitoring of, 321

Mechanical ventilation, during anesthesia, 332, 334–336
  for cardiopulmonary-cerebral resuscitation, 287–290
  in emergency/critical care, of birds, 332
    of reptiles, 577
    of rodents, 510

Meclizine, for rabbits, 438, 458–459

Medetomidine, for pain management, in small mammals, 297, 304

Mediastinal masses, anterior, in ferrets, 493
  in rabbits, 456

Medication administration, routes of, in amphibians, 590–592, 602–603
  in fish, 663–664
  in invertebrates, 626–627
  in reptiles, 560, 567–569
    intracardiac contraindications, 288

Melarsomine, for ferrets, 493

Meloxicam, for pain management, in raptors, 411
  in reptiles, 574
  in small mammals, 297

Mental nerve block, for small mammals, 301

Mentation, as critical care monitoring parameter, 319

Meperidine, for reptiles, 574–575

Mercury poisoning, in raptors, 414

Metabolic acidosis, 341
  in shock syndromes, 284–285, 287

Metabolic alkalosis, 341

Metabolic bone disease, in raptors, 415
  in sugar gliders, 534–535

Metazoan parasites, fish emergencies related to, 670–671
  treatment of, 667–669

Methemoglobin, in pulse oximetry, 336–337

Metoclopramide, for ferrets, 483
  for rabbits, 438

Metronidazole, for exotic mammals, 553
  for ferrets, 483
  for reptiles, 573

Microspridium parasites, fish emergencies related to, 670–671
  treatment of, 667–669

Microsurgical pack, for bird surgery, 428–429

Midazolam, for pain management, in exotic mammals, 549, 553
  in rabbits, 438, 454
  in raptors, 411, 413, 415
  in small mammals, 296, 312
    critically ill surgical patients, 313
    preoperative cesarean section, 312

Millipedes, emergency care of, 633–635

Mite infestations, in invertebrates, arachnids, 632–633
    myriapods, 634–635
  in pet birds, 371

Modified Robert Jones bandage, for birds, 421–422

Molar teeth, malocclusions of, in rabbits, 449

Mollusca, emergency care of, 642–643
 in invertebrate taxonomy, 622–623

Molting process, in hermit crabs, 637–638
 in tarantulas, 632

Monitoring techniques, for blood pressure. See *Blood pressure*.
 for cardiovascular systems, 318–326
 for raptors, 399–400
 for respiratory systems, 336–342
 in critical care, **317–344**. See also *Critical care monitoring*.

Monkeypox, in prairie dogs, emergency procedures for, 534, 536–537

Morphine, for reptiles, 574–575
 for small mammals, 297, 308, 312–313

Moths, emergency care of, 635–637

Mouse/mice, emergency and critical care of, **501–531**. See also *Rodents*.
 physiologic parameters for, 501–502

Mucoid enteritis, in rabbits, 455

Mucolytic therapy, nebulized, for pet birds, 357
 for rodents, 512

Mucous membrane color, as critical care monitoring parameter, 319

Multimodal analgesia, for small mammals, 294

Musculoskeletal system, of ferrets, differential disease diagnoses, 468, 470
 emergency/critical care for diseases of, 497
 examination of, 468, 470, 473, 479
 of rodents, emergency/critical care for diseases of, 522–523
 examination of, 504

Mycobacterial infections, in amphibians, 615

Myiasis, in rabbits, 459

Myofascitis, idiopathic, in ferrets, 497

Myriapods, anatomy of, 634
 emergency care of, 633–635

N

Naloxone, for analgesia reversal, in small mammals, 298–299

Nasal disorders, in rodents, 504

Nasal flush analysis, for pet birds, 352, 356, 360

Nasogastric tubes. See also *Enteral feeding*.
 for rabbits, 442–445, 448

Nausea, emergency procedures for, in ferrets, 469–470, 484
 in pet birds, 382–384

Nebulizers/nebulization, for pet birds, 356–357
 for rodents, 511–512

Necropsy, for amphibian mortality, 608
 for fish mortality, 662

Nematode infections, in amphibians, 614
 in arachnids, 632

Neoplasia, emergency/critical care for, in African hedgehogs, 535
 in ferrets, 468, 470, 490–491
 dermatologic, 491
 in pet birds, coelomic, 365
 in prairie dogs, 534, 537
 in rabbits, 449–450, 456
 in rodents, 521

Nerve blocks, for pain management, in small mammals, 301–304

Neurologic abnormalities, in African hedgehogs, 534, 536
 in pet birds, 347
 heavy metal intoxication and, 380–381
 hypocalcemia syndrome as, 381–382
 proventricular dilatation disease as, 381
 seizures as, 380
 spinal disease and, 379–380
 trauma-related, 378–379
 in rabbits, 457
 in raptors, 415
 in rodents, 504, 522–523
 in sugar gliders, 551–552
 reptile emergencies involving, 577
 toxicity-related. See *Toxins/toxicities*.

Neurologic function, as resuscitation goal, 286–287

Newts, emergency medicine of, **587–620**. See also *Amphibians*.

Niacin, for atherosclerosis, in pet birds, 390

Nitrites, in aquatic fish environment, 648–650
 toxicity of, 665–666

Nitrogen balance, in rabbits, 445–446

Nitroglycerin, for ferrets, 492

NMDA antagonists, for pain management, in small mammals, 296, 305–307

Nociception, pain and, 294

Nonsteroidal anti-inflammatory drugs (NSAIDs), caution with, in ferrets, 484
for airway disease, in pet birds, 364–365
for pain management, in amphibians, 604
in birds, 312, 369–370
in fish, 661
in reptiles, 575
in rodents, 520–521, 523
in small mammals, 297, 299–300
postoperative, 313–314

Normal sinus rhythm, in birds vs. small mammals, 328–330

Normothermia. See *Temperature regulation.*

Nutritional secondary hyperparathyroidism. See also *Metabolic bone disease.*
in amphibians, 617–618
in reptiles, 577–578

Nutritional support, for critically ill patients, amphibians as, 603–604
birds as, 433–434
exotic mammals as, 538–539, 547–548
fish as, 651–652, 664–665
pet birds as, 358
rabbits as, 437, 439, 442–445
BMR requirements vs., 445–446
raptors as, 404–405
reptiles as, 572–574
rodents as, 517–518, 528

O

Octopi, emergency care of, 642–643

Ocular disorders, in rodents, 504, 518–520

Ocular proptosis, in African hedgehogs, 536

Oil contamination, of raptors, 413–414

Omega-3 fatty acids, for atherosclerosis, in pet birds, 390

Ophryocystis elektroscirrha infestation, of butterflies, 636–637

Ophthalmologic disease, in ferrets, 498

Opioids, for pain management, in amphibians, 604
in birds, 312
in fish, 661
in reptiles, 574–575
in small mammals, 295–296, 298–299
local anesthetics with, 300–301

Opisthosoma, in tarantulas, 633

Oral administration, of emergency treatments, in amphibians, 590–592, 602
in fish, 663
in invertebrates, 626–627
in raptors, 401
in rodents, 515

Oral examination, for emergency/critical care, of rabbits, 437, 449–450
of rodents, 504–505, 508, 523

Oscillometric method, for blood pressure monitoring, 321–322

Osmolarity, plasma, in reptiles, with dehydration, 566
with shock, 562
water, for aquatic amphibian species, 602

Osmotic stress, in fish, 656–657

Otitis media, in rabbits, 458–459

Ovarian remnant syndrome, in ferrets, 469, 488–489

Overfeeding, of fish, 651

Overstocking, of fish tanks, 651

Oviduct, in birds, salpingohysterectomy of, 433–435
in pet birds, egg removal surgery on, 376–378
inducement of contractions for egg laying, 374–375
prolapse of, 377–378

Ovocentesis, for egg binding, in pet birds, 376

Oxygen, arterial concentration of, in respiratory monitoring, 340–341
dissolved, in aquatic fish environment, 647–648
low level of, 666

Oxygen therapy, for cardiopulmonary-cerebral resuscitation, 287–290
for emergency stabilization, in hypovolemic shock, 281
of birds, 332–333
of pet birds, 358, 363
of raptors, 398, 413
respiratory disease and, 407
of reptiles, 576–577

of rodents, 503, 510–512, 521–522
in mechanical ventilation, during anesthesia, 334–336

Oxyglobin, for fluid resuscitation, of shock, 280, 282, 284, 565

Oxytocin, for rabbits, 438

Oysters, emergency care of, 642–643

P

P-QRS-T complex, ECG measurement of, 331

P waves, ECG evaluation of, 331
in birds vs. small mammals, 328–329

Packed cell volume (PCV), in critically ill raptors, 400, 402

Pain assessment, in birds, 293–294
in ferrets, 481
in small mammals, 293–294

Pain management, in amphibians, 604
in birds, **293–315**
analgesic drugs for, 311–312
anesthetic drugs for, 311–312
inhalants for, 307
intubation techniques for, 310–311
multimodal analgesia for, 294
options for, 294–295
overview of, 293–294
in exotic mammals, 549, 553
in fish, 661
in pet birds, 369–370, 374
in rabbits, 446–447, 457
in raptors, 398–399, 405, 407
in reptiles, 574–575
in rodents, 518, 520–521, 523
in small mammals, **293–315**
analgesic drugs for, 295–305
anesthesia induction and, 304, 306–307
anesthetic drugs for, 296–305
constant rate infusions for, 305–306, 313–314
dental block techniques for, 301–304
epidural drugs for, 300, 307–309
ferrets as, 481
for cesarean section, 312–313
for critically ill surgical patient, 313–314
inhalants for, 307
intubation techniques for, 309–310

multimodal analgesia for, 294
options for, 294–295
overview of, 293–294

Palantine nerve block, for small mammals, 303

Palpation, for emergency assessments, of ferrets, 472–473

Papillary light reflex (PLR), cardiopulmonary resuscitation and, 287

Paralysis, in amphibians, 609, 611
in pet birds, 379–380
in rabbits, 457–458

Paraphimosis, in rodents, 525–526

Parasites, emergencies related to, in amphibians, 609, 614
in fish, 667–671
in invertebrates, 632, 634, 636–637, 641
in raptors, 415

Parenchymal disease, in ferrets, emergencies involving, 472
in pet birds, air sac physiology in, 366–367
emergencies involving, 367–369
lung anatomy in, 366–367

Parenteral administration, of emergency treatments, in fish, 663
venous. See *Intravenous (IV) access/catheterization.*

Paresis, in amphibians, 609, 611
in pet birds, 379–380
in rabbits, 457–458
in reptiles, 577
in rodents, 522–523

Pasteurella multocida, in rabbits, 458

Patient assessment. See *Physical examination.*

Penicillamine, for raptors, 411

Perfusion deficits, in renal failure, rabbits and, 452
in rodents, 512–513
in shock, 275–277, 283–285
reptile assessment for, 565–566

Perfusion parameters, cardiopulmonary resuscitation and, 289–290
in critical care monitoring, 317–326

Peritonitis, in pet birds, 365

Personal protective equipment, for physical assessment, of amphibians, 591
of raptors, 396–397

Pesticide exposures, emergency/critical care
for, in fish, 666, 668
in raptors, 409, 413–414
Pet birds, emergency and critical care of, **345–394**
common reasons for, 358–391
gastrointestinal disease, 382–384
hypertension, 387–391
mites, 371
neurologic disease, 378–382
renal disease, 384–387
reproductive-related, 372–378
respiratory-related, 358–369
trauma, 369–372
diagnostic testing in, 347–354
history taking for, 346
overview of, 345, 391
physical examination for, 346–347
procedures for, 354–358
treatment protocols for, 369–372
triage in, 345–346
renal function in, 384–385
respiratory system of, 359–369
air sacs, 366–369
coelomic cavity, 364–366
glottis, 360–362
infraorbital sinus, 359–360
large airway, 360–362
larynx, 360–362
lungs, 366–369
small airway, 362–364
trachea to the syrinx, 360–362
upper airway, 359–360
pH, in aquatic environment, for corals and anemones, 640–641
for fish, 648, 650, 652–653
in blood gas analysis, 341
in shock syndromes, 284

Pharyngostomy tube, for rabbits, 445

Phenobarbital, for raptors, 411
for rodents, 522

Phosphorus, serum, in ferrets, 474
in pet birds, 350

Physical assessment. See *Physical examination*.

Physical examination, for emergency/critical care, of amphibians, 595–596
of anemones and corals, 638–639
of ferrets, 471–473
restraint for, 466–467, 475
of fish, 654–655
restraint for, 654, 657–658
of invertebrates, 623–624
of pet birds, 346–347, 352
of rabbits, 437, 439–440
of raptors, 397–399
restraint for, 396–397
of reptiles, 558–559
of rodents, 503
restraint for, 502–503, 507

Plasma osmolarity, in reptiles, with dehydration, 566
with shock, 562

Plastic spica bandage, for birds, 420–421, 423

Pleural space disease, in ferrets, emergencies involving, 472

Pneumonia, bacterial, in ferrets, 493
in rabbits, 456
in reptiles, 572, 577
in rodents, 520

Point-of-care laboratory testing, for blood chemistries, 340–341
for blood gas analysis, 340

Poisonings. See *Toxins/toxicities*.

Polydipsia, in pet birds, 385

Polyuria, in pet birds, 385
in rodents, 527

Positive-pressure ventilation (PPV), for anesthesia, 334–336
for birds, 332
for cardiopulmonary-cerebral resuscitation, 287–289
for reptiles, 577
for rodents, 510

Posture examination, of pet birds, 346, 378–379

Prairie dogs, blood chemistry data for, 550
emergency and critical care of, **501–531**. See also *Rodents*.
common reasons for, 534, 536–538
nutrition for, 538–539, 547–548
stabilization principles for, 539–548
therapeutic drug dosages for, 552–553
hematologic data for, 549–550
physiologic data for, normal, 541–542

Pralidoxime, for raptors, 411

Praziquantel, for fish, 668

Predator trauma, in exotic mammals, 534–537

Prednisolone, for ferrets, 483
  for raptors, 411
Prednisone, for ferrets, 483, 493
Preferred optimal temperature zone (POTZ), for reptiles, 559, 563
Pregnancy toxemia, in rabbits, 459
  in rodents, 525
Preoperative drugs, for small mammals, cesarean section and, 312–313
    critically ill surgical, 313
Pressure-controlled ventilators, 335
Prokinetics, for rabbits, 449
Prolapse emergencies, in amphibians, cloacal, 609, 613
    rectal, 609, 614
  in pet birds, cloacal, 376–378
    oviduct, 377–378
  in reptiles, cloacal, 580
  in rodents, rectal, 525
    vaginal or uterine, 525–526
Proliferative bowel disease, in ferrets, 485–486
Propofol, for pain management, in small mammals, 296, 306, 312
Proprioception evaluation, in pet birds, 346, 378–379
Proptosis, globe, in rodents, 519–520
Prostaglandin therapy, for egg binding, in pet birds, 374–375
Prostatic disease, in ferrets, 494, 496
Protein electrophoresis, plasma, for pet birds, 349
Protozoal diseases, emergencies related to, in fish, 669–670
    treatment of, 667–669
  in invertebrates, 636–637
Proventricular dilatation disease (PDD), in pet birds, 381
Proventriculotomy, in birds, 435–436
Pseudo-odontoma, in prairie dogs, 534, 537–538
    emergency procedures for, 552
Psittacosis, in pet birds, 368
Pulmonary anatomy. See *Respiratory system*.
Pulmonary arrest. See *Cardiopulmonary arrest*.

Pulmonary edema, in rodents, 520–521
Pulse check/quality, in cardiopulmonary-cerebral resuscitation and, 286–287, 289–290
  in raptors, 399–400
  in rodents, 512–514
Pulse oximetry, for respiratory monitoring, 336
    in amphibians, 604
    in birds, 337
    in reptiles, 571
    in small mammals, 337
Pumps, for aquatic fish environment, 648–649
    in immediate emergency response, 652–653
    portable, 654

Q

QRS complexes, ECG evaluation of, 331
  in birds vs. small mammals, 329

R

R waves, ECG evaluation of, 330–331
Rabbits, blood pressure monitoring in, 322–323, 325–326
  critical care of, **437–461**
    common reasons for, acute respiratory distress, 456
      anorexia, 444, 447–449
      cardiac disease, 456–457
      diarrhea, 454–455
      head tilt, 458–459
      heat stress, 459
      myiasis, 459
      neoplasia, 449–450, 456
      neurologic signs, 457
      paresis/paralysis, 457–458
      pregnancy toxemia, 459
      red urine, 455–456
      renal disease, 451–452
      urethral obstruction, 454
      urolithiasis, 453–454
      uterine disorders, 449–451
    diagnostic approaches to, 440–442
    dietary history in, 439
    drugs for, 437–439
    emergency stabilization importance in, 437–439
    physical examination for, 439–440
    therapeutic techniques for, 442–447

Rabbits (continued)
  pain management in, analgesic drugs for, 295–305
    anesthetic drugs for, 296–305
      local administration of, 300–301
      dental block techniques for, 301–304
      epidural anesthesia for, 297, 300, 307–309
      inhalants for, 307
        intubation techniques for, 309–310
      options for, 294
  shock in, **275–291**
    cardiopulmonary-cerebral resuscitation for, 288–290
    effectiveness of, 286–287, 289
    fluid resuscitation for, for dehydration deficits, 285
      plan for, 277–278, 282–284
      types of fluids in, 278–281
    glucocorticoids in, 284
    pathophysiology of, 275–276
    phases of, 276–277
    sodium bicarbonate in, 284–285

Radiography, in emergency/critical examinations, for cardiac evaluation, 326
  of amphibians, 608
  of exotic mammals, 550–551
  of ferrets, 476–477
    contrast indications for, 477
  of fish, 661
  of pet birds, 352–353, 373, 380, 383
  of rabbits, 442, 453
  of raptors, 400–401
  of reptiles, 571–572
  of rodents, 507–508

Radiosurgery equipment, for birds, 430

Ranitidine, for ferrets, 483

Raptors, emergency care of, **395–418**
  bandaging for, 402, 404
  common reasons for, 395, 405–409
    emaciation, 414
    infectious disease, 409, 415
    other presentations, 415
    respiratory disease, 407–409, 413
    toxin exposures, 409, 413–414
    trauma, 400–401, 405–407, 409
  drug formulary for, 407, 410–412
  euthanasia for, 415
  fluid administration sites for, 401–402
  fluid therapy for, 398–399, 402
  handling for, 395–396
  hospitalization for, 397
  monitoring techniques for, 399–400
  nutritional support for, 404–405
  overview of, 395, 415–416
  pain control for, 405
  patient assessment for, 397–399
  radiographs for, 400–401
  restraint for, 396–397
  sample collection for, 400
  stabilization therapies in, 398–399, 404
  transfusion medicine for, 400, 402–403
  triage for, 397–400
  wound care for, 399, 402, 404

Rats, emergency and critical care of, **501–531**. See also *Rodents*.
  physiologic parameters for, 501–502

Rectal prolapse, in amphibians, 609, 614
  in rodents, 525

"Red bug," in corals, 641–642

Red urine, in rabbits, 455–456

Reflexes, evaluation of, in cardiopulmonary-cerebral resuscitation, 287
  in pet birds, 378–379

Regulations, on invertebrate ownership, 621–622

Regurgitation, emergency procedures for, in pet birds, 382–384
  in reptiles, 579

Rehydration, for dehydration. See *Fluid support*.
  for shock. See *Fluid resuscitation*.

Renal biopsy, in pet birds, 385–386

Renal disease, emergencies involving, acute. See *Acute renal failure*.
  in amphibians, 618–619
  in ferrets, 474
  in pet birds, 384–387
    hypertension related to, 388
  in rabbits, 451–452

Renal function, hypovolemic shock impact on, 276
  in ferrets, 474
  in pet birds, 384–385

Renal secondary hyperparathyroidism, in
    amphibians, 617–618
    in reptiles, 577–578

Reproductive function, in amphibians, 588

Reproductive-related emergencies, in pet
        birds, 372–378
    chronic egg laying as, 372
    cloacal prolapse as, 376–378
    egg binding as, 372–376
    oviduct prolapse as, 377–378
    in rabbits, 449–451, 459
    in reptiles, 580–581
    in rodents, 525–526

Reptiles, emergency care of, **557–585**
    analgesia for, 574–575
    anesthetics for, 575–576
    biologic concepts in, 557–558
    blood pressure in, 562–565
    cardiopulmonary-cerebral
        resuscitation in, 558–562
    drugs for, 560, 562
    clinical tests for, 570–572
    common reasons for, 576–581
        cardiovascular, 577
        cloacal prolapse, 580–581
        gastrointestinal, 578–579
        integumental, 579–580
        neurologic, 577
        nutritional, 577–578
        renal, 577–578
        reproductive, 580–581
        respiratory, 576–577
        septicemia, 581
    dehydration in, 565–567
    drug administration in, 567
    fluid resuscitation as, 562–565
    goals of, 572
    history taking for, 558
    nutritional support in, 572–574
    overview of, 557, 581
    physical examination for,
        558–559
    shock in, 562–565
    vascular access for, 567–570
    taxonomy of, 557–558

Respiration, fish examination for, 654

Respiratory acidosis, 341

Respiratory alkalosis, 341

Respiratory disease, emergency/critical care
        for, in ferrets, 493–494
    diagnosis of, 469–472
    drugs in, 482–483
    in pet birds, 359–369
        coelomic cavity conditions,
            364–366

infraorbital sinus
    conditions, 359–360
large airway conditions,
    360–362
parenchymal, 366–369
small airway conditions,
    362–364
upper airway conditions,
    359–360
in raptors, 407–409
in reptiles, 576–577

Respiratory distress, acute management of,
    in ferrets, 471–472, 492
    in pet birds, 356–358
    in rabbits, 456
    in raptors, 409, 413
    in reptiles, 576–577
    in rodents, 508–512

Respiratory minute volume (RMV), in
    positive-pressure ventilation,
    334–335

Respiratory monitors, 337–338

Respiratory muscles, in birds, 332, 347

Respiratory system, of birds, 332–333
    monitoring during anesthesia,
        336–342
    of ferrets, 471–472
    of invertebrates, 624–625, 634
    of pet birds, 359–369
        air sacs, 366–369
        coelomic cavity, 364–366
        glottis, 360–362
        infraorbital sinus, 359–360
        large airway, 360–362
        larynx, 360–362
        lungs, 366–369
        small airway, 362–364
        trachea to the syrinx, 360–362
        upper airway, 359–360
    of small mammals, 333
        monitoring during anesthesia,
            336–342
    reptile emergencies involving, 576–577

Respirometry, 338

Responsiveness, fish examination for, 654

Restraint, for emergency/critical care, of
        exotic mammals, 550–551
    of ferrets, 466–467, 475
    of fish, 654, 657–658
    of pet birds, 346–347, 352
    of raptors, 396–397
    of rodents, 502–503, 507

Resuscitation, cardiopulmonary, goal of,
    286

Resuscitation (*continued*)
  cardiopulmonary-cerebral. See *Cardiopulmonary-cerebral resuscitation (CPCR)*.
  fluid. See *Fluid resuscitation*.
  of fish, 655–656

Retractors, for bird surgery, 430

Rewarming techniques, for critically ill patients, 320
  exotic mammals as, 546–547
  hypovolemic shock and, 283–284
  reptiles as, 561

Roaches, emergency care of, 635–637

Robert Jones bandage, modified, for birds, 421–422

Rodents, emergency and critical care of, **501–531**
  common presentations for, 518–528
    cardiac disease, 522
    gastrointestinal, 523–525
    miscellaneous conditions, 528
    neurologic, 522–523
    renal failure, 527–528
    reproductive, 525–526
    respiratory disease, 521–522
    trauma, 518–521
    urinary obstruction, 526–527
  diagnostic approaches to, 505–508, 521
  general supportive measures in, 513–518
  history taking for, 503
  overview of, 501–502, 528
  patient handling for, 502–503
  physical examination for, 503–505
  radiography for, 507–508
  restraint techniques for, 502–503
  sample collection for, 505–507, 521
  triage for, 508–513
  physiologic parameters for, 501–502
  taxonomy of, 508

Routes of administration, for emergency treatments, in amphibians, 590–592, 597–603
  in fish, 663–664
  in invertebrates, 626–627
  in reptiles, 560, 567–569
  in rodents, 515–517
    intracardiac contraindications, 288

S

S waves, ECG evaluation of, 330–331

Salamanders, emergency medicine of, **587–620**. See also *Amphibians*.

Salinity, in aquatic environment, for corals and anemones, 640
  for fish, 648, 650, 652–653
    restoring balance of, 656–657

Salpingohysterectomy, in birds, 433–435
  in pet birds, 376–378

Scaly mites, in pet birds, 371

Schoeder-Thomas splint, for birds, 422, 424

Scorpions, emergency care of, 630–633. See also *Invertebrates*.

Secondary hyperparathyroidism. See also *Metabolic bone disease*.
  nutritional (renal), in amphibians, 617–618
  in reptiles, 577–578

Sedation, for emergency/critical care, general systemic. See *Anesthesia/anesthetic drugs*.
  of exotic mammals, 550–551
  of raptors, 413
  of rodents, 502, 515, 521

Seizures, in amphibians, 596
  in pet birds, 380
  in rabbits, 380, 457
  in raptors, 415
  in reptiles, 577
  in rodents, 522
  in sugar gliders, 551–552

Selamectin, for ferrets, 483

Self-defense behavior/weapons, in anemones and corals, 639
  in arachnids, 630–631
  in raptors, 395–396

Self-mutilation, emergency/critical care for, in octopi, 643
  in pet birds, 368, 370
  in sugar gliders, 534–535

Sepsis, in amphibians, 615

Septicemia, in reptiles, 581

Sevoflurane, for anesthesia, in birds, 311, 333
  in exotic mammals, 548
  in invertebrates, 625
  in small mammals, 307, 313
  for sedation, in exotic mammals, 551
  for seizures, in raptors, 415

Sexing, of ferrets, 473

Shock, **275–291**
    cardiopulmonary-cerebral
        resuscitation for, 286–290
        drugs for, 286–287
        effectiveness of, 286–287
            algorithm for evaluating,
                288–289
        goal of, 286
        in birds, 287–289
        in small mammals, 288–290
    definition of, 275
    Doppler monitoring of, 282,
        321–322
    emergency procedures for, in birds,
            275–288
        in exotic mammals, 549–550
        in raptors, 398–399
        in small mammals, 275–290, 323
    fluid resuscitation for, 277–285
        during surgery, 282
        for dehydration deficits, 285
        in birds, 281–282
        in reptiles, 562–565
        in small mammals, 282–284
        plan for, 277–278
        types of fluids in, 278–281
    glucocorticoids in, 284
    heart rate response to, 318–319
    hypovolemic, pathophysiology of,
        275–276
    in amphibians, 595
    metabolic response to, 341
    pathophysiology of, 275–276
    phases of, 276–277
    sodium bicarbonate in, 284–285

Signalment, in emergency care, of ferrets,
    467, 470

Silver sulfadiazine, for raptors, 411

Sirens, emergency medicine of, **587–620**. See
    also *Amphibians*.

Skin scrapes, of amphibians, 607–608
    of fish, 659

Skin tumors, in ferrets, 491

Skin wounds. See also *Ulcers*.
    in fish, 671–672
    in reptiles, 579–580

Slugs, emergency care of, 642–643

Small airway, of ferrets, emergency/critical
        care for, 472
    of pet birds, anatomy and physiology
            of, 362
        emergency/critical care for,
            362–364

Small mammals, blood group typing in, 281
    critical care monitoring of, **317–344**
        blood pressure measurements,
            322–323, 325–326
        cardiac evaluation in, 326–332
        cardiovascular system
            components in, 318–326
        overview of, 317–318, 342–343
        perfusion parameters in, 317–326
        respiratory system during
            anesthesia, 332–342
    pain assessment in, 293–294
    pain management in, **293–315**
        analgesic drugs for, 295–305
        anesthesia induction agents for,
            304, 306–307
        anesthetic drugs for, 296–305
        constant rate infusions for,
            305–306, 313–314
        dental block techniques for,
            301–304
        epidural drugs for, 307–309
        for cesarean section, 312–313
        for critically ill surgical patient,
            313–314
        inhalants for, 307
            intubation techniques for,
                309–310
        multimodal analgesia for, 294
        options for, 294–295
        overview of, 293–294
    respiratory system components in, 333
    shock in, **275–291**
        cardiopulmonary-cerebral
            resuscitation for, 288–290
            effectiveness of, 286–287,
                289
        fluid resuscitation for, for
            dehydration deficits, 285
            plan for, 277–278, 282–284
            types of fluids in, 278–281
        glucocorticoids in, 284
        pathophysiology of, 275–276
        phases of, 276–277
        sodium bicarbonate in, 284–285

Snails, emergency care of, 642–643

Snakes, emergency care of, **557–585**. See
    also *Reptiles*.

Soaking solutions, for amphibians, 592,
    598–600

Sodium, plasma, in dehydration, 566

Sodium acetate, for fish resuscitation, 656

Sodium bicarbonate, emergency indications
        for, in fish, 656
    in raptors, 411
    metabolic acidosis as, 284–285

Sodium chloride, for fish infections, 667
Sodium thiosulphate, for fish resuscitation, 656
Sphygmomanometer, for blood pressure monitoring, 322
  in rodents, 513–514
  in small mammals, 323
Spiders, emergency care of, 630–633. See also *Invertebrates.*
  handling of, 630–631
Spinal disease, emergencies involving, in pet birds, 379–380
Spinal nerve roots, degeneration of, in rodents, 522–523
Spleen, in ferrets, aspiration of, 479
  examination of, 473
Splint(s), for birds, leg, 420–421, 423
  tape, 420–421
  Thomas-Schoeder, 422, 424
Squash preparations, for fish necropsy, 662
Squid, emergency care of, 642–643
ST segment, ECG evaluation of, 331
  in birds vs. small mammals, 329
Stabilization principles, in emergency/critical care, for hypovolemic shock, 281
  of birds, 332–333, **419–436**
  of exotic mammals, 539–548
  of pet birds, 358, 363
  of rabbits, 437–439
  of raptors, 398–399, 404, 407, 413
Statins, for atherosclerosis, in pet birds, 390
Stress response, in fish emergencies, 656–657
Stroke volume, critical care monitoring of, 317–318
Subcutaneous emphysema, in raptors, 413
Subcutaneous fluid administration, for critically ill patients, amphibians as, 600–601
  exotic mammals as, 543
  raptors as, 401
  rodents as, 515
Subluxations, in rabbits, 457
  in raptors, 399
Sucralfate, for ferrets, 483
Sudden death, in amphibians, 609, 611
Sugar gliders, blood chemistry data for, 550
  emergency and critical care of, common reasons for, 534–535, 551–552
    nutrition for, 539, 547–548
    stabilization principles for, 539–548
    therapeutic drug dosages for, 552–553
  hematologic data for, 549–550
  physiologic data for, normal, 541–542
  seizures in, 551–552
Supportive emergency care, fluids as. See *Fluid support.*
  for amphibians, 596–597
  for rodents, 513–518
  nutritional. See *Nutritional support.*
  pain control as. See *Pain management.*
  respiratory. See *Oxygen therapy.*
Surgery, anesthesia for. See *Anesthesia/anesthetic drugs.*
  emergency indications for. See *specific disorder, procedure, or species.*
  exploratory, in amphibians, 609
  laparoscopic, in fish, 661
  pain control for. See *Analgesia/analgesia drugs; Pain management.*
  shock resuscitation during, 282
Surgical drapes, for bird surgery, 430
Surgical equipment, for birds, 428–430
Swimming behavior, fish examination for, 654
Syrinx, in bird respiratory system, 332, 360–361
  emergencies involving, 361–362
Systemic vascular resistance (SVR), direct monitoring of, 321

T

Ta wave, ECG evaluation of, in birds, 328–329
Tanks, for fish, animal introductions into, 651–652
  maintenance of. See *Water environment.*
  hospital, for amphibians, 592
Tape splint, for birds, 420–421
Tarantulas, anatomy of, 625
  emergency care of, 630–633. See also *Invertebrates.*
  handling of, 630–631
  molting process in, 632

Taxonomy, of amphibians, 587–589
of ferrets, 463–464
of invertebrates, 622–623, 633
of reptiles, 557–558
of rodents, 508

Tegastes acroporanus infestation, of corals, 641–642

Temperature, core. See *Body temperature.*

Temperature probes, for exotic mammals, 319–320, 546
for rabbits, 437
for reptiles, 559
for rodents, 504

Temperature regulation, in emergency/critical care, aquatic environment and, of amphibians, 593–594
of fish, 648, 650–652
of exotic mammals, 546–547
of reptiles, 558–559, 563
of rodents, 514

Terbinafine, for raptors, 412–413

Terbutaline, nebulized, for ferrets, 483
for pet birds, 356–357, 363
for rodents, 511–512

Thermal support. See *Heaters; Temperature regulation.*

Thermal wounds, in pet birds, 368–369, 371
in reptiles, 579–580
in rodents, 518, 520–521

Thermometers, for exotic mammals, 319–320, 546
for rabbits, 437
for reptiles, 559
for rodents, 504

Thomas-Schoeder splint, for birds, 422, 424

Thoracic emergencies, in ferrets, examination of, 471–472
intervention for, 481
in rodents, 521–522

Thoracocentesis, in ferrets, 481

Thrombocytopenia, in ferrets, 491

Thymoma, in rabbits, 456

Ticarcillin/clavulanic acid, for raptors, 412
for reptiles, 573, 580

Tissue necrosis, rapid, in corals, 640–641
in pet birds, 377

Tissue samples. See *Biopsy(ies).*

Toads, emergency medicine of, **587–620.** See also *Amphibians.*

Topical wound treatments, for pet birds, 370

Torticollis, in rabbits, 458–459

Toxemia, pregnancy, in rabbits, 459
in rodents, 525

Toxins/toxicities, emergency/critical care for, in fish, 652, 665–666, 668
in invertebrates, 627–628
in pet birds, 364, 380–381, 383
in rabbits, 457
in raptors, 409, 413–414
in rodents, 523

Trachea, in bird respiratory system, 332, 361

Trachea to the syrinx, of pet birds, 360–361
biopsy of, 363
emergency/critical care for, 361–362, 364

Tracheal endoscopy, in birds, 426

Tracheal obstruction, in ferrets, 472
in raptors, 408–409

Tracheal trauma, in raptors, 413

Tracheal wash, in ferrets, 479
in reptiles, 572, 577

Tracheotomy, for cardiopulmonary-cerebral resuscitation, 288

Tramadol, for pain management, in small mammals, 296, 299, 313

Tranquilizers, for raptors, 410
for rodents, 522
for small mammals, 296, 306–307

Transport, for corals and anemones, 640–641
for fish emergencies, 654

Trauma, emergency procedures for, in amphibians, 618
in birds, 419–425, 430
in exotic mammals, 534–537
in ferrets, 469, 496–497
in fish, 671–672
in invertebrates, arthropods as, 628–629
mollusks as, 643
in pet birds, 365–372
in raptors, 400–401, 405–407, 409
in reptiles, 576
in rodents, 518–521

Treefrog, lungworm infection in, 606

Triage, for emergency/critical care, of pet birds, 345–346

Triage (*continued*)
  of raptors, 397–400

Tricaine methanesulfonate (MS-222), for anesthesia, in amphibians, 604
  in fish, 657–658

Trichlorfon, for fish, 667

Trimethoprim/sulfamethoxazole, in emergency/critical care, of exotic mammals, 553
  of ferrets, 483
  of fish, 667
  of rabbits, 438

Tumors. See *Mass(es);Neoplasia.*

U

Ulcers, in amphibians, 609, 612
  in fish, 671–672
  in pet birds, 370

Ultrasonic nebulizers, for pet birds, 357
  for rodents, 511

Ultrasound, in emergency/critical examinations, for heart function, 326–328
  of amphibians, 608
  of birds, 326–328
  of ferrets, 478, 496
  of fish, 661
  of pet birds, 353, 373
  of rabbits, 442
  of rodents, 508
  of small mammals, 327

Upper airway, of ferrets, emergency/critical care for, 472
  of pet birds, anatomy and physiology of, 359
    emergency/critical care for, 359–360
  of rabbits, emergency/critical care for, 456

Upper gastrointestinal endoscopy, in birds, 427

Upper respiratory endoscopy, in birds, 426–427

Urethral obstruction, in ferrets, 470
  emergency catheterization for, 494–496
  in rabbits, 454

Urgent care, of rabbits, 437–439

Uric acid concentration, in pet birds, 350

Urinalysis, in ferrets, 476, 496
  in pet birds, 351
  in rabbits, 441–442, 452
  in reptiles, 571

Urinary catheterization, in ferrets, 477, 479–481
  emergency placement of, 494–496
  in rabbits, 441–442
  in rodents, 526–527

Urinary obstruction, in rodents, 526–527

Urinary tract disease, in ferrets, 470, 494–496

Urogenital system, in ferrets, emergency care of diseases of, 470, 494–496
  examination of, 473

Urolithiasis, in rabbits, 453–454
  in rodents, 526–527

Uroliths, struvite, in ferrets, 470

Urticating hairs, of tarantulas, 631, 633

Uterine disorders, emergency/critical care for, in rabbits, 449–451
  in rodents, 525–526

V

Vaccine reactions, in ferrets, 497

Vaginal prolapse, in rodents, 525–526

Vascular support, critical indications for, in exotic mammals, 540–543, 549

Vasopressin, for cardiopulmonary-cerebral resuscitation, 286, 288–290

Vasopressors, for hypovolemic shock, 284

Vena cava puncture, in rodents, 505–507

Venipuncture. See *Blood sample collection.*

Venous access, for critically ill patients. See *Intravenous access/catheterization.*

Venous aneurysms, endometrial, in rabbits, 450

Ventriculotomy, in birds, 435–436

Vertebral fractures, in rabbits, 457

Veterinary care, owner goals for, 590

Viral diseases, emergencies related to, in fish, 667–671
  in invertebrates, 635–636
  in raptors, 415
  in amphibians, 617
  in ferrets, 467, 469, 493–494

Vitamin B, for amphibians, 597

Vitamin C, for guinea pigs, 518

Vitamin K, for raptors, 412, 414

Volume-controlled ventilators, 334–335

Vomiting, emergency procedures for, in ferrets, 467, 469
　in pet birds, 382–384
　in reptiles, 579

Vulvar swelling, in ferrets, 470, 473

W

Warming techniques, for aquatic fish environment, 648, 651
　for blood transfusions, 281
　for critically ill patients, 320
　　exotic mammals as, 546–547
　　in shock, 281–284
　　reptiles as, 558–559, 563, 565

"Water conditioners," for fish environment, 651–652

Water environment, for amphibians, 592–594
　for corals and anemones, 639–640
　for fish, common emergencies of, 665–668
　　health dependent on, 647–648
　　health factors of, 651, 672
　　quality maintenance equipment for, 648, 650–651
　　water parameters for, 648–650

"Water mold," in amphibians, 616

Water osmolarity, for aquatic amphibian species, 602

Water parameters, for aquatic fish environment, 648–650
　emergency management of, 663
　history taking of, 651–652
　in immediate emergency response, 652–653

Water pump, for aquatic fish environment, 648–649
　in immediate emergency response, 652–653

Weight, accurate determination of, in amphibians, 591
　in rabbits, 452
　in raptors, 398
　in rodents, 504, 524

Weight loss, in amphibians, 609–610

Wellness care, for amphibians, 590

Wobbly hedgehog syndrome (WHS), 534, 536

Wound care, for emergency presentations, in amphibians, 609, 612, 615, 618
　in pet birds, 368–370
　in raptors, 399, 402, 404
　in rodents, 518–519

Wound samples, in reptiles, 571

"Wry neck," in rabbits, 458–459

Z

Zoonotic disease, in African hedgehogs, 534, 536
　in raptors, 415

Moving?

Make sure your subscription moves with you!

To notify us of your new address, find your **Clinics Account Number** (located on your mailing label above your name), and contact customer service at:

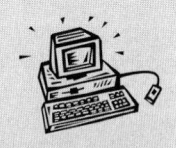

E-mail: elspcs@elsevier.com

800-654-2452 (subscribers in the U.S. & Canada)
407-345-4000 (subscribers outside of the U.S. & Canada)

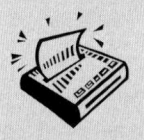

Fax number: 407-363-9661

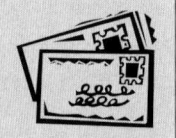

Elsevier Periodicals Customer Service
6277 Sea Harbor Drive
Orlando, FL 32887-4800

*To ensure uninterrupted delivery of your subscription, please notify us at least 4 weeks in advance of move.

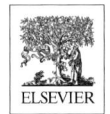

ELSEVIER